MASTERING
Medical
Terminology

MASTERING
Medical
Terminology
3rd edition

Sue Walker, BAppSc (MRA), GradDip (Public Health), MHlthSc
Maryann Wood, BBus (Health Admin), MHlthSc
Jenny Nicol, BBus (Health Admin), MPH, Cert IV TAE

ELSEVIER

ELSEVIER

Elsevier Australia. ACN 001 002 357
(a division of Reed International Books Australia Pty Ltd)
Tower 1, 475 Victoria Avenue, Chatswood, NSW 2067

ISBN: 978-0-7295-4333-0

National Library of Australia Cataloguing-in-Publication Data

A catalogue record for this book is available from the National Library of Australia

Content Strategist: Melinda McEvoy
Content Project Manager: Shruti Raj
Edited by Matt Davies
Proofread by Annabel Adair
Permissions Editing and Photo Research: Sathya Narayanan
Cover and internal design by Lisa Petroff
Index by SPi Global
Typeset by Toppan Best-set Premedia Limited
Printed in China by 1010 Printing International Limited

Last digit is the print number: 9 8 7 6 5 4 3

Contents

Preface   xi
Acknowledgments   xii
Reviewers   xiii
How to use this book   xiv

Module 1: Introduction

Chapter 1 Basic Word Structure   2
Objectives   2
Introduction   3
Basic word structure   3
  Word root   3
  Prefix   4
  Suffix   4
  Combining vowel   4
  Combining form   4
  Reading and interpreting a medical term   5
Important points to note about word
  elements and basic word structure   5
New word elements   6
  Combining forms   6
  Prefixes   7
  Suffixes   8
Exercises   9

Chapter 2 Building a Medical Vocabulary   16
Objectives   16
Introduction   17
Pronunciation of terms   17
Spelling conventions   17
Forming plurals   18
Eponyms   19
  Diseases and syndromes   19
  Body structures   20
  Procedures or tests   20
  Instruments   20
Mnemonics   21
Exercises   22

Module 2: The Body as a Framework

Chapter 3 The Human Body   28
Objectives   28
Introduction   29
New word elements   29
  Combining forms   29
  Prefixes   30
  Suffixes   31

Vocabulary   31
Abbreviations   32
Structural organisation of the body   32
The anatomical position   34
Body cavities   34
Abdominopelvic regions and quadrants   34
Divisions of the spinal column   37
Positional and directional terms   37
Planes of the body   38
Exercises   40

Chapter 4 Musculoskeletal System   47
Objectives   47
Introduction   48
Bones   48
  New word elements relating to bones   48
  Vocabulary relating to bones   52
  Abbreviations relating to bones   52
  Functions and structure of bones   52
  Pathology and diseases relating to bones   53
Joints   56
  New word elements relating to joints   56
  Vocabulary relating to joints   57
  Abbreviations relating to joints   57
  Functions and structure of joints   57
  Pathology and diseases relating to joints   57
Muscles   61
  New word elements relating to muscles   61
  Vocabulary relating to muscles   62
  Abbreviations relating to muscles   62
  Functions and structure of muscles   62
  Pathology and diseases relating to
    muscles   65
Tests and procedures   67
Exercises   70

Chapter 5 Integumentary System   80
Objectives   80
Introduction   81
New word elements   81
  Combining forms   81
  Prefixes   82
  Suffixes   82
Vocabulary   82
Abbreviations   83
Functions and structure of the
  integumentary system   83

Pathology and diseases	85
Common skin lesions	85
Symptomatic skin conditions	87
Skin infections	87
Specific skin disorders	89
Skin cancers	94
Tests and procedures	95
Removal of skin lesions	95
Other tests and procedures on the integumentary system	96
Exercises	98

Module 3: Internal Workings of the Body

Chapter 6 Haematology	**108**
Objectives	108
Introduction	109
New word elements	109
Combining forms	109
Prefixes	110
Suffixes	110
Vocabulary	111
Abbreviations	111
Functions and composition of blood	112
Functions of blood	112
Composition of blood	112
Blood cells	113
Blood types or blood groups	114
Analysis of blood samples	116
Pathology and diseases	116
Blood dyscrasias	117
Clotting disorders	120
Tests and procedures	121
Exercises	125

Chapter 7 Lymphatic and Immune Systems	**135**
Objectives	135
Introduction	136
New word elements	136
Combining forms	136
Prefixes	136
Suffixes	137
Vocabulary	137
Abbreviations	137
Functions and structure of the lymphatic and immune systems	138

Pathology and diseases	140
Tests and procedures	143
Exercises	144

Chapter 8 Endocrine System	**153**
Objectives	153
Introduction	154
New word elements	154
Combining forms	154
Prefixes	155
Suffixes	155
Vocabulary	156
Abbreviations	156
Functions and structure of the endocrine system	157
Pituitary gland	158
Thyroid gland	159
Parathyroid glands	159
Adrenal glands	159
Pancreas	159
Gonads	159
Pineal gland	160
Thymus gland	160
Pathology and diseases	161
Pituitary gland	161
Thyroid gland	163
Parathyroid glands	166
Pancreas	166
Adrenal glands	168
Tests and procedures	169
Exercises	170

Chapter 9 Cardiovascular System	**180**
Objectives	180
Introduction	181
New word elements	181
Combining forms	181
Prefixes	182
Suffixes	182
Vocabulary	183
Abbreviations	184
Functions and structure of the cardiovascular system	185
Heart	185
Arteries, veins and capillaries	186
Pathology and diseases	189
Pathological conditions of the heart	189
Pathological conditions of blood vessels	193

Tests and procedures   197
Exercises   202

Chapter 10 Respiratory System   212
Objectives   212
Introduction   213
New word elements   213
  Combining forms   213
  Prefixes   214
  Suffixes   214
Vocabulary   215
Abbreviations   216
Functions and structure of the respiratory
  system   217
  Nose   217
  Pharynx   217
  Larynx   219
  Trachea   219
  Lungs   219
  Bronchi   219
  Alveoli   219
Pathology and diseases   219
Tests and procedures   226
Exercises   231

Chapter 11 Digestive System   241
Objectives   241
Introduction   242
New word elements   242
  Combining forms   242
  Prefixes   243
  Suffixes   244
Vocabulary   244
Abbreviations   245
Functions and structure of the digestive
  system   246
  Mouth (buccal cavity)   246
  Pharynx and oesophagus   246
  Stomach   246
  Small intestine   247
  Large intestine   248
  Anus   248
  Liver   249
  Pancreas   249
  Gallbladder   249
Pathology and diseases   249
  Diseases of the oral cavity   249
  Diseases of the salivary glands   250
  Diseases of the oesophagus   250

Diseases of the stomach   250
Diseases of the small intestine and
  associated organs   252
Diseases of the large intestine   255
Diseases of the rectum and anus   258
Tests and procedures   259
Exercises   264

Chapter 12 Nervous System   272
Objectives   272
Introduction   273
New word elements   273
  Combining forms   273
  Prefixes   274
  Suffixes   274
Vocabulary   275
Abbreviations   276
Functions and structure of the nervous
  system   276
  Central nervous system   278
  Brain   278
  Spinal cord   279
  Peripheral nervous system   280
  Neurons   281
Pathology and diseases   282
  Degenerative and motor disorders   282
  Episodic neurological disorders   284
  Inflammatory and infectious diseases   284
  Neoplasms   285
  Disorders of nerves   285
  Disorders due to trauma   285
  Paralysis   286
  Vascular disorders   287
  Miscellaneous conditions   288
Tests and procedures   288
Exercises   291

Chapter 13 The Senses   300
Objectives   301
Introduction   301
New word elements for the sense of sight   301
  Combining forms   301
  Prefixes   302
  Suffixes   303
Abbreviations for the sense of sight   303
Functions and structure of the eye –
  the sense of sight   303
  The orbit   304
  Eyelids and eyelashes   304

Sclera   304
Conjunctiva   304
Cornea   304
Anterior chamber   305
Iris and pupil   305
Posterior chamber, lens and ciliary body   306
Vitreous cavity   306
Retina, macula and choroid   306
Optic nerve   306
Pathology and diseases for the sense of
    sight   306
New word elements for the sense of
    hearing   309
    Combining forms   309
    Prefixes   310
    Suffixes   310
Abbreviations for the sense of hearing   310
Functions and structure of the ear –
    the sense of hearing   311
    Outer ear   312
    Middle ear   312
    Inner ear   312
Pathology and diseases for the sense of
    hearing   312
New word elements for the sense of smell   314
    Combining forms   315
    Prefixes   315
Functions and structure of the nose –
    the sense of smell   315
New word elements for the sense of taste   315
    Combining forms   315
Functions and structure relating to the
    tongue – the sense of taste   315
New word elements for the sense of
    touch   316
    Combining forms   316
Functions and structure relating to the
    sense of touch   316
Vocabulary for the senses   316
Tests and procedures for the senses   317
Exercises   321

Chapter 14 Urinary System   331
Objectives   331
Introduction   332
New word elements   332
    Combining forms   332
    Prefixes   332
    Suffixes   333

Vocabulary   333
Abbreviations   334
Functions and structure of the urinary
    system   334
    The kidneys   334
    Ureters   336
    Bladder   336
    Urethra   336
    Urinary sphincters   336
Pathology and diseases   336
    Disorders of the kidneys   338
    Disorders of the bladder   340
    Disorders of the ureter and urethra   342
Tests and procedures   342
    Urinalysis   347
Exercises   348

Chapter 15 Male Reproductive System   358
Objectives   358
Introduction   359
New word elements   359
    Combining forms   359
    Prefixes   360
    Suffixes   360
Vocabulary   360
Abbreviations   361
Functions and structure of the male
    reproductive system   361
    External reproductive structures   361
    Internal reproductive structures   363
Pathology and diseases   363
Tests and procedures   367
Exercises   368

**Chapter 16 Female Reproductive
System   378**
Objectives   378
Introduction   379
New word elements   379
    Combining forms   379
    Prefixes   380
    Suffixes   380
Vocabulary   380
Abbreviations   381
Functions and structure of the female
    reproductive system   381
    Follicular phase   382
    Ovulation   382
    Luteal phase   383

Menstrual phase   383
Female reproductive organs   383
Pathology and diseases   385
    Benign conditions   385
    Malignant tumours   386
    Other gynaecological disorders   387
Tests and procedures   388
Exercises   392

Chapter 17 Obstetrics and Neonatology   401
Objectives   401
Introduction   402
New word elements   402
    Combining forms   402
    Prefixes   403
    Suffixes   403
Vocabulary   403
Abbreviations   404
Functions and structure related to
    obstetrics and neonatology   405
    First trimester   405
    Second trimester   406
    Third trimester   407
    Labour and delivery   407
    Presentation for delivery   408
    Definitions related to obstetrics and
        neonatology   409
Pathology and diseases   409
    Pathological conditions and diseases
        related to obstetrics   410
    Pathological conditions and diseases
        related to neonatology   411
Tests and procedures   415
Exercises   420

Chapter 18 Mental Health   429
Objectives   429
Introduction   430
New word elements   430
    Combining forms   430
    Prefixes   431
    Suffixes   431
Vocabulary   431
Abbreviations   432
Mental health disorders   432
Glossary of mental health terms   433
Specific mental health disorders   434
    Disorders usually first diagnosed in
        infancy, childhood or adolescence   434

Delirium, dementia and amnesic and
    other cognitive disorders   434
Substance-related disorders   435
Schizophrenia and other psychotic
    disorders   435
Mood disorders   436
Anxiety disorders   437
Some common (and not so common)
    phobias   438
Factitious disorders   438
Dissociative disorders   439
Sexual and gender identity disorders   439
Eating disorders   440
Personality disorders   440
Therapeutic interventions   441
    Psychological and psychosocial therapies   441
    Psychopharmacology   442
    Other therapeutic methods   443
Exercises   443

Module 4: Systemic Conditions

Chapter 19 Oncology   452
Objectives   452
Introduction   453
New word elements   453
    Combining forms   453
    Prefixes   454
    Suffixes   454
Vocabulary   454
Abbreviations   455
Cancers and tumours   456
    Differences between malignant and
        benign tumours   456
    Primary tumours versus metastatic
        (secondary) tumours   458
    Common sites for metastatic
        spread   458
    Causes of cancer   458
    Types of cancers   458
    Grading and staging systems   460
    Cancer in Australia and New Zealand   461
Tests and procedures   462
    Diagnostic tests and procedures   462
    Surgical interventions   464
    Radiotherapy   464
    Chemotherapy   465
    Immunotherapy   466
Exercises   467

Chapter 20 Infectious and Parasitic Diseases 475

Objectives 475
Introduction 476
New word elements 476
  Combining forms 476
  Prefixes 476
  Suffixes 476
Vocabulary 477
Abbreviations 477
Types of infections 478
  Viruses 478
  Bacteria 478
  Parasites 478
  Mycoses 478
  Opportunistic infection 478
  Modes of transmission 478
  Outbreaks of disease, disease control and monitoring 479
Pathological descriptions of some specific infectious and parasitic diseases 481
  Vaccine-preventable diseases 482
  Vector-borne diseases 484
  Other infectious and parasitic diseases 485
Tests and procedures 485
Exercises 488

Chapter 21 Radiology and Nuclear Medicine 495

Objectives 495
Introduction 496
New word elements 496
  Combining forms 496
  Prefixes 496
  Suffixes 497
Vocabulary 497
Abbreviations 497
Radiology 498
  Characteristics of x-rays 498
  Diagnostic techniques 499
  Positioning 501
Nuclear medicine 502
  Nuclear medicine techniques 504
Radiotherapy 505
  Radiotherapy techniques 505
Exercises 506

Chapter 22 Pharmacology 513
Objectives 513
Introduction 514
New word elements 514
  Combining forms 514
  Prefixes 515
  Suffixes 515
Abbreviations 515
Glossary of commonly used pharmacological terms 516
How drugs are named 518
Regulation and registration of medications in Australia and New Zealand 518
Administration of drugs 519
Terminology of drug action 520
Drug classes 521
Anaesthesia 522
ASA (American Society of Anesthesiologists) Physical Status Classification 522
Exercises 523

Module 5: Special Applications

Chapter 23 Complementary and Alternative Therapies 532
Objectives 532
Introduction 533
Complementary medicines 533
Complementary therapies 534
Glossary of terms 534

Chapter 24 Public Health, Epidemiology and Research Terms 537
Objectives 537
Introduction 538
Glossary of terms 538

Word element glossary 546
Glossary of medical terms 561
Specific word elements 575
Normal reference values for haematological testing 578
Abbreviations 584
Answer Guide 593
Picture credits 660
Index 664

Preface

Welcome to *Mastering Medical Terminology: Australia and New Zealand, 3rd edition*. This text has been written to provide a medical terminology book that will be relevant to an audience in Australia and New Zealand. Australian terminology, perspectives, examples and spelling have been included and Australian pronunciation specified. Where appropriate, specific references to New Zealand examples have also been included.

The textbook provides instructional materials, a pronunciation guide and practice exercises to reinforce learning about each body system and specialty area. Examples and practical applications show medical terms in context. Diagrams and illustrations enhance understanding of the words you will read.

We hope this textbook will demonstrate the importance of the correct use of medical terminology in communicating information about clinical care. We have developed the textbook using British spelling as seen in Australian and New Zealand health care. It should be noted that many other textbooks incorporate American spelling. Both forms of spelling are equally correct but different countries prefer to use one form over the other. Most countries that have been part of the British Commonwealth at some point in their history choose to use British spelling.

There are two terms that cause a lot of confusion for students and practitioners alike. First, there seems to be a significant misunderstanding with the spelling of the medical term 'fetus'. Although many medical terms with the letter 'e' have the digraph 'oe' when spelled the British way, *fetus* is an exception. According to the *Chambers Guide to Grammar and Usage* by George Davidson (1998), the term originates from the Latin *ferare* meaning to conceive, and not *foetere* meaning to give birth, thus adding an 'o' to the word 'fetus' is actually a grammatical over-correction. To reiterate, the correct spelling is 'fetus'. 'Foetus' is incorrect. It would be useful to make a note of this now.

Similarly, there is often confusion about the correct use of the suffix *-cele*, the suffix *-coele* and the word root *coel/. -coele* and *coel/* mean a cavity of the body, while *-cele* refers to a hernia or swelling. Again, it would be useful to make a note of this information.

Where there has been any question about the appropriate spelling for a medical term, we have deferred to that recommended in *Mosby's Dictionary of Medicine, Nursing & Health Professions* (revised 3rd Australian and New Zealand edition) by Harris P, Nagy S and Vardaxis N.

Throughout *Mastering Medical Terminology*, review of medical terminology as it is used in clinical practice is highlighted. Features of the textbook include:

- simple, non-technical explanations of medical terms
- explanations of clinical procedures, laboratory tests and abbreviations used in Australian clinical practice, as they apply to each body system and specialty area
- pronunciation of terms and spaces to write meanings of terms
- exercises that test your understanding of terminology as you work through the text chapter by chapter
- ample space to write answers to exercises
- a comprehensive glossary and appendices for reference as you study and then later as you use medical terminology
- links to other useful references such as websites and textbooks.

Our goal in creating the third edition of *Mastering Medical Terminology* is to help students learn and to help instructors teach medical terms that are relevant to the Australian and New Zealand healthcare environments. Using an interactive, logical, interesting and easy-to-follow process of instruction, you will find that medical terminology comes 'alive' and begins to make sense. We cannot deny that studying medical terminology is like learning a foreign language. It requires commitment and hard work, but ultimately you will see the benefits. The knowledge that you gain will be valuable for your career in the health workplace and will help you for years to come.

Acknowledgments

We appreciate the guidance and support of our editorial team at Elsevier. It has been great to have you helping us and keeping us on track as we have worked through the revision of this textbook.

We extend our thanks to the reviewers of our work, whose interest in the text and constructive comments have been extremely useful in shaping the final product. We hope you will find the outcome beneficial in your own teaching and learning.

Finally, we would like to thank our families, friends and workmates for their support, encouragement, advice and good humour during the writing of the third edition of this textbook. It has been several years of hard work, but we think you will agree that it has been worthwhile.

Reviewers

Carolyn Allison MHA
Health Information Manager, OTEN (TAFE NSW),
  Sydney, NSW, Australia

Luellen Colquhoun BAL&D (Monash)
Teacher, Business Administration (Medical),
  Chisholm Institute, Frankston & Dandenong
  Campus, Melbourne, Victoria, Australia

Amanda Müller PhD, GradCert TESOL, GradCert
  Education (Higher Ed)
Lecturer, English for Specific Purposes, School of
  Nursing & Midwifery, Flinders University (Sturt
  Campus), Adelaide, South Australia, Australia

Judy Norris TAE/Cert IV Bus Admin, Cert III Bus
  Admin (Medical)
Consultant, Adept Training Pty Ltd,
  Parramatta, NSW, Australia
Medical Administration Trainer & Assessor,
  TAFE South Western Sydney Institute,
  Liverpool College, NSW, Australia
Trainer/Assessor (Online Training), Macarthur
  Community College, Cartwright, NSW, Australia
Trainer/Assessor (Distance Training), Lesley Graham
  Training & Consulting (via Camden Have
  Community College), Laurieton, NSW, Australia

Janette Williams RN, BA, MNsg (UNE),
  DNE (Syd)
Private practice (Education and Training), Sydney,
  NSW, Australia

Technical Reviewers

Peter Harris
Senior Lecturer in Clinical Education
University of New South Wales, Sydney, 2052

Joanne Williams AssocDip (MRA), Cert IV TAE,
  CHIM
Team Leader, Medical Terminology, Education
  Services, Health Information Management
  Association of Australia Ltd, North Ryde, NSW,
  Australia

How to use this book

This book contains 24 chapters divided into five modules. The first module provides an introduction to medical terminology by looking at the basic structure of medical words and how medical terms can be constructed and deconstructed using word roots, prefixes, suffixes and combining vowels. Module 2 gives a general overview of the body as a framework, focusing on the body as a whole, followed by the musculoskeletal and integumentary systems. Module 3 covers each of the internal body systems. The order in which these chapters are completed is not critical. They can be studied in the sequence provided or in any other order, but we believe the structure of the book is in a logical format from an educational perspective. The fourth module provides details about systemic conditions, such as oncology and infectious diseases, followed by chapters relating to radiology and nuclear medicine, and pharmacology. The final module relates to special applications of medical terminology and provides glossaries of terms used for alternative and complementary therapies and in public health, epidemiology and clinical research. The appendices provide useful lists of abbreviations, a word element glossary, a glossary of medical terms and normal reference values for haematological testing.

To facilitate your learning within each body system chapter, the text has been divided into sections as is relevant to that system:

- Objectives
- Introduction
- New word elements
- Combining forms
- Prefixes
- Suffixes
- Vocabulary
- Abbreviations
- Functions and structure of the body system
- Pathology and diseases
- Tests and procedures
- Exercises.

This textbook should not be used as the only reference when learning medical terminology. You will need to use a comprehensive medical dictionary, such as *Mosby's Dictionary of Medicine, Nursing & Health Professions (revised 3rd Australian and New Zealand edition)* by Harris P, Nagy S & Vardaxis N. We also encourage students to be curious – to read more about the medical conditions and procedures in these books. We also recommend using the internet, although care needs to be taken to ensure websites used are current, trustworthy and reputable. Websites such as the Australian Government's *healthdirect* (www. healthdirect.gov.au) and the Victorian Government's Better Health Channel (www.betterhealth.vic.gov.au) are highly regarded.

Medical abbreviations can be confusing, so we suggest you refer to the Health Information Management Association of Australia's useful reference *The Australian Dictionary of Clinical Abbreviations, Acronyms and Symbols*, 7th edition (www.himaa.org.au).

For additional information about therapeutic drugs and chemicals used in the Australian healthcare environment, we suggest accessing the *Monthly Index of Medical Specialties*, known as MIMS. This drug and product information reference is accessible in print, electronically and online (www.mims.com.au). MIMS contains detailed information about drug usage such as dosage, adverse reactions and drug interactions. New Zealand has an equivalent drug reference known as *MIMS New Zealand* (www.mims.co.nz).

It is important that students of medical terminology are diligent in their study. There is a lot to learn but, with repetition and practice, the basic medical terminology building blocks will fall into place. We recommend that students attempt to learn 10 word elements every day, rather than attempting to learn a whole chapter at once. Learning should become easier as you start to remember word elements and are able to create medical terms from them. There are four basic guidelines to keep in mind as you study medical terminology:

1. Analyse words by dividing into their component parts:
   - root
   - prefix
   - suffix
   - combining vowel
   - combining form.
2. Relate the medical terms to the structure and function of the human body.
3. Be aware of spelling inconsistencies, pronunciation problems and formation of plurals.
4. Practise reading, writing and pronouncing medical words at every opportunity.

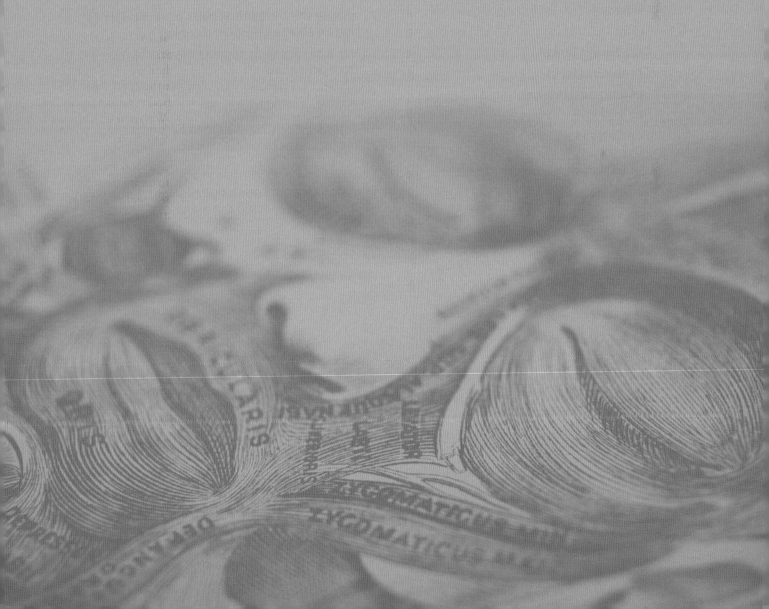

MODULE 1

Introduction

CHAPTER 1

Basic Word Structure

Contents

OBJECTIVES   2

INTRODUCTION   3

BASIC WORD STRUCTURE   3

  Word root   3

  Prefix   4

  Suffix   4

  Combining vowel   4

  Combining form   4

  Reading and interpreting a medical term   5

IMPORTANT POINTS TO NOTE ABOUT WORD ELEMENTS AND BASIC WORD STRUCTURE   5

NEW WORD ELEMENTS   6

  Combining forms   6

  Prefixes   7

  Suffixes   8

EXERCISES   9

Objectives

After completing this chapter, you should be able to:

1. identify and define the main word elements: word roots, prefixes, suffixes, combining vowels and combining forms

2. analyse the component parts of medical terms and be able to give their meaning

3. use word elements to build medical terms from definitions

4. understand the rules associated with the formation of medical terms

5. apply what you have learned by interpreting medical terminology in practice.

Demonstrate your knowledge of the basic word structure by completing the exercises at the end of this chapter.

INTRODUCTION

Medical terminology is the words that have been developed over many centuries to describe anatomical structures, diseases, procedures, treatments, medications and instruments associated with medicine. Medical terminology is the language used to facilitate communication in the medical field. Most medical terms have their origins in Latin and Greek, but there are some terms that come from Arabic, French, German and Anglo-Saxon origins.

Before learning about medical terminology today, it is probably useful to look at how it has developed over time. There are cave paintings from many ancient cultures that depict medical procedures and treatments. These could be described as the earliest forms of medical documentation. However, it was not until about 2700 BC in Egypt that the earliest written records of health care were created. These records were written on papyrus and described the treatments that were performed at the time as well as describing what the ancient Egyptians knew about diseases. By 500–400 BC in Greece there was a more scientific basis to medicine and the use of an appropriate language became more important. Basic medical terminology developed alongside medicine to describe diseases and the instruments and techniques used to treat illness and medical conditions.

Over the next millennium, Latin remained the common language of scholars. New terms to describe medical conditions and procedures continued to be developed in Latin or Greek. These are still the basis of the language of medicine today. It is important to remember that medical terminology is a dynamic, living language that changes and grows over time to meet the needs of each generation of scholars and clinicians and take account of advances in our understanding of medicine and surgery. Many medical terms in current common usage were not even thought of a century ago.

At first, studying medical terminology may seem overwhelming. The words may seem long and complex and totally unpronounceable. It may appear to be a foreign language. That's because it is! But do not be discouraged. Like any language, medical terminology adheres to a set of fairly simple rules.

Basic word elements occur repeatedly in various combinations and will soon become familiar. Most seemingly complex medical terms are simply combinations of much smaller subsets of word parts. These are much easier to learn than whole words. You do not have to remember all the words you come across. This is a critically important concept to understand. Learning the basic structure of medical terms allows you to break down and build up medical terms quite easily. Some rote learning will be required at first, but eventually it will get easier.

This book will give you the skills necessary to understand the terms, use them appropriately and finally demystify this complex but beautiful language called medical terminology.

BASIC WORD STRUCTURE

Understanding medical terminology will be much easier if you learn how to break down each word into its separate elements. If you know the meaning of each of the word elements you will be able to deduce the meaning of even the most complex words. Most medical terms consist of two or more parts. The meaning of each term is the 'sum of its parts'. These word parts will include two or more of the following fundamental elements:

- word root
- prefix
- suffix
- combining vowel
- combining form.

In general, each medical term is formed from one or more word roots. The word root normally provides an overall indication of what the word is about or specifies a part of the body. Added to the word root may be a prefix, which modifies the meaning of the medical term by providing information about location, place, time, shape, size or direction. A medical term may also contain a suffix after the word root. Adding a suffix also creates a new medical term, commonly indicating a disease action or type of test.

Word root

Most medical terms contain at least one word root. The root is the foundation of a word and conveys its central meaning. It is generally a noun or naming word. A word root can be found at the beginning of the medical term or it can form the basis to which a prefix and a suffix may be attached. For example, bronchitis can be divided into a word root and a suffix. The word root *bronch/* means bronchus and the suffix *-itis* means inflammation. Putting it all together, the whole word *bronchitis* means inflammation of the bronchus.

bronch	itis
W R	S

The word hemicolectomy can be divided into a prefix, word root and a suffix. The prefix *hemi-* means half, the word root *col/* means colon and the suffix *-ectomy* means excision or surgical removal. Putting it all together, the whole word *hemicolectomy* means excision or surgical removal of half the colon.

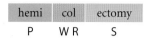

hemi	col	ectomy
P	W R	S

In this book, a word root will be written with a slash (/) after it when a medical term is broken up into its component parts.

Prefix

A prefix is found at the beginning of the word, preceding the word root. It can never be used alone. It must always be used with a word root and/or suffix. It adds to or modifies the meaning of a word or creates a new word. Prefixes are similar to prepositions or adjectives – they tell you more about the word root, such as its location, place, time, shape, size or direction. For example, sublingual can be divided into a prefix, word root and a suffix. The prefix *sub-* means under or below, the word root *lingu/* means tongue and the suffix *-al* means pertaining to. Putting it all together, the whole word means pertaining to under the tongue.

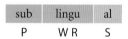

sub	lingu	al
P	W R	S

Remember, not all medical terms will have a prefix.

In this book, prefixes will be documented with a hyphen after the prefix (-).

Suffix

A suffix follows the word root and is found at the end of the word. It is added to alter, modify or give essential meaning to a term. Suffixes generally refer to a type of condition, investigation or procedure and can help identify if a term is a noun or an adjective. For example, hysterectomy can be divided into a word root and a suffix. The word root *hyster/* means uterus and the suffix *-ectomy* means an excision or surgical removal. Putting it all together, the whole word *hysterectomy* means an excision or surgical removal of the uterus.

hyster	ectomy
W R	S

In this textbook, a suffix is written with a hyphen (-) before it.

Combining vowel

A combining vowel (sometimes called a connecting vowel) is a vowel that links parts of a word together. It may link a word root to a suffix or two word roots together. Its purpose is to aid pronunciation. The most common combining vowel is 'o', and 'i' is the next most common. When linking a word root with a suffix, it is normal practice to drop the combining vowel when the suffix starts with a vowel. For example, in the medical term opt/ic the suffix *-ic* begins with a vowel, therefore a combining vowel is not required. This rule does not apply when linking two word roots, the second of which starts with a vowel. For example, in the medical term oste/o/arthr/itis the combining vowel is retained at the end of *oste/o* even though the word root *arthr/* starts with a vowel. Note, however, that the combining vowel has been dropped at the end of *arthr/* because the suffix *-itis* starts with a vowel.

oste	o	arthr	itis
W R	C V	W R	S

Use the list of word elements at the end of this chapter to work out what the medical terms in the preceding paragraph mean. Check the meaning in your medical dictionary to confirm you are correct.

Combining form

A word root plus a combining vowel are known together as a combining form. When learning medical terminology, it is common to use combining forms rather than word roots and combining vowels individually. For example, the medical term erythrocyte can be divided into a word root plus a combining vowel (a combining form) and a suffix. The combining form *erythr/o* consists of the word root *eryth/* and the combining vowel *o*. This combining form means red. The suffix *-cyte* means cell. Putting it all together, the whole word *erythrocyte* means a (blood) cell which is red.

erythr	o	cyte
W R	C V	S
	C F	

The word angioplasty can be divided into a word root plus a combining vowel (a combining form) and a suffix. The combining form *angi/o* means vessel (blood), and the suffix *-plasty* means surgical or plastic repair. Putting it all together, the word *angioplasty* means the surgical or plastic repair of a (blood) vessel.

angi	o	plasty
W R	C V	S
	C F	

As you can see in these examples of combining forms, they are written with the word root followed by a slash (/) then the vowel.

Reading and interpreting a medical term

When giving the meaning of a medical term, the suffix is generally stated first. For example:

mast/ectomy: *mast/* is a word root meaning breast, *-ectomy* is a suffix meaning excision or surgical removal. When used together, the term means an excision or surgical removal of the breast.

psych/o/logy: *psych/* is a word root meaning mind, *o* is the combining vowel and *-logy* is a suffix meaning a study of. When used together the term means the study of the mind.

dermat/itis: *dermat/* is a word root that means skin, *-itis* is a suffix meaning inflammation of. So the term *dermatitis* means an inflammation of the skin.

IMPORTANT POINTS TO NOTE ABOUT WORD ELEMENTS AND BASIC WORD STRUCTURE

A medical term need not contain all the word elements. For example:

electr/o/cardi/o/gram: contains two word roots and a suffix. *Electr/o* means electricity, *cardi/o* means heart, *-gram* means a recording, so the whole term *electrocardiogram* means a recording of the electricity of the heart

myel/oid: contains a word root and a suffix. *Myel/o* means bone marrow, *-oid* means derived from or resembling, so the term *myeloid* means derived from or resembling bone marrow

par/enter/al: contains a prefix, a word root and a suffix. In this term, the prefix *par-* means apart from or other than, the word root *enter/* refers to the intestine and the suffix *-al* means pertaining to. The full term *parenteral* refers to something that is taken into the body other than through the digestive tract/intestine. For example, it might be a drug administered by injection under the skin or into a muscle.

The meanings of word elements do not change no matter how they are used. For example, the combining form *gastr/o* means stomach. It can be used with many different prefixes, suffixes and other combining forms to create different medical terms. Some examples are gastr/o/scopy (a process of viewing the stomach), epi/gastr/ic (pertaining to above the stomach) and gastro/enter/itis (inflammation of the stomach and intestine). It does not matter how or where the combining form *gastr/o* is used, the meaning remains identical. This is the same for all word elements.

Some combining forms have the same meaning but come from different origins. This is often because both Latin (L) and Greek (G) terms developed over time and are still in use. For example, *uter/o* (L), *hyster/o* (G) and *metr/o* (G) all mean uterus. It is important to note, however, that these combining forms are not always interchangeable. Experience and practice will teach you which to use in a particular context. If in doubt, refer to a medical dictionary.

It may be possible to sense the basic meaning of a term from analysing its component parts but not its specific meaning; for example, peri/card/itis. By analysing the meaning of all the word elements, this term literally means inflammation surrounding the heart. However, in a medical context it actually means inflammation of the pericardium – the membranous sac surrounding the heart. This demonstrates why it is important to make use of your medical dictionary when studying medical terminology.

When identifying the meaning of medical terms, the definition based on individual word elements, or origin, may seem to be at odds with the actual meaning. For example, the word artery comes from the Greek word *arteria*, which means windpipe. This is because the ancient Greeks, who could only examine bodies postmortem, thought that arteries were 'air ducts' because they do not contain blood after death. However, it is now known that arteries are responsible for carrying blood. Once again, this demonstrates why it is important to make use of your medical dictionary.

When identifying the meaning of medical terms, parts of the definition may be understood without being explicitly expressed. For example, when the word an/aem/ia is broken down, it literally means a condition of no blood. However, in a medical context, it really means a reduction in the number of erythrocytes in the blood.

In some circumstances, the order of the components determines the meaning of the term. For example:

haemat/ur/ia: condition of blood in urine

ur/aemia: condition of urea in blood

In these examples, the component parts of the terms are the same – *haem/* and *aem/* are word roots that mean blood, *ur/* is a word root that means urea or urine and the suffix *-ia* refers to a process or condition. The order in which the word parts are used changes the meaning of the term.

In other circumstances, however, the order of the word components does not alter the meaning of a term. For example, hysterosalpingectomy and salpingohysterectomy both mean excision of the uterus and fallopian tubes. Both contain the word roots salping/ (fallopian tube) and hyster/ (uterus) and the suffix -ectomy (excision or surgical removal). In this case the order of the word roots does not affect the meaning of the term – an excision of the uterus and one or both fallopian tubes.

Do not be too concerned about these inconsistencies at this stage. As you work through this textbook and become more familiar with medical terminology you should be able to recognise the most common format for terms.

NEW WORD ELEMENTS

Listed below are some commonly used word elements, their meanings and examples of medical terms using each of the word elements. Break down each medical term into its individual word elements. Write the meaning of the medical term in the space provided. You may need to check the meaning in a medical dictionary. As an example:

adenoma
aden/ = WR = gland
-oma = S = tumour, collection, mass or swelling
Meaning = tumour in a gland
Note: The combining vowel 'o' is dropped because the suffix starts with a vowel.

Most of the word elements which you will need to provide the meaning of the medical terms are in the lists below. If not, please refer to the Glossary of medical terms on page 561.

Combining forms

Combining Form	Meaning	Medical Term	Meaning of Medical Term
angi/o	vessel	haemangioma	
arteri/o	artery	arteriosclerosis	
arthr/o	joint	arthroscopy	
bronch/o	bronchus	bronchogenic	
cardi/o	heart	cardiomyopathy	
cephal/o	head	encephalograph	
cerebr/o	cerebrum, brain	cerebrospinal	
chondr/o	cartilage	chondrosarcoma	
cis/o	to cut	incision	
col/o	colon, large intestine	colectomy	
cyst/o	bladder, cyst, sac	cystoscopy	
cyt/o	cell	cytology	
derm/o	skin	dermal	
dermat/o		dermatologist	
electr/o	electricity, electrical activity	electrocardiogram	
encephal/o	brain	encephalitis	
enter/o	intestine (usually small)	gastroenterologist	
erythr/o	red	erythroderma	
fibr/o	fibre	fibreoptic	
gastr/o	stomach	gastritis	
haem/o	blood	haemostasis	
haemat/o		haematoma	
hepat/o	liver	hepatitis	
hyster/o	uterus	hysterectomy	
lapar/o	abdomen	laparoscopic	
lingu/o	tongue	lingual	
lymph/o	lymphoid tissue, lymph gland	lymphocytic	
mast/o	breast	mastectomy	
metr/o	uterus	metritis	
morph/o	form, shape	morphology	

Table continued

Combining Form	Meaning	Medical Term	Meaning of Medical Term
my/o	muscle	myocardial	
myel/o	bone marrow, spinal cord	myelogram	
nephr/o	kidney	nephritis	
neur/o	nerve	neural	
opt/o	eye, vision	optic	
oste/o	bone	ostectomy	
phleb/o	vein	phlebitis	
pneum/o	air, lungs, respiration	pneumoconiosis	
pneumon/o		pneumonia	
psych/o	mind	psychology	
pyel/o	renal pelvis	pyelonephritis	
rhin/o	nose	rhinoplasty	
salping/o	fallopian tube, eustachian (auditory) tube	salpingectomy	
thorac/o	chest, thorax	thoracotomy	
trache/o	trachea	tracheotomy	
ur/o	urine, urinary tract, urea	urolithiasis	
uter/o	uterus	uterotomy	
vas/o	vessel, duct	vasoplasty	

Prefixes

Prefix	Meaning	Medical Term	Meaning of Medical Term
an-	no, not, without, absence of	anaemic	
ante-	before, forward	anteverted	
auto-	self	autosomal	
bi-	two, twice, double	bipolar	
circum-	around, about	circumcision	
di-	double, twice	dicephaly	
dia-	through, across	diarrhoea	
dys-	bad, painful, difficult	dyspnoea	
endo-	within, inside, inner	endometrium	
epi-	above, upon, on	epidermis	
hemi-	half	hemiplegia	
hyper-	above, excessive	hyperactive	
hypo-	below, under, deficient, less than normal	hypoglycaemia	
inter-	between	intercostal	
par-	aside, beyond, apart from, other than, near, against	parenteral	
peri-	around, surrounding	perinatal	
post-	after, behind	postoperative	
pre-	before, in front of	premature	

Table continued

Prefix	Meaning	Medical Term	Meaning of Medical Term
retro-	backward, behind	retrograde	
semi-	half	semicircular	
sub-	under, below	subcutaneous	
super-	above, excessive	supernumerary	
sym-	together, with	symphysis	
syn-		syndactyly	
trans-	across, through, over	transverse	

Suffixes

Suffix	Meaning	Medical Term	Meaning of Medical Term
-aemia	blood (condition of)	hyperglycaemia	
-al	pertaining to, drug action	renal	
-algia	pain (condition of)	arthralgia	
-cyte	cell	erythrocyte	
-derma	skin	leucoderma	
-ectomy	excision, surgical removal	appendicectomy	
-genic	pertaining to formation, producing	carcinogenic	
-gram	record, writing	cardiogram	
-graph	instrument for recording	encephalograph	
-graphy	process of recording	pyelography	
-ia	process, condition	haematuria	
-iac	pertaining to	cardiac	
-ic	pertaining to, drug action	dyspeptic	
-ist	one who specialises in	gynaecologist	
-itis	inflammation	dermatitis	
-logy	study of	histology	
-oid	derived from, resembling	polypoid	
-oma	tumour, collection, mass or swelling	carcinoma	
-osis	abnormal condition	erythrocytosis	
-ous	composed of, pertaining to, relating to	mucinous	
-pathy	disease process	osteopathy	
-plasty	surgical, plastic repair	uteroplasty	
-scope	instrument to view	ophthalmoscope	
-scopy	process of viewing	endoscopy	
-sis	state of	diagnosis	
-tomy	incision, cut into	osteotomy	

Exercises

EXERCISE 1.1: WORD ANALYSIS

Break up the medical terms below into their component parts (prefixes, suffixes, word roots, combining vowels, combining forms). Use a slash (/) in between each word part.

Example:

chondr / o / clast / ic   pertaining to the destruction of cartilage
  WR   CV
        WR   S
    CF

splen / o / megaly   enlargement of the spleen
  WR   CV
         S
    CF

peri / card / itis   inflammation around the heart (i.e. the pericardium)
  P   WR   S

1.	therm o graph ic	pertaining to the record of heat
2.	gastr o enter itis	inflammation of stomach and intestines
3.	bronch o scopy	visual examination of bronchus
4.	an aesthes ia	condition of without feeling or sensation
5.	angi o gram	record of a vessel
(Now it gets a bit harder … you need to divide the word up yourself!)		
6.	laparotomy	incision into the abdominal wall
7.	blepharoplasty	surgical repair of eyelid
8.	atherosclerosis	hardening of blood vessels due to fatty plaque
9.	hepatomegaly	enlargement of the liver
10.	colostomy	process of creating a new opening into the colon

EXERCISE 1.2: IDENTIFYING PREFIXES

Identify the prefix in each of the medical terms below. Give the meaning of the term as a whole.

Example:
supramaxillary

supra/maxillary

supra = above

supramaxillary = above the maxilla (or upper jaw bone)

1. apnoea _____

_____

_____

2. anteflexion _____

_____

_____

3. postmenopausal _____

_____

_____

4. supernumerary _____

_____

_____

5. hemigastrectomy _____

_____

_____

6. transurethral _____

_____

_____

7. hypocalcaemia _____

_____

_____

8. epidermal _____

_____

_____

9. dysphagia _____

_____

_____

10. pericardium _____

_____

_____

EXERCISE 1.3: IDENTIFYING SUFFIXES

Identify the suffix in each of the medical terms below. Give the meaning of the term as a whole.

Example:
osteomalacia

osteo/malacia

malacia = condition of softening

osteomalacia = condition of softening of bone

1. arthralgia _____

_____

_____

2. cholecystitis _____

_____

_____

3. carcinoid _____

_____

_____

4. craniotomy _____

_____

_____

5. osteogenic _____

_____

_____

6. hyperglycaemia _____

_____

_____

7. cystoscopy _____

_____

_____

8. gastroscope _____

_____

_____

9. rhinoplasty _____

_____

_____

10. haematologist _____

_____

_____

EXERCISE 1.4: WORD ROOTS AND COMBINING FORMS

Select the correct response from the choices provided for each question.

1. Which vowel is the most common combining vowel?
    a) a
    b) e
    c) i
    d) o

2. The word root is the _____ of the word.
    a) foundation
    b) meaning
    c) ending
    d) modifier

3. Which word contains a combining vowel between two word roots?
    a) erythrocyte
    b) hysterectomy
    c) salpingitis
    d) gastroenterology

4. Which of the following combining forms means gland?
    a) aden/o
    b) lapar/o
    c) cephal/o
    d) lip/o

5. Chondroplasty is the surgical repair of a _____.
    a) nerve
    b) herniated disc
    c) vertebra
    d) cartilage

6. Which of the following means vein?
    a) vas/o
    b) phleb/o
    c) angi/o
    d) lymph/o

7. A myelogram is an x-ray of the _____ after injection of a contrast medium.
    a) spinal cord
    b) brain
    c) blood vessels
    d) nerves

8. Which word means pain in a nerve or nerves?
    a) neuralgia
    b) nephralgia
    c) fibralgia
    d) myalgia

9. The combining form erythr/o means _____.
    a) haemoglobin
    b) skin
    c) red
    d) brain

10. Cardiology is the study of the _____.
    a) heart
    b) brain
    c) kidneys
    d) urinary tract

11. Encephalitis refers to inflammation of the _____.
    a) brain
    b) head
    c) intestines
    d) eyes

12. Which word means an abnormal condition of the liver?
    a) hepatitis
    b) hepatosis
    c) arthritis
    d) arthrosis

13. Which test would be performed to visually diagnose a stomach ulcer?
    a) gastroscopy
    b) gastroscope
    c) bronchoscopy
    d) bronchoscope

14. A general term for an incision into bone is called a/an _____.
    a) craniotomy
    b) craniectomy
    c) osteoectomy
    d) osteotomy

15. Someone who specialises in the study of blood is a _____.
    a) haematologist
    b) haemologist
    c) phlebotomist
    d) cardiologist

EXERCISE 1.5: WORD BUILDING

Using the following table of word elements, build medical terms for the list of definitions.

Prefixes	Meaning	Suffixes	Meaning	Word Roots	Meaning
a-	no, not, without, absence of	-aemia	blood (condition of)	cardi/o	heart
an-	no, not, without, absence of	-al	pertaining to	cephal/o	head
brady-	slow	-algia	pain (condition of)	cyst/o	bladder, cyst, sac
dys-	bad, painful, difficult	-ectomy	excision, surgical removal	dactyl/o	fingers, toes
endo-	within, inside, inner	-gram	record, writing	derm/o	skin
epi-	above, upon, on	-ia	process, condition	dermat/o	skin
hypo-	below, under, deficient, less than normal	-ic	pertaining to	electr/o	electricity, electrical activity
oligo-	scanty, deficiency, few	-ism	state of	encephal/o	brain
post-	after, behind	-itis	inflammation	enter/o	intestine (usually small)
syn-	together, with	-ium	structure, tissue	gastr/o	stomach
		-logy	study of	glyc/o	sugar
		-meter	instrument used to measure, measurement	haem/o	blood
		-osis	abnormal condition	haemat/o	blood
		-pathy	disease	hepat/o	liver
		-scope	instrument to view	therm/o	heat
		-y	process, condition	ur/o	urine, urinary tract, urea

1. Record of the heart's electrical activity _____

2. Condition of two or more fingers or toes joined together _____

3. Condition of a painful intestine _____

4. Condition of a slow heart (rate) _____

5. Instrument for measuring temperature _____

6. Condition of scanty urine (output) _____

7. Instrument to view the bladder _____

8. Condition of low blood sugar _____

9. Inflammation of the skin _____

10. Study of blood _____

11. Abnormal condition of the liver _____

12. Condition of no blood _____

13. Disease of the brain _____

14. Surgical removal of the intestine _____

15. Pertaining to above the stomach _____

16. Tissue inside the heart _____

17. Pertaining to the head _____

18. Pain in the stomach _____

19. (An injection described as given) below the skin _____

20. Condition of urea in the blood _____

EXERCISE 1.6: CROSSWORD PUZZLE

Complete the puzzle by providing the medical term for each of the clues below.

ACROSS

4. Word root plus a combining vowel (9, 4)
7. Found at the beginning of a word (6)
8. Foundation of a word (4, 4)
9. Found at the end of a word (6)
10. Pertaining to the skin (6)

DOWN

1. A language that is the foundation of medical terminology (5)
2. Links parts of a word together (9, 5)
3. Incision into the uterus (11)
5. Describes anatomical structures, diseases, procedures, treatments, medication and instruments associated with medicine (7, 11)
6. Flow or discharge through (9)

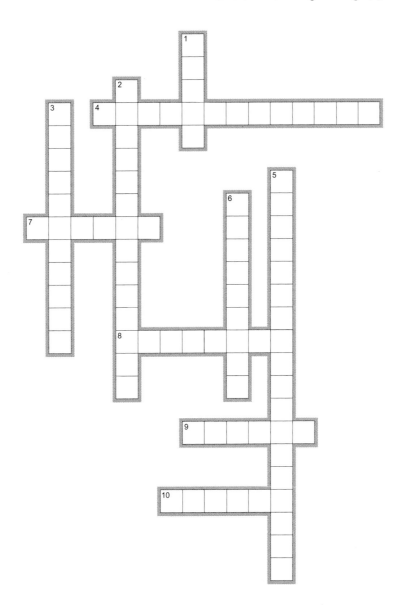

CHAPTER 2
Building a Medical Vocabulary

Contents

OBJECTIVES   16

INTRODUCTION   17

PRONUNCIATION OF TERMS   17

SPELLING CONVENTIONS   17

FORMING PLURALS   18

EPONYMS   19

   Diseases and syndromes   19

   Body structures   20

   Procedures or tests   20

   Instruments   20

MNEMONICS   21

EXERCISES   22

Objectives

After completing this chapter, you should be able to:

1. understand the rules of pronunciation and be able to pronounce medical terms correctly

2. understand spelling conventions specific to medical terminology

3. understand how to form plurals of medical terms

4. understand what an eponym is and be able to define some in common usage

5. understand the application of mnemonics to aid learning medical terminology

6. apply what you have learned by interpreting medical terminology in practice.

Demonstrate your knowledge of vocabulary building by completing the exercises at the end of this chapter.

INTRODUCTION

This chapter builds on what you learned in Chapter 1. Your skills in word analysis will be enhanced by introducing additional word elements and you will start to learn about word elements in practice.

Sometimes medical terms can seem very complex and consequently difficult to pronounce. This chapter provides some basic rules of pronunciation. It is important to understand these rules and to be able to apply them. In subsequent chapters, phonetic pronunciation of many medical terms will be given. Medical words can also be challenging to spell. This chapter contains some important spelling guidelines to help you. Forming plurals of medical terms can also be quite difficult at first. Specific guidelines on how to do this are provided.

The concept of eponyms in medical terminology will be discussed, and some of the more common ones will be identified. The concept of mnemonics as a method for remembering some aspects of anatomy and physiology will be explained and some examples provided.

PRONUNCIATION OF TERMS

When first confronted with a medical term, trying to pronounce it correctly can seem difficult. In this textbook, phonetic spelling has been provided to help you pronounce many of the medical terms that are included. Wherever lists of terms or medical conditions are provided, the pronunciation is also included. Each word or term is written using the correct spelling, followed by the phonetic spelling. The syllable on which the pronunciation stress falls is written in capital letters and the rest of the syllables are in lower case. You should practise pronouncing each term whenever you see the phonetic spelling provided.

For example:

biology is written phonetically as **bi-OL-o-jee**

endoscopy is written phonetically as **en-DOS-kop-ee**

cardiac is written phonetically as **KAH-dee-ak**

gastroenterology is written phonetically as **gas-tro-ENT-er-OL-o-jee**

While some medical terms are quite easy to pronounce, there are some that seem to be more difficult. The following rules of pronunciation will help you. As with anything, practice makes perfect, so remember to say all the terms out loud as you work through the book.

Pronunciation Rule	Examples
ae and *oe* are usually pronounced like *ee*	anaemia, oestrogen
c is pronounced like an *s* before the letters *e**, *i* and *y* (*exception: cephalic, which may be pronounced with a hard *c* sound like the letter *k*)	cervix, cilia, cytoplasm
c is pronounced like a *k* before the letters *a*, *o* and *u*	colon, cavity, cure
ch is sometimes pronounced like *k*	chronic, chromosome
e at the end of a word is often pronounced as a separate syllable *ee*	syncope, systole
es at the end of a word is often pronounced as a separate syllable *eez*	nares, appendices
eu at the start of a word is pronounced *yoo*	euphoria, euthanasia
g is pronounced like *j* before the letters *e*, *i* and *y** (*exception: terms with the word root *gynae/* are pronounced with a hard *g* sound)	generic, giant, gyrus
g is pronounced with a hard *g* sound before the letters *a*, *o* and *u*	ganglion, gonad, gurgle
i at the end of a word (as a plural form) is often pronounced like *eye*	alveoli, glomeruli
ph is pronounced like *f*	phobia, physical
pn is pronounced like *n*	pneumonia
ps is pronounced like *s*	psychiatry, psoriasis
pt is pronounced like *t*	ptosis, pterygium
rh and *rrh* are pronounced like *r*	rheumatic, diarrhoea
x is pronounced like *z* when the first letter of a word	xanthoma, xenograft

Some medical terms can have more than one agreed pronunciation. For example, the term *cephalic* can be pronounced with either a soft or a hard *c* sound. Both are correct, and usage is often determined by where the health professional was educated. When in doubt about how to pronounce a word, use your dictionary, read through this textbook and review the pronunciation provided or ask a health professional.

SPELLING CONVENTIONS

Many medical terminology books are written using American spelling conventions. It is important to realise that this textbook uses only Australian/British spelling conventions. Both forms of spelling are equally correct, but different countries prefer to use one form over the other. Most countries that have been part of the British Commonwealth at some point in their history choose to use British spelling. That is the case in Australia and New Zealand. The differences are too numerous to discuss here, but there are many sources available that discuss them.

Accurate spelling of medical words is an essential part of studying medical terminology. In some instances, correct spelling is extremely important to the meaning of the term. Sometimes words sound the same, or very similar, but have a completely different meaning. For example:

ilium	the hip bone	ileum	part of the small intestine
abduct	move away from	adduct	move towards
arteritis	inflammation of an artery	arthritis	inflammation of a joint
dysphagia	difficulty in swallowing	dysphasia	difficulty in speaking

This example demonstrates that by changing just one letter in a word, the meaning can be entirely different. Therefore, it is very important to get the spelling correct so the meaning of the word in context is also correct. If in doubt, always check the spelling in your medical dictionary. Many words have a Greek origin. Sometimes these words contain silent letters. For example, in the words pneumonia, ptosis and psychology, the letter *p* is silent but still must be included when the word is spelled.

As mentioned in Chapter 1, when joining a combining form with a suffix, as a general rule, if the suffix begins with a vowel, drop the combining vowel. For example:

haemat/o and -oma = haematoma

When a prefix ends in a vowel and a word root begins with one, options for joining them are to use one only, use both or hyphenate the two. For example:

microphthalmia
microorganism
retro-ocular

Check your medical dictionary to see which is correct or commonly used for a particular word. Sometimes more than one option is possible.

The prefixes *syn-* and *sym-* both mean together or with, but which is used in building a medical term depends on the first letter of the word root. *Sym-* is used before the letters *b*, *p* and *m*, for example in the words symbiosis, symphysis and symmetry. *Syn-* is used in most other circumstances – for example, in syndactylism and synthesis.

FORMING PLURALS

Forming plurals of medical terms can sometimes be challenging. Mostly plurals of medical terms are formed following normal English language conventions. For example, adding *s* or *es* to the end of a word (bone/bones) or changing the letter *y* to *ies* (biopsy/biopsies). However, there are exceptions. The following table demonstrates how to make plurals from singular terms based on word endings.

Singular Ending	Example of Singular Word	The Plural Rule	Example of Plural Word	Exceptions to the Rule
a	fibula	Retain the *a* and add an *e*	fibulae	
ax	thorax	Drop the *x* and add *ces*	thoraces	
en	lumen	Drop the *en* and add *ina*	lumina	
ex	index	Drop the *ex* and add *ices*	indices	
is	diagnosis	Drop the *is* and add *es*	diagnoses	iris/irides, epididymis/epididymides
ix	appendix	Drop the *ix* and add *ices*	appendices	
ma	carcinoma	Retain the *ma* and add *ta*	carcinomata	Can also add an *s* to form the plural – carcinomas
nx	phalanx	Drop the *x* and add *ges*	phalanges	

Table continued

Singular Ending	Example of Singular Word	The Plural Rule	Example of Plural Word	Exceptions to the Rule
on	ganglion	Drop the *on* and add *a*	ganglia	
um	diverticulum	Drop the *um* and add *a*	diverticula	
us	stimulus	Drop the *us* and add *i*	stimuli	virus/viruses, sinus/sinuses
y	deformity	Drop the *y* and add *ies*	deformities	
yx	calyx	Drop the *x* and add *ces*	calyces	

EPONYMS

In medical language an eponym is a disease, syndrome, body structure, instrument, procedure or test that is named after the person who first identified the disease, syndrome or structure or developed the instrument, procedure or test bearing the name. In the past, a possessive ('s) was included after the name of the person (for example, Crohn's disease), but this practice is slowly beginning to be dropped (for example, Down syndrome). This textbook reflects current common usage in Australia.

There are some significant problems with using eponyms. The name may be used to describe more than one entity, leading to confusion among health workers. The use of eponyms is not universal between countries and even between health facilities. This also leads to misunderstanding. The name is not descriptive, so it is difficult to derive the meaning or context of the eponym without prior knowledge.

Although using eponyms is discouraged, there are still many commonly in use today. Listed below are a small number of eponyms to raise your awareness of the concept.

Diseases and syndromes

Eponym	Pronunciation	Named after	Definition
Alzheimer's disease	ALZ-hy-merz diz-EEZ	Alois Alzheimer (1864–1915)	This degenerative disease was first described in 1906 by Dr Alois Alzheimer. It is characterised initially by the person's inability to acquire new facts. Ongoing symptoms include confusion, irritability, aggression, mood swings, language breakdown and long-term memory loss.
Burkitt's lymphoma	BURR-kitz lim-FOH-ma	Denis Parsons Burkitt (1911–1993)	Burkitt's lymphoma is a cancer of the lymphatic system first described in Africa in 1956 by Dr Denis Parsons Burkitt.
Creutzfeldt-Jakob disease (CJD)	KROYTZ-feld YAH-kob diz-EEZ	Hans Gerhad Creutzfeldt (1885–1964) and Alfons Maria Jakob (1884–1931)	CJD is a degenerative neurological disorder from the transmissible spongiform encephalopathies. It can be transmitted in contaminated harvested human growth hormone products, immunoglobulins, corneal grafts, dural grafts or electrode implants. It can also be inherited.
Crohn's disease	KROHNZ diz-EEZ	Burrill Bernard Crohn (1884–1983)	Crohn's disease is an autoimmune disease in which the body's immune system attacks the gastrointestinal tract causing inflammation that results in abdominal pain, diarrhoea, vomiting and weight loss.
Cushing's syndrome	KOOSH-ingz SIN-drohm	Harvey Cushing (1869–1939)	Cushing's syndrome is a hormone disorder caused by high levels of cortisol in the blood, resulting from taking glucocorticoid drugs, or by tumours that produce cortisol or adrenocorticotropic hormone. It results in hyperglycaemia, hypertension, obesity and facial oedema.

Table continued

Eponym	Pronunciation	Named after	Definition
Down syndrome	down SIN-drohm	John Langdon Down (1828–1896)	Down syndrome is also known as trisomy 21. It is a chromosomal abnormality that results in distinctive physical abnormalities such as sloping forehead, flat nose, low-set ears and retarded growth, as well as mild to severe mental retardation. It results from the presence of all or part of an additional 21st chromosome.
Hodgkin lymphoma	HOJ-kin lim-FOH-ma	Thomas Hodgkin (1798–1866)	Previously known as Hodgkin's disease, Hodgkin lymphoma is a type of lymphatic cancer characterised by the presence of large cells called Reed-Sternberg cells. Symptoms of the disease include lymphadenopathy, splenomegaly and enlargement of other lymphoid tissue.
Parkinson's disease	PAH-kin-sonz diz-EEZ	James Parkinson (1755–1824)	Parkinson's disease is a degenerative disease of the central nervous system characterised by impairment of cognitive processes and motor skills.

Body structures

Eponym	Pronunciation	Named after	Definition
Bartholin's glands	BAH-thol-inz glandz	Caspar T Bartholin (1655–1738)	The Bartholin's glands are a pair of glands next to the vaginal opening. They produce lubricating secretions.
Cowper's gland	KOW-purrs gland	William Cowper (1666–1709)	Also known as the bulbourethral gland, the Cowper's gland is located beneath the prostate gland in a male. It produces a secretion that makes up part of the semen.
Fallopian tubes	fa-LOH-pee-an tyoobz	Gabriele Falloppio (1523–1562)	The fallopian tubes carry ova from the ovaries to the uterus.

Procedures or tests

Eponym	Pronunciation	Named after	Definition
Nissen fundoplication	NISS-en fun-doh-pli-KAY-shun	Rudolph Nissen (1896–1981)	A Nissen fundoplication is a surgical procedure used to treat GORD (gastro-oesophageal reflux disease) and hiatus hernia. The upper part of the stomach (gastric fundus) is wrapped around the lower end of the oesophagus and stitched in place to reinforce the lower oesophageal sphincter.
Papanicolaou (Pap) smear (test)	pap-a-NIK-a-loh smeer	George Nicholas Papanicolaou (1883–1962)	The Pap smear or test is a gynaecological screening test to detect pre-malignant or malignant cells in the ectocervix.
Shirodkar suture	sheer-ODD-kar soo-cha	Vithalrao Shirodkar (1899–1971)	A Shirodkar suture is inserted into the cervical canal to prevent a spontaneous abortion in women with a history of an incompetent cervix.

Instruments

Eponym	Pronunciation	Named after	Definition
Penrose drain	PEN-roze drayn	Charles Penrose (1862–1925)	A Penrose is a type of drain inserted into a surgical wound to remove fluids to reduce the risk of infection.
Wrigley's forceps	RIG-leez for-sepz	Arthur Wrigley (1904–1984)	Wrigley's forceps are used to deliver a baby when its head is on the perineum and only a small amount of traction is needed.

MNEMONICS

A mnemonic (nem-ON-ik) is a learning technique for aiding memory. It assists in information retention by linking what needs to be remembered with clues for its recall. Common techniques used include creating acronyms or memorable phrases. These work on the principle that we more easily remember spatial, personal or humorous information than abstract or impersonal information. You may find this a useful learning technique as you work towards building your knowledge of medical terminology. Below are several examples of mnemonics, but you can also create your own.

What we are trying to remember	Mnemonic	Translation
Order of parts of the small and large intestines (proximal to distal)	Dow Jones Industrial Average Closing Stock Report	Duodenum Jejunum Ileum Appendix Colon Sigmoid Rectum
Cranial bones	Pest of 6 (the six represents the six bones)	Parietal Ethmoid Sphenoid Temporal Occipital Frontal
Respiratory passages	(Airflow is prominent in) mouthy people who are loud talkers	Mouth Pharynx Larynx Trachea
Divisions of the spinal column	Charlie Thomas likes sweet chocolates	Cervical Thoracic Lumbar Sacral Coccygeal
Number of vertebrae in sections of the spinal column	Breakfast (7 am), Lunch (12 noon) and Dinner (5 pm)	Cervical 1–7 Thoracic 1–12 Lumbar 1–5

Exercises

EXERCISE 2.1: SPELLING

Select the correctly spelled term from the choices provided for each question.

1. An elderly man was diagnosed with _____, which is characterised by abnormal hardening of the arteries.
   a) venosclerosis
   b) angiosclerosis
   c) arteriosclerosis

2. A five-year-old boy was admitted for the surgical removal of his tonsils. The procedure is called a _____.
   a) tonsilectomy
   b) tonsillectomy
   c) tonsilloectomy

3. An injection into a muscle can also be called an _____ injection.
   a) intermuscular
   b) intramuscular
   c) inmuscular

4. An _____ was performed to bypass an intestinal obstruction.
   a) ilieostomy
   b) iliotomy
   c) ileostomy

5. An increased level of urea in the blood is called _____.
   a) haematuria
   b) ureemia
   c) uraemia

6. The period before birth is termed the _____ period.
   a) antenatal
   b) antinatal
   c) antnatal

7. The 59-year-old woman was experiencing urinary tract symptoms. She underwent a _____, which revealed a normal functioning urinary bladder.
   a) cytography
   b) cystography
   c) cholecystography

8. A surgical puncture of the abdominal cavity to remove excess fluid is termed an _____.
   a) adbominocentesis
   b) abdomenocentesis
   c) abdominocentesis

9. A patient who has undergone removal of half of their stomach has had a _____.
   a) hemigastrectomy
   b) hemigastrotomy
   c) semigastroectomy

10. _____ lymph nodes are located in the armpits.
    a) auxillary
    b) ancillary
    c) axillary

EXERCISE 2.2: SPELLING AND CONTEXT

Some medical terms are very similar in spelling and pronunciation but have different meanings. It is very important to use the correct word in the correct context. Define the following pairs of similar terms.

Medical Term	Meaning	Medical Term	Meaning
haematuria		uraemia	
ilium		ileum	
ureter		urethra	
stomatitis		infected stoma site	
poliomyelitis		osteomyelitis	

EXERCISE 2.3: FORMING PLURALS AND SINGULAR TERMS

Provide the plural or singular form of each of the medical terms below.

Medical Term Singular	Medical Term Plural
bacterium	
calyx	
phalanx	
calculus	
ecchymosis	
chalazion	
sinus	

Medical Term Plural	Medical Term Singular
spermatozoa	
ova	
varices	
metastases	
ganglia	
epididymides	
rhonchi	
vertebrae	

EXERCISE 2.4: EPONYMS – WHAT AM I?

Provide the meaning for each of the eponyms below.

1. Foley catheter _____

_____

2. Parkinson's disease _____

_____

3. Snellen chart _____

_____

4. Bell's palsy _____

_____

5. Colles' fracture _____

_____

6. Alzheimer's disease _____

_____

7. APGAR score _____

_____

8. Legionnaires' disease _____

_____

9. Daltonism _____

_____

10. Papanicolaou smear _____

_____

EXERCISE 2.5: PRONUNCIATION AND COMPREHENSION

Read the following paragraph aloud to practise your pronunciation. Using your textbook and a medical dictionary, find the meanings of the underlined medical terms.

Mrs Xavier was 41 years old when admitted with a 6-week history suggestive of <u>hypoadrenalism</u> of unclear cause – query due to inadequate <u>Fludrocortisone</u> replacement. She was first <u>diagnosed</u> as having <u>Addison's disease</u> in 2001. She had a previous history of <u>thyrotoxicosis</u> 20 years ago managed with <u>medication</u>, with normal <u>thyroid function tests</u> since then. She also had an <u>anterior myocardial infarction</u> in 2004 due to a <u>coronary artery spasm</u>. Over the past 6 weeks she has become progressively more <u>lethargic</u> and weak, culminating in this requirement for admission. There has been no history of <u>fevers</u> or any suggestion of <u>infection</u>.

EXERCISE 2.6: ANAGRAMS

Work out each medical term from the jumbled letters below. Then, using the letters in brackets, determine the medical term that matches the description given.

1. gadahsypi	__ __ __ __ (__) __ __ __ __		difficulty in swallowing
2. tcdbau	__ (__) __ __ __ __		move away from
3. npmeyo	__ __ (__) __ __ __		a term named for the person who discovered it
4. zeersimlah	(__) __ __ __ __ __ __ __ __ __		a form of dementia
5. muiil	__ __ (__) __ __		part of the hip
6. wpseroc	__ __ __ (__) __ __ __		a gland on the side of the prostate

Rearrange the letters in brackets to form a word that means 'an obsessive irrational fear of a specific object or situation'.

__ __ __ __ __ __

EXERCISE 2.7: CROSSWORD PUZZLE

Complete the puzzle by providing the medical term for each of the clues below.

ACROSS

3. Also known as trisomy 21 (4, 8)
6. A procedure used to treat GORD (6, 14)
8. Hormone disorder caused by high levels of cortisol in the blood (8, 8)
9. An inflammatory disease of the intestines (6, 7)

DOWN

1. Gland that produces lubricating secretions (10, 5)
2. Degenerative disease of the central nervous system (10, 7)
4. Suture to prevent spontaneous abortion (10, 6)
5. Drain inserted into a surgical wound (7, 5)
7. A cancer of the lymphatic system (8, 8)

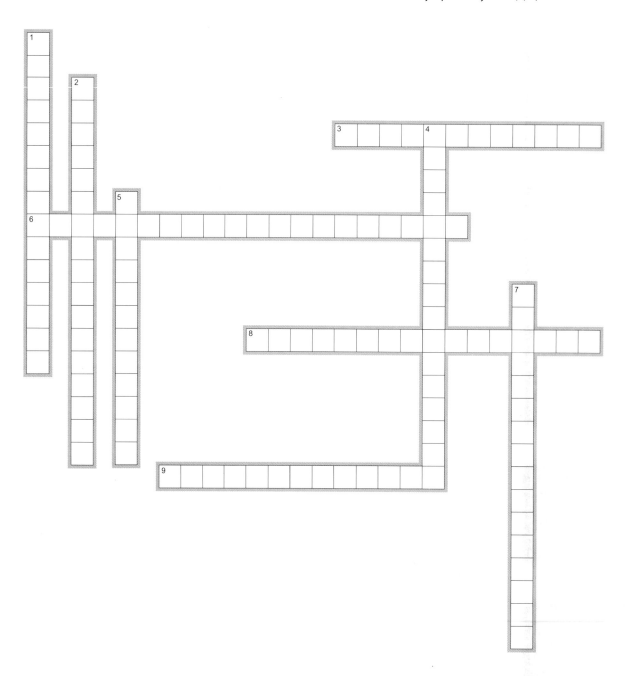

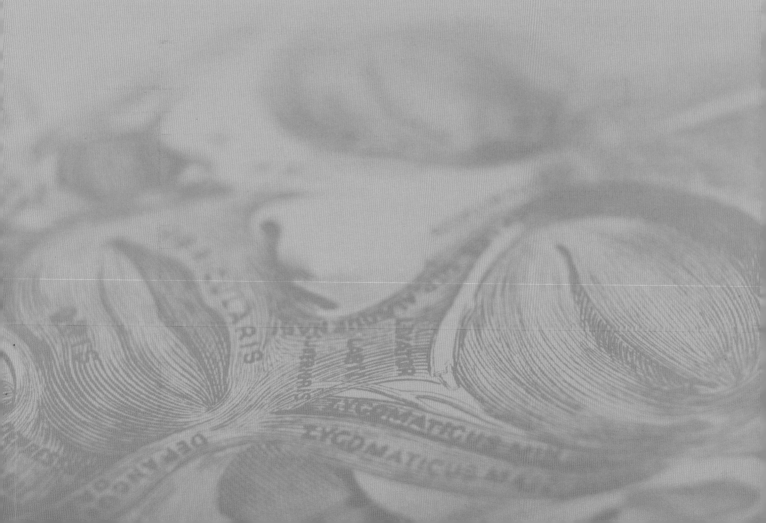

MODULE 2

The Body as a Framework

CHAPTER 3

The Human Body

Contents

OBJECTIVES   28

INTRODUCTION   29

NEW WORD ELEMENTS   29

   Combining forms   29

   Prefixes   30

   Suffixes   31

VOCABULARY   31

ABBREVIATIONS   32

STRUCTURAL ORGANISATION OF
THE BODY   32

   Cells   32

   Tissues   33

   Organs   34

   Body systems   34

THE ANATOMICAL POSITION   34

BODY CAVITIES   34

ABDOMINOPELVIC REGIONS AND
QUADRANTS   34

DIVISIONS OF THE SPINAL
COLUMN   37

POSITIONAL AND DIRECTIONAL
TERMS   37

PLANES OF THE BODY   38

EXERCISES   40

Objectives

When you have completed this chapter, you should be able to:

1. describe the structural organisation of the body

2. identify the location of the body cavities and be able to name the structures in each cavity

3. name the regions and quadrants of the abdominopelvic cavity

4. identify the divisions of the spinal column

5. understand the terms relating to body position and direction

6. identify the body planes

7. apply what you have learned by interpreting medical terminology in practice.

Demonstrate your knowledge of the human body by completing the exercises at the end of this chapter.

INTRODUCTION

Medical terms that are used to describe the structure of the human body are essential knowledge in medical terminology. Some of these terms should be very familiar to you because they are in common English usage, but others will be new and will require learning.

These terms will describe the basic structure of the body, the different body cavities, regions and quadrants and the divisions of the spinal column. There are also specific terms that describe position, direction and the planes of the body.

The purpose of this chapter is to demonstrate the structure of the human body as a whole. It is essential that you understand this before moving on to the subsequent chapters, which discuss specific body systems and specialty areas.

NEW WORD ELEMENTS

Here are some word elements related to the human body as a whole. To reinforce your learning, write the meanings of the medical terms in the spaces provided. Use the Glossary of medical terms on page 561 to help you work out the meanings. You may also need to check the meaning in a medical dictionary, but make an attempt yourself first.

Combining forms

Combining Form	Meaning	Medical Term	Meaning of Medical Term
abdomin/o	abdomen	abdominoplasty	
aden/o	gland	adenitis	
adip/o	fat	adiponecrosis	
aeti/o	cause	aetiology	
anter/o	front	anterior	
bi/o	life	biology	
blast/o	embryonic, developing cell	blastocyte	
caud/o	tail, downward	caudal	
cephal/o	head	cephalic	
cervic/o	neck, cervix uteri	cervicogenic	
chondr/o	cartilage	chondrofibroma	
coccyg/o	coccyx	coccygodynia	
crani/o	cranium, skull	craniotomy	
dist/o	away, far, distant	distal	
dors/o	back of body	dorsolateral	
fibr/o	fibre	fibromyalgia	
granul/o	granules	granuloma	
hist/o	tissue	histology	
histi/o		histiocytosis	
iatr/o	physician, medicine, treatment	iatrogenic	
ili/o	ilium, hip	iliac	
infer/o	below	inferolateral	
inguin/o	groin	inguinal	
kary/o	nucleus	karyocyte	
later/o	side	lateral	
leuc/o	white	leucocyte	
leuk/o		leukaemia	
(Note that the CF leuk/o is used in Australia for the word leukaemia (and derivative terms) only)			

Table continued

Combining Form	Meaning	Medical Term	Meaning of Medical Term
lip/o	fat	lipoma	
lumb/o	loins, lower back	lumbar	
lymph/o	lymphoid tissue, lymph gland	lymphadenitis	
medi/o	middle	medial	
melan/o	black	melanoderma	
my/o	muscle	myocardium	
necr/o	death, dead	necrosis	
neur/o	nerve	neurogenic	
o/o	egg, ovum	oocyte	
ov/i		ovicide	
ov/o		ovoid	
oste/o	bone	osteoarthritis	
path/o	disease	pathology	
pelv/i	pelvis	pelvic	
poster/o	behind, back	posteroanterior	
proxim/o	near, nearest	proximal	
sacr/o	sacrum	sacroiliac	
sarc/o	flesh	sarcoidosis	
somat/o	body	somatomegaly	
sperm/o	spermatozoa, sperm	aspermia	
spermat/o		spermatolysis	
spin/o	spine, thorn	spinal	
stom/o	mouth	stomal	
stomat/o		stomatitis	
super/o	above, excessive	superior	
thorac/o	thorax, chest	abdominothoracic	
tox/o	poison, toxin	toxaemia	
toxic/o		toxicology	
troph/o	nourishment, development	trophoblastic	
umbilic/o	umbilicus, navel	umbilical	
ventr/o	front, belly side	ventral	
vertebr/o	vertebra, spinal column	vertebrocostal	
viscer/o	internal organs	visceral	

Prefixes

Prefix	Meaning	Medical Term	Meaning of Medical Term
ab-	away from	abnormal	
ad-	towards	adrenal	
antl-	against	antibiotic	
bi-	two, twice, double	bilateral	
infra-	inferior to, below	infracostal	
macro-	large	macrocytic	
meta-	beyond, change	metamorphosis	

Table continued

Prefix	Meaning	Medical Term	Meaning of Medical Term
micro-	small	microcytic	
neo-	new	neoplasia	
poly-	many, much	polycystic	
uni-	one	unilateral	

Suffixes

Suffix	Meaning	Medical Term	Meaning of Medical Term
-blast	embryonic or developing cell	osteoblast	
-cyte	cell	lymphocyte	
-gen	producing, originating, causing	antigen	
-genesis	pertaining to formation, producing	pathogenesis	
-iasis	condition or state	hypochondriasis	
-ior	pertaining to	inferior	
-lysis	separation, destruction, breakdown, dissolution	histolysis	
-oma	tumour, collection, mass, swelling	haematoma	
-ose	pertaining to, full of, sugar	adipose	
-osis	abnormal condition	leucocytosis	
-pathy	disease process	myopathy	
-plasia	formation, development, growth	hypoplasia	
-plasm	growth, formation, substance	neoplasm	
-trophy	nourishment, development	hypertrophy	

VOCABULARY

The following list provides many of the medical terms used for the first time in this chapter. Pronunciations are provided with each term. As you read the rest of the chapter, make sure you identify each of these terms and understand their meanings.

Term	Pronunciation
abdominopelvic	ab-DOM-in-oh-PEL-vik
anterior	an-TEER-ee-a
cell membrane	sel MEM-brayn
central nervous system	SEN-tral NER-vus sis-tem
cervical	ser-VYK-el
chromosome	KROME-oh-some
coccygeal	kok-si-JEE-al

Table continued

Term	Pronunciation
connective tissue	kon-NEK-tiv TISH-oo
cranial	KRAY-nee-al
cytoplasm	SY-toh-plazm
distal	DIS-tel
deoxyribonucleic acid (DNA)	dee-OK-see-ry-boh-nyoo-KLEE-ik A-sid
dorsal	DAW-sal
epigastric region	ep-ee-GAS-trik REE-jen
epithelial	ep-ee-THEEL-ee-al
fascia	FASH-ee-a
frontal	FRUN-tal
hypochondriac region	hy-poh-KON-dree-ak REE-jen
hypogastric region	hy-poh-GAS-trik REE-jen

Table continued

Term	Pronunciation
inferior	in-FEER-ee-a
inguinal region	IN-gwin-al REE-jen
intervertebral	in-ter-VER-te-bral
lateral	LAT-er-al
ligament	LIG-a-ment
lumbar	LUM-bah
medial	MEE-dee-al
mitochondria	my-toh-KON-dree-ah
nucleus	NYOO-klee-us
peripheral nervous system	pe-RIF-er-al NER-vus SIS-tem
pituitary gland	pit-YOO-it-ar-ee gland
posterior	pos-TEER-ee-a
prone	prohn
proximal	PROK-sim-al
quadrants	KWAD-rantz
sacral	SAK-ral
sagittal	SAJ-it-al
spinal cord	SPY-nal kord
superficial	soo-per-FISH-al
superior	soo-PEER-ee-a
supine	SOO-pyn
tendon	TEN-don
thoracic	thaw-RAS-ik
transverse	TRANZ-vers
umbilical region	um-BIL-ee-kel REE-jen
ventral	VEN-tral
vertebra	VERT-e-bra

ABBREVIATIONS

The following abbreviations are commonly used in the Australian healthcare environment. Because some abbreviations can have more than one meaning, check the context in which the abbreviation is used before assigning a meaning to it.

Abbreviation	Definition
C	cervical – there are 7 cervical vertebrae: C1–C7
L	lumbar – there are 5 lumbar vertebrae: L1–L5
LLQ	left lower quadrant
LUQ	left upper quadrant
RLQ	right lower quadrant

Table continued

Abbreviation	Definition
RUQ	right upper quadrant
S	sacral – the sacrum consists of 5 fused vertebral bones: S1–S5
T	thoracic – there are 12 thoracic vertebrae: T1–T12

STRUCTURAL ORGANISATION OF THE BODY

The human body is made up of classes of structures, ranging from the smallest units of the body called cells, through to groups of cells called tissues, to arrangements of related tissues into organs and finally to groups of organs with specific functions, known as body systems. These are the body systems covered in this textbook:

- cardiovascular system
- digestive system
- respiratory system
- musculoskeletal system
- integumentary system
- endocrine system
- urinary system
- lymphatic system
- immune system
- nervous system
- reproductive systems (male and female).

In this textbook, you will find a chapter relating to each body system and detailed information about the organs and their functions and the terminology associated with each system.

Cells

Cells are generally considered the smallest living units of the human body and constitute every part of it. They are formed from atoms that bond to create molecules, which in turn combine to form cells. In the human body, there are around 100 trillion cells, each of which is invisible to the eye. Although there are many types of cells, they all have much the same basic structure. Each cell is specialised to perform a particular function.

All cells are surrounded by cell membranes. The membrane has several important functions: it holds the contents of the cell together but it also functions to identify the type of cell to other cells and to selectively allow substances, such as those produced by the body or drugs introduced into it, to pass into and out of the interior of the cell. The two major parts of the inside of the cell are the cytoplasm and the nucleus (Fig. 3.1).

Figure 3.1 Parts of a human body cell

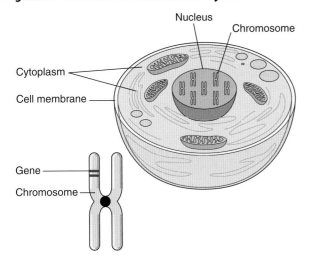

The cytoplasm is a clear substance with a jelly-like consistency. It consists mainly of water but also includes enzymes, salts, organelles such as mitochondria and ribosomes and certain organic molecules. Its principal activities are to dissolve wastes created by the cell and to move materials around inside the cell. It also permits the cells to carry out their specialised functions such as transmitting impulses or storing fats and is therefore vital to effective functioning of the human body. The various organelles contained in the cytoplasm are responsible for maintaining the cell. The mitochondria in the cytoplasm are the site of cellular respiration, which generates energy to enable the cell to function. Within the cytoplasm of most cells are a series of membranous channels known as the endoplasmic reticulum. The role of the endoplasmic reticulum relates to the production, processing and transport of proteins and lipids. The membranes of the endoplasmic reticulum differ in size and structure from cell to cell. For example, some cells, such as erythrocytes, do not have any endoplasmic reticulum, whereas other cells, particularly those that have an important role in synthesising proteins, need more endoplasmic reticulum.

The nucleus acts as the centre for administration and information and regulates the activities of the cell. In humans the nucleus also contains the chromosomal materials (deoxyribonucleic acid or DNA) and controls cell growth and reproduction. There are 46 chromosomes, consisting of 23 matched pairs, in all cells of the body except for the egg cells in the female and sperm cells in the male. These two types of cells have 23 chromosomes, which combine at the time of conception.

The chromosomes contain large numbers of genes in a specific order. The genes contain information about the composition of particular cells in the body to instruct them to grow in a specific way. Genes pass inherited materials to offspring, corresponding to various biological traits. Examples of such hereditary traits are blood type, hair and eye colour. If something goes wrong with a gene or the way it behaves, this is known as a mutation. Some genes that have mutations are responsible for causing defects and illnesses in the body. If the gene mutation exists in either an ovum or a sperm cell or both, the defect may be passed on to, or be inherited by, a child whose parents have the mutated gene. Diseases can occur due to a defect in a single gene or in a set of genes.

Tissues

A group of cells from the same origin that work together to carry out a particular function in the body is known as body tissue. There are four types of tissue in the human body: epithelial tissue, muscle tissue, nervous tissue and connective tissue.

- **Epithelial tissue** covers all external surfaces of the body. It also lines internal body cavities and organs and forms the basis for certain glands. Epithelial tissue has several important roles, including protecting underlying body tissues, secreting various chemicals and hormones into the blood and recognising sensation. Epithelial tissue provides a selective permeable membrane and all substances that enter the body or organ must pass through it.
- **Muscle tissue** can be classified into three types: skeletal, smooth and cardiac muscle. The primary functions of muscle tissues are to provide motion, maintain the body's posture and produce heat.
- **Nervous tissue** is responsible for controlling and coordinating body functions. Nervous tissue senses stimuli and sends impulses to different parts of the body to create a response. Nervous tissue makes up the central nervous system, which consists of the brain and spinal cord, and the peripheral nervous system, which covers all other nervous tissue. The function of the peripheral nervous system is to gather signals from all parts of the body and send them to the central nervous system, which then determines an appropriate reaction to the signal and responds back through the peripheral nervous system, directing a particular action.
- **Connective tissue** is found between the cells, acting to connect, support, insulate and stabilise organs of the body. Made primarily of collagen, there are four types of connective tissue: loose connective tissue, dense connective tissue, cartilage and other tissue. Loose connective tissue is the most common type, and it has a role in connecting epithelial tissue to underlying

structures, surrounding blood vessels and nerves and holding organs in fixed positions. This type of tissue is found underneath mucous membranes in areas such as the digestive tract and can also be found at the point of connection between skin and muscles. Dense connective tissue is made up of flexible collagen fibres and is very strong. Tendons, ligaments and fascia are examples of dense connective tissue. Cartilage is made up of various percentages of chondrocytes, elastin and collagen. Its purpose is to provide structure and support to other tissues. It also provides a form of padding in the joints. The other category of connective tissue includes bone or osseous tissue, blood and lymphatic tissue.

Organs

Organs are the next level of organisation in the body. Organs are composed of several different types of tissue that work together to perform a special function. There are many organs within the body, such as the heart, lungs, kidneys and skin.

Body systems

Two or more organs that perform collaboratively to undertake a common function are called a body system. This is the highest level of organisation in the human body and is the way that it is generally studied. As an example, the digestive system is responsible for receiving and digesting food and excreting waste. It consists of several organs from the mouth down to the anus including the stomach, small and large intestines, the pancreas, liver and gall bladder.

THE ANATOMICAL POSITION

This is a standard point or frame of reference that describes the human body when it is standing erect, facing forward, feet flat on the floor pointing forward and slightly apart, the arms slightly raised from the sides with the palms facing forward. When the position of an organ or body structure is described, the body is always considered as being in the anatomical position. When an organ is described as being on the right, it refers to the right side from the perspective of the person in the anatomical position. Similarly, something described as being on the left refers to the left of the body when it is in the anatomical position (Fig. 3.2).

BODY CAVITIES

The inside of the human body consists of five cavities or hollow spaces located within two main cavities,

called the dorsal cavity and the ventral cavity. Each of the cavities contains specific organs. The dorsal cavities are at the back of the body and are also called the posterior cavities. Included here are the cranial cavity, which contains the brain and the pituitary gland, and the spinal cavity, containing the nerves of the spinal cord (Fig. 3.3).

The ventral or anterior cavities are at the front of the body. The three ventral cavities are the thoracic cavity, the abdominal cavity and the pelvic cavity. The thoracic cavity contains the heart, lungs, oesophagus, trachea, bronchi, thymus gland and the aorta. Within the abdominal cavity are the peritoneum, stomach, intestines, spleen, pancreas, liver, kidneys and gall bladder. The pelvic cavity contains small parts of the intestines, the rectum, bladder, urethra and ureters. In females, the uterus and vagina also form part of the pelvic cavity. The abdominal and pelvic cavities are frequently considered together and are called the abdominopelvic cavity.

ABDOMINOPELVIC REGIONS AND QUADRANTS

Because of the location of various organs within the abdominopelvic cavity, clinicians often divide the cavity into quadrants (quarters), each of which contains specific organs and therefore may be affected by particular diseases. This assists with making a provisional diagnosis. The quadrants are the right upper quadrant (RUQ), right lower quadrant (RLQ), left upper quadrant (LUQ) and left lower quadrant (LLQ) (Fig. 3.4).

To more specifically locate diseased organs, the abdominopelvic region can be further divided into a grid, with nine regions (Fig. 3.5). Remember that right and left refer to the body when it is in the anatomical position.

The regions are:

Region	Location
umbilical region	middle of the abdomen, surrounding the umbilicus
epigastric region	above (superior to) the stomach and umbilical region
hypogastric region	below (inferior to) the stomach and umbilical region
right inguinal (or right iliac) region	right side of the hypogastric region
right hypochondriac region	right of the epigastric region
left hypochondriac region	left of the epigastric region

Figure 3.2 Anatomical position

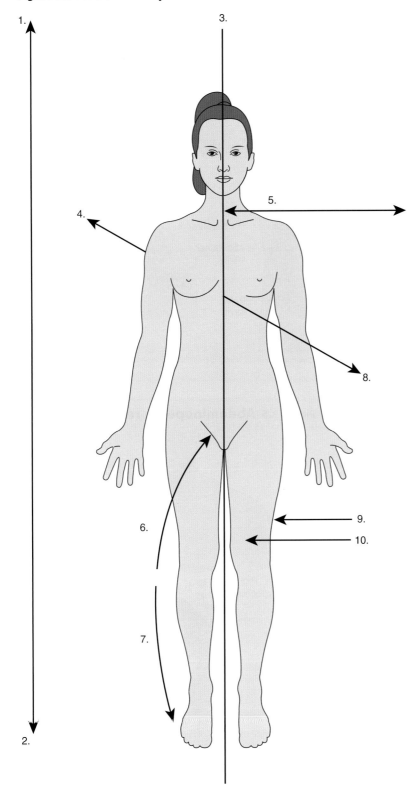

1. Superior
2. Inferior
3. Median line
4. Posterior/dorsal – back
5. Medial – lateral
6. Proximal
7. Distal
8. Anterior/ventral – front
9. Superficial
10. Deep

Figure 3.3 **Body cavities**

(Based on Salvo 2007)

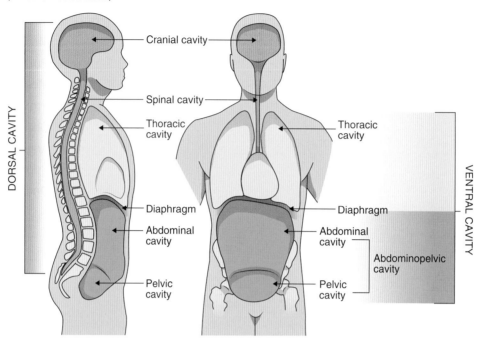

Figure 3.4 **Abdominopelvic quadrants**

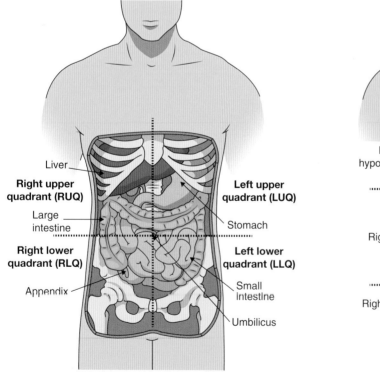

Figure 3.5 **Abdominopelvic regions**

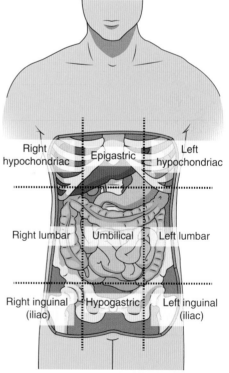

Table continued

Region	Location
left inguinal (or left iliac) region	left side of the hypogastric region
right lumbar region	lateral to the umbilical region on the right side
left lumbar region	lateral to the umbilical region on the left side

DIVISIONS OF THE SPINAL COLUMN

The spinal column consists of 33 bones, some of which are fused. Each spinal bone is known as a vertebra (plural: vertebrae). The spinal column is generally considered to consist of five divisions (Fig. 3.6). The divisions are:

cervical	Consists of 7 vertebrae, labelled C1–C7 and located in the neck region
thoracic	Consists of 12 vertebrae, labelled T1–T12 and located in the chest region
	Each of the 12 pairs of ribs is attached to a thoracic vertebra
lumbar	Consists of 5 vertebrae, labelled L1–L5 and located in the flank region (the area between the ribs and the hip bone)
sacral	Consists of 5 vertebrae, labelled S1–S5
	These bones are fused to form the sacrum
coccygeal	Consists of 4 fused bones that form the coccyx or tailbone

It is important to make a distinction between the spinal column, which is made up of bone tissue, and the spinal cord, which consists of nervous tissue.

Each vertebra is separated by an intervertebral space which contains a small disc made up of water and cartilage. The purpose of the disc is to act as a cushioning mechanism for the vertebrae as well as a stabiliser, and to ensure flexibility and movement of the spinal column. An intervertebral space is labelled or identified based on the location of the vertebrae either side of the space. For example, intervertebral space T12/L1 is the space between the last thoracic vertebra (T12) and the first lumbar vertebra (L1).

POSITIONAL AND DIRECTIONAL TERMS

Provided below is a list of common terms used in medical terminology to describe the location of an organ or body structure in relation to another.

Figure 3.6 Divisions of the spinal column
(Mosby's Dictionary 2014)

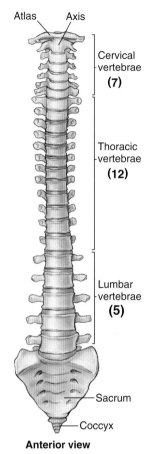

Atlas · Axis

Cervical vertebrae **(7)**

Thoracic vertebrae **(12)**

Lumbar vertebrae **(5)**

Sacrum

Coccyx

Anterior view

Remember that when describing positions or directions the body is considered to be in the anatomical position. Refer back to Fig. 3.2 for guidance in understanding the terms. The terms have been paired with their opposing term to also aid in your understanding.

Position	Explanation	Example
anterior	Also known as ventral and refers to being in front of an organ or at the front of the body.	The nose is on the anterior side of the body.
posterior	Also known as dorsal and refers to being behind an organ or at the back of the body.	The rectum lies posterior to the uterus.
deep	Refers to being further or well away from the surface of the body.	The knife penetrated deep into the thoracic cavity.

Table continued

Position	Explanation	Example
superficial	Refers to on or close to the surface of the body.	The patient sustained superficial cuts to the hands which did not require sutures.
proximal	Refers to locations that are close to the point of origin of a structure or attachment to the body.	The tibia and fibula articulate proximally with the femur at the knee.
distal	Refers to locations that are further away from the point of origin of a structure or attachment to the body.	The ulna and radius are distal to the humerus.
inferior	Refers to organs or structures that are below another.	The heart lies inferior to the head.
superior	Refers to organs or structures that are above another.	The liver lies superior to the bladder.
medial	Refers to organs or structures closer to the midline of the body.	The heart lies medial to the arms.
lateral	Refers to organs or structures that are further away from the midline of the body.	The ears lie lateral to the nose.
supine	Refers to a person lying face up.	The supine position allows for palpation of the abdomen and testing the effect of leg raising during a physical examination.

Table continued

Position	Explanation	Example
prone	Refers to a person lying face down.	The patient was placed in the prone position to allow for a better examination of the back wound.

PLANES OF THE BODY

Often sections of the body are referred to in terms of anatomical planes, which are imaginary lines that are drawn through a body in the anatomical position. Use Fig. 3.7 to guide you in understanding the following terms.

Plane	Explanation
frontal	A vertical line that runs lengthwise through the body, dividing the body or structure into anterior and posterior sections; also known as the coronal plane.
sagittal	A vertical line that runs lengthwise through the body, dividing the body or structure into left and right sides. The mid-sagittal plane divides the body into equal right and left halves; also known as the lateral plane.
transverse	A plane that runs horizontally through the body or structure and divides it into superior and inferior sections; also known as the axial or cross-sectional plane.

Figure 3.7 Planes of the body

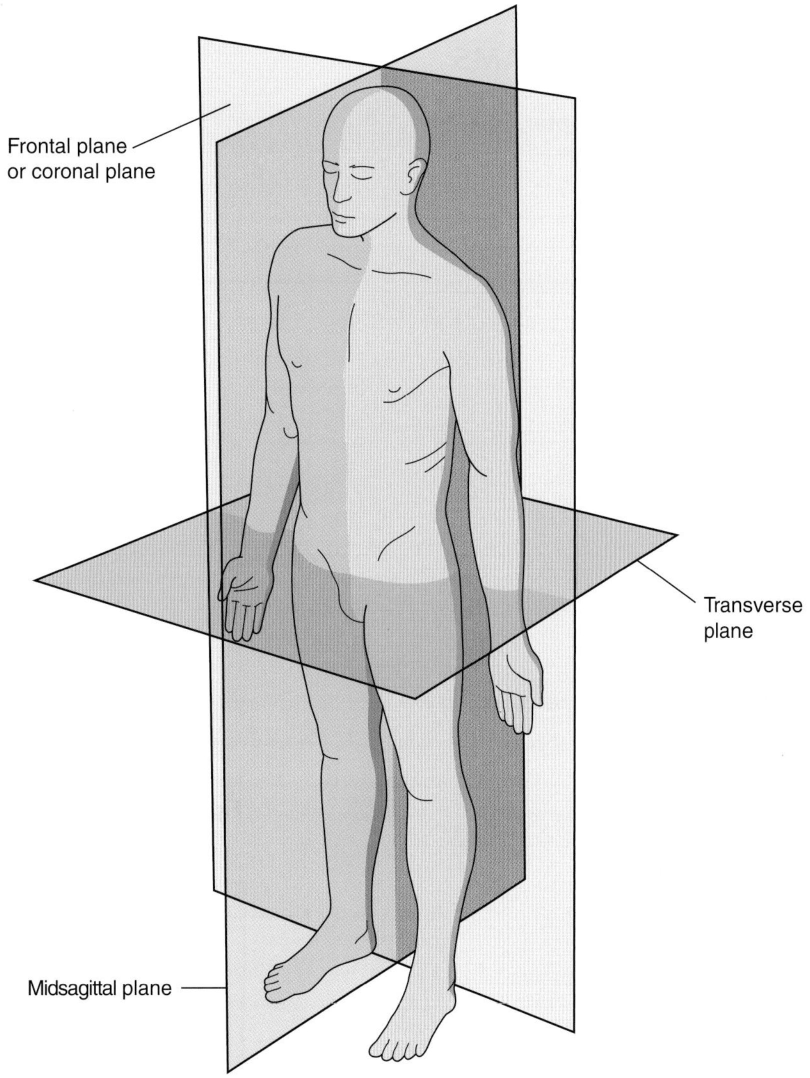

Frontal plane or coronal plane

Transverse plane

Midsagittal plane

Exercises

EXERCISE 3.1: LABEL THE DIAGRAMS

Using the information provided in this chapter, label the anatomical parts in the figures below.

1 _____

2 _____

3 _____

4 _____

5 _____

6 _____

7 _____

8 _____

9 _____

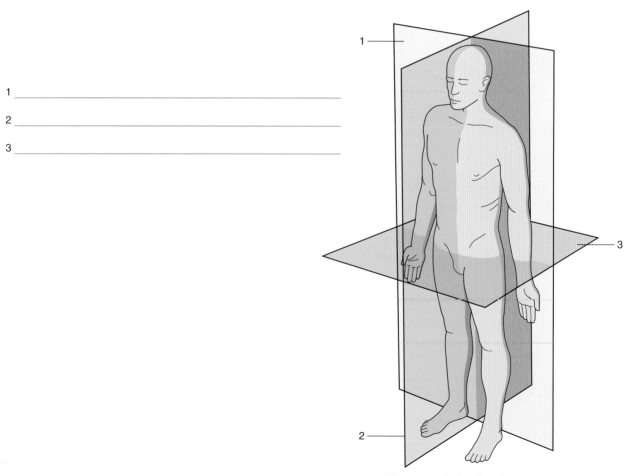

Figure 3.8 Abdominopelvic regions

1 _____

2 _____

3 _____

Figure 3.9 Planes of the body

1 _____

2 _____

3 _____

4 _____

5 _____

6 _____

7 _____

8 _____

9 _____

10 _____

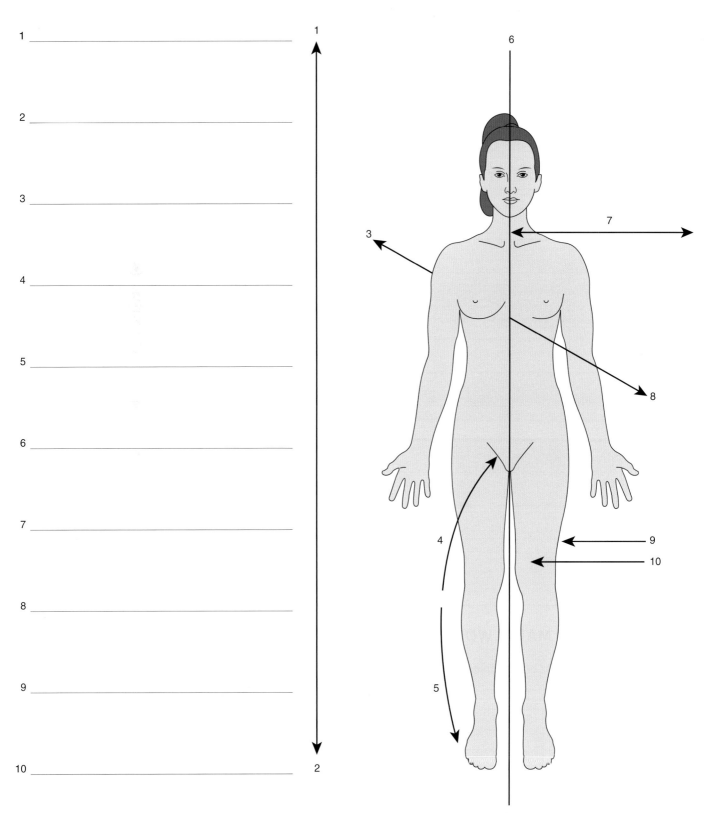

Figure 3.10 Anatomical position

EXERCISE 3.2: WORD ELEMENT MEANINGS AND WORD BUILDING

Define each of the word elements, then use each element correctly in a medical term.

Word Element	Meaning	Medical Term
anter/o		
coccyg/o		
cervic/o		
cyt/o		
hist/o		
inguin/o		
proxim/o		
thel/o		
vertebr/o		
cata-		
hypo-		
inter-		
epi-		
-ose		
-plasm		

EXERCISE 3.3: MATCH WORD ELEMENTS AND MEANINGS

Match the prefix, suffix or combining form in Column A with its meaning from Column B.

Column A	Answer	Column B
1. crani/o		A. ilium
2. meta-		B. egg
3. -eal		C. formation
4. sacr/o		D. excision
5. viscer/o		E. pertaining to
6. adip/o		F. navel
7. ili/o		G. internal organs
8. -plasia		H. nucleus
9. -ectomy		I. fat
10. umbilic/o		J. skull
11. ov/o		K. change
12. kary/o		L. sacrum

EXERCISE 3.4: WORD ANALYSIS AND MEANING

Break up the medical terms below into their component parts (prefixes, suffixes, word roots, combining vowels). Provide the meaning for each word element and each term as a whole.

Example:
osteosarcoma

oste / o / sarc / oma
WR   CV WR   S

Meaning: tumour of bones and flesh

1. abdominopelvic

_____ / _____ / _____ / _____

Meaning:

2. posterolateral

_____ / _____ / _____ / _____

Meaning:

3. thoracic

_____ / _____

Meaning:

4. hypogastric

_____ / _____ / _____

Meaning:

5. vertebral

_____ / _____

Meaning:

6. inguinal

_____ / _____

Meaning:

7. pleural

_____ / _____

Meaning:

8. craniotomy

_____ / _____ / _____

Meaning:

EXERCISE 3.5: VOCABULARY BUILDING

Provide the medical term for each of the definitions below.

1. The plane that divides the body into anterior and posterior sections: _____

2. The stomach is located in this cavity: _____

3. Tissue that connects, supports, stabilises and provides insulation to organs: _____

4. Pertaining to further away from the body or a structure: _____

5. Lying on the back with face up: _____

6. The cavity above the abdomen that contains the heart and lungs: _____

7. Tissue composed of fat cells: _____

8. The five bones S1–S5 form the: _____

9. Removal of a section of the skull: _____

10. This structure controls how a cell operates: _____

EXERCISE 3.6: BUILDING MEDICAL TERMS

Complete the medical terms below using the correct word elements.

1. Hypo_____ refers to the left and right upper abdominal regions.

2. _____al cavity contains the spinal cord.

3. Epi_____ cell is a skin and lining cell.

4. Inter_____ discs provide cushioning between the bones of the spine.

5. _____al pertaining to at the front of a structure or organ.

6. _____ior referring to being above a structure or organ.

EXERCISE 3.7: EXPAND THE ABBREVIATIONS

Expand the abbreviations to form correct medical terms.

Abbreviation	Expanded Abbreviation
RUQ	
C1	
LUQ	
T12–L1	
LLQ	

Abbreviation	Expanded Abbreviation
DNA	
RLQ	
AP	

EXERCISE 3.8: APPLYING MEDICAL TERMINOLOGY

Referring to Fig. 3.9 Planes of the body and Fig. 3.10 Anatomical directions (i.e. standing facing forwards with palms facing the front) in Exercise 3.1, complete the following sentences with terms illustrating the spatial relationship of these body parts.

1. The leg is _____ to the foot.

2. A _____ plane divides the body into right and left halves.

3. The cheeks are _____ to the nose.

4. The mouth is _____ to the cheeks.

5. The chest is _____ to the abdomen.

6. The wrist is _____ to the elbow.

7. A _____ plane through the arm divides the hand from the shoulder.

8. A _____ plane separates the face from the rest of the head.

9. The skin is _____ to the muscles.

10. The waist is _____ to the neck.

EXERCISE 3.9: APPLYING MEDICAL TERMINOLOGY

From smallest to largest, what are the different classes of structures that make up the human body? Fill in the blanks in the boxes below.

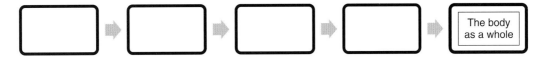

EXERCISE 3.10: PRONUNCIATION AND COMPREHENSION

Read the following paragraphs aloud to practise your pronunciation. Using your textbook and a medical dictionary, find the meanings of the underlined medical terms.

Mr Watson, a 62-year-old man, presented to an emergency department with a 24-hour history of <u>right iliac fossa pain</u>. He had no other significant past medical history.

On examination he had a low-grade temperature with <u>maximal tenderness</u> and <u>guarding</u> in the <u>RIF</u>. His <u>white cell count</u> was 19.5. A diagnosis of <u>acute appendicitis</u> was made, and he was taken to theatre that evening. Acute <u>gangrenous</u> appendicitis was found during an emergency laparoscopic <u>appendicectomy</u>, which was performed under a <u>general anaesthetic</u> (<u>ASA = 1E</u>).

Postoperatively he received several days of <u>IV antibiotics</u> and gradually settled. Mr Watson was discharged home with oral antibiotics and is to be followed up in surgical <u>outpatients</u>.

EXERCISE 3.11: CROSSWORD PUZZLE

Complete the puzzle by providing the medical term for each of the clues below.

ACROSS

4. To be lying face down (5)
5. The plane also known as frontal (7)
8. The space between two vertebrae (14)

DOWN

1. The head is said to be this to the neck (8)
2. This cavity contains the bladder (6)
3. The smallest unit of life (4)
6. The study of the structure of the body (7)
7. Basic DNA molecule that determines inheritance (4)

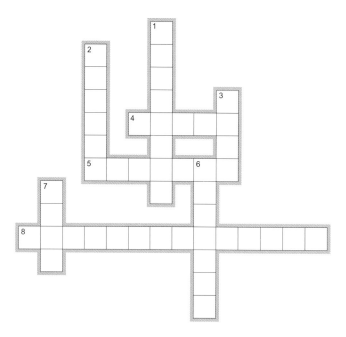

EXERCISE 3.12: ANAGRAMS

Work out each medical term from the jumbled letters below. Then, using the letters in brackets, determine the medical term that matches the description given.

1.	lemdai	— — — (_) — —	towards the midline of the body or structure
2.	tavnler	(_) — — — — — —	also known as anterior
3.	emeoptirnu	— — — — (_) — — — — —	serous membrane covering the abdominal wall
4.	ylraxn	— — — (_) — —	voice box
5.	aohdncorm	(_) — — — — — — — —	a benign tumour of the cartilage
6.	nsgora	— — — (_) — —	structures composed of tissues and cells that perform particular functions

Rearrange the letters in brackets to form a word that means 'a hollow space within the body that contains organs'.

— — — — — —

CHAPTER 4

Musculoskeletal System

Contents

OBJECTIVES 47

INTRODUCTION 48

BONES 48

New word elements relating to bones 48

Vocabulary relating to bones 52

Abbreviations relating to bones 52

Functions and structure of bones 52

Pathology and diseases relating to bones 53

JOINTS 56

New word elements relating to joints 56

Vocabulary relating to joints 57

Abbreviations relating to joints 57

Functions and structure of joints 57

Pathology and diseases relating to joints 57

MUSCLES 61

New word elements relating to muscles 61

Vocabulary relating to muscles 62

Abbreviations relating to muscles 62

Functions and structure of muscles 62

Pathology and diseases relating to muscles 65

TESTS AND PROCEDURES 67

EXERCISES 70

Objectives

After completing this chapter you should be able to:

1. state the meanings of the word elements related to the musculoskeletal system

2. build words using the word elements associated with the musculoskeletal system

3. recognise, pronounce and effectively use medical terms associated with the musculoskeletal system

4. expand abbreviations related to the musculoskeletal system

5. describe the structure and functions of the musculoskeletal system including the bones, joints, tendons and muscles

6. describe common pathological conditions associated with the musculoskeletal system

7. describe common laboratory tests and diagnostic and surgical procedures associated with the musculoskeletal system

8. apply what you have learned by interpreting medical terminology in practice.

Demonstrate your knowledge of the musculoskeletal system by completing the exercises at the end of this chapter.

INTRODUCTION

Musculoskeletal is a general term defined as relating to muscles and the bones of the skeleton. The musculoskeletal system comprises bones, joints, cartilage, bursae, tendons, muscles and ligaments. It is the system that moves the body and maintains its form. Study of this system consists of osteology (the study of bones), arthrology (the study of joints) and myology (the study of muscles).

The musculoskeletal system does not work in isolation. It is closely linked with many other systems in the body including the nervous system, genitourinary system, circulatory system, immune system, respiratory system, digestive system and endocrine system.

Other than the Tests and Procedures section, all topics in this chapter have been divided into three sections: those pertaining to bones, those pertaining to joints and those pertaining to muscles.

BONES

New word elements relating to bones

To reinforce your learning, write the meanings of the medical terms in the spaces provided. Use the Glossary of medical terms on page 561 to help you work out the meanings. You may also need to check the meaning in a medical dictionary, but make an attempt yourself first.

Combining forms relating to bones

Combining Form	Meaning	Medical Term	Meaning of Medical Term
calc/i	calcium	hypercalcaemia	
calc/o		calcinosis	
condyl/o	condyle	condyloid	
kyph/o	humpback	kyphoscoliosis	
lamin/o	lamina	laminotomy	
lord/o	curve, sway-back	lordosis	
lumb/o	loins, lower back	lumbosacral	
myel/o	bone marrow, spinal cord	myelopoiesis	
orth/o	straight, upright	orthopaedic	
osse/o	bone	osseous	
oste/o		osteomyelitis	
scoli/o	crooked, bent	scoliosis	
spondyl/o *(used for disorders)*	vertebra	spondylitis	
vertebr/o *(used for structures)*	vertebra, spinal column	vertebrocostal	

The following combining forms refer to specific bones in the body. As well as knowing the meanings of each of the combining forms, make sure you can identify the location of each of the bones on a picture of the skeleton, as in Fig. 4.1.

Combining Form	Meaning	Medical Term	Meaning of Medical Term
acetabul/o	acetabulum	acetabular	
brachi/o	arm	brachial	
calcane/o	calcaneus	calcaneodynia	
carp/o	carpal	carpectomy	
cervic/o	neck, cervix uteri	cervicothoracic	
clavic/o	clavicle	clavicectomy	
clavicul/o		supraclavicular	
cleid/o		cleidocostal	

Combining Form	Meaning	Medical Term	Meaning of Medical Term
cost/o	rib	intercostal	
crani/o	cranium, skull	craniotomy	
dactyl/o	finger, toe	syndactyly	
disc/o	intervertebral disc	discectomy	
femor/o	femur	femoral	
fibul/o	fibula	fibulotibial	
humer/o	humerus	humeroradial	
ili/o	ilium, hip	iliac	
ischi/o	ischium	ischial	
malleol/o	malleolus, little hammer	malleolar	
mandibul/o	mandible, lower jaw	submandibular	
maxill/o	maxilla, upper jaw	maxillofacial	
metacarp/o	metacarpal	metacarpophalangeal	
metatars/o	metatarsal	metatarsalgia	
olecran/o	olecranon	olecranal	
patell/o	patella	patellectomy	
pelv/i	pelvis	pelvimetry	
phalang/o	phalanx	phalangeal	
pub/o	pubis	pubiotomy	
radi/o	radius	radial	
scapul/o	scapula	scapular	
stern/o	sternum	sternocleidomastoid	
tars/o	tarsal	tarsalgia	
thorac/o	thorax, chest	thoracic	
tibi/o	tibia	tibial	
uln/o	ulna	ulnar	

Suffixes relating to bones

Suffix	Meaning	Medical Term	Meaning of Medical Term
-blast	embryonic or developing cell	osteoblast	
-clast	to break	osteoclast	
-listhesis	slip or slide	retrolisthesis	
-lysis	separation, destruction, breakdown, dissolution	osteolysis	
-malacia	condition of softening	osteomalacia	
-physis	growth	diaphysis	
-tome	instrument to cut	osteotome	

Figure 4.1 Bones of the body and the axial and appendicular skeleton
(Mosby's Dictionary 2014)

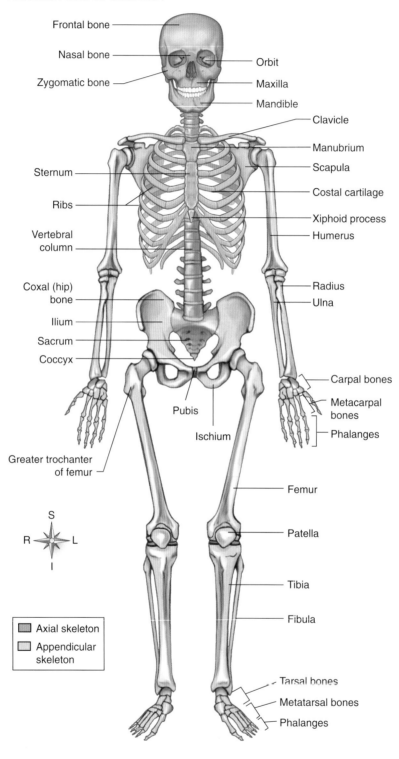

ANTERIOR VIEW OF SKELETON

Frontal bone

Nasal bone

Zygomatic bone

Orbit

Maxilla

Mandible

Clavicle

Manubrium

Sternum

Scapula

Ribs

Costal cartilage

Xiphoid process

Vertebral column

Humerus

Coxal (hip) bone

Radius

Ulna

Ilium

Sacrum

Coccyx

Pubis

Ischium

Carpal bones

Metacarpal bones

Phalanges

Greater trochanter of femur

Femur

Patella

Tibia

Fibula

Axial skeleton

Appendicular skeleton

Tarsal bones

Metatarsal bones

Phalanges

S

R ⟵✦⟶ L

I

Figure 4.1, cont'd

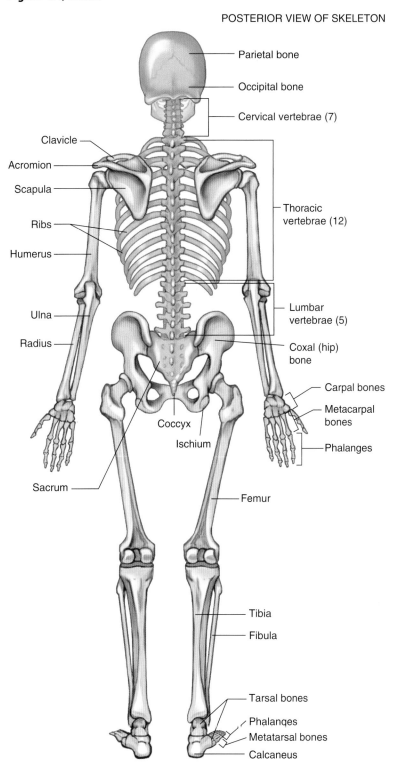

POSTERIOR VIEW OF SKELETON

Parietal bone

Occipital bone

Cervical vertebrae (7)

Clavicle

Acromion

Scapula

Ribs

Humerus

Thoracic vertebrae (12)

Ulna

Lumbar vertebrae (5)

Radius

Coxal (hip) bone

Carpal bones

Metacarpal bones

Coccyx

Phalanges

Ischium

Sacrum

Femur

Tibia

Fibula

Tarsal bones

Phalanges

Metatarsal bones

Calcaneus

Vocabulary relating to bones

The following list provides many of the medical terms used for the first time in this chapter. Pronunciations are provided with each term. As you read the rest of the chapter, make sure you identify each of these terms and understand their meanings.

Term	Pronunciation
appendicular skeleton	a-pen-DIK-yoo-lah skel-e-ton
axial skeleton	AKS-ial skel-e-ton
cancellous bone	KAN-sel-us bohn
collagen	KOL-a-jen
compact bone	KOM-pakt bohn
fracture	FRAK-sha
herniated intervertebral disc	HER-nee-ay-ted in-ter-VER-teb-ral disk
kyphosis	ky-FOH-sis
lordosis	lor-DOH-sis
osseous tissue	OS-ee-us TISH-oo
ossification	os-if-i-KAY-shun
osteomalacia	os-tee-oh-ma-LAY-see-a
osteoporosis	os-tee-oh-pe-ROH-sis
scoliosis	sko-lee-OH-sis

Abbreviations relating to bones

The following abbreviations are commonly used in the Australian healthcare environment. Because some abbreviations can have more than one meaning, check the context in which the abbreviation is used before assigning a meaning to it.

Abbreviation	Definition
AKA	above knee amputation
BKA	below knee amputation
C1–C7	cervical vertebrae 1–7
Ca	calcium
Fx, fx,#	fracture
L1–L5	lumbar vertebrae 1–5
NOF	neck of femur
OA	osteoarthritis
ORIF	open reduction internal fixation (of fracture)
POP	plaster of Paris
RIF/LIF	right iliac fossa / left iliac fossa
S1–S5	sacral vertebrae 1–5
T1–T12	thoracic vertebrae 1–12

Functions and structure of bones

In the first weeks after conception, the skeleton is represented by a matrix of flexible cartilage. As the fetus grows, ossification takes place as the cartilage is gradually replaced by hard deposits of calcium, phosphorus and collagen, which make up the bones. In newborn babies the body has 270 bones, but many of these fuse and ossification continues to occur as the child grows. The adult human body has 206 bones. The smallest bones are the ossicles in the middle ear and the largest bones are the right and left femurs, or thigh bones. Around 12–15% of the body's total weight is made up of bone. There are certain differences in the bones of males and females, primarily in the pelvic region because of the requirement of the female pelvis to accommodate pregnancy and childbirth.

The two main divisions of the bones of the body are called the **axial** skeleton and the **appendicular** skeleton, as can be seen in Fig. 4.1. The axial skeleton is made up of the skull, rib cage and vertebral column. The remainder of the skeleton, including the extremities, is known as the appendicular skeleton. It is called appendicular because these bones are appended or attached to the axial skeleton.

Bones are classified into five types: **long bones** (such as femur, tibia, humerus, radius), **short bones** (such as the bones in the ankles and wrists), **flat bones** (sternum, cranium, scapula, ribs), **irregular bones** (vertebrae, hips, bones of the face) and **sesamoid bones** (round bone masses embedded in tendons, such as the patella).

The functions of bones are to:

- provide a framework to shape and support the body and a place for tendons and muscles to attach
- enable movement by acting as levers in collaboration with muscles and joints
- provide protection for the body's most vital and delicate organs – the brain, heart and lungs among others
- create blood cells through a process called haematopoiesis – this takes place in the bone marrow
- store minerals such as calcium and iron
- help regulate certain hormones including those that assist with maintaining blood sugar levels and depositing fats.

There are two types of osseous tissue making up bones: compact or hard bony tissue (also known as cortical tissue) and cancellous or spongy tissue (Fig. 4.2). The difference lies in the denseness of the cells. Hard bone is made up of closely packed cells that have thin canals running through it for blood vessels to pass through. This compact tissue is usually located on the outside of bones and gives bones

Figure 4.2 **Bone structure**
(Thibodeau & Patton 2010)

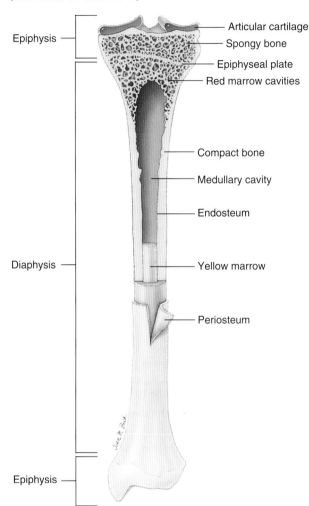

Epiphysis

Diaphysis

Epiphysis

- Articular cartilage
- Spongy bone
- Epiphyseal plate
- Red marrow cavities
- Compact bone
- Medullary cavity
- Endosteum
- Yellow marrow
- Periosteum

their characteristic hard, smooth, white appearance. Cancellous bone has spaces in between the cells, giving it a lattice-like appearance. This type of osseous tissue is generally found on the inside of bones, is highly vascular and generally houses the bone marrow where haematopoiesis takes place.

Pathology and diseases relating to bones
The following section provides a list of some common diseases and pathological conditions relevant to bone.

Curvature of the spine

Term	Pronunciation	Definition
kyphosis	ky-FOH-sis	Kyphosis is an abnormal convex or posterior curvature of the thoracic spine. It is also called hunchback or humpback.
lordosis	lor-DOH-sis	Lordosis is an abnormal concave or anterior curvature of the lumbar spine. It is also called a sway-back.
scoliosis	skol-ee-OH-sis	Scoliosis is a lateral S-shaped curvature of the spine.

Fractures

Term	Pronunciation	Definition
fracture	FRAK-sha	A fracture is a break or crack in a bone. Fractures are caused by trauma such as a fall or motor vehicle accident, through overuse or repetitive movements as may occur in athletes, or as a result of a disease process such as osteoporosis that weakens the bones. Fractures are classified by type and whether they are open or closed (Fig. 4.3).
		Open fracture: an open fracture occurs when there is an open wound communicating with the fracture, exposing the underlying bone. There is an increased risk of infection with an open fracture.
		Closed fracture: in a closed fracture the bone is broken, but there is no open wound.
		Different types of fractures (Fig. 4.3):
		Avulsion: an avulsion fracture is a closed fracture that occurs when a strong muscle contraction pulls a tendon free, resulting in a fragment of bone being broken off. Avulsion commonly occurs in athletes.
		Buckle: a buckle fracture is an incomplete fracture where one side of the bone bulges or buckles without causing a disruption to the other side of the bone. It appears more commonly in children.

Table continued

Term	Pronunciation	Definition
		Complete: a complete fracture occurs when bone fragments at the fracture site are completely separated.
		Complicated: a complicated fracture involves injury to bones and other organs such as blood vessels, brain and lungs.
		Compound: a compound fracture is another name for an open fracture.
		Compression: a compression fracture is a closed fracture that occurs when bones are forced into each other, crushing them. It commonly occurs to the bones of the spine and may be caused by a heavy landing onto the feet or falling into a sitting position, or as a result of advanced osteoporosis.
		Comminuted: a comminuted fracture occurs when a bone is broken into multiple fragments.
		Greenstick: a greenstick fracture is an incomplete break, a bending of the bone. This most often occurs in children.
		Impacted: an impacted fracture is a closed fracture that occurs when force is applied to both ends of a bone, driving them into each other.
		Incomplete: an incomplete fracture occurs when bone fragments at the fracture site are partially joined.
		Oblique: an oblique fracture is where the fracture occurs diagonally across the bone shaft as a result of angled force to the bone.
		Pathological: a pathological fracture is caused because bones have been weakened by a disease process such as osteoporosis, metastatic neoplasm or Paget's disease. Usually, no significant trauma or injury occurs to cause the fracture. A gentle bump or rolling over in bed may be enough force to cause the diseased bone to fracture.
		Segmental: a segmental fracture occurs in two places on the same bone, resulting in the bone fragment floating.
		Simple: a simple fracture is a closed nondisplaced fracture that does not require manipulation.
		Spiral: in a spiral fracture, part of the bone has been twisted. The fracture runs around the long axis of the affected bone.
		Stress: a stress fracture is a closed fracture, often just a hairline crack that occurs as a result of repetitive movements that cause strain on a body part. It is common in athletes such as runners and ballet dancers.
		Transverse: in a transverse fracture, the fracture is in a straight line across the affected bone.
		Fractures are diagnosed by clinical history, x-ray and sometimes by CT scan or MRI. Treatment involves administering analgesic medication and immobilisation by a plaster cast or splint. Treatment sometimes involves surgery.

Figure 4.3 **Types of fractures**

(Griffith 1994)

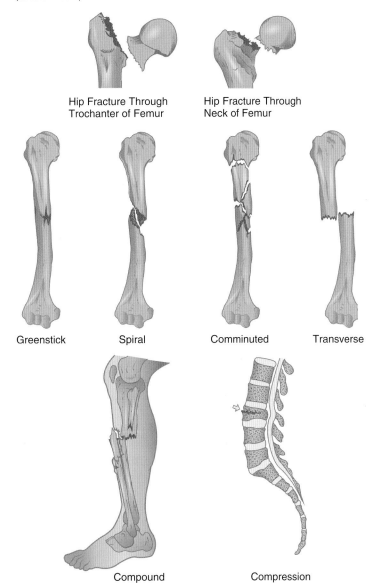

Hip Fracture Through Trochanter of Femur

Hip Fracture Through Neck of Femur

Greenstick   Spiral   Comminuted   Transverse

Compound   Compression

Other conditions

Term	Pronunciation	Definition
herniated intervertebral disc	HER-nee-ay-ted in-ter-VER-teb-ral disk	Intervertebral discs are pillows of fibrocartilagenous tissue located between the vertebrae of the spine. Sometimes as a result of an acute injury to the spine or because of degenerative wear and tear to a disc, a disc bulges, splits or ruptures. When this happens, the inner gel-like substance (nucleus pulposus) leaks out into the spinal canal. This is called a herniation of the nucleus pulposus or a herniated disc.
		A herniated disc is often referred to as a slipped disc, but this terminology is erroneous because a disc cannot actually slip. The most common site for a herniated disc is in the lumbar spine, especially at L4–L5. Symptoms will vary depending on the site and degree of the herniation but can include **paraesthesia** (pa-ress-THEEZ-ee-a), **sciatica** (sy-AT-ik-a) and back pain. Some patients will not experience any pain at all. Many cases will resolve spontaneously with bed rest, analgesics and physiotherapy, but if the condition persists, more invasive treatment such as discectomy or laminectomy may be required.

Table continued

Term	Pronunciation	Definition
osteomalacia	os-tee-oh-ma-LAY-see-a	Osteomalacia is a softening of the bones due to a lack of vitamin D or a problem with the body's ability to metabolise and absorb this vitamin. Adequate amounts of vitamin D are essential for the body to be able to absorb calcium and phosphorous into the bloodstream. Vitamin D deficiency may be caused by a lack in the diet, limited exposure to sunlight (which produces vitamin D in the body) or malabsorption by the intestines. Treatment involves vitamin D, calcium and phosphorous supplements. In children, osteomalacia is called rickets.
osteoporosis	os-tee-oh-pe-ROH-sis	Osteoporosis occurs when there is a decrease in bone density due to bones losing minerals, such as calcium, more quickly than the body can replace them. Bones become porous and brittle, resulting in an increased likelihood of fractures. While any bone can be affected by osteoporosis, the most common sites for osteoporotic fractures are the hip, spine, ribs, pelvis, wrist and upper arm. Although it is most frequently seen in postmenopausal women due to decreased levels of oestrogen, osteoporosis can occur in younger women and in men.

JOINTS

New word elements relating to joints

To reinforce your learning, write the meanings of the medical terms in the spaces provided. Use the Glossary of medical terms on page 561 to help you work out the meanings. You may also need to check the meaning in a medical dictionary, but make an attempt yourself first.

Combining forms relating to joints

Combining Form	Meaning	Medical term	Meaning of Medical Term
ankyl/o	crooked, bent, stiff	ankylosis	
arthr/o	joint	haemarthrosis	
articul/o	joint	articular	
burs/o	bursa	bursitis	
chondr/o	cartilage	chondrodysplasia	
ligament/o	ligament	ligamental	
menisc/o	meniscus, crescent	meniscectomy	
rheumat/o	watery flow	rheumatology	
synov/o	synovial membrane or fluid	synovectomy	
synovi/o		synoviosarcoma	

Suffixes relating to joints

Suffix	Meaning	Medical Term	Meaning of Medical Term
-clasis	break	arthroclasis	
-desis	to bind, surgical fixation, fusion	arthrodesis	
stenosis	narrowing, stricture	craniostenosis	

Vocabulary relating to joints

The following list provides many of the medical terms used for the first time in this chapter. Pronunciations are provided with each term. As you read the rest of the chapter, make sure you identify each of these terms and understand their meanings.

Term	Pronunciation
arthritis	arth-RY-tis
articulation	ah-tik-yoo-LAY-shun
ball and socket joint	ball and SOK-et joynt
bunion	BUN-yun
bursitis	bur-SY-tis
cartilage	KAH-til-aj
cartilaginous joint	kah-til-AJ-en-us joynt
condyloid joint	KON-di-loyd joynt
coronal suture	kor-OH-nal SOO-cha
dislocation	dis-loh-KAY-shun
fibrous joints	FY-brus joynt
gouty arthritis (gout)	GOW-tee arth-RY-tis
hinge joint	hinj joynt
lambdoid suture	lam-DOYD SOO-cha
meniscus tear	me-NISS-kus tear
osteoarthritis	os-tee-o-arth-RY-tis
pivot joint	PIV-ot joynt
rheumatoid arthritis	ROO-ma-toyd arth-RY-tis
rotator cuff syndrome	roh-TAY-ta kuf SIN-drohm
saddle joint	sa-del joynt
sagittal suture	SAJ-i-tel SOO-cha
sprain	sprayn
synovial fluid	sy-NOH-vee-al FLOO-id
synovial joint	sy-NOH-vee-al joynt
synovial membrane	sy-NOH-vee-al MEM-brayn

Abbreviations relating to joints

The following abbreviations are commonly used in the Australian healthcare environment. As some abbreviations can have more than one meaning, check the context in which the abbreviation is used before assigning a meaning to it.

Abbreviation	Definition
ACL	anterior cruciate ligament
CTS	carpal tunnel syndrome
DJD	degenerative joint disease
DMARD	disease-modifying antirheumatic drugs

Table continued

Abbreviation	Definition
OA	osteoarthritis
NSAID	non-steroidal anti-inflammatory drug
RA	rheumatoid arthritis
ROM	range of movement
THR	total hip replacement
TKR	total knee replacement
TMJ	temporomandibular joint

Functions and structure of joints

Joints are the location where two or more bones come together to create body movement or articulation. The three types of joints are fibrous, cartilaginous and synovial, classified according to the amount of movement they permit and the type of tissue present in the joint.

Fibrous joints are fixed and unable to move because thick membranous collagen fibres hold the bones together. Also known as sutures, this type of joint is found in the skull where the coronal suture joins the frontal and parietal bones; the sagittal suture joins the two parietal bones from the front to the back and the lambdoid suture joins the parietal bones with the occipital bone.

As the name suggests, **cartilaginous joints** have cartilage between them. Although they allow movement, this is far more restricted than the movement of synovial joints. The joints of the vertebral column and the pelvis are examples of this type of joint.

Synovial joints permit the greatest range of movement. In between the bones are spaces covered with synovial membrane, which fill with synovial fluid. These are called the joint capsule. The fluid in the capsule lubricates and protects the bones as they move. Synovial joints include ball and socket joints (such as the shoulders and hips), hinge joints (such as the ulnar part of the elbows and the knees), gliding joints (also known as plane joints), which allow bones to glide across each other (such as in the ankles and wrists), condyloid joints, which allow movement but not rotation (such as in the jaw or the fingers and toes), pivot joints, which allow both rotation and twisting (such as in the radius part of the elbow and the neck) and saddle joints, which permit side to side and forward and backward movement but not rotation (such as in the thumb) (Fig. 4.4).

Pathology and diseases relating to joints

The following section provides a list of some common diseases and pathological conditions relevant to joints.

Figure 4.4 Types of synovial joints

(Hansen 2019)

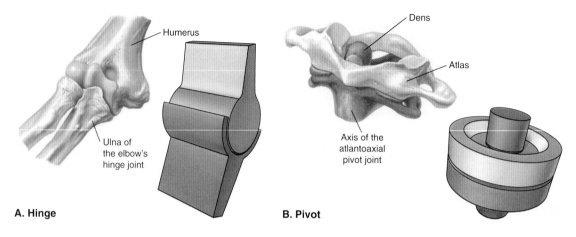

A. Hinge

B. Pivot

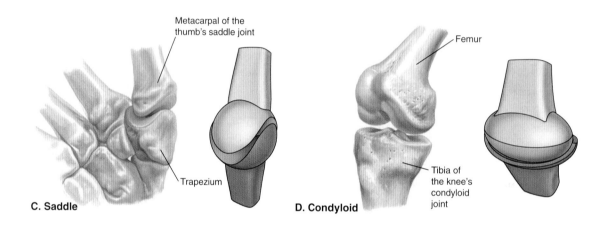

C. Saddle

D. Condyloid

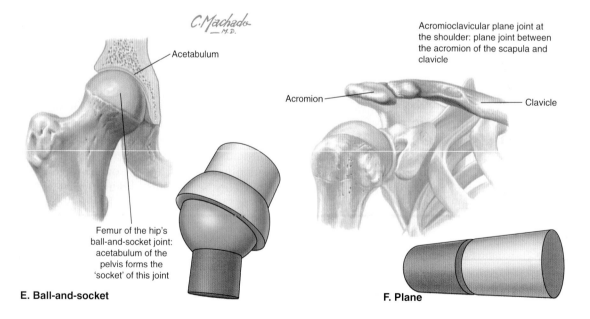

E. Ball-and-socket

F. Plane

Term	Pronunciation	Definition
arthritis	arth-RY-tis	Arthritis is inflammation of a joint resulting in pain, swelling and alteration to structure and function. There are several types of arthritis with different aetiologies.
– osteoarthritis	os-tee-o-arth-RY-tis	Osteoarthritis is a progressive, degenerative joint disease characterised by loss of articular cartilage, the presence of osteophytes (bony projections) and hypertrophy of bone. This leaves the ends of the bones unprotected, and the joint loses its ability to move smoothly and becomes painful and stiff. Osteoarthritis occurs mainly in the hips and knees (Fig. 4.5). It is diagnosed by clinical history and x-ray. Treatment consists of analgesic medication such as aspirin or NSAIDs and physiotherapy. As the disease progresses, joint replacement surgery may be necessary.

Figure 4.5 Osteoarthritis of the knee

(Based on LaFleur Brooks 2005)

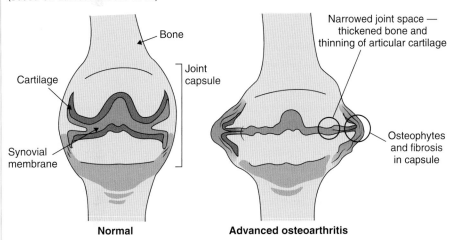

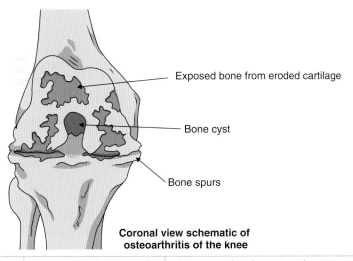

Coronal view schematic of osteoarthritis of the knee

– rheumatoid arthritis	ROO-ma-toyd arth-RY-tis	Rheumatoid arthritis is a chronic autoimmune disease in which the body's immune system attacks the synovium, the thin membrane that lines each joint. As a result, fluid builds up in the joints, causing pain and inflammation. Joint deformity and stiffness often result. The hands, feet and knees are most commonly affected. There is no cure, but rheumatoid arthritis can be managed with NSAID medication to reduce pain, DMARDs to stop disease progression and physiotherapy. Complementary therapies such as acupuncture and massage may help some patients.

Table continued

Term	Pronunciation	Definition
– gouty arthritis (gout)	GOW-tee arth-RY-tis	Gouty arthritis is caused by hyperuricaemia (a build-up of uric acid in the blood), resulting in the formation of tiny crystals of urate in body tissues. When the crystals form in joints, acute arthritis results. The feet, ankles, wrists and fingers can be affected, but the big toe is the most common site. Repeated bouts of gouty arthritis can damage the joint and lead to chronic arthritis. A diet high in fats and alcohol and a family history are possible causes of gout. Men are more likely to develop gouty arthritis than are women. While gout is a progressive disease, there are effective treatments to lower uric acid levels and prevent inflammation. Dietary restrictions to reduce intake of fats and alcohol are required.
bunion	BUN-yun	A bunion (hallux valgus) is an abnormal swelling of the medial aspect of the joint between the big toe and the first metatarsal bones. It is a common disorder that is caused by degenerative joint disease or pressure from poorly fitting shoes. It can be hereditary. Treatment involves wearing wide-toed shoes with cushioned lining. If the bunion is severe, a bunionectomy may be performed.
bursitis	bur-SY-tis	Bursitis is inflammation of a bursa, which is a fibrous fluid-filled sac between a tendon and bone. Normally, the bursa provides a slippery surface that assists movement and reduces friction. When a bursa becomes inflamed it results in joint pain, stiffness and swelling around the affected joint. Bursitis is caused by chronic overuse, trauma and infection. The most commonly affected joints are the shoulder, elbow, knee and hip. Treatment consists of administering NSAIDs such as ibuprofen, physiotherapy and rest as required. In some cases, an injection of a corticosteroid into the joint is required.
dislocation	dis-loh-KAY-shun	A dislocation (also called a luxation) is the displacement of two bones from their normal position where they articulate in a joint. It usually occurs as the result of trauma. Ligaments in the joint are usually injured as well. A subluxation is a partial dislocation. An x-ray is required to identify if a fracture has also occurred. Any dislocation needs to be reduced urgently to prevent complications such as ischaemia.
meniscus tear	men-IS-kus tear	A tear to the meniscus may be a traumatic injury, commonly seen in athletes, when a knee joint is bent then twisted. It often occurs in conjunction with an anterior cruciate and medial cruciate ligament tear. It can also be non-traumatic and part of the degenerative process in older patients who have more brittle cartilage. The most common symptoms of a meniscus tear are swelling and pain in the knee, tenderness on palpation of the meniscus, popping or clicking within the knee and limited range of motion of the knee joint. A tear is diagnosed by MRI or by an arthroscopy. Treatment consists of ice packs and rest (conservative treatment) or meniscus repair.
rotator cuff syndrome	roh-TAY-ta kuf SIN-drohm	Rotator cuff syndrome occurs when there is a tear or impingement of the tendons or muscles in the shoulder. The supraspinatus tendon is the most common one to tear. This is part of the rotator cuff on the back of the shoulder. The tear is often a result of an acute trauma or age related degeneration. In some patients there is no pain, while in some patients it feels like a dull ache in the shoulder that may make sleep difficult. Others again experience severe debility. Impingement syndrome may cause pain when raising the arm to the front or to the side. In this condition, the rotator cuff tendons are sporadically trapped and squeezed against the bones during shoulder movement. Conservative treatments such as analgesic medication, rest, hot/cold packs and physiotherapy are the initial treatment options. If the condition persists, a surgical procedure to repair the rotator cuff may be performed.

Table continued

Term	Pronunciation	Definition
sprain	sprayn	A sprain occurs when a ligament is overstretched or torn due to trauma to the joint. The most common site affected is the ankle. There is no fracture or dislocation present. It can result in pain, swelling, joint instability and loss of function. Rest, application of ice and a compression bandage are effective treatments.

MUSCLES

New word elements relating to muscles

To reinforce your learning, write the meanings of the medical terms in the spaces provided. Use the Glossary of medical terms on page 561 to help you work out the meanings. You may also need to check the meaning in a medical dictionary, but make an attempt yourself first.

Combining forms relating to muscles

Combining Form	Meaning	Medical Term	Meaning of Medical Term
clon/o	turmoil	clonic	
dors/o	back (of the body)	dorsodynia	
fasci/o	fascia (a band)	fasciectomy	
fibr/o	fibre	fibromyalgia	
fibros/o	fibrous connective tissue	fibrosis	
kinesi/o	movement, motion	kinesiologist	
lei/o	smooth, smooth muscle	leiodermia	
leiomy/o		leiomyoma	
muscul/o	muscle	muscular	
my/o	muscle	myofascial	
myos/o		myositis	
plant/o	sole of the foot	plantar	
rhabd/o	rod-shaped, striated (skeletal)	rhabdomyosarcoma	
tax/o	order, coordination	ataxia	
ten/o	tendon	tenorrhaphy	
tend/o		tendolysis	
tendin/o		tendinitis	
ton/o	tone, tension, pressure	myotonia	
tort/i	twisted	torticollis	

Prefixes relating to muscles

Prefix	Meaning	Medical Term	Meaning of Medical Term
ab-	away from	abductor	
ad-	towards	adductor	
dorsi-	back	dorsiflect	
poly-	many, much	polymyalgia	

Suffixes relating to muscles

Suffix	Meaning	Medical Term	Meaning of Medical Term
-asthenia	condition of weakness	myasthenia	
-trophy	development, nourishment	atrophy	

Vocabulary relating to muscles

The following list provides many of the medical terms used for the first time in this chapter. Pronunciations are provided with each term. As you read the rest of the chapter, make sure you identify each of these terms and understand their meanings.

Term	Pronunciation
aponeurosis	ap-on-yoo-ROH-sis
cardiac muscle	KAH-dee-ak MUS-el
fascia	FASH-ee-a
fibromyalgia	fy-broh-my-AL-jee-a
involuntary muscle	in-VOL-un-terry MUS-el
muscular dystrophy	MUS-kyoo-lah DIS-troh-fee
myasthenia gravis	my-as-THEEN-ee-ah GRA-vis
polymyositis	pol-ee-my-oh-SY-tis
skeletal muscle	ske-LEE-tal MUS-el
smooth muscle	smooth MUS-el
strain	strayn
striated	stry-AY-ted
tendon	TEN-don
voluntary muscle	VOL-un-terry MUS-el

Abbreviations relating to muscles

The following abbreviations are commonly used in the Australian healthcare environment. Because some abbreviations can have more than one meaning, check the context in which the abbreviation is used before assigning a meaning to it.

Abbreviation	Definition
ANA	antinuclear antibody (test)
CK	creatine kinase (test)
CT	computed tomography
DMD	Duchenne's muscular dystrophy
EMG	electromyogram
ESR	erythrocyte sedimentation rate
IM	intramuscular
MD	muscular dystrophy
MRI	magnetic resonance imaging
RF	rheumatoid factor (test)
SLE	systemic lupus erythematosus

Functions and structure of muscles

There are more than 650 muscles in the human body, which together compose 30–40% of the body weight of the average human (Fig. 4.6). Muscle tissue is made up of cells called fibres. Depending on their purpose, the size and shape of the fibres differ. The fibres are surrounded by connective tissue and are enclosed in fascia, a type of strong connective tissue. As the muscle fibres contract and relax, they produce movement in the body. Many body movements are a result of several muscles working collaboratively. Muscles are often grouped in pairs, where a contraction of one muscle moves a bone in a particular direction, and a contraction of the other muscle moves the bone in the opposite direction. The biceps and triceps muscles of the upper arm are a good example of this mechanism. When the central nervous system instructs the biceps muscle to contract, a corresponding impulse relaxes the triceps muscle, and vice versa. Occurring at the same time, these impulses allow for movement in both directions.

Muscles can be attached to bones, to skin or to other muscles by tendons and aponeuroses. Tendons are thick fibrous bands of tissue, whereas aponeuroses are more like flat ribbons, having fewer blood vessels and nerves than tendons. The body regions with aponeuroses are in the ventral abdominal region, the dorsal lumbar region and in the palm of the hand.

Humans have three different kinds of muscle (Fig. 4.7):

Skeletal muscles attach to bones by tendons across connecting joints, which allows the muscles to pull on bones and create movement. Skeletal muscle is striated in appearance; that is, the cell fibres have alternating light and dark bands (known as striations). Skeletal muscles are under the conscious control of the body – in other words, they are voluntary muscles. These muscles hold the skeleton together, give the body shape, and help it with everyday movements by contracting or tightening. Skeletal muscles vary considerably in size, shape and arrangement of fibres. The smallest muscles in the body are found in the inner ear and the largest and most bulky is the muscle in the buttock.

Smooth muscles are commonly involved in involuntary movements – movements over which we have no conscious control. Smooth muscles are formed from thin layers or sheets made up of cells and are found in the walls of the internal organs such as the stomach, intestine, bladder and blood vessels (excluding the heart).

Figure 4.6 Muscles of the body

(Mosby's Dictionary 2014)

ANTERIOR VIEW

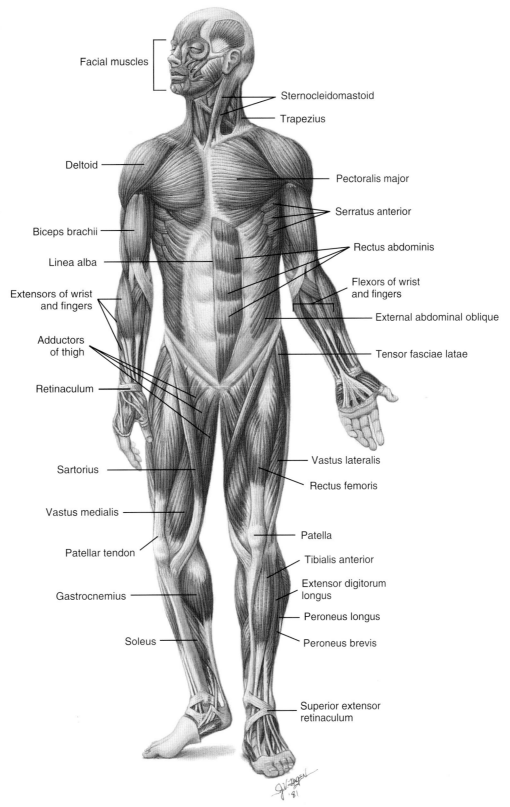

Facial muscles

Sternocleidomastoid

Trapezius

Deltoid

Pectoralis major

Serratus anterior

Biceps brachii

Rectus abdominis

Linea alba

Flexors of wrist
and fingers

Extensors of wrist
and fingers

External abdominal oblique

Adductors
of thigh

Tensor fasciae latae

Retinaculum

Vastus lateralis

Sartorius

Rectus femoris

Vastus medialis

Patella

Patellar tendon

Tibialis anterior

Extensor digitorum
longus

Gastrocnemius

Peroneus longus

Peroneus brevis

Soleus

Superior extensor
retinaculum

Continued

Figure 4.6, cont'd

POSTERIOR VIEW

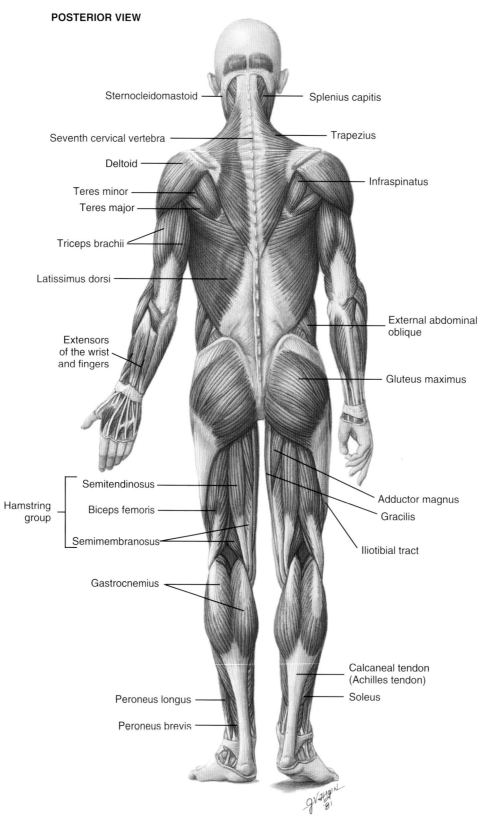

Figure 4.7 Types of muscle tissue

(Thibodeau & Patton 2003)

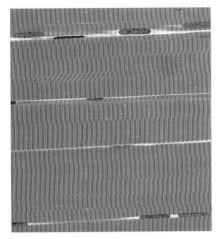

Skeletal muscle

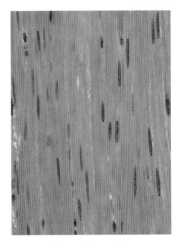

Smooth muscle

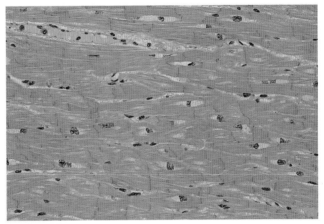

Cardiac muscle

Cardiac muscles are unique in that they are striated in appearance but involuntary in action. As the name implies, cardiac muscles are found in the myocardium of the heart and largely make up the heart wall. This type of muscle contracts to force blood out of the heart into the blood vessels and relaxes to allow the heart to fill with blood.

Pathology and diseases relating to muscles

The following section provides a list of some common diseases and pathological conditions relevant to the muscles.

Term	Pronunciation	Definition
fibromyalgia	fy-bro-my-AL-jee-a	Fibromyalgia is a term used to describe a common syndrome in which people experience long-term, widespread pain and tender points in joints, muscles, tendons and other soft tissues. It also results in disturbed sleep and exhaustion. The cause is unknown, but possible triggers include viral infection, physical and emotional stress. It tends to be more common in people with pre-existing lupus, rheumatoid arthritis or ankylosing spondylitis. There is no cure, but symptomatic treatment can help some patients.

Table continued

Term	Pronunciation	Definition
muscular dystrophy	MUS-kyoo-lah DIS-troh-fee	Muscular dystrophy refers to a group of hereditary diseases that weaken different muscle groups in various ways. A person affected with muscular dystrophy has a genetic mutation that prevents the repair of muscle tissue. This muscle weakening occurs gradually over time. Symptoms may start at any time from infancy through to adulthood.
		The most common form of muscular dystrophy is Duchenne's muscular dystrophy (DMD). It is caused by a genetic defect, which results in the body's failure to produce a specific protein called dystrophin, which strengthens muscle tissue. It predominantly affects boys between the ages of 2 and 6 years. By age 10–12 years these children will often be in a wheelchair. This disease also affects other body systems, so patients need regular respiratory and cardiac assessment. It is likely that these patients will eventually need a ventilator to breathe. People with DMD usually do not survive beyond their late teens or early adulthood.
myasthenia gravis	my-as-THEEN-ee-a GRA-vis	Myasthenia gravis is an autoimmune, neuromuscular disorder that causes weakness of the voluntary (skeletal) muscles. The flow of impulses between nerves and muscles is compromised. It can occur at any age but predominantly affects young women and older men. Muscle weakness becomes worse with activity but improves with rest. Patients with myasthenia gravis will experience dyspnoea, dysphasia, dysphagia, facial paralysis, diplopia, blepharoptosis and general fatigue. There is currently no cure, but treatment can help alleviate some of the symptoms. Medications, plasmapheresis, intravenous immunoglobulins and lifestyle adjustments to allow for more rest can all improve quality of life.
polymyositis	pol-ee-my-oh-SY-tis	Polymyositis is an inflammatory muscle disease that results in muscle weakness. The cause is unknown; however, it is thought to be triggered by environmental agents such as viruses. Other research indicates an autoimmune or genetic aetiology. Polymyositis is often associated with autoimmune diseases such as rheumatoid arthritis and lupus erythematosus. It is more common in females than males and tends to develop between the ages of 50 and 70 years.
		Most patients experience an improvement of their symptoms with treatment such as corticosteroids, although there may be some long-term muscle weakness. It is rarely fatal, but it has been linked with respiratory and cardiac conditions, as well as an increased risk of certain cancers such as bladder cancer and non-Hodgkin lymphoma.
strain	strayn	A strain occurs when a muscle and/or tendon is overstretched or torn. There is no fracture or dislocation present. Pain, weakness and muscle spasms are common symptoms experienced after a strain occurs. Rest, application of ice and a compression bandage are effective treatments.

TESTS AND PROCEDURES

The following section provides a list of common diagnostic tests, procedures and clinical and surgical interventions that are performed on the musculoskeletal system.

Test/procedure	Pronunciation	Definition
amputation	amp-yoo-TAY-shun	An amputation is the surgical or traumatic removal/excision of an extremity (arm, hand, finger, leg, foot, toe). In addition to traumatic amputations, some of the common reasons leading to the need for amputation include diabetes, peripheral vascular disease and cancer.
antinuclear antibody test	an-tee-NYOO-klee-a AN-tee-bod-ee test	An antinuclear antibody test is a diagnostic test used in patients with systemic lupus erythematosus (SLE or lupus) to detect antibodies present in the patient's serum.
arthrocentesis	arth-roh-sen-TEE-sis	An arthrocentesis is also known as joint aspiration. A needle is inserted into the joint to withdraw synovial fluid to relieve joint pain and swelling or for analysis to identify conditions such as infection, rheumatoid arthritis and gout.
arthrography	arth-ROG-raf-ee	An arthrography involves injecting contrast material containing iodine into a joint to allow for an x-ray called a fluoroscopy to be performed. It is used to identify abnormalities with the function and structure of a joint and to determine the need for further treatment and surgery.
arthroplasty	ARTH-roh-plas-tee	An arthroplasty is a surgical procedure that leads to reconstructing or replacing joint structures with artificial devices. The procedure is performed to relieve the symptoms of pain from conditions such as osteoarthritis. Arthroplasty of the knee or hip are the most common. Total or partial replacement may be performed; for example, a hemiarthroplasty is commonly performed for a fractured neck of femur.
arthroscopy	arth-ROS-kop-ee	An arthroscopy is a procedure to view a joint using an arthroscope (Fig. 4.8). The procedure is used both as a diagnostic process and as a method of entry to allow for more complex procedures such as a meniscectomy. **Figure 4.8 Arthroscopy** (Leonard 2005) Quadriceps femoris / Head of femur / Synovial space
bone density test	bohn DEN-sit-ee test	A bone density test is a diagnostic procedure used to identify decreased bone density. The test identifies conditions such as osteoporosis and osteopenia. Generally, x-rays of the spinal column, pelvis and wrist are taken to measure the density of the bones.

Table continued

Test/procedure	Pronunciation	Definition
bone scan	bohn skan	A bone scan is a diagnostic test used to identify abnormalities in bones resulting from conditions such as primary bone cancers, bony metastases and bone inflammation (Fig. 4.9). The patient receives an injection of a small amount of radioactive material and then is scanned using a gamma camera. Bones with an abnormality will have a greater uptake of the radioactive material.
computed tomography (CT)	kom-PYOO-ted to-MOG-raf-ee	A CT is a diagnostic test performed to identify disorders of the soft tissues, bone and muscle. Cross-sectional images are taken using a computer in conjunction with x-ray beams.
C-reactive protein	see ree-ak-tiv PRO-teen	A C-reactive protein test is an examination of blood to identify the presence of inflammation and infection and to assess a patient's response to treatment for such conditions. It can also assist with differentiating a viral infection from a bacterial infection. It is often used to diagnose certain types of arthritis, most commonly rheumatoid arthritis.
electromyography (EMG)	ee-LEK-troh-my-OG-raf-ee	An EMG is a diagnostic test used to identify neuropathic and myopathic disorders. Electrodes are placed on the muscle and are used to record motor unit activity at rest and during muscle contraction.

Figure 4.9 Technetium-99m bone scan

showing an area of increased radioactive uptake on the left femur that indicates a bone tumour

(Orkin et al 2009)

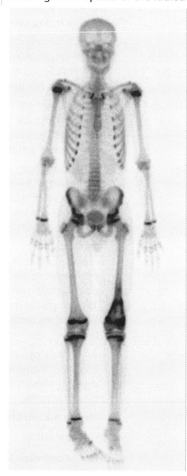

Table continued

Test/procedure	Pronunciation	Definition
erythrocyte sedimentation rate (ESR)	e-REETH-roh-syt SED-ee-men-TAY-shun rayt	ESR is a measure to determine the rate at which erythrocytes settle out of plasma in a test tube. In conditions such as infections, joint inflammation and tumours that increase the immunoglobulin content of blood, the sedimentation rate is altered.
joint injection	joynt in-JEK-shun	A joint injection is a method of treatment using a hypodermic needle to inject anti-inflammatory agents into a joint to treat such conditions as arthritis, gout and tendonitis.
laminectomy	lam-in-EK-tom-ee	A laminectomy is a surgical procedure that involves incising a vertebra to allow access to the spinal cord to remove herniated intervertebral discs and tumours. It is also used to relieve pressure on a spinal nerve.
magnetic resonance imaging (MRI)	mag-NET-ik REZ-on-ans IM-a-jing	An MRI is a diagnostic test that creates images of soft tissue using radio waves and a magnetic field.
meniscectomy	men-i-SEK-toh-mee	A meniscectomy is a surgical procedure that involves removing damaged meniscal tissue in the knee. The route for entry is generally via arthroscopy.
muscle biopsy	MUS-el BY-op-see	A muscle biopsy is a diagnostic procedure involving excising a sample of muscle for laboratory examination.
reduction and fixation	re-DUK-shun and fik-SAY-shun	This group of procedures generally refers to the manipulation of a bone or joint to correct its position following a fracture or dislocation, and the subsequent process of securing the structure with screws, wires, pins or plates. The reduction can be accomplished either as a closed procedure (non-surgical) or open procedure (a surgical incision is required to access the fracture or dislocation). For those fractures and dislocations that require fixation, the procedure can include internal or external fixation. Internal fixation involves the use of fixators such as pins, bone screws, wires, rods and plates that are attached directly to the bone or joint and used to support the structure while healing occurs. External fixation involves placing pins and screws that are then secured to a frame on the outside of the skin.
rheumatoid factor test (RF)	ROO-ma-toyd FAK-ta test	An RF test is a diagnostic test used in patients with rheumatoid arthritis to detect antibodies present in the patient's serum.
serum calcium (Ca)	SEE-rum KAL-see-um	A serum Ca test is a diagnostic test to identify the levels of calcium in serum. It is used to identify the presence of hypercalcaemia or hypocalcaemia.
serum creatine kinase (CK)	SEE-rum kree-AT-in KY-naze	A serum CK test is a diagnostic test to identify increased levels of the enzyme creatine kinase in serum that is present in the conditions polymyositis, muscular dystrophy and traumatic muscular injuries.

Exercises

EXERCISE 4.1: LABEL THE DIAGRAMS

Using the information provided in this chapter, label the anatomical parts in Figs 4.10a and 4.10b.

1 _____
2 _____
3 _____
4 _____
5 _____
6 _____
7 _____
8 _____
9 _____
10 _____
11 _____
12 _____
13 _____
14 _____
15 _____
16 _____
17 _____
18 _____
19 _____
20 _____
21 _____
22 _____
23 _____
24 _____
25 _____
26 _____
27 _____
28 _____
29 _____
30 _____
31 _____
32 _____
33 _____
34 _____
35 _____
36 _____

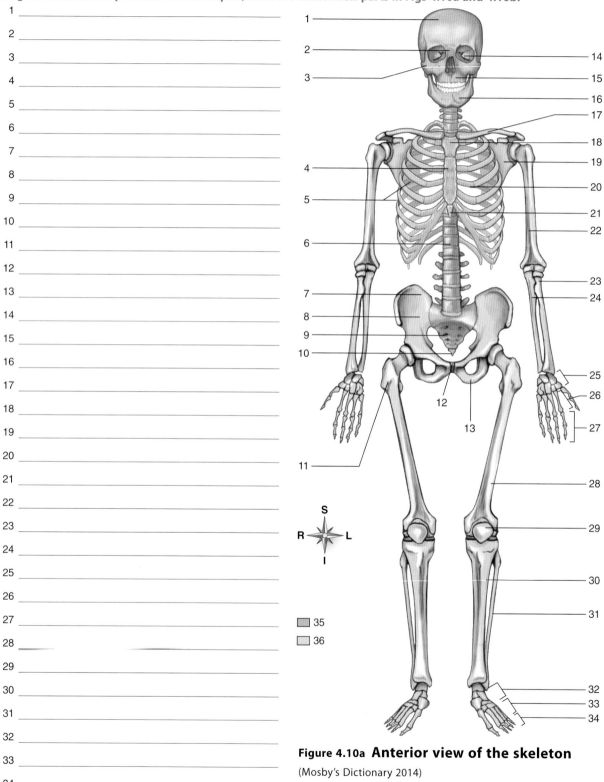

Figure 4.10a Anterior view of the skeleton
(Mosby's Dictionary 2014)

1 _____

2 _____

3 _____

4 _____

5 _____

6 _____

7 _____

8 _____

9 _____

10 _____

11 _____

12 _____

13 _____

14 _____

15 _____

16 _____

17 _____

18 _____

19 _____

20 _____

21 _____

22 _____

23 _____

24 _____

25 _____

26 _____

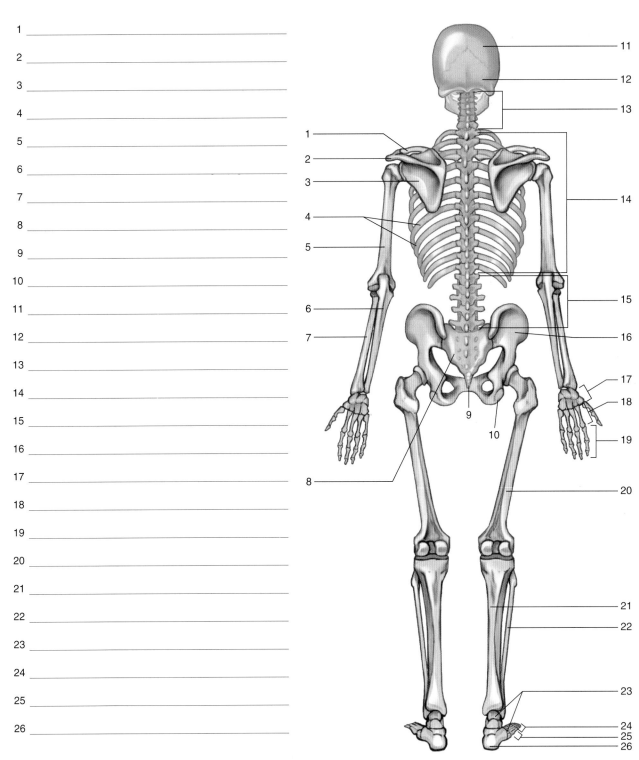

Figure 4.10b Posterior view of the skeleton

(Mosby's Dictionary 2014)

EXERCISE 4.2: WORD ANALYSIS AND MEANING

Break up the medical terms below into their component parts (prefixes, suffixes, word roots, combining vowels). Provide the meaning for each word element and each term as a whole.

Example:
osteomalacia

oste/o/malacia

oste/o = bone

malacia = pertaining to softening

Meaning = pertaining to softening of bone

1. costovertebral _____

_____

_____

2. arthroscopy _____

_____

_____

3. osteogenic _____

_____

_____

4. bursitis _____

_____

_____

5. meniscectomy _____

_____

_____

6. polymyositis _____

_____

_____

7. intervertebral _____

_____

_____

8. fibromyalgia _____

_____

_____

9. dyskinesia _____

_____

_____

10. lordosis _____

_____

_____

EXERCISE 4.3: MATCH WORD ELEMENTS AND MEANINGS

Match the prefix, suffix or combining form in Column A with its meaning from Column B.

Column A	Answer	Column B
1. spondyl/o		A. clavicle
2. -listhesis		B. joint
3. scoli/o		C. to bind, surgical fixation or fusion
4. lei/o		D. vertebra
5. -desis		E. slip or slide
6. articul/o		F. rod-shaped, striated
7. rhabd/o		G. crooked or bent
8. cleid/o		H. narrowing or stricture
9. tort/i		I. smooth
10. lumb/o		J. weakness
11. -stenosis		K. loins, lower back
12. -asthenia		L. twisted

EXERCISE 4.4: MATCH MEDICAL TERMS AND MEANINGS

Match the medical term in Column A with its meaning in Column B.

Column A	Answer	Column B
1. metatarsals		A. kneecap
2. radius		B. bones of the toes
3. occipital bone		C. thigh bone
4. fibula		D. breastbone
5. patella		E. lower jaw
6. ischium		F. cheekbone
7. femur		G. back of the skull
8. calcaneus		H. outer, thinner bone of lower leg
9. zygoma		I. part of the nasal cavity
10. sternum		J. part of the pelvis
11. mandible		K. outer bone of the forearm
12. ethmoid		L. heel

EXERCISE 4.5: EXPAND THE ABBREVIATIONS

Expand the abbreviations to form correct medical terms.

Abbreviation	Expanded Abbreviation
ACL	
CT scan	
CTS	
MRI	
NOF	
NSAID	
OA	
ORIF	
T1–T12	
TKR	

EXERCISE 4.6: APPLYING MEDICAL TERMINOLOGY

Fill in the blank or select the correct medical term or word element.

1. Which of the following is a term for involuntary contraction and relaxation of skeletal muscles?
   a) rigor
   b) spasm
   c) tetany
   d) tremor

2. Osteomyelitis is a condition of the bone and bone marrow causing _____.
   a) decreased bone density
   b) vitamin D deficiency
   c) atrophy of skeletal muscles
   d) inflammation

3. Which of the following means stiff?
   a) lord/o
   b) scoli/o
   c) ankyl/o
   d) rhabd/o

4. _____ provide(s) a protective covering for internal organs and produces body heat.
   a) skeleton
   b) tendons
   c) cartilage
   d) muscles

5. Which of the following is not an inflammation of the musculoskeletal system?
   a) bursitis
   b) chondromalacia
   c) myositis
   d) epiphysitis

6. Softening of the bone is termed _____.
   a) osteoporosis
   b) osteomyalgia
   c) osteomalacia
   d) osteosclerosis

7. The clavicle is part of the _____ skeleton.
   a) appendicular
   b) axial

8. A surgical repair of damaged cartilage is _____.
   a) arthroplasty
   b) chondritis
   c) chondroplasty
   d) osteoplasty

9. A fracture in which the ends of the bones are crushed is a _____ fracture.
   a) compound
   b) comminuted
   c) simple
   d) greenstick

10. What term means slowness of movement?
    a) hypotonia
    b) myotonia
    c) dyskinesia
    d) bradykinesia

EXERCISE 4.7: CORRECT THE SPELLING AND IDENTIFY THE INCORRECT TERMS

Identify the medical terms spelled incorrectly or words used inappropriately. Provide the correct terms.

1. There had clearly been atrofy of the upper extremity muscles since the patient's last attendance at the authopedic clinic.

2. Spinal x-ray revealed spondilosis and there was forward slipping of the fifth vertebrae of the lumber spine onto the saccrum.

3. Mrs Jones had bylateral carple tunnel sindrome. Surgical division of the ligament in the left wrist was undertaken to compress the middle nerve.

4. Her arteritis of the knee was so debilitating that she had to have a prosthotic device implanted.

5. The spinel fracture was reduced at open surgery and an internal fixation device was inserted into the tibia to maintain alignment.

EXERCISE 4.8: PRONUNCIATION AND COMPREHENSION

Read the following paragraphs aloud to practise your pronunciation. Using your textbook and a medical dictionary, find the meanings of the underlined medical terms.

Mrs Lennane was an elderly lady who was admitted to hospital after slipping on a wet path at her home. On admission she was <u>disoriented</u> and in considerable pain. An <u>indwelling catheter</u> was inserted. She was sent for x-rays, which confirmed the presence of an <u>intertrochanteric fracture of her left neck of femur</u>. There was also significant <u>soft tissue injury</u> around the fracture site. She was sent to theatre where an <u>ORIF</u> using pins and plate was performed under a GA. Her ASA score was 3NE.

Postoperatively she progressed slowly. Unfortunately, on day 3 she fell out of bed and <u>dislocated</u> her right shoulder and sustained a <u>laceration</u> to her right forearm. She was taken back to theatre where the shoulder dislocation was <u>reduced</u> and her forearm was <u>sutured</u> under a light GA. There were no further complications but <u>re-mobilisation</u> was slow.

She was transferred to the <u>rehabilitation</u> unit for intensive <u>physiotherapy</u>. After 2 weeks she was discharged home into the care of her daughter. On discharge she was mobile with the assistance of a walking frame.

EXERCISE 4.9: CROSSWORD PUZZLE

Complete the puzzle by providing the medical term for each of the clues below.

ACROSS

2. Tear or impingement of the tendons or muscles in the shoulder (7, 4, 8)
4. A break or crack in a bone (8)
5. Connective tissue that provides structure and support to other tissue (9)
8. The process of formation of bone (12)
9. An inflammatory muscle disease that results in muscle weakness (12)
10. Fixed immovable joint (7)

DOWN

1. Cell fibres having alternating light and dark bands (8)
3. Fibrous connective tissues that attach muscles to bone, bind muscle together or to other tissue at their point of origin or insertion (11)
6. Inflammation of a joint (9)
7. S-shaped curvature of the spine (9)

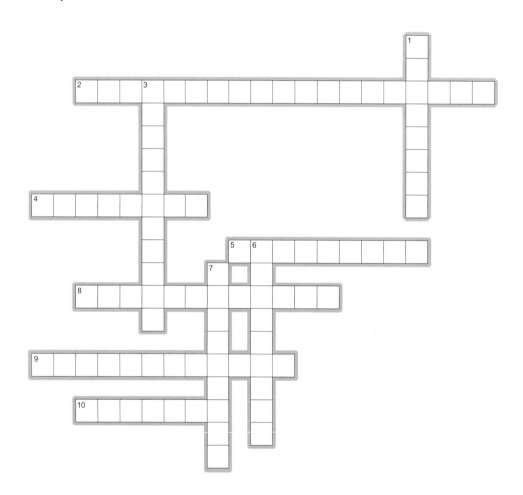

EXERCISE 4.10: ANAGRAMS

Work out each medical term from the jumbled letters below. Then, using the letters in brackets, determine the medical term that matches the description given.

1. aemltngi	__ __ __ __ __ __ __ (__)	a band of connective tissue that connects joints
2. ylaagim	__ __ __ __ __ (__) __	pain in a muscle
3. xtbalsniouu	(__) __ __ __ __ __ __ __ __ __ __	an incomplete displacement of a joint
4. xnefoil	__ __ __ __ (__) __ __	bending a limb
5. aieblnmd	__ (__) __ __ __ __ __ __	the lower jaw
6. valeiccl	__ __ __ __ __ (__) __ __	the combining form cleid/o refers to this bone
7. csfiaa	__ __ __ (__) __ __	the fibrous connective membrane surrounding a muscle
8. tionucabd	(__) __ __ __ __ __ __ __ __	move away from the midline

Rearrange the letters in brackets to form a word that means 'pain radiating from lower back down the leg'.

__ __ __ __ __ __ __ __

EXERCISE 4.11: DISCHARGE SUMMARY ANALYSIS

Read the discharge summary below and answer the questions.

UNIVERSITY HOSPITAL DISCHARGE SUMMARY	**UR number:** 123456
	Name: Harrison Brown
	Address: 55 Idol Court, Farrowville
	Date of birth: 25/06/1986
	Sex: M
	Nominated primary healthcare provider: Dr Elizabeth French
Episode details **Consultant:** Dr Gamble **Registrar:** Dr Winters **Unit:** Orthopaedics **Admission source:** Elective **Date of admission:** 23/3/2020	**Discharge details** **Status:** Home **Date of discharge:** 28/3/2020
Reason for admission / Presenting problems: Autologous bone graft to non-union of # of right tibia	
Principal diagnosis: Non-union # of right tibia	
Comorbidities: Nil reported	

Previous medical history:

This 33-year-old man presented 3 months after a motor bike accident in which he sustained a fractured right femur, fractured right tibia and fibula and left brachial plexus injury. At the time an ORIF was performed. A recent x-ray had revealed that the fractured tibia had failed to unite.

Clinical synopsis:

- General examination was unremarkable. Right leg examination corroborated the Dx.
- The following morning, under GA, a bone graft was performed on the right tibial fracture site (donor site right iliac crest).
- He was managed with bed rest and was mobilised on crutches.
- Five days post-surgery, the patient was discharged home.

Complications:

Postoperatively, the patient was given IV cloxacillin. He had a hypersensitivity reaction to this antibiotic, which was discontinued with a warning to the patient about taking penicillin therapy in the future.

Clinical interventions:

Bone graft – right tibial fracture site (donor site right iliac crest)

Diagnostic interventions:

Nil reported

Medications at discharge:

Panadol, as required

Ceased medications:

Nil reported

Allergies:

Intravenous cloxacillin

Alerts:

Nil reported

Arranged services:

Recommendations:

He is to be reviewed in the orthopaedic outpatient clinic in 2 weeks' time.

Information to patient/relevant parties:

Patient is to rest at home.

Authorising clinician:

Dr Winters

Document recipients:

Patient

LMO: Dr Elizabeth French

1. **Expand the following abbreviations as found in the discharge summary above.**

    GA

    ORIF

    IV

    Dx

    #

2. **What is non-union of a fracture?**

3. **What is an autologous bone graft?**

4. **What is a brachial plexus injury?**

5. **What does a hypersensitivity reaction mean?**

CHAPTER 5

Integumentary System

Contents

Objectives

OBJECTIVES	80
INTRODUCTION	81
NEW WORD ELEMENTS	81
Combining forms	81
Prefixes	82
Suffixes	82
VOCABULARY	82
ABBREVIATIONS	83
FUNCTIONS AND STRUCTURE OF THE INTEGUMENTARY SYSTEM	83
PATHOLOGY AND DISEASES	85
Common skin lesions	85
Symptomatic skin conditions	87
Skin infections	87
Specific skin disorders	89
Skin cancers	94
TESTS AND PROCEDURES	95
Removal of skin lesions	95
Other tests and procedures on the integumentary system	96
EXERCISES	98

After completing this chapter you should be able to:

1. state the meanings of the word elements related to the integumentary system

2. build words using the word elements associated with the integumentary system

3. recognise, pronounce and effectively use medical terms associated with the integumentary system

4. expand abbreviations related to the integumentary system

5. describe the structure and functions of the integumentary system including the skin, hair, nails and specialised glands

6. describe common pathological conditions associated with the integumentary system

7. describe common laboratory tests and diagnostic and surgical procedures associated with the integumentary system

8. apply what you have learned by interpreting medical terminology in practice.

Demonstrate your knowledge of the integumentary system by completing the exercises at the end of this chapter.

INTRODUCTION

The integumentary system consists of the skin and its appendages, hair, nails, sebaceous glands and sweat glands. The word integumentary literally means pertaining to the integument. An integument is a covering, in this case the skin. The skin is the largest organ in the body.

The integumentary system is one of the most diverse body systems in both form and function – from the thick skin on the soles of the feet to the hair that makes up the eyelashes. It protects the body from the outside environment, prevents water loss, regulates body temperature and senses external surroundings. The skin also contains receptors for the sense of touch.

The female breasts are technically part of the integumentary system because they are modified sweat glands but will be discussed in the chapter on the female reproductive system.

NEW WORD ELEMENTS

Here are some word elements related to the integumentary system. To reinforce your learning, write the meanings of the medical terms in the spaces provided. Use the Glossary of medical terms on page 561 to help you work out the meanings. You may also need to check the meaning in a medical dictionary, but make an attempt yourself first.

Combining forms

Combining Form	Meaning	Medical Term	Meaning of Medical Term
acanth/o	thorny, spiny	acanthoid	
adip/o	fat	adipocyte	
aesthesi/o	sensation, feeling	anaesthesia	
albin/o	white	albinism	
caus/o	burn, burning	causalgia	
cauter/o	heat, burn	cautery	
cutane/o	skin	intracutaneous	
derm/o	skin	hypodermic	
dermat/o		dermatology	
diaphor/o	profuse sweating	diaphoretic	
epitheli/o	epithelium	epithelial	
erythem/o	red	erythema	
erythemat/o		erythematous	
hidr/o	sweat	hidrosis	
hist/o	tissue	histology	
histi/o		histioblast	
ichthy/o	scaly, dry	ichthyoid	
kerat/o	hard, horny tissue, cornea	keratosis	
leuc/o, leuk/o	white	leuconychia	
(Note that leuk/o is used in Australia for the word leukaemia (and derivative terms) only)			
lip/o	fat	lipoma	
melan/o	black	melanoderma	
myc/o	fungus, mould	mycosis	
onych/o	nail	onychotomy	
pil/o	resembling or composed of hair	pilocystic	

Table continued

Combining Form	Meaning	Medical Term	Meaning of Medical Term
rhytid/o	wrinkle, crease	rhytidoplasty	
scler/o	hardening, sclera	sclerodermatitis	
seb/o	sebum	seborrhoeic	
sebace/o		sebaceous	
squam/o	scale	squamous	
stear/o	fat	stearodermia	
steat/o		steatorrhoea	
trich/i	hair	trichilemmoma	
trich/o		trichopathy	
ungu/o	nail	ungual	
xanth/o	yellow	xanthoderma	
xer/o	dry	xeroderma	

Prefixes

Prefix	Meaning	Medical Term	Meaning of Medical Term
epi-	above, upon, on	epidermis	
intra-	within, inside	intradermal	
pachy-	thick	pachyonychia	
par-	near, aside, apart from, other than, beyond, against	paraesthesia	
sub-	under, below	subcutaneous	

Suffixes

Suffix	Meaning	Medical Term	Meaning of Medical Term
-derma	skin	leucoderma	
-lemma	confining membrane, sheath	neurolemma	
-oma	tumour, collection, mass, swelling	xanthoma	
-plakia	condition of plaques	leucoplakia	
-plasty	surgical or plastic repair	dermatoplasty	
-rrhoea	discharge, flow	seborrhoea	
-trophy	nourishment, development	hypertrophy	
-tropic	affinity for	lipotropic	

VOCABULARY

The following list provides many of the medical terms used for the first time in this chapter. Pronunciations are provided with each term. As you read the rest of the chapter, make sure you identify each of these terms and understand their meanings.

Term	Pronunciation
acne	AK-nee
apocrine glands	AP-oh-kryn glandz
basal cell carcinoma	BAY-zal sel kah-sin-OH-ma
burn	bern
cellulitis	sell-u-LY-tis

Table continued

Term	Pronunciation
collagen	KOL-a-jen
dermatitis	der-ma-TY-tis
dermis	DER-mis
eccrine glands	EK-rine glandz
eczema	EKS-ma
elastin	e-LASS-tin
epidermis	ep-ee-DER-mis
flap	flap
furuncle	fur-UN-kil
graft	grahft
hair follicle	hair FOL-i-kel
impetigo	im-pe-TY-goh
keratosis	ker-a-TOH-sis
melanin	MEL-a-nin
melanocyte	MEL-an-oh-syt
melanoma	mel-a-NOH-ma
pilonidal cyst	pye-lon-EYE-dal sist
psoriasis	saw-RY-a-sis
rosacea	roh-ZAY-she-a
sebaceous gland	se-BAY-shus gland
sebum	SEE-bum
squamous cell carcinoma	SKWAH-mus sel kah-sin-OH-ma
squamous epithelium	SKWAH-mus ep-ee-THEE-lee-um
subcutaneous tissue	sub-kyoo-TAY-nee-us TISH-oo
subdermis	sub-DER-mis
sweat gland	swet gland
tinea	TIN-ee-a
verruca	ve-ROO-ka
vitiligo	vi-ti-LY-goh

ABBREVIATIONS

The following abbreviations are commonly used in the Australian healthcare environment. Because some abbreviations can have more than one meaning, check the context in which the abbreviation is used before assigning a meaning to it.

Abbreviation	Definition
ABCDE	characteristics associated with skin cancer: **a**symmetry (shape), **b**order (irregularity), **c**olour (variation within lesion), **d**iameter (> 6 mm), **e**volving (changes in size, shape, colour over time)

Table continued

Abbreviation	Definition
BCC	basal cell carcinoma
Bx, bx	biopsy
FS	frozen section
I&D	incision and drainage
PUVA	psoralen and ultraviolet A therapy
SC	subcutaneous
SCC	squamous cell carcinoma
SLE	systemic lupus erythematosus
SPF	sunscreen protection factor
TBSA	total body surface area
Ung	*unguentum*, ointment
UV	ultraviolet

FUNCTIONS AND STRUCTURE OF THE INTEGUMENTARY SYSTEM

The word integumentary has Latin origins and means cover or enclosure. The integumentary system in the human body consists of the skin and accessory structures, the nails, hair and associated glands. The various organs in this system are disparate, ranging from small, fragile eyelashes through to the tough, horny skin on the soles of the feet. Together they act to provide protection – for example, the skin provides a waterproof, insulating covering for the entire body, which prevents the entry of organisms and provides a barrier against injury. It also reduces the effects of damaging ultraviolet rays from the sun while using them as a source of vitamin D. The skin regulates body temperature, moderates water loss and has a large number of nerves that act as sensory receptors to inform the internal organs about external conditions. These functions assist the body in maintaining homeostasis. The skin is the largest and heaviest organ in the human body, covering around 2 square metres in the average adult and weighing around 3.5 kilograms.

The skin has three layers: the epidermis, the dermis and the subcutaneous layer (Fig. 5.1). The outermost layer is the **epidermis**, which consists of stratified (multilayered) squamous epithelium with four types of cells: keratinocytes, melanocytes, Merkel cells and Langerhans' cells. There are several layers of keratinocytes. As new cells are formed on lower layers, the top layer flakes off and is discarded. The cycle from birth to death of these cells is around 28 days. The number of layers of keratinocytes differs in different parts of the body, with the soles of the feet having the most layers and the eyelids the least.

Figure 5.1 Structure of the skin

(Adkinson 2008)

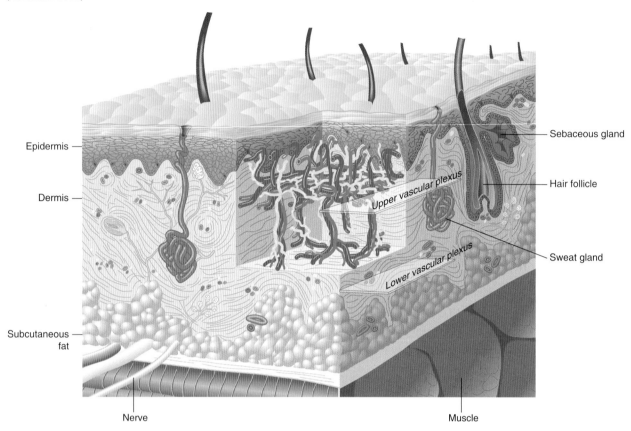

Epidermis

Dermis

Subcutaneous fat

Sebaceous gland

Hair follicle

Upper vascular plexus

Lower vascular plexus

Sweat gland

Nerve

Muscle

Melanocytes are specialised cells found in the deepest layer of the epidermis – the basal layer. They produce a pigment called melanin, which provides some protection against the ultraviolet radiation found in sunlight. The number of melanocytes a person has is approximately the same in all races. Differences in skin colour are due to the level of activity of the melanocytes; in other words, the amount of melanin they produce. The more melanin that is produced, the darker the skin colour. In general, people in hotter and more tropical climates are predisposed to inheriting darker skin. For fairer-skinned people, exposure to strong sunlight creates a sun tan, which is actually the skin's form of protection against the damaging rays.

The body uses the Merkel cells and Langerhans' cells to identify and trigger a response to external agents. Merkel cells are associated with nerve cells that are responsible for the sensation of touch. Langerhans' cells act against antigens seeking to enter and infect the human body.

The epidermis does not contain any blood vessels, lymph vessels or nerve endings. It relies on the blood vessels in the dermis for its nourishment.

Under the epidermis and attached to it, is a layer known as the **dermis** or **corium**, which is composed of dense connective tissue containing collagen and elastin. This layer has many blood vessels that expand or contract to alter the flow of blood in response to external temperatures. The dermis interacts with the brain by providing it with sensations of pain, temperature and touch through the many nerve endings it contains. Also in the dermis are hair follicles and various glands – sweat glands, apocrine glands and sebaceous glands. These three sets of glands have roles in: producing perspiration to lower the body's temperature and to rid it of excess levels of urea and lactate; producing a scented sweat that attracts sexual partners; and secreting sebum, an oily substance that lubricates the skin and hair. The dermal layer allows the body to stretch and be flexible.

The innermost layer of the skin is called the **subdermis** or **subcutaneous tissue**. It connects the dermis to underlying tissues. This layer consists of loose connective tissue and varying amounts of adipose tissue. The adipose tissue cushions the internal organs against injury and provides warmth and insulation. It also provides fuel or fat for the body that can be used in times of privation.

The **hair** is one of the accessory organs of the integumentary system. Hair is produced by layers of cells arising from the dermis. The hair root is embedded in follicles in the dermis, with the shaft of each hair pushing out through the skin. The follicles have a number of associated blood vessels and nerve fibres. Small muscles called arrector pili muscles are attached to each hair follicle. If stimulated to contract, they pull the follicles upright, causing goosebumps. Body hair, particularly that on the head, also serves to maintain warmth and prevent heat loss as well as helping to provide protection against sunlight and injury. Hair in the eyebrows stops sweat from running into the eyes, and the hairs in the nose and ears filter particles from the air.

Nails also form in the epidermis and protect the sensitive ends of the fingers and toes. They consist of the nail body, nail bed, nail root and free edge (Fig. 5.2).

The nail body is the visible portion of the nail. It consists of a hard keratin plate that extends from the nail root to the free edge. The nail bed is a highly vascular layer of epithelium upon which the nail body sits. The nail root is at the base of the nail and is embedded underneath the skin. It is protected by the eponychium or cuticle and is attached to an active growth layer called the matrix. The free edge is the end portion of the nail plate that extends from the tip of the finger or toe. At the base of the nail is the lunula or half-moon. The lunula is usually whitish in colour as a result of the epidermis being thicker underneath the matrix, blocking the pink colour from the blood vessels below.

As well as protecting the ends of the digits, nails assist us to pick up small objects and allow us to scratch.

Figure 5.2 **Parts of the nail**
(Leonard 2009)

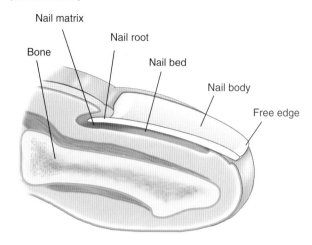

PATHOLOGY AND DISEASES

The following section provides a list of some of the most common diseases and pathological conditions relevant to the integumentary system.

Common skin lesions

A skin lesion can be defined as any abnormality such as a growth or marking on the surface of the skin that differs from the surrounding area (Fig. 5.3). Some of the most common skin lesions are:

Term	Pronunciation	Definition
bulla	BULL-a	A bulla is a fluid-filled lesion > 0.5 cm in size. Also called a blister.
cicatrix	SIK-a-trix	Commonly called a scar, a cicatrix is the result of damage or injury to the dermis left after healing has occurred.
cyst	sist	A cyst is a sac containing liquid or semi-solid material.
fissure	FISH-a	A fissure is a cleft or crack extending from the surface of the skin to the dermis.
keloid	KEE-loyd	A keloid scar is a thick, irregular, raised scar.
macule	MAK-yool	A macule is a flat circular lesion < 1 cm in size that differs in colour from surrounding skin – for example, a freckle or flat mole. When the macule is > 1 cm in size, it is called a patch.
naevus	NEE-vus	A naevus is also called a mole or a birthmark. The actual definition depends on the type of naevus.
nodule	NOD-yool	A nodule is a solid lesion with defined borders, a deep-seated papule.
papule	PAP-yool	A papule is a raised lesion < 1 cm in size with distinct borders. The surface of the papule may be crusty or scaly in texture, as in psoriasis.
polyp	POL-ep	A polyp is also called a skin tag and is a growth protruding from the surface of the skin. Polyps also occur in other organs such as the bladder, nose and colon.

Table continued

Term	Pronunciation	Definition
plaque	plark	Plaque is a palpable flat lesion > 0.5 cm.
pustule	PUST-yool	A pustule is a raised lesion that contains pus – for example, a boil or impetigo.
telangiectasia	tel-an-jee-ek-TAY-zee-a	Dilated superficial blood vessels on the surface of the skin are called telangiectasia. They are often a symptom of other conditions such as rosacea.
ulcer	UL-sa	Ulcer is the term given to an erosion of the epidermis and dermis due to infection or injury.
vesicle	VEE-sik-el	A vesicle is a raised lesion < 0.5 cm in size filled with clear fluid – for example, a sunburn blister or herpes blister. A large vesicle is a bulla.
wheal	weel	A wheal is an area of pruritic swelling in the epidermis often due to an allergic reaction such as an insect bite or a hive.

Figure 5.3 Types of skin lesions

(Talley & O'Connor 2009)

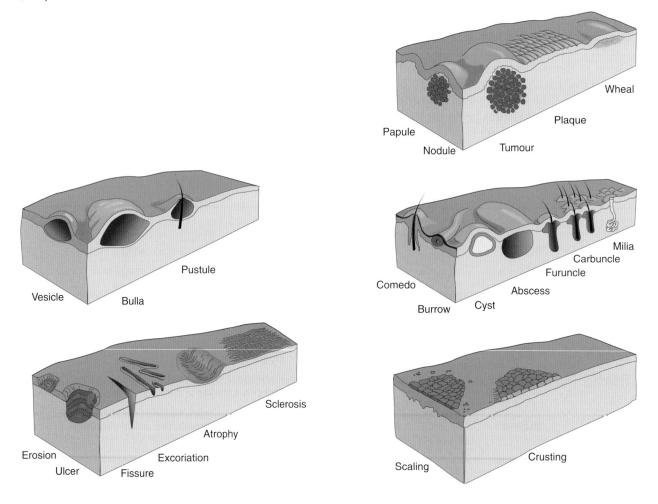

Symptomatic skin conditions

Term	Pronunciation	Definition
erythema	e-rith-EE-ma	Erythema is redness of the skin due to dilation of capillaries.
pruritus	proo-RY-tus	Pruritus is itchiness of the skin.
urticaria	ur-tik-AIR-ee-a	Urticaria are raised, pruritic areas on the skin usually due to an allergic reaction such as hives.

Skin infections

Term	Pronunciation	Definition
acne	AK-nee	Acne is a very common skin disease characterised by pimples, comedones (blackheads), whiteheads and cysts that develop on the face, chest, shoulders and back. Although it can affect people at any age, acne usually begins at puberty and worsens during adolescence. A pimple is caused by a blockage of the opening of sebaceous glands that become infected. Blackheads are plugs of oily sebum in a hair follicle, which darken when exposed to air. If the blockage is deeper in the tissue, cysts may develop. These may leave significant scarring on healing. In mild cases, treatment involves keeping the skin clean by washing with a gentle cleanser to reduce the amount of sebum. In more severe cases, antibiotics and some topical medications such as cleansing solutions, creams and gels applied directly to the skin may be prescribed.
cellulitis	sell-u-LY-tis	Cellulitis is a bacterial infection affecting the dermis and subcutaneous tissue (Fig. 5.4). The bacteria enters through a cut or tear in the skin. It is characterised by redness, swelling, tenderness or pain and heat in the affected region (generally the leg, but any part of the body can be affected). It is most commonly caused by group A β-*haemolytic Streptococci* and *Staphylococcus aureus*. Treatment involves administering oral or intravenous antibiotics. **Figure 5.4 Cellulitis** (Black & Hawks 2009)
furuncle	fur-UN-kil	A furuncle (also called a boil) is a deep, severe infection of a hair follicle and associated sebaceous gland resulting in the formation of a core of pus or slough. It is commonly due to infection with the *Staphylococcus aureus* bacterium. A **carbuncle** is a group of furuncles in adjacent follicles. Treatment methods will vary depending on the severity. Oral and/or topical antibiotics may be required. Radiant heat and a paste to encourage drainage may be helpful. Treatment should continue until the pus-filled core separates. Lancing is occasionally necessary.

Table continued

Term	Pronunciation	Definition
impetigo	im-pe-TY-goh	Impetigo is a highly contagious, pruritic skin condition caused by infection with *Streptococcus pyogenes* or *Staphylococcus aureus* bacteria or a combination of the two. It results in pus-filled blisters that ooze fluid and eventually crust over (Fig. 5.5). Because impetigo often occurs in young children, it is commonly known as school sores. Treatment involves cleansing frequently with an antibacterial soap and the application of an antibiotic cream. **Figure 5.5 Impetigo** (Habif 2009) 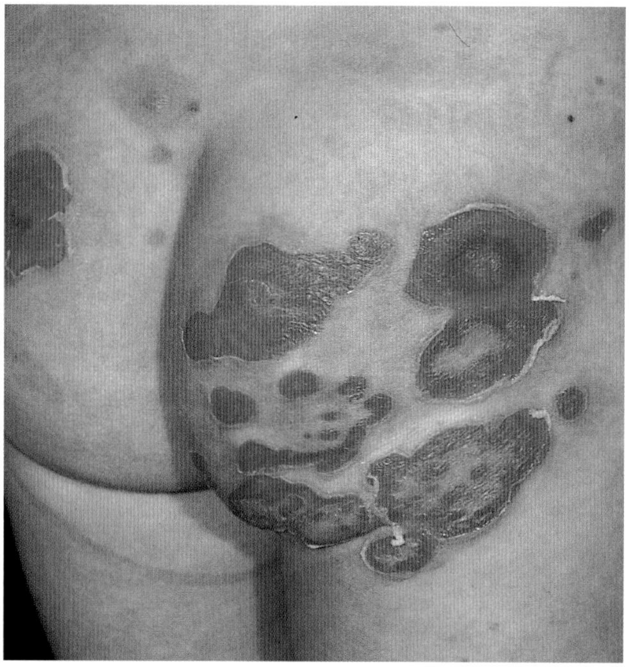
pilonidal cyst	pye-lon-EYE-dal sist	A pilonidal cyst (or sinus) is a cyst or abscess usually found in the coccygeal region that commonly contains skin debris or hair. It is not clear how the cysts form, but current assumptions are that small groups of hair and skin debris are trapped in skin pores and form a sinus or cavity in the skin that may become infected, forming an abscess. It is most common in those aged 15–34 years of age and in people whose occupations or lifestyle involve excessive sitting (e.g. truck drivers or students).
tinea	TIN-ee-a	Tinea is a common fungal infection of the skin. There are several different types of tinea: tinea corporis (also called ringworm) affects the skin on the body (Fig. 5.6), tinea capitis affects the scalp, tinea cruris (also called jock itch) affects the skin in the groin area, tinea unguium (also called onychomycosis) affects nails, and tinea pedis (also called athlete's foot) affects the skin on the feet. Tinea is very contagious and can be spread by skin-to-skin contact or indirect contact (e.g. sharing towels) and using public showers and change rooms. Tinea usually responds well to treatment with antifungal creams and oral antifungal medications.

Table continued

Term	Pronunciation	Definition
		Figure 5.6 Tinea (Gawkrodger 2008)
verruca	ve-ROO-ka	A verruca, commonly known as a wart, is a skin lesion caused by infection with the human papillomavirus (HPV), which infects the surface layer of the skin. Verrucae are highly contagious. There are many different types of verrucae including common warts (hands), plantar warts (soles of the feet), genital warts (pubic and genital areas), flat warts (face) and subungual warts (under the nails). Removal is by cryosurgery, electrocautery or application of salicylic acid.

Specific skin disorders

Term	Pronunciation	Definition
burn	bern	A burn is an injury to tissues caused by contact with intense heat, flame, liquid or steam, gases, radiation, certain chemicals (such as acids) or electricity. Burns are classified according to their depth or severity (Fig. 5.7). **Erythema (previously called first degree)** This is a minor burn affecting only the epidermis. The burned area is painful, red and slight swelling may be present but there are no blisters. An example is sunburn. **Partial thickness burn (previously called second degree)** In this type of burn, the epidermis and the upper region of the dermis are damaged. The burned area is red, painful and blistered. If infection is prevented, this type of burn will heal without permanent scarring. **Full thickness burn (previously called third degree)** This is a severe burn which involves destruction of both the epidermis and dermis and usually damage to the subcutaneous layer of the skin. Blood vessels and nerve endings are destroyed and therefore the burn is not painful. The area will appear waxy white or black in colour. Muscle tissue and underlying bone may also be damaged in severe cases. The risk of infection is high. Skin grafting will be required and there will be permanent scarring.

Table continued

Term	Pronunciation	Definition

Figure 5.7 Burn injuries by depth of burn

(Mosby's Dictionary 2014)

Epidermal burn: damaged epidermis and oedema

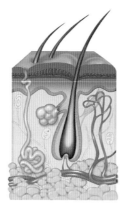 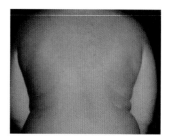

Superficial dermal burn

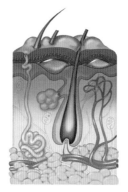 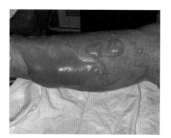

Mid-dermal burn

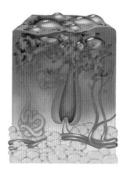 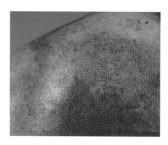

Deep dermal full-thickness burn

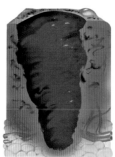 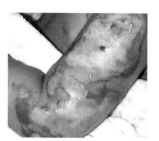

(Photos reproduced with permission
from Burn Injury Network,
NSW Agency for Clinical Innovation)

Table continued

Term	Pronunciation	Definition
		Two factors will determine a patient's prognosis: the depth of their burn (erythema, partial thickness, full thickness) and the extent of their body burned.
		Treatment protocols require health practitioners to be able to quickly determine the total body surface area (TBSA) that has been burned. The **rule of nines** is one way to do this (Fig. 5.8). The rule of nines divides the body into sections that each represent approximately 9% or multiples of 9% of the TBSA. Different percentages are used in paediatrics because the surface area of the head and neck relative to the surface area of the limbs is typically larger in children than adults. Therefore this method of calculation should be used for adults only.
		For example, in an adult who has been burned, the percentage of the body involved can be calculated as follows:
		If both legs (18% × 2 = 36%), both arms (9% × 2 = 18%), the groin (1%) and the face (4.5%) were burned, the burns would involve 59.5% of the body.

Figure 5.8 Rule of nines

(Mosby's Dictionary 2014)

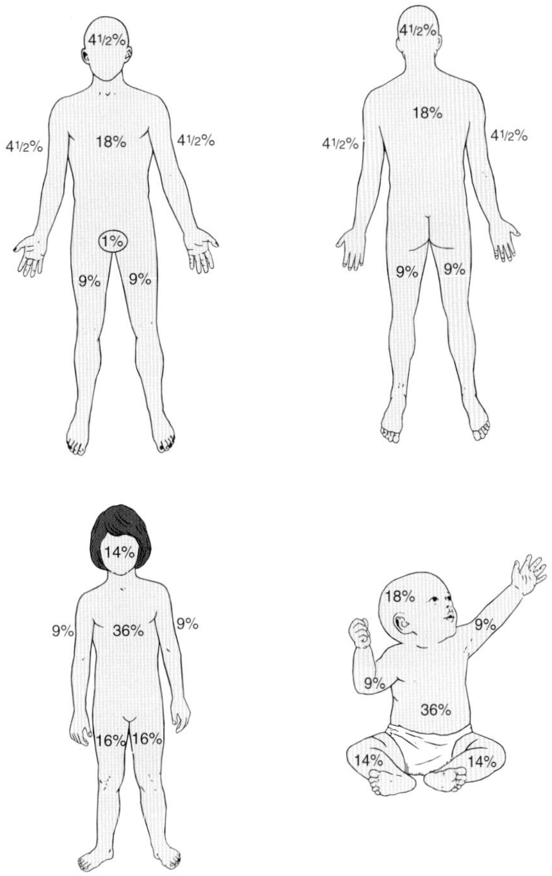

Table continued

Term	Pronunciation	Definition
dermatitis	der-ma-TY-tis	Dermatitis is an inflammation of the skin characterised by a pruritic, erythematous rash (Fig. 5.9). People with a genetic tendency to allergies, frequently including dermatitis, are said to suffer from atopy. Atopic dermatitis occurs when antibodies are developed in response to exposure to common allergens in the environment. The most common types of dermatitis are contact/allergic and seborrhoeic. Contact dermatitis occurs when a person touches a substance to which they are allergic or sensitive. Common allergens include plants, perfumes, soaps, cosmetics. Seborrhoeic dermatitis occurs mainly in areas where the skin has more sebum, such as on the face and scalp. Dandruff (adults) and cradle cap (infants) are forms of non-inflammatory seborrhoeic dermatitis. Treatment of dermatitis includes application of topical creams and steroids, UV therapy, antihistamines and the removal of the causative agent.

Figure 5.9 Dermatitis

A. Acute dermatitis; **B.** Typical acute dermatitis with erythema and tiny vesicles, some of which have burst as a result of scratching

(Stevens et al 2009)

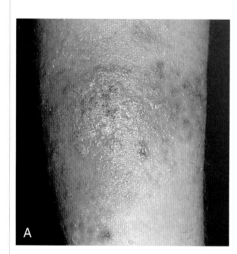

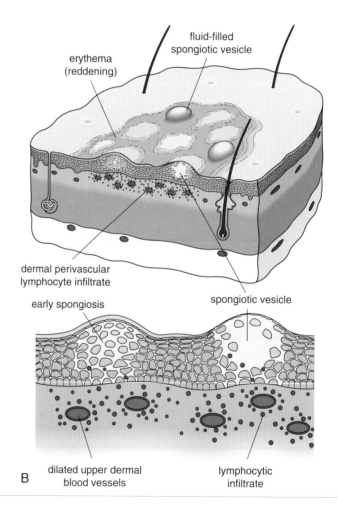

Table continued

Term	Pronunciation	Definition
eczema	EKS-ma	Eczema is a general term used to describe many types of pruritic, inflammatory skin conditions such as chronic dermatitis and allergic skin rashes. It occurs most frequently in children and often occurs in conjunction with asthma and hay fever. The words eczema and dermatitis are often used synonymously. See **dermatitis** for details.
keratosis	ker-a-TOH-sis	Keratosis develops from excessive proliferation of epidermal cells. There are several different types of keratosis, but the most commonly occurring types are: **Seborrhoeic keratoses** are non-malignant tumours or growths that occur on the skin of older persons. While not dangerous in any way, they do have an unsightly appearance ranging from large blackened growths to smaller raised lesions on the epidermal surface of the skin. It is medically acceptable to leave them alone, but many patients request to have a seborrhoeic keratosis removed because of cosmetic appearances or because it becomes itchy. Removal is usually performed by cryotherapy or shaving the lesion off. **Solar keratoses** are also known as actinic keratoses or sunspots. They appear as roughened, red, scaly patches on skin that has had overexposure to UV radiation from the sun over an extended period of time. Solar keratoses commonly appear on the face, scalp, back of hands and forearms. It can take many years after sun exposure for the lesions to appear. While not malignant themselves, solar keratoses have the propensity to change into squamous cell carcinomas if not treated. They are treated by cryotherapy, creams or excision.
psoriasis	saw-RY-a-sis	Psoriasis is a common skin disorder characterised by red patches on the skin covered with silvery scales (Fig. 5.10). The most common sites affected are the elbows, knees, trunk, buttocks and scalp. Normally, skin cells mature approximately every 28 days. Psoriasis causes skin cells to mature in about 7 days, resulting in a rapid build-up of skin at the affected sites. The cause is unknown but there is a family history in about one-third of patients. Treatments such as topical steroids, tar baths and creams and even exposure to sunlight or UV radiation can help to alleviate the symptoms, but there is no permanent cure and relapses are likely particularly during cold weather and times of stress. Psoriasis comes from the Greek word *psorian* meaning an itching.

Figure 5.10 Psoriasis
A. Guttate psoriasis; **B.** Generalised pustular psoriasis; **C.** Erythrodermic psoriasis

(Schwarzenberger et al 2009)

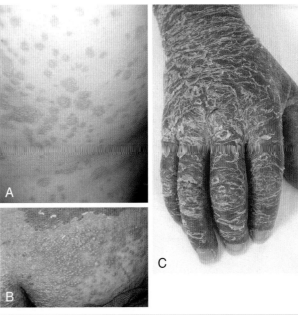

Table continued

Term	Pronunciation	Definition
rosacea	roh-ZAY-she-a	Rosacea is a chronic inflammatory skin disorder most commonly occurring on the central face. Skin appears erythematous and is covered in small pustules and telangiectasia. Eyes are often watery and irritated. Rosacea mostly affects fair-skinned Caucasians. Treatment includes antibiotics, topical medications and avoidance of triggers such as alcohol and spicy foods. There is no cure.
vitiligo	vi-ti-LY-goh	Vitiligo is a skin disorder where a decrease in the number of melanocytes results in a decrease in the production of melanin. This results in the formation of milky white patches on the skin (Fig. 5.11). Synonyms for this disorder are leucoderma and piebald skin. It can affect any ethnicity but is more common in people living in the tropics and more obvious in people with darker skin. The cause of vitiligo is unknown, but it is thought to be a type of autoimmune disease in which the body targets and destroys its own cells and tissues. There is no cure for vitiligo. Using tinted cosmetics can help blend the white areas with the surrounding normal skin, giving a more even appearance. **Figure 5.11 Vitiligo** (Callen et al 2000)

Skin cancers

Skin cancers are the most common malignancy in Australia and the most treatable if diagnosed early. The cause of most skin cancers is not known, but overexposure to UV radiation in sunlight during early years of life is a significant risk factor. Skin cancers are classified according to the type of cell in which they arise.

Term	Pronunciation	Definition
basal cell carcinoma (BCC)	BAY-zal sel kah-sin-OH-ma	A BCC is the most common type of skin cancer. It arises in the basal cells in the epidermis and can then spread locally into the dermis and subcutaneous layer. It is rare for a BCC to metastasise. BCCs occur most commonly on sun-exposed areas of the body such as the face, ears, the backs of the hands and the arms.

Table continued

Term	Pronunciation	Definition
melanoma	mel-a-NOH-ma	A melanoma is a malignant tumour that begins in the melanocytes in the epidermis. Melanomas often arise in a naevus. Over time, the naevus may change colour to bluish black, increase in size and develop an irregular margin (Fig. 5.12). In addition to invading surrounding tissues, a melanoma can metastasise to other sites especially the brain, bones, lungs and liver. Melanomas occur more frequently in fair-skinned people who have been sunburnt. Another significant risk factor is genetics. Early diagnosis is the key to long-term survival. The primary treatment for a melanoma is surgical removal and regional lymphadenectomy. If the melanoma has metastasised, the prognosis is poorer. **Figure 5.12 Melanoma** (Marks & Miller 2006)
squamous cell carcinoma (SCC)	SKWAH-mus sel kah-sin-OH-ma	An SCC is a malignant tumour that arises in the squamous epithelial cells in the epidermis. On the skin, an SCC presents as a small, scaly lump with a crusty centre. If not removed, an SCC will metastasise to adjacent lymph nodes. Similar to a BCC, an SCC usually occurs on sun-exposed skin such as the face, ears, hands and arms. However, SCCs can also be found in the lungs, bladder, larynx and other internal structures where there is epithelial tissue.

TESTS AND PROCEDURES

The following section provides a list of common diagnostic tests and procedures and clinical interventions and surgical procedures that are undertaken for the integumentary system.

Removal of skin lesions

Several methods are used to remove skin lesions. The following table provides a summary.

Test/Procedure	Pronunciation	Definition
cryosurgery	kry-oh-SER-ja-ree	Cryosurgery involves freezing a lesion using a cryogen such as liquid nitrogen, which destroys the tissue.
curettage	kyoo-ret-AHJ	Curettage is a procedure that involves using an instrument with a circular cutting loop (curette) that is scraped across a lesion in successive strokes until it is removed.
electrodessication	ee-lek-tro-des-i-KAY-shun	Electrodessication involves removing a skin lesion by destroying the tissue using electric currents.

Table continued

Test/Procedure	Pronunciation	Definition
excision of skin lesion	ek-SI-shun ov skin LEE-shun	A skin excision is a procedure that is generally performed in a general practitioner's surgery, outpatient clinic or as a day procedure in hospital. A local anaesthetic is injected around the site and then the skin lesion is excised using a scalpel. A small margin of normal looking skin is also removed. The procedure may be performed to remove a lesion that has previously been biopsied where the pathology indicates a malignancy and the need to remove the remainder of the lesion. Alternatively, it may be performed to undertake a biopsy of the lesion and therefore is known as an excisional biopsy.
Moh's surgery	mohz SER-ja-ree	Moh's surgery is used to treat malignant lesions by removing the lesion in thin layers. After each layer is removed, the margins are examined under the microscope. If the margins are not clear, then the surgeon will continue removing layers until the examination under microscope identifies clear margins.

Other tests and procedures on the integumentary system

Test/Procedure	Pronunciation	Definition
bacterial analysis	bak-TEER-ee-al a-NAL-e-sis	A bacterial analysis is a diagnostic test to identify microorganisms that may be present on skin or in purulent (pus-filled) skin exudates. Samples are sent for laboratory examination.
dermabrasion	derm-a-BRAY-shun	Dermabrasion is a procedure that involves using sandpaper and wire brushes to remove the epidermal layers of the skin to eradicate scars, lines and tattoos.
excisional debridement	ek-SI-shun-al de-BRYD-ment	Excisional debridement is important in the healing process for people with burns and serious wounds. It involves removing dead (necrotic), damaged or infected tissue from the wound site using a scalpel or scissors.
flap	flap	A surgical flap involves transplanting skin from one site to another. Flaps differ from grafts in that they contain their own blood supply and, in some cases, include muscle. The flaps are used to cover skin defects. For example, a local flap is used when a portion of skin is able to be rotated, transposed or advanced from the donor site to an adjacent site without complete removal of the flap from the donor site. A free flap is the transplant of a flap from one part of the body to another site. For example, a flap may be taken from the leg to cover a defect in the neck. The vessels in the flap are connected to the vessels in the defect site to ensure continued blood supply in the donor flap.
fungal test	FUN-gal test	A fungal test is a diagnostic test that uses skin scrapings, hair or nails to identify the presence of fungal infection.

Table continued

Test/Procedure	Pronunciation	Definition
graft	grahft	A skin graft involves transplanting healthy skin from one part of the body to another. A graft can be either split thickness (epidermis and part of the dermis) or full thickness (the entire epidermis and dermis). Donor grafts can be: **Autograft:** where donor skin is taken from a site on the same patient's body (Fig. 5.13). **Heterograft:** where donor skin is transplanted from one animal species to another. **Homograft or allograft:** where donor skin is transplanted from one human to another. **Figure 5.13 Epithelial autograft** Thin sheets of skin attached to gauze backing. (McCance & Huether 2002) 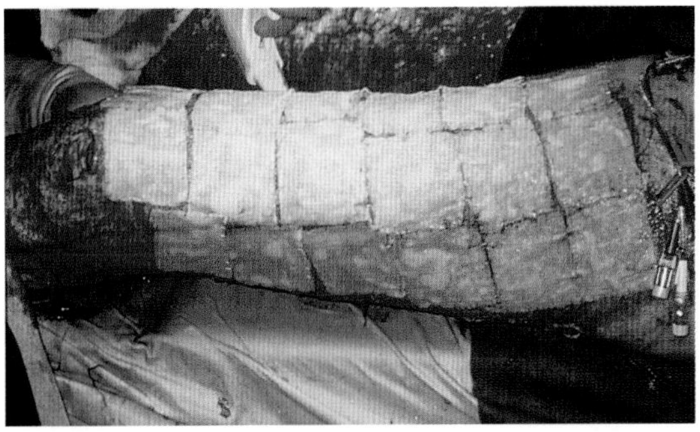
incision and drainage (I&D)	in-si-SHUN and DRAYN-aj	Incision and drainage is a procedure used to treat conditions such as an abscess or boil where there is a build-up of pus or pressure under the skin. A small incision is made into the skin using a needle, scalpel or lancet, releasing the fluid through the incision site.
skin biopsy	skin BY-op-see	A skin biopsy involves removing a sample of skin using either a punch or shave technique for laboratory examination of a lesion. The shave biopsy involves using a scalpel to shave the top off the lesion. A punch biopsy involves using a small circular instrument that is rotated into the lesion to remove a core or sample of the lesion. The punch may also be used to remove an entire small suspect lesion.
skin test	skin test	Skin tests are performed to identify a substance that causes allergies or other reactions in a person or to detect the presence of disease. In the case of allergy testing, a patch or scratch test will be performed. The scratch test involves applying a small amount of the allergen to scratches made in the skin. The patch test applies gauze or filter paper containing the allergen to the skin. Skin tests used to identify the presence of disease include the Mantoux and purified protein derivative tests for tuberculosis.

Exercises

EXERCISE 5.1: LABEL THE DIAGRAM

Using the information provided in this chapter, label the anatomical parts in Fig. 5.14.

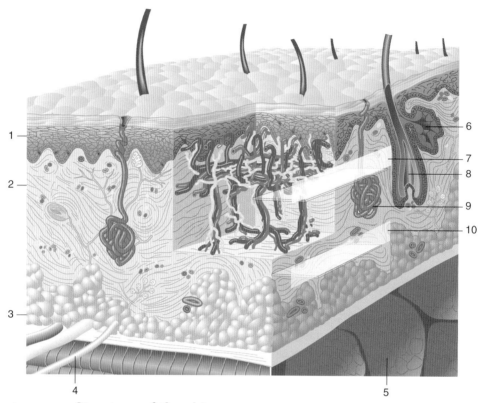

Figure 5.14 Structure of the skin

(Adkinson 2008)

1 _____	6 _____
2 _____	7 _____
3 _____	8 _____
4 _____	9 _____
5 _____	10 _____

EXERCISE 5.2: WORD ANALYSIS AND MEANING

Break up the medical terms below into their component parts (prefixes, suffixes, word roots, combining vowels). Provide the meaning for each word element and each term as a whole.

Example:
melanoma

melan/o = black

oma = tumour

Meaning = tumour of black (cells)

1. subungual _____

2. blepharoplasty _____

3. onychomycosis _____

4. dermatofibroma _____

5. xanthoderma _____

6. trichophytosis _____

7. hidradenitis _____

8. albinism _____

9. xenograft _____

_____

_____

10. rhytidectomy _____

_____

_____

EXERCISE 5.3: MATCH WORD ELEMENTS AND MEANINGS

Match the prefix, suffix or combining form in Column A with its meaning from Column B.

Column A	Answer	Column B
1. pachy-		A. nourishment, development
2. pil/o		B. skin
3. erythem/o		C. surgical or plastic repair
4. -trophy		D. within, inside
5. cutane/o		E. affinity for
6. diaphor/o		F. red
7. acanth/o		G. thick
8. intra-		H. thorny, spiny
9. -plasty		I. resembling or composed of hair
10. -tropic		J. profuse sweating

EXERCISE 5.4: MATCH MEDICAL TERMS AND MEANINGS

Match the medical term in Column A with its meaning in Column B.

Column A	Answer	Column B
1. alopecia		A. intense itchiness
2. ecchymosis		B. hardening of the skin
3. icterus		C. bruise
4. keloid		D. a wart
5. melanoma		E. overgrowth of scar tissue
6. nodule		F. dilation of superficial capillaries
7. scleroderma		G. baldness
8. telangiectasia		H. tumour of the pigmented cells of the skin
9. urticaria		I. small palpable node
10. verruca		J. yellow skin

EXERCISE 5.5: VOCABULARY BUILDING

Provide the medical term for each of the definitions below.

1. A malignant tumour of squamous epithelium sometimes called an SCC: _____

2. Inflammation of the skin: _____

3. An abnormal condition of hard horny tissue: _____

4. Flow of sebum: _____

5. A procedure to remove a lesion using heat and electricity: _____

6. A graft between individuals of the same species: _____

7. An abnormal condition where the patient does not produce sweat: _____

8. A fat cell: _____

9. A swelling or tumour of the nose: _____

10. Dry skin: _____

EXERCISE 5.6: EXPAND THE ABBREVIATIONS

Expand the abbreviations to form correct medical terms.

Abbreviation	Expanded Abbreviation
ABCDE	
BCC	
Bx	
FS	
I&D	
PUVA	
SCC	
SLE	
SPF	
UV	

EXERCISE 5.7: APPLYING MEDICAL TERMINOLOGY

Fill in the blank or select the correct medical term or word element.

1. Cyanosis means what kind of discolouration of the skin?
   a) reddish
   b) yellowish
   c) bluish
   d) brownish

2. A subcutaneous injection is _____.
   a) within the skin
   b) under the muscle
   c) under the skin
   d) within the vein

3. The integumentary system helps regulate _____.
   a) bowel movement
   b) kidney excretion
   c) body temperature
   d) heart rate

4. An example of a papule is a _____.
   a) vesicle
   b) wart
   c) vitiligo
   d) hive

5. A _____ is most often associated with communicable disease.
   a) pruritus
   b) comedo
   c) rash
   d) naevus

6. Which of the following skin conditions is commonly known as a boil?
   a) carbuncle
   b) abscess
   c) furuncle
   d) impetigo

7. The technique used to excise tumours of the skin by removing fresh tissue layer by layer until a tumour-free plane is reached is known as _____ surgery.
   a) Moh's
   b) Mah's
   c) dermashave
   d) skin curettage

8. Removal of an entire lesion for histological examination is called a/an _____.
   a) excisional biopsy
   b) frozen section
   c) incisional biopsy
   d) shave biopsy

9. Which of the following surgical procedures is used to remove scars and tattoos?
   a) electrocautery
   b) debridement
   c) laser surgery
   d) curettage

10. Which of the following skin disorders is characterised by a decrease in the number of melanocytes resulting in white patches on the skin?
    a) dermatitis
    b) eczema
    c) psoriasis
    d) vitiligo

EXERCISE 5.8: VOCABULARY BUILDING

Provide the meaning of each of the medical terms below. Use your dictionary if you are unsure.

Term	Meaning	Term	Meaning
alopecia		cellulitis	
decubitus ulcer		eczema	
epidermophytosis		impetigo contagiosa	

Term	Meaning	Term	Meaning
hyperpigmentation		petechiae	
papule		pustule	
paronychia		verruca	
psoriasis		ecchymosis	
pyogenic		lipoma	
subcutaneous		curettage	
vesication		proliferation	

EXERCISE 5.9: CROSSWORD PUZZLE

Complete the puzzle by providing the medical term for each of the clues below.

ACROSS

2. Structure within the dermis that produces sweat (5, 5)
6. A malignant tumour that begins in the melanocytes in the epidermis (8)
8. The transplantation of healthy skin from one part of the body to another (5)
10. Sweat gland that promotes cooling (7, 5)

DOWN

1. Skin disorder characterised by the formation of milky white patches on the skin (8)
3. Also called the corium (6)
4. Chronic inflammatory skin disorder most commonly occurring on the central face (7)
5. An oily substance that lubricates the hair and skin (5)
7. Skin disease characterised by pimples, comedones (blackheads), whiteheads and cysts (4)
9. Surgical procedure to transplant skin that contains its own blood supply from one site to another (4)

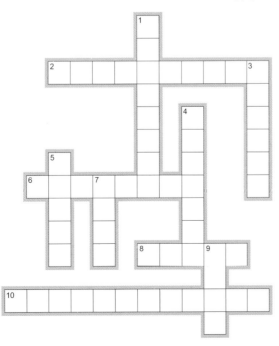

EXERCISE: 5.10: ANAGRAMS

Work out each medical term from the jumbled letters below. Then, using the letters in brackets, determine the medical term that matches the description given.

1. lkdeoi	__ __ __ __ __ (__)	scar tissue
2. ebums	__ __ __ __ (__)	an oily substance secreted by sebaceous glands
3. lceru	__ __ __ __ (__)	a skin erosion
4. htameery	__ __ __ __ __ (__) __ __	redness of skin
5. lpaaieco	__ __ __ __ __ __ (__) __	baldness
6. iisssaorp	__ __ __ __ __ __ __ __ (__)	silver grey scales and red patches on the skin

Rearrange the letters in brackets to form a word that means 'one of the layers of skin'.

__ __ __ __ __ __

EXERCISE 5.11: DISCHARGE SUMMARY ANALYSIS

Read the discharge summary below and answer the questions.

UNIVERSITY HOSPITAL DISCHARGE SUMMARY	**UR number:** 678910
	Name: Clarice Smithson
	Address: 5/56 Bird Way, Billington
	Date of birth: 3/11/1923
	Sex: F
	Nominated primary healthcare provider: Dr Francis Kelly
Episode details **Consultant:** Dr Summer **Registrar:** Dr Carrington **Unit:** Surgical **Admission source:** Elective **Date of admission:** 12/7/2020	**Discharge details** **Status:** Home **Date of discharge:** 15/7/2020
Reason for admission / Presenting problems: Elective admission for SCC excision	
Principal diagnosis: Poorly differentiated SCC of skin of lower lip	
Comorbidities: Nil reported	
Previous medical history: Nil reported	

Clinical synopsis:

This 96-year-old lady was an elective admission for excision of a SCC of the lower lip that had been present for the past 4 months. It was noted to be increasing in size.

On examination, a 1.5 cm diameter, probably infiltrating, SCC was noted on the lower lip. Mrs Smithson made an unremarkable postoperative recovery and was able to be discharged home.

Complications:

Nil

Clinical interventions:

A full thickness wedge excision of 50% of the lower lip was performed under LA (ASA = 2NE). This was then closed in a Y fashion.

Diagnostic interventions:

The histology report revealed a moderately to poorly differentiated SCC, extending into muscle.

There was no lymphatic or perineural invasion identified, and the margins of excision were noted to be clear.

Medications at discharge:

Nil reported

Ceased medications:

Nil reported

Allergies: Nil reported

Alerts: Nil reported

Arranged services: Meals on Wheels

Recommendations: Nil reported

Information to patient/relevant parties: Nil reported

Authorising clinician: Dr Carrington

Document recipients:

Patient

LMO: Dr Francis Kelly

1. **Expand the following abbreviations as found in the discharge summary above.**

   SCC

   LA

   ASA

   LMO

2. **What is a full thickness wedge excision?**

3. **What does 'closed in a Y fashion' mean?**

4. **What does 'margins of excision were noted to be clear' mean?**

5. **What does 'moderately to poorly differentiated' mean?**

MODULE 3

Internal Workings of the Body

CHAPTER 6

Haematology

Contents

Objectives

OBJECTIVES   108

INTRODUCTION   109

NEW WORD ELEMENTS   109
   Combining forms   109
   Prefixes   110
   Suffixes   110

VOCABULARY   111

ABBREVIATIONS   111

FUNCTIONS AND COMPOSITION
OF BLOOD   112
   Functions of blood   112
   Composition of blood   112
   Blood cells   113
   Blood types or blood groups   114

ANALYSIS OF BLOOD SAMPLES   116

PATHOLOGY AND DISEASES   116
   Blood dyscrasias   117
   Clotting disorders   120

TESTS AND PROCEDURES   121

EXERCISES   125

After completing this chapter you should be able to:

1. state the meanings of the word elements related to haematology

2. build words using the word elements associated with haematology

3. recognise, pronounce and effectively use medical terms associated with haematology

4. expand abbreviations related to haematology

5. describe the structure and functions of blood including blood cells, blood groups and the clotting process

6. describe common pathological conditions associated with haematology

7. describe common laboratory tests and diagnostic and surgical procedures associated with haematology

8. apply what you have learned by interpreting medical terminology in practice.

Demonstrate your knowledge of haematology by completing the exercises at the end of this chapter.

INTRODUCTION

Haematology (haemat/o = blood, -logy = study of) is the study of blood. Blood is essential to life. It is a specialised fluid composed of several different types of cells suspended in an intercellular substance called plasma. The primary functions of blood are to transport nutrients and oxygen around the body and to remove waste products from the body cells. Blood also has an important role to play in transporting hormones, regulating body temperature, mediating the immune response and in defending the body against infection. The actions of blood result in homeostasis or internal balance in the body.

Because blood flows around the entire body, through all organs and tissues, its disorders often have a systemic effect on the body. Blood is the most commonly tested part of the body, and changes in blood composition can help detect many diseases.

This chapter will look at the blood itself, how it is created and the way it is transported around the body. The study of blood is closely linked with the study of the cardiovascular and the lymphatic systems.

NEW WORD ELEMENTS

Here are some word elements related to haematology. To reinforce your learning, write the meanings of the medical terms in the spaces provided. Use the Glossary of medical terms on page 561 to help you work out the meanings. You may also need to check the meaning in a medical dictionary, but make an attempt yourself first.

Combining forms

Combining Form	Meaning	Medical Term	Meaning of Medical Term
agglutin/o	clumping, gluing, sticking together	agglutination	
bas/o	base, basis	basophil	
blast/o	embryonic, developing cell	blastogenesis	
chrom/o	colour	hypochromia	
chromat/o		chromatism	
coagul/o	clotting	anticoagulant	
cyt/o	cell	cytology	
embol/o	embolism, plug	embolectomy	
eosin/o	red, dawn, rosy	eosinophil	
erythr/o	red	erythrocyte	
granul/o	granules	agranulocytosis	
haem/o	blood	haemostasis	
haemat/o		haematoma	
haemoglobin/o	haemoglobin	haemoglobinopathy	
home/o	same, alike	homeostasis	
is/o	same, equal	isoagglutination	
kary/o	nucleus	karyomegaly	
leuc/o, leuk/o (Note that leuk/o is used in Australia for the word leukaemia (and derivative terms) only)	white	leucopenia leukaemoid	
morph/o	shape, form	dysmorphic	
myel/o	bone marrow, spinal cord	myeloid	
neutr/o	neutral	neutropenia	
nucle/o	nucleus	nuclear	
phag/o	eat, swallow	phagocytosis	
phleb/o	vein	phlebotomy	

Table continued

Combining Form	Meaning	Medical Term	Meaning of Medical Term
poikil/o	varied, irregular	poikilocyte	
reticul/o	net-like	reticulocyte	
sangui/o	blood	sanguiferous	
sanguin/o		exsanguination	
sider/o	iron	sideroblastic	
spher/o	globe, round	spherocytosis	
splen/o	spleen	splenomegaly	
thromb/o	clot	thrombophlebitis	
thym/o	thymus gland	thymectomy	

Prefixes

Prefix	Meaning	Medical Term	Meaning of Medical Term
aniso-	unequal, asymmetrical, dissimilar	anisocytosis	
macro-	large	macrophage	
micro-	small	microcythaemia	
mono-	one, single	monocyte	
pan-	all, entire	pancytopenia	
poly-	many, much	polymorphonuclear	
trans-	across, through, over	transfusion	

Suffixes

Suffix	Meaning	Medical Term	Meaning of Medical Term
-aemia	condition of blood	anaemia	
-apheresis	removal, carry away	plasmapheresis	
-blast	embryonic or developing cell	myeloblast	
-cyte	cell	lymphocyte	
-cytosis	abnormal condition of cells	erythrocytosis	
-globin	protein	haemoglobin	
-globulin		immunoglobulin	
-lytic	pertaining to destruction, drug that breaks down	thrombolytic	
-oid	resembling, derived from	lipoid	
-osis	abnormal condition	thrombosis	
-penia	deficiency	neutropenia	
-phage	eat, swallow	macrophage	
-phagia		dysphagia	
-phil	affinity for, attraction for	neutrophil	
-philia		neutrophilia	
-poiesis	formation, production of	erythropoiesis	
-rrhage	bursting forth, excessive discharge or flow	haemorrhage	
-rrhagia		menorrhagia	
-stasis	stop, control, stand still	haemostasis	

VOCABULARY

The following list provides many of the medical terms used for the first time in this chapter. Pronunciations are provided with each term. As you read the rest of the chapter, make sure you identify each of these terms and understand their meanings.

Term	Pronunciation
agglutination	ay-gloo-tin-AY-shun
albumin	AL-byoo-min
anaemia	a-NEEM-ee-a
antibody	AN-tee-bod-ee
antigen	AN-tee-jen
basophil	BASS-o-fil
bilirubin	bill-ee-ROO-bin
bone marrow	bohn MA-roh
coagulation	ko-ag-yoo-LAY-shun
differentiation	diff-er-en-shee-AY-shun
electrophoresis	ee-lek-tro-for-EE-sis
eosinophil	ee-o-SIN-o-fil
erythrocyte	e-REETH-ro-syt
erythropoietin	e-REETH-ro-poy-EE-tin
fibrin	FIB-rin
fibrinogen	fib-RIN-o-jen
formed elements	formed EL-e-mentz
globin	GLOW-bin
globulin	GLOB-yoo-lin
granulocyte	GRAN-yoo-loh-syt
haeme	heem
haemoglobin	HEEM-oh-glow-bin
heparin	HEP-ar-in
immune reaction	im-yoon re-AK-shun
immunoglobulin	im-yoon-o-GLOB-yoo-lin
leucocyte	LOO-koh-syt
lymphocyte	LIM-foh-syt
macrophage	MAK-roh-fahj
megakaryocyte	meg-a-KARE-ee-o-syt
monocyte	MON-oh-syt
myeloid	MY-el-oyd
neutrophil	NEWT-roh-fil
pancytopenia	pan-syt-oh-PEE-nee-a
phlebotomy	fleb-OT-oh-me
plasma	PLAZ-ma
plasmapheresis	plaz-ma-fer-EE-sis
platelet	PLAYT-let
prothrombin	pro-THROM-bin

Table continued

Term	Pronunciation
reticulocyte	re-TIK-yoo-loh-syt
Rh factor	R H FAK-ta
serum	SEE-rum
spleen	spleen
stem cell	STEM sell
thrombin	THROM-bin
thrombocyte	THROM-boh-syt
thromboplastin	THROM-boh-plass-tin
transfusion	trans-FYOO-shun

ABBREVIATIONS

The following abbreviations are commonly used in the Australian healthcare environment. Because some abbreviations can have more than one meaning, check the context in which the abbreviation is used before assigning a meaning to it.

Abbreviation	Definition
Ab	antibody
ABO	three main blood types: A, B and O
Ag	antigen
ALL	acute lymphocytic leukaemia, acute lymphoblastic leukaemia
AML	acute monocytic leukaemia, acute myelocytic leukaemia, acute myeloblastic leukaemia, acute myeloid leukaemia
AMML	acute myelomonocytic leukaemia
AST	aspartate aminotransferase
BMT	bone marrow transplant
CLL	chronic lymphocytic leukaemia
CML	chronic myelogenous leukaemia, chronic myeloid leukaemia, chronic myelocytic leukaemia
CMML	chronic myelomonocytic leukaemia
DIC	disseminated intravascular coagulation or coagulopathy
diff.	differential count (white blood cells)
EBV	Epstein-Barr virus
EPO	erythropoietin
ESR	erythrocyte sedimentation rate
FBC	full blood count
Fe	iron
GVH	graft-versus-host

Table continued

Abbreviation	Definition
GVHD	graft-versus-host disease
Hb, Hgb	haemoglobin
Hct	haematocrit
HDN	haemolytic disease of the newborn
HLA	human leucocytic antigen
IgA	immunoglobulins
IgD	
IgE	
IgG	
IgM	
IM	infectious mononucleosis
INR	international normalised ratio
ITP	immune (idiopathic) thrombocytopenic purpura
MCH	mean corpuscular haemoglobin
MCHC	mean corpuscular haemoglobin concentration or count
MCV	mean corpuscular volume
mono	monocyte
PMN	polymorphonuclear neutrophil (leucocyte)
PMNL, poly	polymorphonuclear leucocyte
PT	prothrombin time
PTT	partial thromboplastin time
RBC	red blood cell
RCC	red cell count
WBC	white blood cell
WCC	white cell count

FUNCTIONS AND COMPOSITION OF BLOOD

Functions of blood

Blood provides a transportation system for the body. It transfers:

- gases, such as oxygen and carbon dioxide, to and from the lungs and the rest of the cells of the body
- nutrients from the gastrointestinal organs to other parts of the body
- waste products to the urinary system to be excreted
- hormones from the endocrine glands to the organs on which they act
- heat to the skin to help regulate body temperature.

Blood also has a role in protecting the body through its component white blood cells, antibodies and platelets, which act to fight infections and to initiate blood clotting. Blood has a regulatory role, transferring water to and from body tissues and helping to maintain electrolyte balance.

Composition of blood

Components of blood

The body of a normal adult human contains about 5 litres of blood, making up 7–8% of total body weight. Blood has a slightly thick, sticky consistency and is around five times more viscous than water. This level of viscosity or stickiness is necessary because if blood flows too quickly or too slowly through the blood vessels, it can put stress on the cardiovascular system. Approximately one-third of the total volume is made up of a straw-coloured fluid known as plasma and the remainder consists of formed elements called cells. Blood cells (erythrocytes, some leucocytes, platelets) arise in the bone marrow. Bone marrow is found in the interior of spongy bones and in the centre of long bones. All cells begin as undifferentiated stem cells, and these then mature into the various types of cells. Bone marrow contains two types of stem cells: haematopoietic (which produce blood cells) and stromal (which produce fat, cartilage and bone). Bone marrow consists of two types: yellow and red. Both types of bone marrow contain many blood vessels and capillaries. At birth, all bone marrow is red, but with increasing age, some of the red bone marrow is converted into the yellow type. Adults generally have about half red and half yellow bone marrow.

Red bone marrow

This is the functioning part of the bone marrow, acting to create the various blood components. Erythrocytes, platelets and most leucocytes arise in red marrow, which is also called myeloid tissue. The process of creating new blood cells is called haematopoiesis. Red bone marrow is principally found in the hip bone, breast bone, skull, ribs, vertebrae and shoulder blades, and in the cancellous (spongy) material at the proximal ends of the long bones such as the femur and humerus.

Yellow bone marrow

Yellow bone marrow is red bone marrow that has largely turned into fat. Haematopoiesis is not a function of this type of bone marrow. Yellow bone marrow stores the fat that the body uses when exposed to extreme privation. In cases of severe anaemia or blood loss, the body can turn the yellow bone marrow into red bone marrow to help maintain homeostasis. Yellow marrow is mainly found in the body's long bones, principally in the upper and lower limbs.

Blood cells

The cellular portions of the blood are often called the formed elements and consist of three major types of cells: erythrocytes, leucocytes and thrombocytes (Fig. 6.1).

Erythrocytes

Erythrocytes (*erythr/o* = red, *-cyte* = cell) are red blood cells, the most common type of cell, comprising approximately 43% of total blood volume. The active constituent of erythrocytes is haemoglobin, an iron-containing protein that transports oxygen from the lungs to every cell in the body and collects waste gases, such as carbon dioxide, and returns them to the lungs for expiration. Normal haemoglobin levels differ between males and females. A healthy adult male should have a haemoglobin level between 130 and 180 g/L (grams per litre). Women usually have a slightly lower haemoglobin level of between 115 and 165 g/L. These levels may vary slightly depending on the laboratory reference used.

Erythrocytes are a flat circular shape with a thumb-print depression in the centre. This shape provides greater surface area to the cell, which assists with the transport of gases around the body. Erythrocytes live for approximately 120 days, becoming increasingly fragile as they age. They are destroyed by phagocytic cells in the liver and the spleen and are replaced by new cells arising in the red bone marrow.

Leucocytes

Leucocytes (*leuc/o* = white, *-cyte* = cell) are white blood cells that live for between a few hours to a few days, although some can exist for many years. They consist of two types: **granulocytes** and **agranulocytes**. Granulocytes consist of neutrophils, eosinophils and basophils and have a typical granular appearance under a microscope. In contrast, agranulocytes do not look granular. There are two types of agranulocytes called lymphocytes and monocytes.

Neutrophils help to destroy bacteria through phagocytosis. They are also capable of releasing chemicals that can kill or slow the growth of bacteria. Once a neutrophil ingests a pathogen, it cannot survive. Neutrophils are the main constituent of pus and are responsible for its white colour. Neutrophils exist in the bloodstream until called to a site of infection by various chemicals in the body. They are fast acting, arriving at the site of infection within an hour to begin their work.

Eosinophils live predominantly in the body's submucosal tissue and act against inflammation, allergies and immune reactions in the body.

Basophils release histamine and heparin in response to an inflammation, the presence of an allergen or a suspected infection. Normally there are very few circulating basophils in the blood. However, an active infection or allergic response, such as occurs in asthma, causes the number of basophils in the blood to rise.

Figure 6.1 Blood smear

(Based on Hutton 2002)

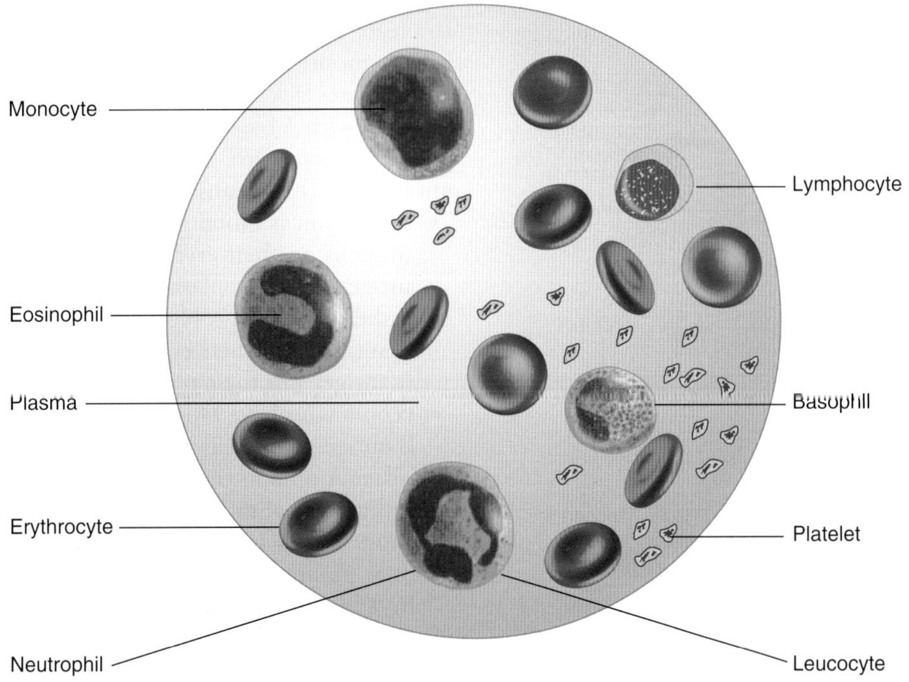

Lymphocytes are mainly responsible for the body's immune reaction and circulate through the body in the lymphatic fluid as well as in the blood. Lymphocytes make up 20–40% of the leucocytes in the body. There are two predominant types of lymphocytes: B cells and T cells. The B cells attack bacteria and toxins through the creation of antibodies, while T cells attack the body's own cells if they have been invaded by viruses or have become cancerous.

Monocytes make up 1–3% of the body's leucocytes. Monocytes can turn into either dendritic cells or macrophages. Dendritic cells assist T cells before they are fully developed, helping them to recognise an antigen. Macrophages are cells that eat other cells, including bacteria or viruses. This function also provides the body with an antigen so that it will be able to recognise the foreign material in the future. Macrophages can eat cells in the body that have been infected by a pathogen to slow or halt the spread of the pathogen.

Thrombocytes

Thrombocytes (*thromb/o* = clot, *-cyte* = cell) are also known as platelets. The role of thrombocytes is to help with clotting of the blood, a process also known as coagulation (Fig. 6.2). Agents such as calcium ions (CA^{2+}) are also required for this process. This prompts haemostasis, the process that stops blood loss from a damaged vessel. The platelets produce a plug (fibrinogen) to stop the bleeding and begin repair of

the damaged vessel. If there are too few thrombocytes, haemostasis may not be possible, and uncontrolled or prolonged bleeding may result. If the blood contains too many thrombocytes, abnormal blood clot formation or thrombosis may result, and this may cause a life-threatening situation if normal blood vessels are blocked.

Plasma: If the erythrocytes, leucocytes, platelets and any other cellular components of blood are removed, what is left is a clear, light yellow-coloured fluid. This is the blood plasma, the liquid component of blood that makes up approximately 55% of total blood volume. Plasma consists of water, salts, enzymes, antibodies, clotting factors and other proteins. It is responsible for transporting nutrients, hormones and proteins around the body. Waste products from the cells are also transported away in the plasma. Blood plasma carries immune system cells (antibodies) and delivers them to the site of an infection in the body. It also delivers clotting factors to support blood coagulation where there is damage to a vessel.

Blood types or blood groups

Although there are many blood group systems with several sub-types, the two best-known ways of classifying blood are the ABO group system and the rhesus (Rh) type system. In the former, there are four main blood groups, known as types A, B, AB and O, which are identified based on combinations of inherited antigens and antibodies present on the surface of erythrocytes. Known as the ABO system, the blood types are determined by the presence or absence of two different proteins, known as A and B antigens, on the erythrocytes. Antigens are proteins that cause the body to create antibodies to foreign substances. By the age of six months, antibodies against the antigens the erythrocytes lack are formed in the plasma. For instance, a person with A blood type will form anti-B antibodies, and a person with B blood type will have anti-A antibodies. This means:

- If a person is blood group A, they will have A antigens on their erythrocytes and antibodies to B antigens in their plasma.
- If the individual is blood group B, they will have B antigens on their erythrocytes and antibodies to A antigens in their plasma.
- People who have blood type AB have both A and B antigens on their erythrocytes and do not have either A or B antibodies in their plasma.
- Individuals with blood type O have no A or B antigens and have both A and B antibodies in their plasma.

In addition to the blood groups, there are also inherited antigens knowns as the Rh antigens found on the surface of erythrocytes. There are five known

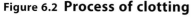

Figure 6.2 **Process of clotting**

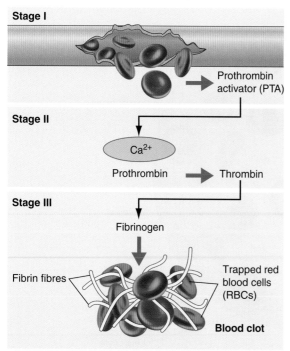

Stage I

Prothrombin activator (PTA)

Stage II

Ca²⁺

Prothrombin → Thrombin

Stage III

Fibrinogen

Fibrin fibres

Trapped red blood cells (RBCs)

Blood clot

Rh antigens – C, c, D, E, e – but the most important of these is the Rh D. People with the D antigen on their red blood cells have Rh positive (+) blood. Blood without the Rh D antigen is called Rh negative (-). The presence or absence of the rhesus factor, or Rh factor as it is also called, was first identified in the blood of rhesus monkeys. These small monkeys were often used for medical experimentation.

The ABO blood group system was first identified by an Austrian scientist, Dr Karl Landsteiner, in 1901. Dr Landsteiner recognised the reactions between the blood antigens and certain antibodies in the plasma that caused the blood serum of some people to clump. After further experimentation, he formally identified the four mutually incompatible blood groups (A, B, AB, O; see Table 6.1) based on the presence or absence of the two specific antigens, A and B. Later in his career, Landsteiner also identified the Rh factor.

A blood transfusion is the transfer of blood or blood products from a donor to a recipient. It may be given to replace the blood of a patient following haemorrhage, surgery, injury or certain illnesses such as anaemia. The blood used in a transfusion must be compatible with the blood type of the recipient; otherwise the antibody reaction called agglutination will result. This is the clumping that Landsteiner noted. It is always preferable for patients to be transfused with blood of the same ABO and Rh groups as they have themselves. If a person undergoing transfusion of blood has a blood group that does not have any antibodies against the antigens present in the donor blood, all will be well. However, if the recipient's blood has antibodies that match the antigens in the donated blood, agglutination or binding of the erythrocytes in the donated blood will occur. In an emergency, however, if the required blood group is not available, it is possible for a patient to be given a different group as follows.

A person with type O blood is known as the universal donor. Type O blood can be given to a person with any blood type because type O blood has no A or B antigens. However, a person with type O blood can only receive type O blood. A person with type AB blood is known as the universal recipient because they can receive type A, B, AB or O blood. A person with type A blood can receive a transfusion of types A and O blood. For a type B recipient, the blood transfusion must be type B or type O. In normal circumstances, people with Rh-negative blood should not receive Rh-positive blood. They will experience a severe immune system reaction because their body creates antibodies against the foreign protein in the Rh-positive blood. This can occur during a mismatched transfusion or through the placenta during a second or subsequent pregnancy where the mother is Rh negative and the baby inherits Rh-positive blood from its father. During a first pregnancy, the antibodies usually do not cause problems because the baby generally is born before many of the antibodies develop. The mother's blood is sensitised to the presence of the Rh-positive factor and will develop antibodies in a future pregnancy if the mismatch in blood type occurs again. Rh (D) immunoglobulin (also known as anti-D) is given prophylactically to Rh-negative mothers to prevent future antibody development. If there is a subsequent pregnancy and anti-D has not been given, the baby is at risk of developing haemolytic disease of the newborn, which causes complications such as severe anaemia and brain damage and can sometimes be fatal.

However, if transfusion of an Rh-positive blood product to an Rh-negative patient is unavoidable, it is

Table 6.1 ABO blood groups

(Australian Red Cross Lifeblood 2018)

		Donor's Blood Type							
		O−	O+	B−	B+	A−	A+	AB−	AB+
Recipient's Blood Type	AB+	x	x	x	x	x	x	x	x
	AB−	x		x		x		x	
	A+	x	x			x	x		
	A−	x				x			
	B+	x	x	x	x				
	B−	x		x					
	O+	x	x						
	O−	x							

possible to avoid major problems through administering anti-D immunoglobulin, which prevents the antibody formation.

A blood transfusion may consist of whole blood, containing both the plasma and cellular components of blood, or only the red cells known as packed cells. In the latter case, most of the plasma has been removed prior to the transfusion. This type of transfusion is normally given to a patient who is lacking erythrocytes because of anaemia.

The frequency of the various blood groups in the Australian population is shown in Fig. 6.3.

ANALYSIS OF BLOOD SAMPLES

As previously discussed in this chapter, haematology is a general term for the study of blood. Within the specialty of haematology, there are several different categories of blood tests that a laboratory might perform. All tests compare a patient's results against a reference range. The reference range represents the average value for a 'normal' population group, generally with any expected variation that may be seen (usually plus or minus 2 standard deviations from the average).

Figure 6.3 Distribution of blood types among first time Australian blood donors

(Australian Red Cross Lifeblood 2018)

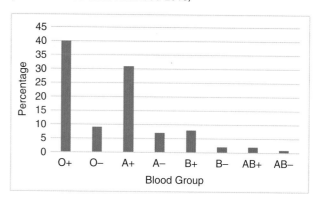

Reference ranges are set by the laboratory that provides the test results, and different laboratories use varying equipment and testing methods. That means each laboratory has its own reference ranges, and these may differ from laboratory to laboratory. Therefore, results from one laboratory cannot always be compared with those from another laboratory. See page 578 for examples of standard haematological values.

Category of blood test	What is tested
biochemistry	Biochemistry assesses the levels of chemicals in the body to determine if a disease is present or not. Biochemistry tests include electrolytes, liver function tests, cholesterol, triglycerides, lipids, blood glucose and drug levels.
cytogenetics	Cytogenetics is an area of study that examines genes and chromosomes. It is concerned with genetic testing and cancer diagnosis. Cytogenetic tests can be performed on blood, bone marrow, fetal specimens and body tissues.
haematology	Haematology specifically looks at blood and bone marrow to identify cancers of the blood (such as leukaemia and lymphoma) and clotting disorders. Blood grouping and antibody testing for blood banking is also done by haematology as is the most commonly ordered test – a full blood count (FBC). An FBC identifies the number and type of cells in the blood: erythrocytes, leucocytes and platelets. Abnormalities in any of these cells suggest that disease is present.
microbiology	Microbiology looks for infections such as viruses, bacteria, parasites in blood and other body tissues.
serology	Serology examines blood serum for antibodies to specific infections such as influenza, rubella, Epstein-Barr virus, Ross River fever and to various allergens. By performing a serology test, it is possible to determine a patient's infection status or if they have responded to an immunisation.

PATHOLOGY AND DISEASES

The following section provides a list of common diseases and pathological conditions relevant to haematology. Blood dyscrasias and clotting disorders will be discussed here. Other haematological disorders such as leukaemia, myeloma and certain infections are discussed in other chapters.

Blood dyscrasias

Term	Pronunciation	Definition
anaemia	a-NEEM-ee-a	Anaemia is the most common haematological disorder. In general terms it is a medical condition in which the number of erythrocytes, the amount of haemoglobin or the volume of packed red cells in the blood is reduced (Fig. 6.4). This leads to a diminished capacity for erythrocytes to transport oxygen to the body tissues. There are many types of anaemia. All are very different in their causes and treatments. The following entries in this table describe some of the main types of anaemia.

Figure 6.4 Erythrocytes in anaemic conditions

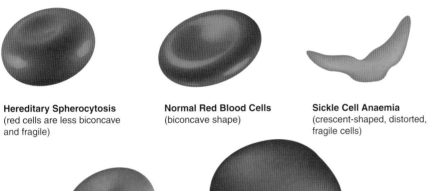

Hereditary Spherocytosis
(red cells are less biconcave and fragile)

Normal Red Blood Cells
(biconcave shape)

Sickle Cell Anaemia
(crescent-shaped, distorted, fragile cells)

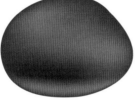

Thalassaemia
(haemoglobin concentration is low)

Pernicious Anaemia
(large, immature, megaloblasts)

Term	Pronunciation	Definition
– aplastic anaemia	ay-PLAS-tik a-NEEM-ee-a	In aplastic anaemia there is a suppression of bone marrow function. This results in pancytopenia, in particular a decrease in the production of erythrocytes. The cause of the anaemia can be acquired or inherited; however, the cause is idiopathic in more than half the cases diagnosed. Acquired aplastic anaemia may be due to exposure to toxins such as pesticides and benzene, radiation and chemotherapy, viruses such as Epstein-Barr virus, human immunodeficiency virus (HIV) and hepatitis and autoimmune diseases such as lupus and rheumatoid arthritis. Aplastic anaemia that is inherited, such as Fanconi's anaemia, is very rare. Treatment is often multimodal, and the aim is to prevent or limit complications, relieve symptoms and improve quality of life. It may include blood transfusions to keep blood cell counts at acceptable levels, antibiotics to prevent secondary infections, bone marrow or stem cell transplantation to potentially cure the anaemia in some patients and immunosuppressant drugs to prevent rejection.

Table continued

Term	Pronunciation	Definition
– haemolytic anaemia	heem-oh-LIT-ik a-NEEM-ee-a	Haemolytic anaemia is a rare form of anaemia that results from the premature destruction (haemolysis) and removal of erythrocytes from the blood. In haemolytic anaemia, the bone marrow increases production of erythrocytes to replace the haemolysed blood cells, but it cannot produce them fast enough to meet the body's needs. There are several different types of haemolytic anaemia. Autoimmune haemolytic anaemia is the most common type. Antibodies produced by the immune system destroy erythrocytes. This is often associated with disorders such as systemic lupus erythematosus and lymphoma. In infants, blood group incompatibility between mother and child is a cause of haemolytic anaemia. Another example of haemolytic anaemia is hereditary spherocytosis. This is characterised by spherical shaped erythrocytes, which are extremely fragile and tend to haemolyse. Treatments include corticosteroids, blood transfusions, splenectomy and bone marrow transplantation. Immunosuppressive drugs may be required.
– iron deficiency anaemia	EYE-on de-FISH-en-see a-NEEM-ee-a	Anaemia that is due to low iron levels is called iron deficiency anaemia. Iron is the major component of haemoglobin, which is responsible for transporting oxygen around the body. It is also responsible for fighting some toxins and infections in the blood. Chronic blood loss due to long-term internal bleeding is the main cause. Women are more likely than men to have iron deficiency anaemia because of the loss of blood each month through normal menstruation. Iron deficiency anaemia can also be due to small amounts of repeated bleeding from the gastrointestinal tract – for instance, from a tumour in the colon or from a stomach ulcer. In young children, the elderly and vegetarians, iron deficiency anaemia is most often due to a diet lacking iron. Iron supplements, an improved dietary intake or transfusion of blood products are common treatments.
– macrocytic anaemia	mak-roh-SIT-ik a-NEEM-ee-a	Macrocytic anaemia occurs when the body's erythrocytes are abnormally large but relatively few in number. Because they are scarce, they also carry less haemoglobin, causing a lack of oxygen in the blood. Most commonly, the condition is caused by a lack of vitamin B_{12} or folate or the inability to utilise these. It can also indicate an underlying condition such as alcoholism, liver disease, hypothyroidism and myelodysplastic syndromes.
– microcytic anaemia	myk-roh-SIT-ik a-NEEM-ee-a	Microcytic anaemia occurs when there is a decrease in the number of erythrocytes present. These erythrocytes are abnormally small and often hypochromic. Microcytic anaemia is caused when the body produces an insufficient amount of haemoglobin. Iron deficiency is the most common cause of microcytic anaemia.
– pernicious anaemia	per-NISH-us a-NEEM-ee-a	Pernicious anaemia is usually caused by a lack of the protein, intrinsic factor, which is normally found in the stomach. Intrinsic factor is necessary for vitamin B_{12} absorption. Vitamin B_{12} is found in most meats, eggs and some seafood but it requires adequate amounts of intrinsic factor for it to be absorbed into the bloodstream. Vitamin B_{12} is required by the body for the production and maturation of erythrocytes. Lifelong vitamin B_{12} injections are the usual treatment for pernicious anaemia. Oral vitamin B_{12} supplements may also be used as pernicious anaemia treatment, but they are not as effective as B_{12} injections.

Table continued

Term	Pronunciation	Definition
– **post-haemorrhagic anaemia**	poh-st hem-oh-RAY-jik a-NEEM-ee-a	Post-haemorrhagic anaemia results from the body losing a large quantity of blood, and therefore erythrocytes, at one time – for example, in trauma where a patient haemorrhages a large volume of blood. When many erythrocytes are lost in a short timeframe, the body will compensate by using all reserves of iron and nutrients in the body, resulting in anaemia. Treatment of post-haemorrhagic anaemia includes instigating immediate measures to stop the haemorrhage, restoring blood volume with transfusion and fluids and preventing shock.
– **sickle cell anaemia**	SIK-el sel a-NEEM-ee-a	Sickle cell anaemia is a serious inherited disorder occurring primarily in people of African descent but also in those from India and Mediterranean regions. Normal erythrocytes are disc-shaped, but in patients with sickle cell anaemia, their erythrocytes are shaped like the old agricultural tool called a sickle – hence the name of the disease. These erythrocytes have a shortened lifespan of 10–20 days, resulting in anaemia. Normal erythrocytes live for approximately 120 days. They can bend easily, but sickle cell erythrocytes tend to be inflexible, forming clumps that get stuck in the smaller blood vessels. These small blood vessels easily become blocked, preventing oxygen from getting through and causing severe pain and damage to organs. There is no cure for sickle cell anaemia, but bone marrow transplants have been successful for some patients because they can provide a source of normal cells. However, the transplant must be performed before there is any permanent damage to vital organs.
– **thalassaemia**	thal-a-SEEM-ee-a	Thalassaemia is a genetic blood disorder that results in a fault in the rate of production of haemoglobin. Thalassaemia is usually diagnosed within the first 6 months of life and can be fatal in early childhood without ongoing treatment. There are two major types. Thalassaemia minor is the more common and milder form. People with this type can expect to have a normal lifespan. Thalassaemia major, which is also known as Cooley's anaemia, is much more serious and requires lifelong treatment. Thalassaemia is most common in people of Mediterranean descent. The word thalassaemia comes from the Greek word *thalassa*, which means sea. The treatment for patients with thalassaemia minor will vary depending on the severity of the condition. Some patients will only require iron supplements, while others will require occasional blood transfusions. Patients with thalassaemia major will need regular blood transfusions to build up the amount of haemoglobin in their blood. Splenectomy and bone marrow transplants are currently being investigated as possible treatments for thalassaemia.

Clotting disorders

Term	Pronunciation	Definition
haemophilia	heem-oh-FIL-ee-a	Haemophilia is a rare hereditary bleeding disorder in which the blood does not clot normally. It almost always occurs in males. People born with haemophilia usually have a normal platelet count but have little or no clotting factor. Clotting factors are proteins needed for normal blood clotting. Around 90% of patients will be missing factor VIII.
		People who have haemophilia will bleed for a long time after an injury or accident. They may also bleed spontaneously into joints such as knees, ankles and elbows. This causes pain and, if not treated, can lead to arthritis. Bleeding in the brain is a very serious complication of haemophilia and requires emergency treatment.
		The main treatment is injections of the missing clotting factor into the bloodstream. The different types of haemophilia include haemophilia A (classical haemophilia), which is the most common form resulting from reduced levels of factor VIII, haemophilia B (Christmas disease) due to a reduction in factor IX and haemophilia C (Rosenthal's syndrome) due to factor XI deficiency.
immune (idiopathic) thrombocytopenic purpura (ITP)	im-YOON (id-ee-o-PATH-ik) throm-boh-syt-oh-PEE-nik PER-per-a	ITP, previously known as idiopathic thrombocytopenic purpura, is a rare autoimmune disorder where a person's blood does not clot properly because platelets are destroyed by antibodies. The cause of ITP is unknown (idiopathic) but is thought to be linked to a viral infection that causes the body to produce antibodies to destroy the virus. These antibodies target platelets so the spleen and liver see them as foreign and destroy them. Often ITP is asymptomatic; however, a very low platelet count can lead to visible signs such as purpura, frequent nosebleeds and abnormal menstruation. Treatment will vary depending on the severity of the ITP. It may include a watchful wait to see if the ITP resolves spontaneously, steroid medication to reduce immune activity or plasmapheresis to filter the antibodies from the blood. In severe or chronic cases, a splenectomy may be required.
purpura	PER-per-a	Purpura (from the Latin word meaning purple) is a condition characterised by haemorrhage into the skin, mucous membranes and sometimes the internal organs. Initially purpura appears as red areas that become purple and later brownish-yellow. Purpura usually appears in crops and generally disappears over several days. Small purpura present as pinpoint-sized haemorrhages of capillaries in the skin or mucous membranes and are called **petechiae** (pet-EE-kee-ee). Large purpura present as deeper bleeding beneath the skin and are called **ecchymoses** (ek-ee-MOH-seez), similar to haematomas or bruises. Purpura is a common non-specific sign that can indicate an underlying more serious condition such as a platelet disorder (thrombocytopenia), vascular disorder (vasculitis), a coagulation disorder, malignancy or some infectious diseases. Treatment depends on the cause.

TESTS AND PROCEDURES

The following section provides a list of common diagnostic tests and procedures and clinical interventions and surgical procedures that are undertaken for the haematology system.

Test/procedure	Pronunciation	Definition
antiglobulin test (Coombs' test)	an-tee-GLOB-yoo-lin (kooms) test	A Coombs' test is a diagnostic test used to test for the presence of antibodies that coat and damage erythrocytes. It is helpful to detect if antibodies are present in patients with autoimmune haemolytic anaemia or in infants of Rh-negative women.
apheresis	ay-fer-EE-sis	Apheresis is a non-surgical procedure to remove toxic substances or autoantibodies, or may be used to harvest blood cells. Blood is withdrawn from the body, the target components are removed and the blood is reinfused into the body. Examples of this type of procedure include leucapheresis, plateletapheresis and plasmapheresis.
bleeding time	BLEE-ding tym	Bleeding time is a measure to determine the time it takes for a small puncture wound to stop bleeding, with the normal time being 8 minutes or less. The use of aspirin and the presence of platelet disorders such as thrombocytopenia can lead to prolonged bleeding times. There are several methods for measuring bleeding time, with the most common involving an incision being made as continuous pressure is applied using a sphygmomanometer.
blood transfusion	blud trans-FYOO-shun	A blood transfusion is a non-surgical procedure that involves administering whole blood or components of blood (e.g. plasma) to replenish blood lost through surgery, trauma or disease. The donor blood is tested before transfusion to ensure that blood-borne infections such as hepatitis and HIV are not in the donation. After the donor blood has been tested to ensure it closely matches the blood type, red cells or platelets of the recipient, the blood is transfused into the recipient. This is known as an allogenic transfusion. Recipients can also receive an autologous transfusion, which involves collecting the patient's own blood for reinfusion at a later date.
bone marrow biopsy	bohn MA-roh BY-op-see	A bone marrow biopsy is a procedure that involves removing the marrow from inside a bone to diagnose such conditions as leukaemia, certain infections, some anaemias and other blood disorders. The procedure is performed by inserting a trephine needle into the bone, usually into the posterior iliac crest, and removing a small sample of marrow for microscopic examination to identify abnormal tissue.
bone marrow (or stem cell) transplant	bohn MA-roh TRANZ-plant	A bone marrow (or stem cell) transplant involves transplanting healthy bone marrow that has been treated by irradiation. The transplant is a two-step process that involves aspirating the bone marrow from the patient (autologous transplant) or a compatible donor (a donor whose tissues and blood cells closely match the recipient, allogenic or allogeneic transplant) (Fig. 6.5). The purpose of the transplant is to replace the diseased bone marrow in the recipient with healthy cells. Once the infusion has occurred, the marrow repopulates the patient's marrow space with normal cells. Complications that can occur include infection, graft-versus-host disease and relapse of the original disease.

Table continued

Test/procedure	Pronunciation	Definition

Figure 6.5 Bone marrow harvest and transplant

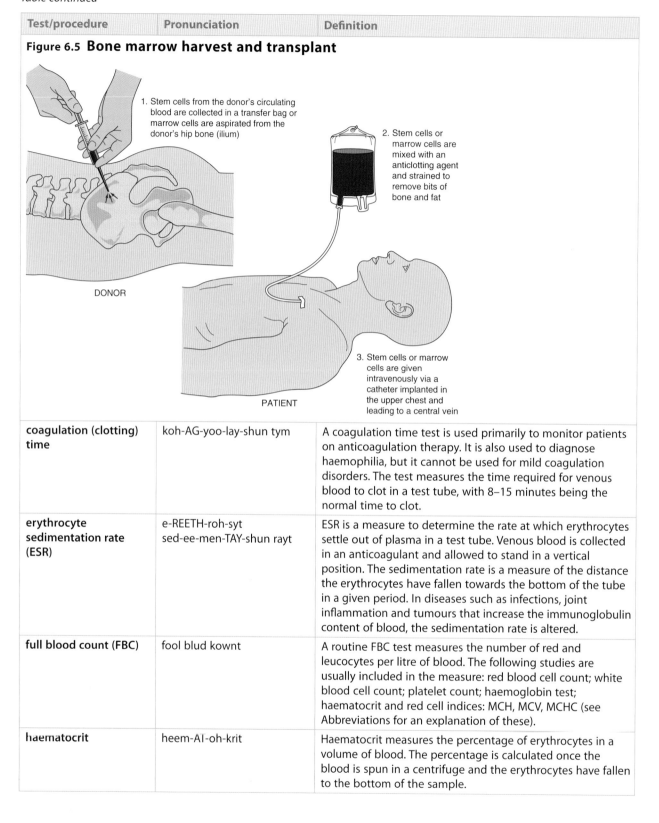

1. Stem cells from the donor's circulating blood are collected in a transfer bag or marrow cells are aspirated from the donor's hip bone (ilium)

DONOR

2. Stem cells or marrow cells are mixed with an anticlotting agent and strained to remove bits of bone and fat

3. Stem cells or marrow cells are given intravenously via a catheter implanted in the upper chest and leading to a central vein

PATIENT

Test/procedure	Pronunciation	Definition
coagulation (clotting) time	koh-AG-yoo-lay-shun tym	A coagulation time test is used primarily to monitor patients on anticoagulation therapy. It is also used to diagnose haemophilia, but it cannot be used for mild coagulation disorders. The test measures the time required for venous blood to clot in a test tube, with 8–15 minutes being the normal time to clot.
erythrocyte sedimentation rate (ESR)	e-REETH-roh-syt sed-ee-men-TAY-shun rayt	ESR is a measure to determine the rate at which erythrocytes settle out of plasma in a test tube. Venous blood is collected in an anticoagulant and allowed to stand in a vertical position. The sedimentation rate is a measure of the distance the erythrocytes have fallen towards the bottom of the tube in a given period. In diseases such as infections, joint inflammation and tumours that increase the immunoglobulin content of blood, the sedimentation rate is altered.
full blood count (FBC)	fool blud kownt	A routine FBC test measures the number of red and leucocytes per litre of blood. The following studies are usually included in the measure: red blood cell count; white blood cell count; platelet count; haemoglobin test; haematocrit and red cell indices: MCH, MCV, MCHC (see Abbreviations for an explanation of these).
haematocrit	heem-AT-oh-krit	Haematocrit measures the percentage of erythrocytes in a volume of blood. The percentage is calculated once the blood is spun in a centrifuge and the erythrocytes have fallen to the bottom of the sample.

Table continued

Test/procedure	Pronunciation	Definition
haemoglobin test	heem-oh-GLOW-bin test	A haemoglobin test measures a sample of peripheral blood to determine the total amount of haemoglobin, which reflects erythrocytes in the blood. Disease conditions such as anaemia, erythrocytosis and sickle cell disease are detected through abnormal levels of haemoglobin.
heparinisation	hep-ar-in-EYE-say-shun	Heparinisation involves administering heparin to either prevent a clot forming or to break down a clot.
international normalised ratio	in-ter-NASH-on-al NOR-mal-ized RAY-shee-oh	An INR is a laboratory test that measures how long it takes for blood to clot. It is also known as a prothrombin test. It is generally used to assess the effectiveness of anticoagulant treatment.
partial thromboplastin time (PTT)	PAH-shal throm-boh-PLAS-tin tym	A PTT test is a measure of the time it takes for a clot to form in test plasma compared with that of normal plasma. Delays in clotting time are an indication of an abnormality in factors that act at early points in the coagulation pathway. The normal range for PTT is between 25 and 45 seconds from the time that a reagent or ionised calcium is added to the plasma.
platelet count	PLAYT-let kownt	A platelet count measures the number of platelets per litre of blood, with the average count ranging between 150 and 400 $\times 10^9$/L. The test is performed on all patients who develop petechiae, spontaneous bleeding or heavy menses and may be used to monitor progress of the diseases thrombocytopenia and bone marrow failure.
prothrombin time test	proh-THROM-bin tym	A prothrombin time test is used to measure the blood's ability to clot and is used for patients using certain anticoagulants. The test is conducted by adding calcium and thromboplastin to a blood sample and measuring how long it takes for a visible clot to appear. Another name for this test is the international normalised ratio (or INR).
red (blood) cell count	red (blud) sel kownt	A red (blood) cell count measures the number of erythrocytes in a specimen of whole blood. Normally there are approximately 4–6×10^{12}/L.
red (blood) cell morphology	red (blud) sel maw-FOL-o-jee	A red (blood) cell morphology test is performed to detect the presence of anisocytosis, poikilocytosis, sickle cells and hypochromia. The shape or form of individual red cells is examined on a stained blood smear.
splenectomy	splen-EK-toh-mee	A splenectomy is a surgical procedure to either partially or completely remove the spleen. It is removed when the spleen has become enlarged due to conditions such as lymphoma or leukaemia, due to trauma or spontaneous rupture and in long-term conditions such as porphyria and severe haemolytic anaemia where the spleen is destroying too many erythrocytes.
venepuncture	VEN-i-punk-cha	A venepuncture involves gaining access to a vein to extract blood, to administer a medication or to begin an intravenous infusion (Fig. 6.6). Access is gained through puncture of the vein.

Table continued

Test/procedure	Pronunciation	Definition
Figure 6.6 Venepuncture (Perry & Potter 2005) 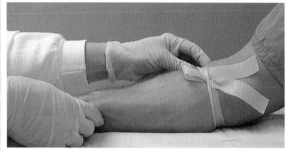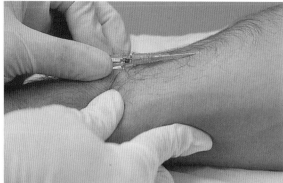		
white (blood) cell count	wyt (blud) sel kownt	A white (blood) cell count measures the number of leucocytes in a specimen of blood. Normally there are approximately $4.5–11 \times 10^9$/L.
white (blood) cell differential	wyt (blud) sel dif-er-ENT-shel	A white (blood) cell differential test is used to determine the count of the different types of leucocytes (both immature and mature forms) in blood. After cells are stained, a minimum of 100 cells are counted to determine the percentage of neutrophils, lymphocytes, monocytes, basophils and eosinophils. When there is an increase in the number of immature neutrophils and a decrease in the mature forms, the term left shift is used.

Exercises

EXERCISE 6.1: LABEL THE DIAGRAM

Using the information provided in this chapter, label the components in Fig. 6.7.

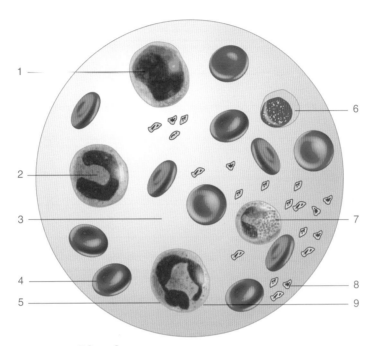

Figure 6.7 Blood smear
(Based on Hutton 2002)

1 _____   6 _____

2 _____   7 _____

3 _____   8 _____

4 _____   9 _____

5 _____

EXERCISE 6.2: WORD ELEMENT MEANINGS AND WORD BUILDING

Define the word elements below then use the element correctly in a medical term.

Word Element	Meaning	Medical Term
chrom/o		
erythr/o		
haem/o		

Word Element	Meaning	Medical Term
leuc/o		
mono-		
myel/o		
phag/o		
phleb/o		
pan-		
poly-		
-aemia		
-blast		
-penia		
-philia		
-rrhage		

EXERCISE 6.3: MATCH WORD ELEMENTS AND MEANINGS

Match the prefix, suffix or combining form in Column A with its meaning from Column B.

Column A	Answer	Column B
1. cyt/o		A. varied or irregular
2. -globin		B. stop or control
3. macro-		C. rupture
4. poikil/o		D. removal, carry away
5. -stasis		E. protein
6. -rrhexis		F. blood
7. -crit		G. small
8. micro-		H. nucleus
9. -apheresis		I. pertaining to formation, producing
10. -genesis		J. cell
11. sangu/i		K. large
12. kary/o		L. to separate

EXERCISE 6.4: VOCABULARY BUILDING

Using the definition as a guide, complete the medical term by writing the missing part in the space provided.

1. _____cyte   white blood cell

2. _____penia   a reduced number of erythrocytes

3. haemato_____   formation or production of blood

4. _____cyte   a cell that clots

5. spleno_____   enlargement of the spleen

6. _____penia   reduced number of neutrophils in the blood

EXERCISE 6.5: WORD ANALYSIS AND MEANING

Break up the medical terms below into their component parts (prefixes, suffixes, word roots, combining vowels). Provide the meaning for each term as a whole.

Example:

embolectomy

embol / ectomy

WR   S

Meaning: excision or surgical removal of an embolism

1. splenorrhexis

_____ / _____ / _____
    WR   CV   S

Meaning:

2. polycythaemia

_____ / _____ / _____ / _____
    P   WR   WR   S

Meaning:

3. erythroblastosis

_____ / _____ / _____ / _____
    WR   CV   WR   S

Meaning:

4. phlebotomy

_____ / _____
    WR   S

Meaning:

5. haemochromatosis

_____ / _____ / _____ / _____
    WR   CV   WR   S

Meaning:

6. leucopenia

_____ / _____ / _____
　　　　WR　　　　　　　　CV　　　　　　　　S

Meaning:

7. haemolysis

_____ / _____ / _____
　　　　WR　　　　　　　　CV　　　　　　　　S

Meaning:

8. anaemia

_____ / _____ / _____
　　　　P　　　　　　　　WR　　　　　　　　S

Meaning:

EXERCISE 6.6: VOCABULARY BUILDING

Provide the medical term for each of the definitions below.

1. Condition in which the sizes of erythrocytes are dissimilar: _____

2. A break in a blood vessel causing a bursting forth of blood: _____

3. A 'tumour', swelling or collection of blood: _____

4. A high level of calcium in the blood: _____

5. A high level of potassium in the blood: _____

6. The process by which cells in bone marrow develop: _____

7. An abnormal condition in which blood is more acidic than normal: _____

8. Stop or control blood: _____

9. The immature form of all blood cells: _____

10. Condition in which erythrocytes have irregular shapes: _____

EXERCISE 6.7: EXPAND THE ABBREVIATIONS AND MATCH WITH THE MEANING

Expand the abbreviations in Column A to form correct medical terms; match the medical term with its meaning from Column B.

Column A	Expanded Abbreviation	Match	Column B
1. AML			A. A blood test for coagulation defects
2. FBC			B. A disease due to autoimmune destruction of platelets resulting in thrombocytopenia
3. EBV			C. Protein iron compound in blood
4. RCC			D. Identification of the number of different types of blood cells in a litre of blood
5. PT			E. A condition where a recipient's tissues react against donor tissues, causing rejection
6. ITP			F. The virus that causes infectious mononucleosis
7. Hb			G. An antibody that protects against bacterial and viral conditions
8. ESR			H. A malignant condition of blood characterised by an abnormality in the number of monocytes or myeloid cells
9. GVH			I. A non-specific blood test that indicates the presence of inflammation
10. IgA			J. Identification of the number of erythrocytes in a litre of blood

EXERCISE 6.8: VOCABULARY BUILDING

Provide the medical term for each of the definitions below.

1. The clear straw-coloured part of blood is called _____.

2. The iron-containing pigment in erythrocytes is called _____.

3. The condition called _____ results from a lack of iron in erythrocytes.

4. _____ are formed in red bone marrow and are essential for the clotting process.

5. _____ is the process where leucocytes engulf and destroy microorganisms in the blood.

6. _____ measures the percentage of erythrocytes in a volume of blood.

7. Administration of whole blood or components of blood to replenish blood lost through surgery, trauma or disease is known as

_____.

8. Leucocytes that fight infection by phagocytosis are called _____.

9. An elevated _____ count may indicate a chronic infection.

10. A blood disorder in which erythrocytes are larger than normal and where there is a deficiency of vitamin B$_{12}$ is called

_____ anaemia.

EXERCISE 6.9: PRONUNCIATION AND COMPREHENSION

Read the following paragraphs aloud to practise your pronunciation. Using your textbook and a medical dictionary, find the meanings of the underlined medical terms.

Immune thrombocytopenic purpura (ITP) is a condition in which the body does not have enough platelets. ITP is an autoimmune disorder where a person's antibodies attack and destroy healthy platelets. The cause is unknown. Symptoms of ITP may include purpura, petechiae, prolonged bleeding time, epistaxis, haematuria and menorrhagia. Some people with mild ITP may be asymptomatic. Diagnosis of ITP is made by taking the patient's history and undertaking a physical examination. Patients will also have blood tests such as a full blood count and a blood smear.

Some patients will recover without any treatment. Other patients may require treatment to increase the number of platelets in their blood. This involves administering prednisone or an immunoglobulin, which is usually given intravenously. If patients do not respond to this treatment, a splenectomy may be required. Some people with ITP may have severe haemorrhaging and will require a platelet transfusion. If treatment regimens are followed, prognosis is usually good.

EXERCISE 6.10: ANAGRAMS

Work out each medical term from the jumbled letters below. Then, using the letters in brackets, determine the medical term that matches the description given.

1. ylytgoco	__ __ __ __ (__) __ __ __	the study of cells
2. dpaeinsireo	(__) __ __ __ __ __ __ __ __ __	deficiency of iron in the blood
3. tatellpe	__ __ (__) __ __ __ __ __	a clotting cell
4. hospalbi	__ __ __ __ (__) __ __ __	a type of white blood cell
5. dimleoy	(__) __ __ __ __ __ __	derived from bone marrow
6. raphnei	__ __ __ (__) __ __ __	an anticoagulant found in blood

Rearrange the letters in brackets to form a word that means 'the fluid part of blood in which cells are suspended'.

__ __ __   __ __ __ __ __

EXERCISE 6.11: CROSSWORD PUZZLE

Complete the puzzle by providing the medical term for each of the clues below.

ACROSS

4. White blood cell associated with allergic reactions (10)
5. A condition characterised by haemorrhage into the skin, mucous membranes and internal organs (7)
9. Deficiency of neutrophils (11)
10. Hereditary disease characterised by lack of factor VIII (11)
11. The pigment produced from haemoglobin (9)
12. Plasma without blood cells (5)

DOWN

1. The oxygen-carrying component of blood (11)
2. Separation of blood into its parts (9)
3. White blood cell (9)
6. A large white blood cell (8)
7. Infection in blood (11)
8. Excessive erythrocytes of unequal size (12)

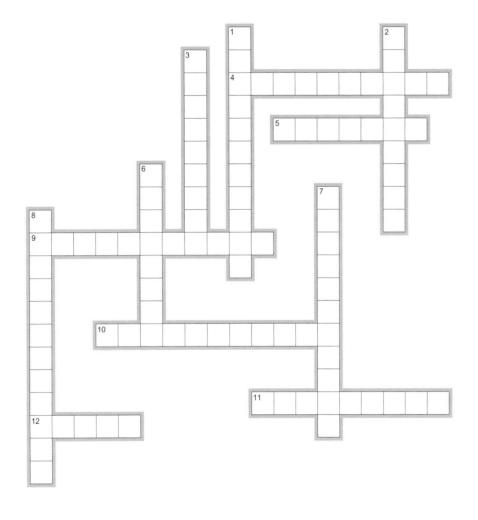

EXERCISE 6.12: APPLYING MEDICAL TERMINOLOGY

Answer the following questions.

1. Name the four blood groups. _____

_____

_____

2. What blood type is considered to be a universal donor, and which is the universal recipient? _____

_____

_____

3. If a patient has type AB⁺ blood, what blood should be given in a transfusion? _____

_____

_____

EXERCISE 6.13: MATCH THE ANAEMIA TYPE WITH THE DESCRIPTION

Match the type of anaemia in Column A with its description from Column B.

Column A	Answer	Column B
1. aplastic anaemia		A. anaemia caused by excessive blood loss
2. haemolytic anaemia		B. a type of haemolytic anaemia characterised by a difficulty in producing haemoglobin, commonly seen in persons of Mediterranean ancestry
3. post-haemorrhagic anaemia		C. an anaemia common in persons of African ancestry where red cells have a distinctive crescent shape
4. sickle cell anaemia		D. anaemia caused by failure of blood cell production in the bone marrow
5. thalassaemia		E. anaemia due to destruction of erythrocytes

EXERCISE 6.14: DISCHARGE SUMMARY ANALYSIS

Read the discharge summary below and answer the questions.

UNIVERSITY HOSPITAL DISCHARGE SUMMARY	**UR number:** 010203 **Name:** Kathy Swifte **Address:** 111 Creek Street, Summer Bay **Date of birth:** 11 January 1950 **Sex:** F **Nominated primary healthcare provider:** Dr Goodhew
Episode details **Consultant:** Dr Barney **Registrar:** Dr Scott **Unit:** Haematology **Admission source:** home **Date of admission:** 11/11/2020	**Discharge details** **Status:** Home **Date of discharge:** 15/11/2020

Reason for admission / Presenting problems:
A 69-year-old woman presenting to this hospital referred from GP with increasing tiredness/fatigue and anaemia due to lack of iron.

Principal diagnosis: Anaemia

Comorbidities:
Chronic anaemia (likely GI loss)
Multiple admissions in recent years for transfusions
Patient refuses further Ix e.g. colonoscopy
End-stage kidney disease
Renal biopsy showed burnt-out crescentic change
Patient refuses haemodialysis or renal transplant therapy
Congestive cardiac failure
Note echo result – normal LV size and function (EF 60%) MI December 2019
Raised cholesterol
COAD/asthma
Emphysema (most recent FV: 0.6)
Mild exertional dyspnoea
Ex-smoker
GORD
Osteoporosis
Rheumatoid arthritis

Previous medical history:
Previous admission 10/4/18 and 27/6/18 with anaemia
Previous admission 10/3/17 with diastolic dysfunction secondary to anaemia/LVH
Previous admission 25/02/16 with anaemia

Clinical synopsis:
Mrs Swifte is a well-known patient who was again admitted for transfusion of blood. She remains refractory to any further intervention, particularly dialysis or colonoscopic investigation, for her chronic blood loss. She responded well to a total transfusion of 4 units over 3 days and was discharged asymptomatic with a haemoglobin of 110. Mrs Swifte is currently in receipt of palliative care services for the ESKD and refuses to accept further treatment.

Complications: Nil reported

Clinical interventions: Blood transfusion

Diagnostic interventions:
On admission: Na 132, K 4.5, Urea 5.6, Creat 0.55
Hb: 21/10 – 73, 23/10 – 85, 25/10 – 81, 27/10 – 89, 29/10 – 110
Chest x-ray

Medications at discharge:

Ceased medications:

Allergies:

Alerts:

Arranged services: Palliative care service

Recommendations:
Mrs Swifte is now receiving assistance at home from several sources including home nursing and the palliative care service and should be able to manage at home with their help. She does not want to be admitted to a palliative care facility and would prefer to stay at home. To enable this, the palliative care team can arrange blood transfusions at home to prevent her from requiring frequent hospitalisations. She will continue to require close monitoring of her haemoglobin. Should the requirement arise, please contact the palliative care team to arrange for a transfusion.

| **Information to patient/relevant parties:** |
| Liaise with palliative care regarding future management; they are happy to arrange transfusions at home. |
| **Authorising clinician:** Dr Scott |
| **Document recipients:** |
| Patient and GP |

1. Expand the following abbreviations as found in the discharge summary above.

   GI

   GORD

   COAD

   LV

   Creat

   Hb

   Na

   Ix

   MI

   LVH

2. What was the diagnosis that brought Mrs Swifte to hospital? Why was her condition treated with a blood transfusion?

3. Why was a chest x-ray performed for Mrs Swifte?

4. It states under In-hospital management that Mrs Swifte 'remains refractory to further intervention'. What does this mean?

5. Mrs Swifte has had her sodium, urea and creatinine levels checked. Which of her comorbidities were being monitored?

CHAPTER 7

Lymphatic and Immune Systems

Contents

OBJECTIVES	135
INTRODUCTION	136
NEW WORD ELEMENTS	136
Combining forms	136
Prefixes	136
Suffixes	137
VOCABULARY	137
ABBREVIATIONS	137
FUNCTIONS AND STRUCTURE OF THE LYMPHATIC AND IMMUNE SYSTEMS	138
PATHOLOGY AND DISEASES	140
TESTS AND PROCEDURES	143
EXERCISES	144

Objectives

After completing this chapter you should be able to:

1. state the meanings of the word elements related to the lymphatic and immune systems

2. build words using the word elements associated with the lymphatic and immune systems

3. recognise, pronounce and effectively use medical terms associated with the lymphatic and immune systems

4. expand abbreviations related to the lymphatic and immune systems

5. describe the structure and functions of the lymphatic and immune systems, including lymph fluid, lymph nodes, lymph vessels and associated organs such as the tonsils, thymus and spleen

6. describe common pathological conditions associated with the lymphatic and immune systems

7. describe common laboratory tests and diagnostic and surgical procedures associated with the lymphatic and immune systems

8. apply what you have learned by interpreting medical terminology in practice.

Demonstrate your knowledge of the lymphatic and immune systems by completing the exercises at the end of this chapter.

INTRODUCTION

The immune system and lymphatic system are both important in the defence of the body against invasion by foreign microorganisms such as bacteria and viruses and for protection against disease. The lymphatic and immune systems include lymph fluid, lymph vessels, lymph ducts, lymph nodes, and associated organs such as the tonsils, thymus and spleen. The immune system is more a functional system rather than an anatomical system. The immune system includes cells known as lymphocytes, which are responsible for producing the immune response. Immunology includes the study of these cells and their specific functions. Both systems are closely linked to elements of the haematology system.

NEW WORD ELEMENTS

Here are some word elements related to the lymphatic and immune systems. To reinforce your learning, write the meanings of the medical terms in the spaces provided. Use the Glossary of medical terms on page 561 to help you work out the meanings. You may also need to check the meaning in a medical dictionary, but make an attempt yourself first.

Combining forms

Combining Form	Meaning	Medical Term	Meaning of Medical Term
aden/o	gland	lymphadenopathy	
adenoid/o	adenoids	adenoidectomy	
agglutin/o	clumping, gluing, sticking together	agglutinogen	
angi/o	vessel	angiogram	
axill/o	armpit	axillary	
cervic/o	neck, cervix uteri	cervical	
immun/o	protection	immunotherapy	
inguin/o	groin	inguinal	
lymph/o	lymphoid tissue, lymph gland	lymphangiography	
phag/o	swallow, eat	phagocytosis	
plas/o	formation	aplastic	
reticul/o	net-like	reticulocyte	
splen/o	spleen	splenomegaly	
thym/o	thymus gland	thymectomy	
tonsill/o	tonsils	tonsillitis	
tox/o	poison, toxin	cytotoxic	

Prefixes

Prefix	Meaning	Medical Term	Meaning of Medical Term
ana-	up, towards, apart	anaphylaxis	
anti-	against	antigen	
auto-	self	autoantigen	
inter-	between	intercellular	
mono-	one, single	mononucleosis	
retro-	backwards, behind	retropharyngeal	

Suffixes

Suffix	Meaning	Medical Term	Meaning of Medical Term
-ation	process, action, condition	agglutination	
-blast	embryonic, developing cell	lymphoblast	
-cyte	cell	phagocyte	
-genesis	pertaining to formation, producing	agenesis	
-genic		allergenic	
-globin	protein	haemoglobin	
-globulin		immunoglobulin	
-oid	derived from, resembling	lymphoid	
-pathy	disease process	lymphadenopathy	
-phylaxis	protection	anaphylaxis	
-poiesis	formation or production of	leucopoiesis	
-stitial	pertaining to standing/ positioned	interstitial fluid	

VOCABULARY

The following list provides many of the medical terms used for the first time in this chapter. Pronunciations are provided with each term. As you read the rest of the chapter, make sure you identify each of these terms and understand their meanings.

Term	Pronunciation
acquired immune deficiency syndrome (AIDS)	ak-wy-ed im-YOON de-FISH-en-see SIN-drohm
acquired immunity	ak-wy-ed im-YOON-i-tee
adenoids	AD-en-oydz
allergy	AL-er-jee
anaphylaxis	ana-fi-LAK-sis
autoimmune disease	or-toh-im-YOON diz-EEZ
bone marrow	bohn ma-roh
CT scan	see-tee skan
ELISA test	e-LYZ-a test
Hodgkin lymphoma	HOJ-kin lim-FOH-ma
immunoelectrophoresis	im-YOON-oh-e-LEK-troh-for-EE-sis
immunotherapy	im-YOON-oh-THER-a-pee
innate immunity	in-AYT im-YOON-i-tee
interstitial fluid	in-ter-STISH-al FLOO-id
lymph	limf
lymph node	limf nohd
lymph vessel	limf VESS-el

Table continued

Term	Pronunciation
lymphadenectomy	limf-ad-en-EK-tom-ee
lymphocyte	LIMF-oh-syt
lymphoedema	limf-oh-DEE-ma
lymphoma	limf-OH-ma
macrophage	MAK-roh-farj
non-Hodgkin lymphoma	non-HOJ-kin lim-FOH-ma
spleen	spleen
thymus gland	THY-mus gland
tonsillectomy	ton-sil-EK-tom-ee
tonsillitis	ton-sil-EYE-tis
tonsils	TON-silz

ABBREVIATIONS

The following abbreviations are commonly used in the Australian healthcare environment. Because some abbreviations can have more than one meaning, check the context in which the abbreviation is used before assigning a meaning to it.

Abbreviation	Definition
AIDS	acquired immunodeficiency syndrome
B-cells	a type of lymphocyte that produces antibodies, which forms and matures in bone marrow
CMV	cytomegalovirus

Table continued

Abbreviation	Definition
ELISA	enzyme-linked immunosorbent assay
HAART	highly active antiretroviral therapy
HIV	human immunodeficiency virus
HSV	herpes simplex virus
IgA, IgD, IgE, IgG, IgM	immunoglobulins
MOAB	monoclonal antibody
NHL	non-Hodgkin lymphoma
NK cells	natural killer cells
PCP	*Pneumocystis* pneumonia
SLE	systemic lupus erythematosus
T4, T8	T-cell lymphocytes
T-cells	lymphocytes, matured in thymus

FUNCTIONS AND STRUCTURE OF THE LYMPHATIC AND IMMUNE SYSTEMS

The lymphatic and immune systems work together with various other systems in the human body. The lymphatic system consists of a series of capillaries, vessels, ducts, nodes and organs that act to filter and remove infectious agents and foreign materials from the circulating clear fluid called lymph (Fig. 7.1). Lymph fluid originates as blood plasma. When blood is conveyed to the capillaries, some of it leaks out as interstitial or intercellular fluid. Interstitial fluid acts as the intermediary between the blood and the body cells, helping to deliver hormones, oxygen and nutrients and to remove waste products. The excess fluid moves into the lymphatic capillaries, then into the lymphatic vessels.

The main functions of the lymphatic and immune systems are to:
- remove excess fluid, waste, debris, dead blood cells, pathogens, cancer cells and toxins from body cells and the spaces in the tissues between the cells by transporting them to the bladder, bowel, lungs and skin for removal
- destroy pathogens and remove waste from the lymphatic fluid before it is returned to the circulatory system
- help the circulatory system to deliver nutrients, oxygen and hormones from the blood to the cells in the rest of the body
- maintain fluid levels in the body by draining excess fluid and preventing oedema caused by

Figure 7.1 Vessels and structures of the lymphatic system
(Mosby's Dictionary 2014)

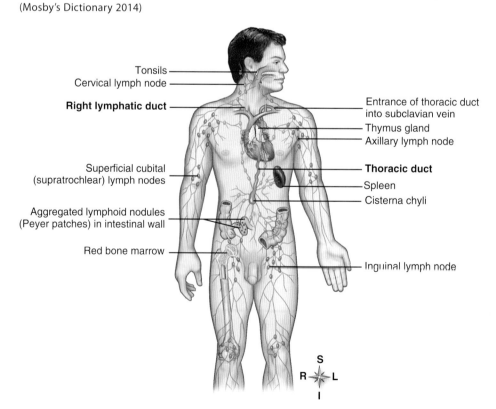

Tonsils
Cervical lymph node
Right lymphatic duct
Superficial cubital (supratrochlear) lymph nodes
Aggregated lymphoid nodules (Peyer patches) in intestinal wall
Red bone marrow

Entrance of thoracic duct into subclavian vein
Thymus gland
Axillary lymph node
Thoracic duct
Spleen
Cisterna chyli
Inguinal lymph node

excess fluid from the blood seeping into body tissues

- carry fats away from the digestive system.

The main organs of the lymphatic system are:

Lymph vessels: carry lymph throughout the body in a similar way to blood vessels carrying blood. Afferent vessels move lymphatic fluid towards lymph nodes and efferent vessels move the fluid away from the nodes. Lymph capillaries move the lymph around the lymphatic system in a one-way direction. Lymphatic ducts return the lymph to the bloodstream. Lymph from the upper right section of the body is drained by the right lymphatic duct (Fig. 7.2). The rest of the body is drained by the thoracic duct.

Lymph nodes: collections of tissue at points along the lymph vessels that contain macrophages and lymphocytes. These cells forage for pathogens, killing and removing bacteria and viruses. Swollen lymph nodes occur due to an increase in the number of cells in the nodes as they react to these infectious agents. Major locations for lymph nodes include the axilla (armpits), cervical region (neck) and inguinal region (groin) (Fig. 7.3).

Tonsils: accumulations of lymphatic tissue found on each side of the back of the throat. The tonsils act as the first line of defence in warding off infections in the gastrointestinal and respiratory tracts.

Adenoids: clumps of lymphoid tissue at the back of the nasopharyngeal region. Adenoids also trap infections and produce antibodies. They are most active in young children, beginning to atrophy by 4–5 years of age.

Spleen: a blood-filled organ that lies in the left upper quadrant of the abdomen lateral to the stomach. All blood cells pass through the spleen, which identifies those cells that are too old or abnormal and destroys them through the activity of its lymphocytes. White blood cells in the spleen act to trap pathogens. As a reservoir, the spleen is also able to supply blood when needed by the body, such as when a haemorrhage occurs.

Thymus: an organ located in the mediastinum (upper thoracic cavity behind the sternum). The role of the thymus is to produce hormones that act to develop immature lymphocytes from the bone marrow into T (for thymus) cells. T-cells tailor the body's immune response to various types of pathogens. B-cells, produced by the bone marrow, also have a role in producing antibodies to fight disease. The thymus is most active in childhood when immunity is developing.

The human body is vulnerable to a variety of infections and toxins. It is the immune system that acts to protect the body against these foreign invaders through innate and acquired immunity. Innate or natural immunity is the body's first line of defence against

Figure 7.2 **Lymphatic drainage**
(Mosby's Dictionary 2014)

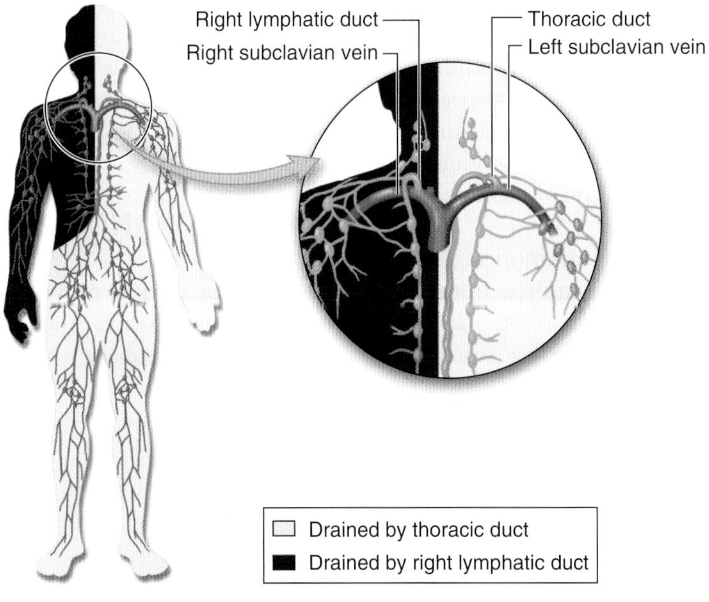

Right lymphatic duct
Right subclavian vein
Thoracic duct
Left subclavian vein

☐ Drained by thoracic duct
■ Drained by right lymphatic duct

Figure 7.3 Lymph node

(Applegate 2011)

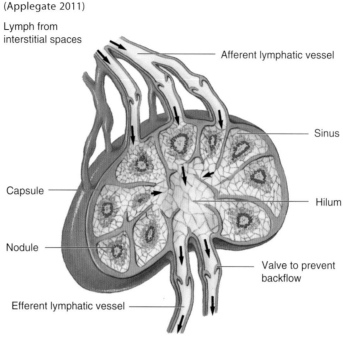

Lymph from interstitial spaces

Afferent lymphatic vessel

Sinus

Capsule

Hilum

Nodule

Valve to prevent backflow

Efferent lymphatic vessel

To subclavian veins

infection and to some cancers, providing a broad, non-specific response that is present from birth and is always ready to be deployed. Active lymphocytes that are part of the innate immune system are called natural killer (NK) cells. The innate immune system does not react specifically to different types of infection but provides a physical barrier – skin, mucous membranes, stomach acid, saliva and tears. It also produces phagocytes that ingest invading microorganisms.

Acquired or adaptive immunity, on the other hand, needs to be sensitised to particular types of infection before its action is triggered and the body produces antibodies in response. By recognising the particular antigen on the surface of a pathogen, the acquired immune system can act against it and produce a maximally effective response. The action of vaccinations also represents acquired immunity.

B-cells and T-cells are the most common types of lymphocytes and have roles in the acquired immune response. Both are produced in the bone marrow and then move into the bloodstream or are stored in the lymph nodes. B-cells are formed as stem cells in the bone marrow and travel through the lymphatic system to lymph nodes. B-cells produce antibodies or immunoglobulins that are set in operation on contact with antigens. They produce antibodies that bind to the invading antigens, producing an infective response. The B-cells retain a 'memory' of the invading pathogen, producing future immunity to the specific type of infection. T-cells are a form of white blood cells that are also produced by the bone marrow but move to the thymus for maturation. T-cells also act in response to specific antigens by stimulating inflammation and also encouraging the production of phagocytes that devour or dissolve the infective agent.

PATHOLOGY AND DISEASES

The following section provides a list of some of the most common diseases and pathological conditions relevant to the lymphatic and immune systems.

Term	Pronunciation	Definition
allergy	AL-er-jee	An allergy is an exaggerated reaction by the immune system in response to contact with certain foreign substances called antigens. Usually these antigens are seen by the body as harmless and no response occurs in non-allergic people. However, susceptible people can have a reaction such as rhinitis, pruritus, urticaria, oedema or asthma. Substances that can trigger an allergy include pollens, dust mites, mould spores, animal dander, some foods, drugs and insect bites. Most allergic reactions are relatively minor and are treated with antihistamines. However, in some cases, an allergic reaction can be life threatening. This is called anaphylaxis.
anaphylaxis	ana-fi-LAK-sis	Anaphylaxis (also called anaphylactic shock) is a severe, life-threatening, generalised allergic reaction that requires immediate medical treatment. It occurs after exposure to an allergen to which the patient is already sensitive. This stimulates a severe immune response and release of histamine. The most common triggers are certain foods (peanuts, eggs, crustaceans), insect venom (e.g. bee or wasp stings) and certain medications. Usually the reaction occurs within 20 minutes of exposure. The reaction will often have a multisystem focus: welts or hives; swelling of the lips, tongue and throat; dyspnoea; tachycardia; loss of consciousness; and potentially death. Treatment is by injection with adrenaline, which can be given via an anaphylaxis autoinjector. While treatment is usually successful if given in time, preventing the reaction is preferable. Therefore, triggers need to be identified and avoided.
autoimmune disease	ort-oh-im-YOON diz-EEZ	Autoimmune diseases occur when the body does not recognise its own tissues and the immune system turns against itself causing the body to produce auto-antibodies that attack and destroy its own tissues. In patients with an autoimmune disease, the immune system cannot distinguish between healthy body tissue and antigens. The associated immune response destroys normal body tissues. There are more than 80 autoimmune diseases. Some of the more common ones are multiple sclerosis, rheumatoid arthritis, systemic lupus erythematosus, Hashimoto's thyroiditis and type 1 diabetes mellitus.
human immunodeficiency virus (HIV) and acquired immune deficiency syndrome (AIDS)	hyoo-man imm-YOO-no-de-FISH-en-see vy-rus; ak-wy-ed im-YOON de-FISH-en-see SIN-drohm	HIV is a virus that is transmitted from person to person through the exchange of body fluids such as blood, semen, breast milk and vaginal secretions. The virus is generally spread through participating in high-risk activities. Unprotected sexual contact is the most common way to spread HIV, but it can also be transmitted by sharing needles when injecting drugs, or during childbirth and breastfeeding. It cannot be spread by casual contact with an infected person. AIDS is a disease of the immune system that results from an infection with HIV. HIV destroys the immune cells called CD4 T-lymphocytes. These lymphocytes are part of the body's defence system that protects against infectious diseases. As HIV progressively destroys these cells, the body becomes increasingly vulnerable to infections. Because there is no cure for the disease, once people are HIV positive, they remain that way for the rest of their lives. In some patients the HIV infection can damage the immune system enough for AIDS to develop. AIDS is a condition that describes an advanced state of HIV infection. It can be diagnosed either when the number of CD4 cells in the blood of an HIV-positive person drops below a certain level or when they have developed an AIDS-related condition or symptom, such as an opportunistic infection, or an AIDS-related cancer or other disease. These illnesses and infections are said to be AIDS defining because they mark the onset of AIDS.

Table continued

Term	Pronunciation	Definition
		AIDS-defining conditions
		There are numerous conditions that are referred to as AIDS-defining conditions when they occur in the presence of HIV. Some of the more common ones include:
		• AIDS-related dementia
		• AIDS wasting syndrome
		• candidiasis
		• cytomegalovirus
		• encephalitis
		• Kaposi's sarcoma
		• lymphoma
		• meningitis
		• *Pneumocystis jiroveci* (formerly known as *Pneumocystis carinii*) pneumonia
		• toxoplasmosis
		• tuberculosis.
		Treatment
		There is no cure for HIV/AIDS, but the progress of the disease can be slowed by taking antiretroviral drugs, which can prolong the time between HIV infection and the onset of AIDS. Modern drug therapy is highly effective, and someone with HIV who is taking treatment could live for the rest of their life without developing AIDS.
lymphoedema	lim-foh-DEE-ma	One of the functions of the lymphatic system is to remove excess fluid from body tissues after an injury of some sort. If this does not occur, a swelling (oedema) of the affected area will result because of the retention of lymphatic fluid (Fig. 7.4). Usually this is only temporary. However, if there is blockage of, or damage to, the lymphatic system and the oedema lasts for more than approximately 3 months, chronic lymphoedema is said to be present in the soft tissues. It can occur anywhere but most commonly occurs in the arms and legs. It may be primary (due to an inefficient lymphatic system) or secondary (as a result of damage to lymphatic vessels after surgery or injury).

Figure 7.4 Lymphoedema

Chronic acquired lymphoedema of the lower extremities. Note severe skin changes **A.** and swelling of the foot **B.** associated with squaring of the toes (Stemmer's sign) and typical peau d'orange **C.** severe lymphoedema with subcutaneous lymph cysts and chronic verrucous superinfection.

(Cronenwett & Johnston 2010)

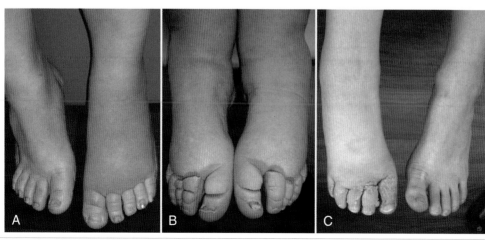

Table continued

Term	Pronunciation	Definition
lymphoma	lim-FOH-ma	Lymphoma is a type of malignancy involving either B- or T-lymphocytes. Lymphomas originate in lymph glands or other lymphoid tissue. Sometimes they can form in tissue other than lymph nodes such as in the brain, bone and colon. These are called extranodal lymphomas. There are many different forms of lymphoma. Two of the most common are Hodgkin lymphoma and non-Hodgkin lymphoma.
		Treatment options will vary depending on the type of lymphoma. In some cases multiple treatment modalities may be required. Options include 'watchful waiting', chemotherapy, radiation therapy, stem cell/bone marrow transplantation or immunotherapy.
- Hodgkin lymphoma	HOJ-kin lim-FOH-ma	Hodgkin lymphoma is a type of lymphoma characterised by lymphadenopathy, splenomegaly and enlargement of other lymphoid tissue. It involves abnormal B-lymphocytes that become damaged and grow and multiply uncontrollably, which causes enlarged lymph nodes. When examined under a microscope, the cells have a specific appearance that is characteristic of Hodgkin lymphoma. These are called Reed-Sternberg cells. Lymphoma cells that do not have that appearance are classified as non-Hodgkin lymphoma.
- non-Hodgkin lymphoma (NHL)	non-HOJ-kin lim-FOH-ma	NHL is sometimes called B-cell lymphoma or T-cell lymphoma, depending on the type of cells affected. NHL is much more common than Hodgkin lymphoma. It presents with similar signs and symptoms and can only be distinguished by microscopic examination of the tumour. The differentiation between Hodgkin lymphoma and non-Hodgkin lymphoma depends on the type of cancer cell. Reed-Sternberg cells are not found in non-Hodgkin lymphoma.

TESTS AND PROCEDURES

The following section provides a list of common diagnostic tests and procedures and clinical interventions and surgical procedures that are undertaken for the lymphatic and immune system.

Test/Procedure	Pronunciation	Definition
CT scan	see-tee skan	A computed tomography or CT scan is a diagnostic test to identify disorders of organs such as lymph nodes, spleen and thymus gland. Images are taken in the transverse plane using a computer in conjunction with x-ray beams.
ELISA test	e-LYZ-a test	The enzyme-linked immunosorbent assay (ELISA) test is used to detect immune responses in the body. The test detects substances such as hormones, antigens and antibodies and is used to identify antibodies to HIV antigens that are of a specific molecular weight.
immunoelectrophoresis	im-YOON-oh-ee-LEK-troh-for-EE-sis	Immunoelectrophoresis is a test that involves separating and identifying proteins in the blood and their reaction to antibodies. For patients with conditions such as multiple myeloma and Waldenstrom's macroglobulinaemia, the test is used to detect an abnormal level of antibodies.
immunotherapy	im-YOON-oh-THER-a-pee	Immunotherapy involves using knowledge of the body's immune response and immune technologies to treat or prevent diseases such as cancer, allergies and transplanted organ rejection. Examples include:
		• Controlled administration of small doses of allergens to desensitise a patient with allergies;
		• Administration of vaccines that train the patient's immune system to recognise tumour cells;
		• Administration of therapeutic antibodies that stimulate the patient's immune system to destroy tumour cells.
lymphadenectomy	limf-ad-en-EK-tom-ee	A lymphadenectomy is a surgical procedure to remove one or more lymph nodes. It is generally performed with other surgical procedures used in managing cancer.

Exercises

EXERCISE 7.1: LABEL THE DIAGRAM

Using the information provided in this chapter, label the anatomical parts in Fig. 7.5.

1 _____

2 _____

3 _____

4 _____

5 _____

6 _____

7 _____

8 _____

9 _____

10 _____

11 _____

12 _____

13 _____

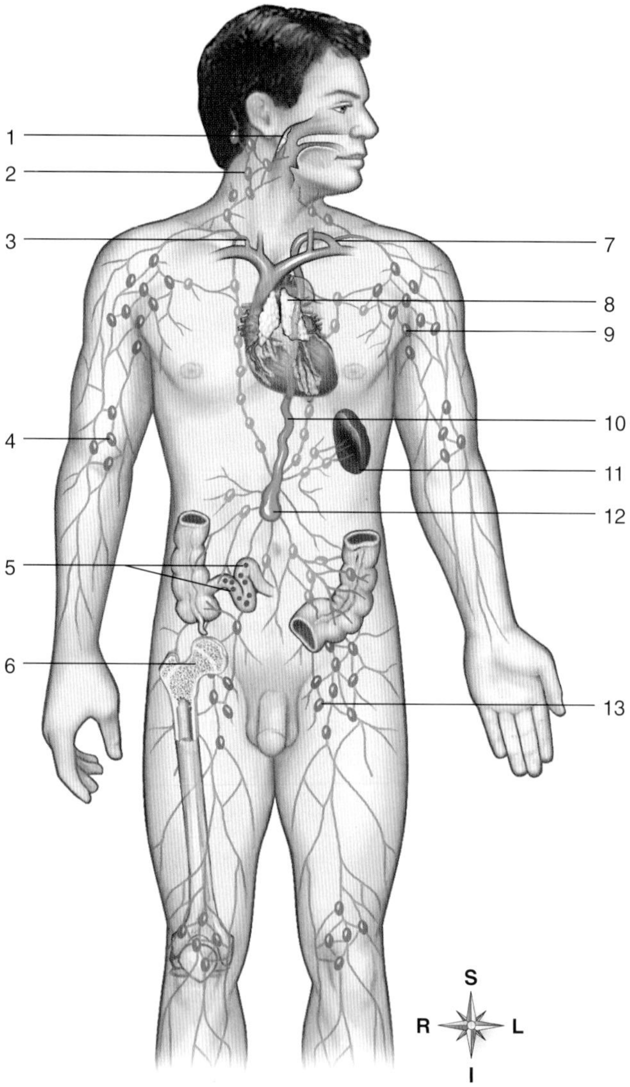

Figure 7.5 Vessels and structures of the lymphatic system

(Mosby's Dictionary 2014)

EXERCISE 7.2: WORD ELEMENT MEANINGS AND WORD BUILDING

Define the following word elements, then use each element correctly in a medical term.

Word Element	Meaning	Medical Term
aden/o		
agglutin/o		
angi/o		
axill/o		
inguin/o		
phag/o		
plas/o		
tox/o		
ana-		
mono-		
-blast		
-genic		
-oid		
-pathy		
-phylaxis		

EXERCISE 7.3: MATCH WORD ELEMENTS AND MEANINGS

Match the prefix, suffix or combining forms in Column A with its meaning from Column B.

Column A	Answer	Column B
1. -poiesis		A. thymus gland
2. anti-		B. cell
3. auto-		C. backwards, behind
4. -stitial		D. formation or production of
5. cervic/o		E. between
6. -cyte		F. protection
7. inter-		G. protein
8. reticul/o		H. self
9. thym/o		I. pertaining to standing/positioned
10. retro-		J. against
11. -globin		K. neck, cervix uteri
12. immun/o		L. not like

EXERCISE 7.4: WORD ANALYSIS AND MEANING

Break up the medical terms below into their component parts (prefixes, suffixes, word roots, combining vowels). Provide the meaning for each term as a whole.

Example:
adenoidectomy
adenoid / ectomy
WR   S

Meaning: surgical removal of the adenoids

1. immunotherapy

_____ / _____ / _____

Meaning:

2. phagocytosis

_____ / _____ / _____ / _____

Meaning:

3. cytotoxic

_____ / _____ / _____ / _____

Meaning:

4. lymphangiography

_____ / _____ / _____ / _____

Meaning:

5. axillary

_____ / _____

Meaning:

6. intercellular

_____ / _____ / _____

Meaning:

7. lymphoid

_____ / _____

Meaning:

8. lymphadenopathy

_____ / _____ / _____ / _____

Meaning:

9. leucopoiesis

_____ / _____ / _____

Meaning:

10. retropharyngeal

_____ / _____ / _____

Meaning:

EXERCISE 7.5: CIRCLE THE CORRECT SPELLING

Circle the correctly spelled medical term from the options provided.

aksillary	axillary	axilary	axsillary
retikulocyte	rheticulocyte	reticulosite	reticulocyte
thymeectomy	thimectomy	thymectomy	thimeectomy
monnonucleosis	mononucleosis	mononoocleosis	mononuclosis
agglutination	aglutination	aggluttination	agglootination
piogenic	pyogenic	pyoginec	phyogenic
immunoglobbulin	imunoglobulin	immunoglobullin	immunoglobulin
intastitial	interstishial	intestitial	interstitial

EXERCISE 7.6: EXPAND THE ABBREVIATIONS

Expand the abbreviations to form correct medical terms.

Abbreviation	Expanded Abbreviation
AIDS	
B-cells	
CMV	
ELISA	
HAART	
HIV	
IgA	
MOAB	
NHL	
NK cells	
PCP	
SLE	
T4, T8	
T-cells	

EXERCISE 7.7: MATCH STRUCTURE WITH FUNCTION

Match the structure in Column A with its function from Column B.

Column A	Answer	Column B
1. macrophages		A. produces a hormone that aids development of immature lymphocytes
2. lymph vessels		B. traps infections and are located at the back of the nasopharyngeal region
3. adenoids		C. carries lymph throughout the body
4. lymph		D. all blood cells pass through this organ
5. thymus gland		E. delivers hormones, oxygen and nutrients to cells
6. spleen		F. fluid originating as blood plasma
7. lymph nodes		G. cells that help remove bacteria
8. interstitial fluid		H. collection of tissue at points along lymph vessels

EXERCISE 7.8: CROSSWORD PUZZLE

Complete the puzzle by providing the medical term for each of the clues below.

ACROSS

5. Cells of the immune system that are called big eaters (11)

6. Act as the first line of defence against infections (7)

9. Delivers hormones, oxygen and nutrients to cells throughout the body and picks up waste products for removal (12, 5)

10. Lymphoid tissue at the back of the nasopharyngeal region that traps infections and produces antibodies (8)

DOWN

1. Cells of the immune system that destroy old and abnormal blood cells in the spleen (11)

2. Produces hormones that aid the development of immature lymphocytes into T-cells (6, 5)

3. A severe generalised allergic reaction (11)

4. A test used to detect immune responses in the body (5, 4)

7. An organ through which all blood cells pass with identification of old cells for destruction by lymphocytes (6)

8. Acquired immune deficiency syndrome (4)

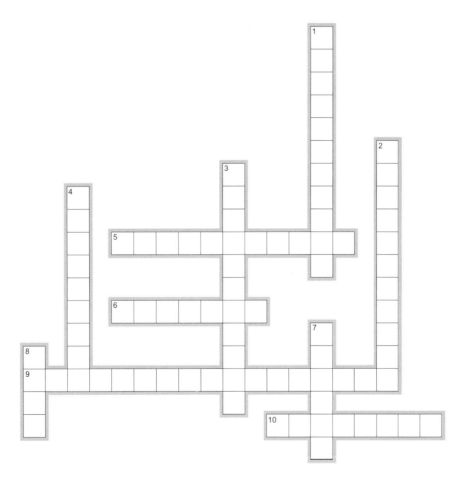

EXERCISE 7.9: ANAGRAMS

Work out each medical term from the jumbled letters below. Then, using the letters in brackets, determine the medical term that matches the description given.

1. nepsle	( )	the largest of the lymphoid organs that stores erythrocytes
2. xtsnio	__ __ __ __ (__) __	another name for poisons
3. gyrlela	__ __ __ (__) __ __ __	a hypersensitivity reaction to a substance
4. selclt	(__) __ __ __ __ __	lymphocytes formed in the thymus gland
5. neddsioa	(__) __ __ __ __ __ __ __	lymphatic tissue located in the nasopharynx
6. galiinnu	(__) __ __ __ __ __ __ __	pertaining to the groin region
7. ndgla	(__) __ __ __ __	the combining form for this structure is aden/o

Rearrange the letters in brackets to form a word that means 'a substance that the body recognises as foreign and results in an immune response'.

— — — — — —

EXERCISE 7.10: DISCHARGE SUMMARY ANALYSIS

Read the discharge summary below and answer the questions.

UNIVERSITY HOSPITAL DISCHARGE SUMMARY	**UR number:** 111213 **Name:** John Jackson **Address:** 3/14 Crisp Terrace, Smithfield **Date of birth:** 9/4/1984 **Sex:** M **Nominated primary healthcare provider:** Dr Peter Williams
Episode details **Consultant:** Dr Jones **Registrar:** Dr Harrison **Unit:** Medical **Admission source:** Emergency department **Date of admission:** 17/9/2020	**Discharge details** **Status:** Home **Date of discharge:** 24/9/2020
Reason for admission / Presenting problems: History of diarrhoea and dehydration	
Principal diagnosis: Superficial gastritis and CMV colitis	
Comorbidities: Late-stage AIDS Oral candidiasis	
Previous medical history: HIV positive dx 12/16	

Clinical synopsis:

This 36-year-old man who is HIV positive was admitted with a 12/7 history of diarrhoea and dehydration.

During his admission, the patient underwent a gastroscopy and colonoscopy under IV sedation (ASA = 3NE). Biopsies taken revealed superficial gastritis and CMV colitis.

The patient is currently being treated with itraconazole for his oral candidiasis.

He was started on a course of ganciclovir for his CMV colitis and discharged home to be reviewed in OPD in 2 weeks' time.

Complications:

Clinical interventions:

Gastroscopy and colonoscopy with biopsy

Diagnostic interventions:

Medications at discharge:

Ganciclovir

Itraconazole

Ceased medications:

Nil reported

Allergies: Nil reported

Alerts: Nil reported

Arranged services: Nil reported

Recommendations:

Outpatient review 2 weeks post discharge

Information to patient/relevant parties:

Outpatient review 2 weeks post discharge

Authorising clinician: Dr Harrison

Document recipients

Patient and LMO: Dr Peter Williams

1. **Expand the following abbreviations as found in the discharge summary above.**

   AIDS

   CMV

   HIV

   IV

   OPD

2. **Is a gastroscopy undertaken from the same entry point as a colonoscopy?**

3. **Provide a brief explanation of CMV.**

4. **Are any of the conditions listed on this summary considered AIDS-defining conditions? If so, list them.**

5. **What is meant by ASA = 3NE when the patient is under IV sedation?**

CHAPTER 8
Endocrine System

Contents

OBJECTIVES 153
INTRODUCTION 154
NEW WORD ELEMENTS 154
    Combining forms 154
    Prefixes 155
    Suffixes 155
VOCABULARY 156
ABBREVIATIONS 156
FUNCTIONS AND STRUCTURE OF
THE ENDOCRINE SYSTEM 157
    Pituitary gland 158
    Thyroid gland 159
    Parathyroid glands 159
    Adrenal glands 159
    Pancreas 159
    Gonads 159
    Pineal gland 160
    Thymus gland 160
PATHOLOGY AND DISEASES 161
    Pituitary gland 161
    Thyroid gland 163
    Parathyroid glands 166
    Pancreas 166
    Adrenal glands 168
TESTS AND PROCEDURES 169
EXERCISES 170

Objectives

After completing this chapter you should be able to:

1. state the meanings of the word elements related to the endocrine system

2. build words using the word elements associated with the endocrine system

3. recognise, pronounce and effectively use medical terms associated with the endocrine system

4. expand abbreviations related to the endocrine system

5. describe the structure and functions of the endocrine system including the glands, hormones, target organs and effects

6. describe common pathological conditions associated with the endocrine system

7. describe common laboratory tests and diagnostic and surgical procedures associated with the endocrine system

8. apply what you have learned by interpreting medical terminology in practice.

Demonstrate your knowledge of the endocrine system by completing the exercises at the end of this chapter.

INTRODUCTION

The endocrine system is one of the most important and complex systems in the body. It controls and integrates several body functions such as growth, reproduction and cellular metabolism by stimulating and regulating the release of hormones from various glands. The hormones are carried by the bloodstream to target organs for specific action. Hormones are generally secreted continuously but at varying levels depending on the body's requirements. A deficiency or excess of levels of any of the hormones will cause an abnormal effect (or pathological condition) in other glands or body systems. The endocrine system has very close links with the nervous system.

NEW WORD ELEMENTS

Here are some word elements related to the endocrine system. To reinforce your learning, write the meanings of the medical terms in the spaces provided. Use the Glossary of medical terms on page 561 to help you work out the meanings. You may also need to check the meaning in a medical dictionary, but make an attempt yourself first.

Combining forms

Combining Form	Meaning	Medical Term	Meaning of Medical Term
aden/o	gland	adenoma	
adren/o	adrenal glands	adrenocortical	
adrenal/o		adrenalectomy	
andr/o	male	androgynous	
calc/i	calcium	hypocalcaemia	
chrom/o	colour	chromatic	
cortic/o	cortex, outer layer of organ	corticoid	
crin/o	secrete	endocrinology	
dem/o	people	endemic	
dips/o	thirst	polydipsia	
gluc/o	glucose, sugar, sweet(ness)	glucogen	
glyc/o		glycaemic	
glycos/o		glycosuria	
gonad/o	gonads, sex glands (ovaries and testes)	gonadoblastoma	
home/o	same, alike	homeostasis	
hormon/o	hormone	hormonal	
insulin/o	insulin	insulinogenic	
iod/o	iodine	iodism	
kal/i	potassium	kaliuresis	
ket/o	ketone bodies	ketogenesis	
keton/o		ketonuria	
lact/o	milk	lactose	
myx/o	mucus	myxopoiesis	
natr/o	sodium	natraemia	
oestr/o	oestrogen, female hormone	oestrogen	
oophor/o	ovary	oophorogenous	
ovar/i		ovarian	
ovari/o		ovariocentesis	

Table continued

Combining Form	Meaning	Medical Term	Meaning of Medical Term
orchi/o orchid/o	testis, testicle	orchitis orchidopexy	
pancreat/o	pancreas	pancreatectomy	
parathyro/o parathyroid/o	parathyroid gland	parathyrotrophic parathyroidectomy	
phae/o	dusky, dark	phaeochromocytoma	
pituitar/o	pituitary gland	hyperpituitarism	
somat/o	body	somatomegaly	
test/o testicul/o	testis, testicle	testosterone testicular	
thym/o	thymus gland	thymoma	
thyr/o thyroid/o	a shield, thyroid gland	thyrogenic hyperthyroidism	
toc/o	childbirth, labour	oxytocin	
tox/o toxic/o	poison, toxin	toxic thyrotoxicosis	
ur/o	urine, urinary tract, urea	diuretic	

Prefixes

Prefix	Meaning	Medical Term	Meaning of Medical Term
acro-	extremities	acromegaly	
endo-	within, inside, inner	endocrinology	
eu-	good, normal	euthyroid	
exo-	outward, outside	exocrine	
oxy-	quick, sharp	oxytocic	
pan-	all, entire	panhypopituitarism	
para-	beside, near, alongside	parathyroid	
tri-	three	triiodothyronine	

Suffixes

Suffix	Meaning	Medical Term	Meaning of Medical Term
-aemia	condition of blood	hypercalcaemia	
-agon	assemble, gather together	glucagon	
-crine	secrete	endocrine	
-in, -ine	made of, having the nature of, relating to	adrenaline	
-megaly	enlargement	pancreatomegaly	
-physis	growth	hypophysis	
-trophin	stimulating the effect of (a hormone)	somatotrophin	
-uria	urination, urine condition, presence of substance in urine	polyuria	

VOCABULARY

The following list provides many of the medical terms used for the first time in this chapter. Pronunciations are provided with each term. As you read the rest of the chapter, make sure you identify each of these terms and understand their meanings.

Term	Pronunciation
acromegaly	ak-roh-MEG-a-lee
Addison's disease	AD-i-sens dis-EEZ
adenomatous goitre	ad-en-O-mat-us GOY-tah
adrenal virilism	ad-REEN-al VI-ril-iz-em
adrenocorticotrophic hormone	ad-REE-noh-KAW-ti-koh-TROH-fik HAW-mohn
amine	am-een
antidiuretic hormone	an-tee-dy-yu-RET-ik HAW-mohn
catecholamines	kat-e-KOL-a-meenz
congenital hypothyroidism	kon-JEN-i-tal hy-po-THY-royd-iz-em
Cushing's syndrome	KOOSH-ings SIN-drohm
diabetes insipidus	dy-a-BEET-eez in-SIP-id-us
diabetes mellitus	dy-a-BEET-eez mel-EYE-tus
dwarfism	DWAW-fiz-em
endemic goitre	en-DEM-ik GOY-tah
endocrine	EN-doh-cryn
exocrine	EX-oh-cryn
follicle-stimulating hormone	FOL-i-kel STIM-yoo-lay-ting HAW-mohn
gigantism	jy-GAN-tiz-em
glucagon	GLOO-ka-gon
goitre	GOY-tah
gonads	GOH-nadz
Graves' disease	GRAYVs dis-EEZ
growth hormone	grohth HAW-mohn
Hashimoto's thyroiditis	hash-ee-MOHT-ose thy-royd-EYE-tis
hormone	HAW-mohn
hypercalcaemia	hy-PER-kal-SEE-mee-a
hyperinsulinism	hy-per-IN-syoo-lin-iz-em
hypocalcaemia	hy-POH-kal-SEE-mee-a
hypothalamus	hy-poh-THAL-a-mus
insulin	IN-syoo-lin
islets of Langerhans	eye-letz of LANG-er-hanz
luteinising hormone	LOO-tin-EYE-zing HAW-mohn
melatonin	mel-a-TOH-nin
myxoedema	mix-e-DEE-mah

Table continued

Term	Pronunciation
oestrogen	EE-stroh-jen
ovaries	OH-vah-reez
oxytocin	ok-see-TOH-sin
pancreas	PAN-kree-as
panhypopituitarism	pan-hy-poh-pit-YOO-i-tah-riz-em
parathyroid gland	pa-ra-THY-royd gland
parathyroid hormone	pa-ra-THY-royd HAW-mohn
peptide	PEP-tyd
phaeochromocytoma	FEE-o-KROH-moh-sy-TOH-ma
pineal gland	PIN-ee-el gland
pituitary gland	pit-YOO-i-tah-ree gland
progesterone	proh-JES-te-rohn
prolactin	proh-LAK-tin
steroid	STE-royd
syndrome of inappropriate ADH	sin-drohm of in-a-PROH-pree-at ay-dee-aych
testes	TES-teez
testosterone	tes-TOS-ter-ohn
thyroid gland	THY-royd gland
thyroid-stimulating hormone	THY-royd STIM-yoo-lay-ting HAW-mohn
thyroxine (T$_4$)	thy-ROK-sin
triiodothyronine (T$_3$)	try-EYE-oh-doh-THY-ron-een

ABBREVIATIONS

The following abbreviations are commonly used in the Australian healthcare environment. Because some abbreviations can have more than one meaning, check the context in which the abbreviation is used before assigning a meaning to it.

Abbreviation	Definition
ACTH	adrenocorticotrophic hormone
ADH	antidiuretic hormone
DI	diabetes insipidus
DM	diabetes mellitus
FBG	fasting blood glucose
FBS	fasting blood sugar
FSH	follicle-stimulating hormone
GH	growth hormone
GTT	glucose tolerance test
hCG	human chorionic gonadotrophin

Abbreviation	Definition
IDDM	insulin-dependent diabetes mellitus
LH	luteinising hormone
MSH	melanocyte-stimulating hormone
NIDDM	non-insulin-dependent diabetes mellitus
RAIU	radioactive iodine uptake test
SIADH	syndrome of inappropriate antidiuretic hormone
T1DM	type 1 diabetes mellitus
T2DM	type 2 diabetes mellitus
TFTs	thyroid function tests
TRH	thyrotrophin-releasing hormone
TSH	thyroid-stimulating hormone

FUNCTIONS AND STRUCTURE OF THE ENDOCRINE SYSTEM

The endocrine system consists of a series of glands that secrete hormones and act to regulate the functioning of body cells and activities (Fig. 8.1). The endocrine system affects body metabolism, growth, mood, tissue function and reproductive processes. The action of hormones is generally slow and occurs over time, unlike the actions of the nervous system, which create an immediate response to environmental factors.

Hormones are chemical messengers that transfer information and instructions from one set of body cells to another to stimulate a response. Hormones are specific in their actions. Although there are many different hormones circulating in the body through the bloodstream, each has only one specific action and has

Figure 8.1 Endocrine glands

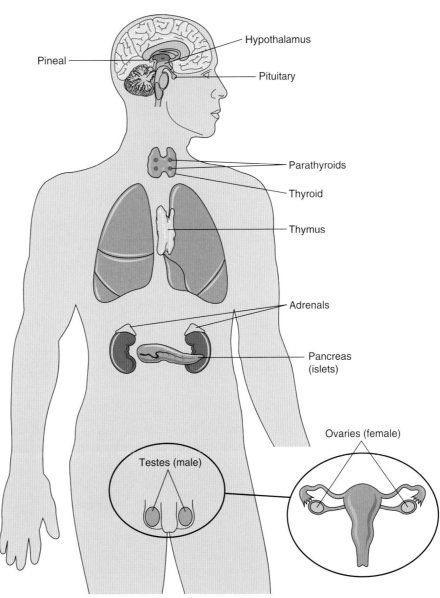

to be recognised by the receptors in its intended target. There are three types of hormones: amines, steroids and peptides. Amines are neurotransmitters that include adrenaline, which mobilises the body for activity. Steroids mainly operate to stimulate sexual maturation and fertility and are produced in the placenta in the prenatal period or by the gonads (testes and ovaries) after birth. Peptides or protein hormones regulate other body activities such as growth, production of energy and other metabolic processes to keep the body in homeostasis.

The glands that make up this body system are classified as endocrine or exocrine. The endocrine glands release their hormones directly into the bloodstream. Examples of endocrine glands include the pituitary gland, ovaries, testes, pancreas, thyroid and adrenal glands. Exocrine glands differ from endocrine glands in that they release hormones into ducts that lead to an internal or external epithelial surface. There are more exocrine glands in the body than endocrine glands. Examples of exocrine glands are the sweat, sebaceous and mammary glands and those glands in the gastrointestinal system that secrete hormones that aid digestion.

Pituitary gland

The pituitary gland, also called the hypophysis, is located at the base of the brain. It is often considered the body's master controller because it produces hormones that in turn control other endocrine glands (Fig. 8.2). The pituitary gland has two lobes: the anterior pituitary or adenohypophysis and the posterior pituitary or neurohypophysis, which is actually an extension of the hypothalamus. The hypothalamus is located between the pituitary gland and the thalamus. It acts to determine the amount of circulating hormones in the body. If it identifies either an increase or decrease in hormone levels, the hypothalamus relays information to the pituitary gland that, in turn, produces hormones and sends them to the appropriate receptors, instructing them to either increase or decrease tissue activities.

The hormones secreted by the anterior lobe of the pituitary gland (adenohypophysis) are:

- thyroid-stimulating hormone (TSH), which acts on the thyroid gland
- adrenocorticotrophic hormone (ACTH), which stimulates the adrenal glands
- follicle-stimulating hormone (FSH) and luteinising hormone (LH), which act to stimulate the production of oestrogen, progesterone and testosterone by the gonads
- prolactin, which stimulates the production of breast milk
- growth hormone (GH), which acts on all the cells of the body
- melanocyte-stimulating hormone (MSH), which regulates the function of melanocytes in the skin.

The posterior lobe of the pituitary gland (neurohypophysis) does not actually synthesise hormones. It stores and releases hormones produced by the hypothalamus as required. The two hormones it stores are:

- antidiuretic hormone (ADH), which regulates urine production
- oxytocin, which helps contract the uterus during labour and delivery.

Figure 8.2 **Hormones of the pituitary gland**

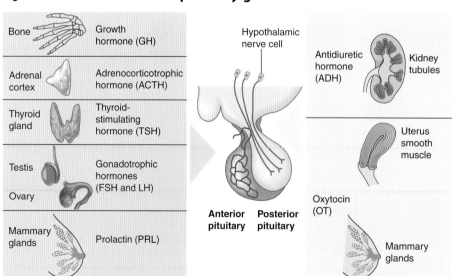

Thyroid gland

The thyroid gland secretes hormones that regulate growth, metabolism and energy use. The thyroid consists of two butterfly-shaped lobes. It is located in the throat inferior to the larynx and anterior to the trachea. The thyroid gland produces a number of hormones. Thyroxine (T_4) and triiodothyronine (T_3) are the main hormones produced. The letter T is followed by a number that refers to the number of iodine atoms in each of the molecules of the hormones. Dietary iodine is vital for producing the thyroid hormones. Thyroid-stimulating hormone produced by the anterior pituitary gland controls the rate of secretion of thyroid hormones. The thyroid gland also produces calcitonin, which regulates the level of calcium in the blood. When the level is too high, calcitonin is released to lower the level and to prevent calcium from being leached from the bones. Calcitonin has the opposite effect to parathyroid hormone.

Parathyroid glands

There are four pea-shaped parathyroid glands in the human body, located on the posterior surface of the thyroid gland. The main function of the parathyroid glands is to produce parathyroid hormone, which acts to regulate levels of calcium and, to some degree, phosphate in the body. Parathyroid hormone controls the amount of calcium within the blood and consequently controls how much calcium is in the bones. As blood filters through the parathyroid glands, the amount of calcium is monitored. If the calcium level is low the gland releases parathyroid hormone. This results in calcium leaching from the bones into the blood. However, if the level of circulating calcium is high, the glands slow or cease production of parathyroid hormone. The thyroid gland will release calcitonin to lower the levels, as discussed previously. An adequate concentration of calcium in the blood is very important for normal functioning of the body.

Adrenal glands

The body contains two adrenal glands, situated above each kidney. The adrenal glands are triangular in shape and consist of an **adrenal medulla** in the centre surrounded by an **adrenal cortex**. The adrenal medulla produces adrenaline (epinephrine) and noradrenaline (norepinephrine), collectively known as the catecholamines. These hormones help the body to react to stress by initiating the fight or flight response. Heart rate and blood pressure are increased, as is blood flow to the muscles. The metabolism of glucose to increase energy levels is stimulated. All of these physiological changes are necessary for the body to respond to a physical or emotional stressor.

The adrenal cortex produces glucocorticoids (e.g. cortisol) and mineralocorticoids (e.g. aldosterone), which promote homeostasis in the body by balancing fluid and electrolyte levels and maintaining adequate blood pressure. It also produces androgen, one of the male sex hormones that promotes the development of secondary sex characteristics.

Pancreas

Located in the abdominal cavity behind the stomach, the pancreas has dual roles in both the endocrine system and the digestive system. When food is partially digested by the stomach and moves into the small intestine, the pancreas releases enzymes through a duct into the duodenum to aid in further digestive action by breaking down fats and carbohydrates and neutralising stomach acids. This is referred to as the exocrine function of the pancreas. In addition, the pancreas has an important endocrine role by producing the hormone insulin. Insulin is produced by the islets of Langerhans, a small clump of cells in the pancreas. The main functions of insulin are to promote the movement of glucose from the blood into cells for energy and to convert the glucose into glycogen. These actions control the levels of blood sugar. The pancreas also produces glucagon. Glucagon is a hormone that aids in controlling blood sugar levels by preventing them from dropping too low. To do this, glucagon stimulates the conversion of glycogen that is stored in the liver to glucose. This is then released into the bloodstream. Glucagon works in conjunction with insulin to control blood sugar levels and keep them within set parameters. Glucagon is released to stop blood sugar levels falling too low (hypoglycaemia), while insulin is released to stop blood sugar levels becoming too high (hyperglycaemia).

Gonads

The gonads produce gametes or sex cells. In males, the gonads are the testes, and in females, the ovaries. The **testes** are located behind the penis in a sac called the scrotum. In addition to producing sperm, they are also the principal source of production of the male hormone testosterone. Testosterone is responsible for characteristic male traits such as body and facial hair, a low voice and broad shoulders. The **ovaries** in females sit above the fallopian tubes on either side of the uterus. The role of the ovaries is to release ova for fertilisation according to a monthly cycle. The ovaries also produce two groups of hormones known as oestrogen and progesterone. Oestrogen creates the typical female characteristics during puberty – development of breasts, body shape and maturation of the reproductive organs. Oestrogen and progesterone, acting on instructions from the pituitary gland, prepare the body for pregnancy or, if fertilisation does not occur, for the menstrual cycle. Levels of oestrogen fall rapidly at the time of menopause.

The testes and ovaries will be discussed in greater detail in Chapter 15 Male Reproductive System and Chapter 16 Female Reproductive System.

Pineal gland

The pineal gland is a small gland tucked in between the two hemispheres of the brain. It secretes the hormone melatonin, which acts to regulate the sleep–wake cycles or the circadian rhythm. The production of melatonin is inhibited by exposure to light and stimulated by darkness.

Thymus gland

The thymus gland is located in the mediastinum, posterior to the sternum between the lungs. The thymus gland is both an endocrine and lymphatic gland. Its lymphatic function is to produce special leucocytes called T-lymphocytes that fight infection and are crucial as a part of the immune system, especially in children. After puberty, the thymus starts to slowly shrink and become replaced by fat. The endocrine function of the thymus is the production of the hormone thymosin, a hormone necessary for T-lymphocyte development and production.

The main functions of the endocrine gland hormones are summarised in Table 8.1.

Table 8.1 Summary of endocrine glands, hormones and functions

Endocrine gland	Hormone	Main function of hormone
anterior lobe of the pituitary gland	thyroid-stimulating hormone (TSH)	stimulates release of thyroxine and triiodothyronine from the thyroid gland
	adrenocorticotrophic hormone (ACTH)	stimulates the adrenal cortex to release hormones particularly cortisol
	luteinising hormone (LH)	females: stimulates ovulation and the secretion of oestrogen males: stimulates the secretion of testosterone from the testes
	follicle-stimulating hormone (FSH)	females: stimulates the development of ova and the growth of the ovarian follicle males: stimulates the production of sperm
	prolactin (PRL)	stimulates the development of breasts and milk production
	growth hormone (GH)	promotes the growth of bones and organs
	melanocyte stimulating hormone (MSH)	regulates the function of melanocytes in the skin
posterior lobe of the pituitary gland (release of hormones is controlled by the hypothalamus)	antidiuretic hormone (ADH), also called vasopressin	stimulates the reabsorption of water by the kidneys, thereby maintaining blood pressure and urine output
	oxytocin	stimulates uterine contractions during labour and stimulates secretion of milk from the breasts
thyroid gland	thyroxine (T_4)	regulates metabolism
	triiodothyronine (T_3)	regulates metabolism
	calcitonin	decreases blood calcium levels when they are high
parathyroid glands	parathyroid hormone (PTH)	increases blood calcium levels when they are low
adrenal medulla	adrenaline and noradrenaline	affects the sympathetic nervous system in times of stress by increasing the heart rate and blood pressure, stimulating glucose metabolism
adrenal cortex	cortisol	promotes homeostasis by balancing fluid and electrolyte levels; also regulates blood pressure and blood glucose levels
	aldosterone	promotes homeostasis by balancing fluid and electrolyte levels
	androgen	promotes the development of secondary sex characteristics

Table 8.1 Summary of endocrine glands, hormones and functions—cont'd

Endocrine gland	Hormone	Main function of hormone
pancreas	insulin	lowers blood glucose levels
	glucagon	raises blood glucose levels
testis	testosterone	promotes the development of male sexual characteristics and spermatogenesis
ovary	oestrogen	promotes the development of female sexual characteristics and regulates the reproductive cycle
	progesterone	promotes the development of female sexual characteristics and maintains the uterus in pregnancy
pineal gland	melatonin	regulates sleep–wake cycles
thymus gland	thymosin	promotes T-lymphocyte development and production

PATHOLOGY AND DISEASES

Pathological conditions and diseases of the endocrine system result from either a hypersecretion or hyposecretion of specific hormones from the endocrine glands. This section will discuss the hypersecretion and hyposecretion of hormones for each of the glands separately, except for pathology and diseases of the testes and ovaries, which will be discussed in Chapter 15 Male Reproductive System and Chapter 16 Female Reproductive System.

Pituitary gland

Term	Pronunciation	Definition	Type of secretion
acromegaly	ak-roh-MEG-a-lee	Acromegaly occurs when there is a hypersecretion of growth hormone after puberty (usually between 30 and 50 years of age at a time when the bony growth plates have fused). Bones in the extremities (hands and feet), face and jaw grow abnormally large (Fig. 8.3). Visceromegaly is also present. Overall stature does not change. Acromegaly usually reduces life expectancy. The most common cause is an adenoma of the pituitary gland. Treatment involves resecting the tumour in conjunction with medication.	**Hypersecretion** from the anterior lobe of the pituitary gland

Figure 8.3 Characteristic facial appearance in acromegaly

(Hochberg et al 2008)

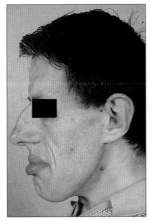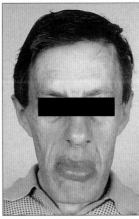

Table continued

Term	Pronunciation	Definition	Type of secretion
gigantism	jy-GAN-tiz-em	Gigantism occurs when there is a hypersecretion of growth hormone before puberty (which is often delayed). This results in abnormal overgrowth of the bones before the epiphyseal growth plates have closed. There may also be a loss of other hormones (TSH, LH, FSH), which may affect target organs. Gigantism is most commonly caused by a benign adenoma of the pituitary gland. Treatment includes resection and irradiation of the tumour. Results are better if there is early diagnosis of the gigantism.	**Hypersecretion** from the anterior lobe of the pituitary gland
dwarfism	DWAW-fiz-em	Dwarfism results from a congenital hyposecretion of growth hormone. Bones remain small and underdeveloped and the person is small all over. Dwarfism is generally defined as an adult height of 147 centimetres or less. It is known as proportionate dwarfism and is caused by a congenital aplasia or hypoplasia of the pituitary gland. Intelligence is not affected. Treatment involves administering growth hormone to try to stimulate bone growth. This type of dwarfism differs from achrondroplastic dwarfism, which has a genetic aetiology rather than an endocrine cause. People with achondroplasia have a problem converting cartilage to bone while growing, especially in the long bones of the arms and legs. Head and trunk are generally normally sized.	**Hyposecretion** from the anterior lobe of the pituitary gland
panhypopituitarism	pan-hy-poh-pit-YOO-i-tah-riz-em	Panhypopituitarism occurs in adults or children when there is a partial or complete failure of the pituitary gland to produce all six of the vital hormones. Functions of target organs are subsequently affected. Panhypopituitarism can be primary or secondary. Primary causes are tumours in the sella turcica region, arterial aneurysms, pituitary infarction, or a partial or complete hypophysectomy. Secondary causes are due to hypothalamus dysfunction as a result of infection, trauma or tumour, or due to idiopathic causes. Treatment is by hormone replacement therapy.	**Hyposecretion** from the anterior lobe of the pituitary gland
syndrome of inappropriate ADH	sin-drohm of in-a-PROH-pree-at ay-dee aych	Syndrome of inappropriate antidiuretic hormone (SIADH) occurs when there is an excessive secretion of antidiuretic hormone (ADH). This results in excess water retention in the body. SIADH is caused by a tumour, drug reaction or head injury. Treatment is by dietary water restriction.	**Hypersecretion** from the posterior lobe of the pituitary gland

Table continued

Term	Pronunciation	Definition	Type of secretion
diabetes insipidus	dy-a-BEET-eez in-SIP-id-us	Diabetes insipidus occurs when a hyposecretion of ADH results in a disorder of water metabolism. Kidney tubules fail to reabsorb needed water and salts. Symptoms include polyuria and polydipsia. Diabetes insipidus may be congenital or caused by a tumour, head trauma or infection, or from idiopathic causes. Treatment involves administering synthetic preparations of ADH, the hormone that instructs the kidneys to retain water. If there is an underlying cause, that must also be treated.	**Hyposecretion** from the posterior lobe of the pituitary gland

Thyroid gland

Term	Pronunciation	Definition	Type of secretion
goitre	GOY-tah	Goitre is a generic term for enlargement of the thyroid gland caused by a tumour, lack of dietary iodine or more commonly by thyroid dysfunction. It presents as a swelling in the anterior neck (Fig. 8.4). **Figure 8.4 Goitre** (Zimmernamm et al 2008) 	**Hypersecretion** from the thyroid gland
– adenomatous goitre	ad-en-OH-ma-tus GOY-tah	Adenomatous or nodular goitre occurs when there is hyperplasia of the thyroid gland with formation of nodules or adenomas in the gland. Thyrotoxic symptoms such as sweating, nervousness, tremors, rapid pulse will be present. Treatment by use of thyroid hormone to suppress thyroid gland functioning will be given.	**Hypersecretion** from the thyroid gland

Table continued

Term	Pronunciation	Definition	Type of secretion
Graves' disease	GRAYVs dis-EEZ	Graves' disease, also called exophthalmic goitre, toxic goitre or thyrotoxicosis, is an autoimmune disorder where hyperplasia of the thyroid parenchyma leads to excess thyroid hormone being produced (Fig. 8.5). There is an increase in the metabolic rate of cells, resulting in thyrotoxic symptoms such as sweating, weight loss, rapid pulse and warm moist skin. Exophthalmos (also called exophthalmia) occurs. Treatment includes drugs or destruction or removal of the thyroid gland. **Figure 8.5 Graves' disease** (Lemmi & Lemmi 2007) 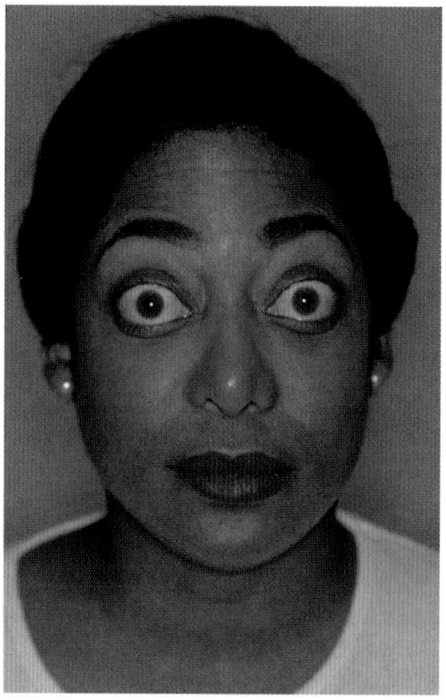 	**Hypersecretion** from the thyroid gland
congenital hypothyroidism	kon-JEN-i-tal hy-po-THY-royd-iz-em	Congenital hypothyroidism (previously called cretinism) is an extreme form of hypothyroidism occurring in infancy and childhood. It results in a lack of normal physical growth and mental development. Skeletal growth is most affected. A child with congenital hypothyroidism will appear short, stocky and obese. Treatment consists of administering thyroid hormone. If given early enough, there may be a reduction in some of the hypothyroid effects.	**Hyposecretion** from the thyroid gland
endemic goitre	en-DEM-ik GOY-tah	Endemic goitre is prevalent in some geographical regions and specific populations in the world. In endemic goitre there is an accumulation of material in the thyroid gland, leading to hypertrophy of the gland. It is caused by a deficiency of iodine in the diet. Treatment consists of providing an increased supply of iodine in the diet, generally via iodised salt.	**Hyposecretion** from the thyroid gland

Table continued

Term	Pronunciation	Definition	Type of secretion
Hashimoto's thyroiditis	hash-ee-MOH-tose thy-royd-EYE-tis	Hashimoto's thyroiditis is also called Hashimoto's disease. It is an autoimmune disorder resulting in an inflammation of the thyroid gland. This leads to hypothyroidism. The symptoms of Hashimoto's thyroiditis are generally similar to those of hypothyroidism. Patients with mild hypothyroidism may have no signs or symptoms. The symptoms generally become more obvious as the condition worsens and are related to a metabolic slowing of the body. Common symptoms are weight gain, fatigue and lethargy, dry skin and hair, bradycardia and depression. There is no cure for Hashimoto's thyroiditis, but thyroid hormone replacement medication will reduce the symptoms.	**Hyposecretion** from the thyroid gland
myxoedema	mix-e-DEE-ma	Myxoedema is a form of advanced hypothyroidism in adults. The thyroid gland atrophies, and little or no thyroid hormone is produced. Skin appears dry and puffy (oedematous) due to mucus-like material under the skin (Fig. 8.6). Patients may also develop bradycardia, atherosclerosis, dry hair, sensitivity to cold and may gain weight. Thyroid hormone is administered as treatment. If given early enough, it is possible for the patient to fully recover. 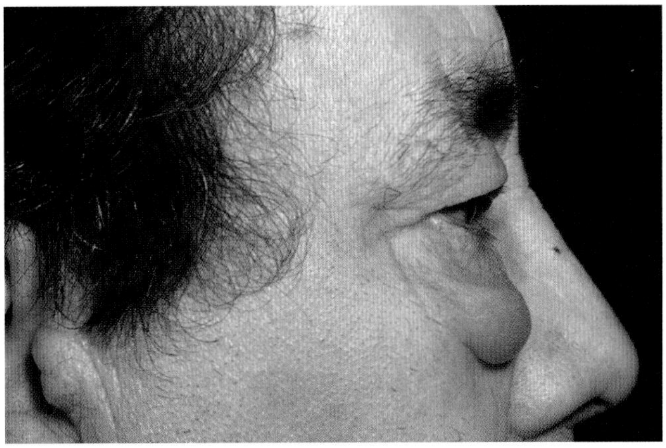	**Hyposecretion** from the thyroid gland

Figure 8.6 Myxoedema

(Kanski 2006)

Parathyroid glands

Term	Pronunciation	Definition	Type of secretion
hyperparathyroidism	hy-PER-pa-ra-THY-royd-iz-em	Hyperparathyroidism occurs when there is an increased activity of one or more of the parathyroid glands, resulting in the hypersecretion of parathyroid hormone. This causes excessive amounts of calcium to leave the bones and enter the bloodstream, causing hypercalcaemia. Bones decalcify, resulting in osteoporosis, fractures and cysts. There is an increased likelihood of renal calculus in these patients. This is the result of the increased level of calcium in the blood, which the kidney tries to remove. Excess calcium may collect in the renal pelvis, clumping into one or more small stones. Hyperparathyroidism is usually due to a tumour in one of the parathyroid glands. Treatment involves removing the tumour.	**Hypersecretion** from the parathyroid glands
hypoparathyroidism	hy-PO-pa-ra-THY-royd-iz-em	Hypoparathyroidism occurs when there is deficient production of parathyroid hormone. This results in a loss of calcium from, or insufficient entry of calcium into, the bloodstream. In turn, this results in muscle and nerve weakness and muscle spasms (tetany). Treatment involves giving calcium and large amounts of vitamin D to prevent further decreases in calcium levels.	**Hyposecretion** from the parathyroid glands

Pancreas

Term	Pronunciation	Definition	Type of secretion
hyperinsulinism	hy-per-IN-su-lin-iz-em	Hyperinsulinism occurs when excess insulin secreted from the pancreas draws glucose out of the bloodstream, leading to hypoglycaemia. This can result in syncope, convulsions and loss of consciousness. It is usually caused by either an overdose of insulin or a tumour such as an adenoma or carcinoma of the pancreas. Treatment depends on the cause but includes medication or surgical resection of the tumour.	**Hypersecretion** from the pancreas

Table continued

Term	Pronunciation	Definition	Type of secretion
diabetes mellitus	dy-a-BEET-eez mel-EYE-tus	Diabetes mellitus occurs when there is a lack of insulin secreted by the pancreas or a problem with the way the body metabolises it. Glucose is prevented from leaving the bloodstream to enter body cells. This leads to hyperglycaemia, glycosuria, polyuria, loss of weight or weight gain and ketonuria. There are two main types of diabetes mellitus: • Type 1 (previously called insulin-dependent diabetes mellitus) most commonly occurs in childhood. It results from an underproduction of insulin caused by an autoimmune reaction of the body to the beta cells in the pancreas. • Type 2 (previously called non-insulin-dependent diabetes mellitus) most commonly occurs in adults who are overweight. In type 2 diabetes, body cells do not react to the presence of insulin (i.e. they become resistant). As a result, the pancreas creates more insulin, but because of the resistance, the insulin remains in the blood, rather than entering the cells to be used for energy. Ultimately the pancreas becomes damaged as it works harder to create sufficient insulin to reduce the level of glucose in the blood. Hyperglycaemia results and this can cause microvascular and macrovascular complications and diabetic ketoacidosis and coma. The insulin resistance results from lifestyle factors such as increased weight, high blood pressure and high cholesterol levels. Treatment depends on factors such as the type of diabetes, severity of disease, age and symptoms. Treatment for type 1 diabetes mellitus is daily administration of insulin. For type 2 diabetes mellitus, treatment includes dietary management and improvements to other lifestyle factors such as quitting smoking and increasing exercise; it may also include administering insulin or other hypoglycaemic drugs. It is very important that treatment is adequate to prevent the occurrence of diabetic complications such as nephropathy, neuropathy, retinopathy and cataracts.	**Hyposecretion** from the pancreas
gestational diabetes mellitus	jes-STAY-shun-al dy-a-BEET-eez mel-EYE-tus	Gestational diabetes mellitus is a transitional diabetes that may occur in pregnancy as a result of the hormones produced by the placenta blocking the action of insulin, and subsequently causing insulin resistance and problems with metabolising carbohydrates. It resolves after delivery but it means the woman is predisposed to developing type 2 diabetes later in life. Treatment is by limiting the amount of carbohydrates eaten, regular exercise and, in a small percentage of women, daily insulin medication.	

Adrenal glands

Term	Pronunciation	Definition	Type of secretion
adrenal virilism	ad-REE-nal VI-ril-iz-em	Adrenal virilism occurs in adult women as a result of excessive output of adrenal androgens. This results in amenorrhoea, hirsutism, acne and deepening of the voice. It Is caused by adrenal hyperplasla or a tumour. Treatment includes drugs to suppress hormone production or an adrenalectomy.	**Hypersecretion** from the cortex of the adrenal glands
Cushing's syndrome	KOOSH-ings SIN-drohm	Cushing's syndrome occurs when there is an increased secretion of cortisol. This results in hyperglycaemia, hypertension, obesity, facial oedema (which gives a 'moon-face' appearance) and a 'buffalo hump' in the upper back due to fat deposits (Fig. 8.7). It is caused by excess stimulation by adrenocorticotrophic hormone (ACTH), a tumour of the adrenal gland or due to medication for other conditions such as rheumatoid arthritis. Treatment includes a subtotal adrenalectomy or pituitary irradiation.	**Hypersecretion** from the cortex of the adrenal glands

Figure 8.7 Cushing's syndrome
Same patient before and after treatment for Cushing's syndrome.

(Zitelli & Davis 1997)

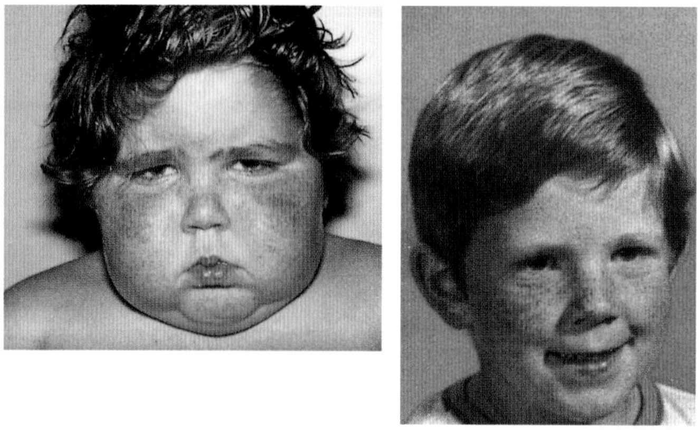

Term	Pronunciation	Definition	Type of secretion
Addison's disease	AD-i-sens-dis-EEZ	Addison's disease occurs when deficient amounts of glucocorticoids and mineralocorticoids are produced by the adrenal glands. This results in hypoglycaemia, hypotension, excess excretion of water and salts, weakness, weight loss and melanin pigmentation of the skin. It is thought to be caused by either an infection or by autoimmune adrenalitis. Treating Addison's disease involves replacing the hormones that are deficient. Hydrocortisone tablets and, for some patients, a form of oral aldosterone replacement may be prescribed. For patients receiving aldosterone replacement, an increase in salt intake is also recommended.	**Hyposecretion** from the cortex of the adrenal glands
phaeochromocytoma	FEE-o-KROH-moh-sy-TOH-ma	A phaeochromocytoma is a benign tumour of the adrenal medulla. Tumour cells produce excessive amounts of adrenaline and noradrenaline, resulting in hypertension, palpitations, severe headaches, sweating, facial flushing and muscle spasms. Treatment includes removing the tumour and administering antihypertensive drugs if required.	**Hypersecretion** from the medulla of the adrenal glands

TESTS AND PROCEDURES

The following section provides a list of common diagnostic tests and procedures and clinical interventions and surgical procedures that are undertaken for the endocrine system.

Test/procedure	Pronunciation	Definition
exophthalmometry	ek-sof-thal-MOM-e-tree	An exophthalmometry test is undertaken to measure the extent of protrusion of the eyeball in patients with exophthalmos.
fasting blood sugar	FAH-sting blud SHOO-ga	A fasting blood sugar test measures the blood sugar concentration or blood glucose level after the patient has refrained from eating and drinking for at least 8 hours. A high level of sugar or glucose is known as hyperglycaemia and persistently high levels can be an indication of diabetes mellitus. Other conditions that can result in elevated blood glucose levels include acromegaly, acute stress, Cushing's syndrome and pancreatic cancer.
glucose test	GLOO-kose test	A glucose test measures the level of glucose (sugar) in a urine sample or capillary blood sample. It is most commonly used to screen for diabetes.
human chorionic gonadotrophin (hCG) test	HYOO-man kaw-ree-ON-ick goh-NAD-oh-troh-fin test	hCG is a hormone produced by the placenta in pregnancy to maintain progesterone levels in order to prevent break down of the corpus luteum. The test is performed to confirm pregnancy.
ketone test	kee-tohn test	A ketone test checks for ketones (substances that result from the body breaking down fat for energy), usually in the urine. Ketones result when the body does not have enough carbohydrates to supply it with energy or when the body is resistant to or not using glucose that is produced correctly.
parathyroid hormone test	pa-ra-THY-royd HAW-mohn test	A parathyroid hormone test measures the level of parathyroid hormone in the blood to identify hyperparathyroidism or to find the cause of abnormal calcium levels.
parathyroidectomy	pa-ra-THY-royd-EK-tom-ee	A parathyroidectomy is a surgical procedure to remove one or more of the parathyroid glands. The procedure is performed to treat hyperparathyroidism from tumours or hyperplasia of the parathyroid gland.
prolactin test	pro-LAK-tin test	A prolactin test is used to identify causes of galactorrhoea, diagnose infertility or prolactinomas and evaluate pituitary gland function. The test measures the level of prolactin in the blood.
radioactive iodine uptake test (RAIU)	ray-dee-oh AK-tiv EYE-O-deen UP-tayk test	An RAIU test is used in conjunction with a thyroid scan to measure the amount of radioactive iodine the thyroid gland absorbs from the blood. The patient swallows 100–200 microcuries (a measure of radioactivity) in the form of a tablet or liquid and the uptake (absorption) is measured at 6 hours and 24 hours. A low uptake is an indication of thyroiditis, a high uptake suggests Graves' disease and an uneven uptake is an indication of the presence of a thyroid nodule.
serum calcium test	see-rum KAL-see-um test	A serum calcium test measures how much calcium is circulating in the blood to identify hypercalcaemia or hypocalcaemia. It is used to diagnose conditions such as kidney stones, bone disease and neurological disorders.
serum cortisol test	see-rum KAW-tee-zol test	A serum cortisol test may be undertaken on the blood and urine to diagnose Cushing's syndrome or Addison's disease. Cortisol is a steroid hormone produced by the adrenal gland in response to stress.
somatomedin C test	soh-MAT-oh-med-in see test	A somatomedin C blood test is used to test for abnormalities in growth hormone production or pituitary gland disorders such as gigantism and short stature.
thyroid function tests	THY-royd FUNK-shun tests	A number of tests are undertaken to measure thyroid function. They include: TSH levels (testing of the level of thyroid-stimulating hormone in the blood, with a high level indicating that the thyroid is not functioning correctly and a low level indicating an overactive thyroid gland), T_3 and T_4 tests (blood tests to determine the presence of hyperthyroidism or hypothyroidism).
total thyroidectomy	TOH-tel THY-royd-EK-tom-ee	A total thyroidectomy is a surgical procedure involving the complete removal of the thyroid gland. The procedure is performed to treat hyperthyroidism, thyroid cancer and compression from an enlarged thyroid gland.

Exercises

EXERCISE 8.1: LABEL THE DIAGRAM

Using the information provided in this chapter, label the anatomical parts in Fig. 8.8.

1 _____

2 _____

3 _____

4 _____

5 _____

6 _____

7 _____

8 _____

9 _____

10 _____

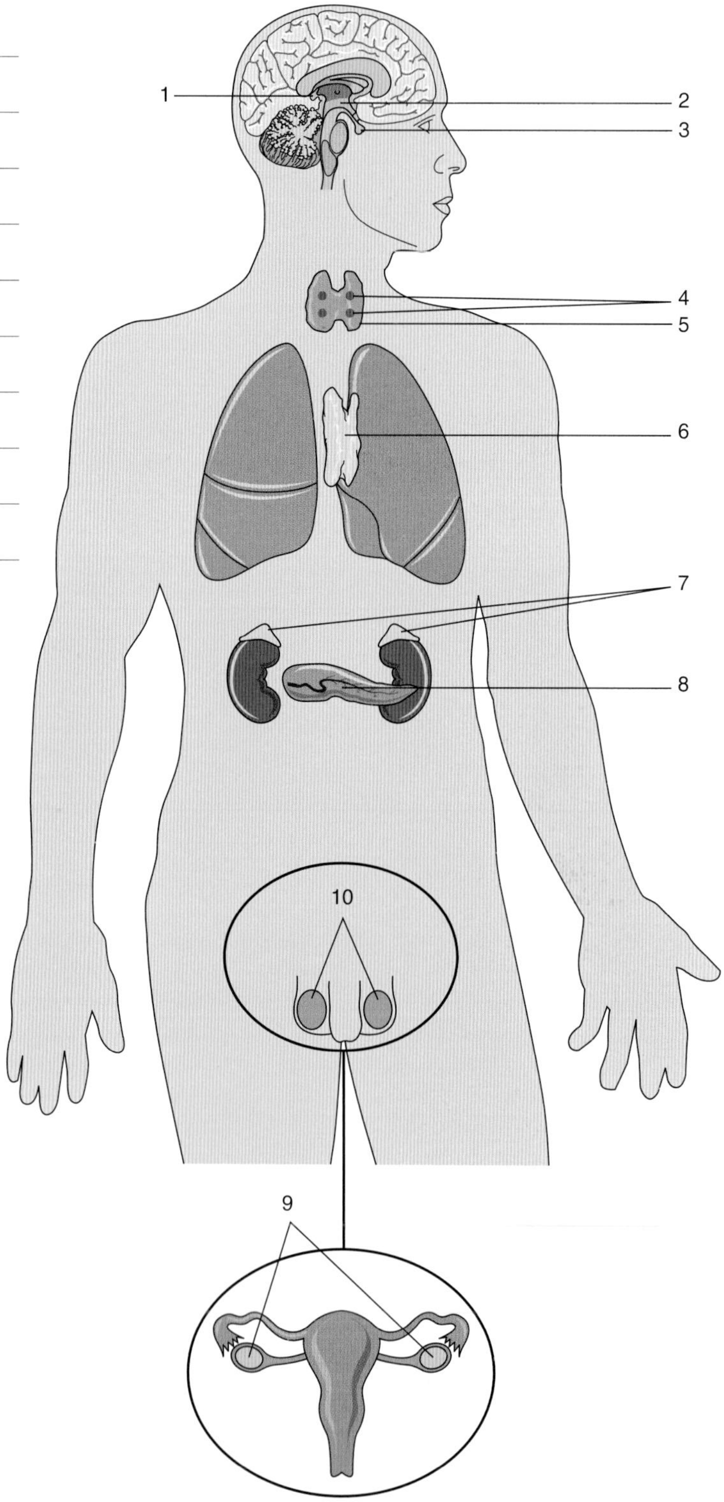

Figure 8.8 Endocrine glands

EXERCISE 8.2: WORD ANALYSIS AND MEANING

Break up the medical terms below into their component parts (prefixes, suffixes, word roots, combining vowels). Provide the meaning for each word element and each term as a whole.

Example:
thyroidectomy

thyroid/o = thyroid

-ectomy = surgical removal or excision

Meaning = excision of thyroid gland

1. thyrochondrotomy _____

_____

_____

2. acromegaly _____

_____

_____

3. pancreatotropic _____

_____

_____

4. hypernatraemia _____

_____

_____

5. polydipsia _____

_____

_____

6. polyuria _____

_____

_____

7. endocrinology _____

_____

8. homeostasis _____

_____

_____

9. ketonuria _____

_____

_____

10. phaeochromocytoma _____

_____

_____

EXERCISE 8.3: MATCH WORD ELEMENTS AND MEANINGS

Match the prefix, suffix or combining form in Column A with its meaning from Column B.

Column A	Answer	Column B
1. endo-		A. good, normal
2. oxy-		B. body
3. gonad/o		C. potassium
4. -crine		D. male
5. eu-		E. stimulating the effect of
6. natr/o		F. quick, sharp
7. andr/o		G. sex glands
8. somat/o		H. within
9. -trophin		I. secrete
10. kal/i		J. sodium

EXERCISE 8.4: SPELLING AND MEANINGS

Identify the correct spelling of the following medical terms by circling the correct word. Then write the meaning of the word on the line that follows.

hersuitism	hersutism	hirsutism	hursutism

thirotoxicoses	thyrotocicosis	thyrotoxicoses	thyrotoxicosis

hyperglycaemia	hyperglykemia	hypaglycemia	hypaglycaemia

pancreatectomy	pancrectomy	pankreatectomy	pankreatotomy

cretenism	cretinism	kretenism	kretinism

| pituitary gland | pituitery gland | pituitry gland | pituitury gland |

| keitoacidosis | keitoacidosus | ketoacidosis | keytoacidosis |

| diabetes mellitis | diabetes mellitus | diabetis mellitis | diabetis mellitus |

| goita | goitar | goyta | goitre |

| mixedema | mixoedema | myxadema | myxoedema |

EXERCISE 8.5: EXPAND THE ABBREVIATIONS

Expand the abbreviations to form correct medical terms.

Abbreviation	Expanded abbreviation
ACTH	
ADH	
FBG	
FSH	
GH	
GTT	
hCG	
T1DM	
T2DM	
TSH	

EXERCISE 8.6: APPLYING MEDICAL TERMINOLOGY

Fill in each of the following blanks with the correct medical term.

1. Masculinisation in women is called_____.
   a) andronism
   b) hirsutism
   c) vitiligo
   d) virilism

2. The _____ gland secretes a hormone that lowers blood calcium levels.
   a) adrenal
   b) thyroid
   c) parathyroid
   d) pancreas

3. The _____ gland secretes a hormone that raises blood calcium levels.
   a) adrenal
   b) thyroid
   c) parathyroid
   d) pancreas

4. Graves' disease is also known as _____.
   a) hypothyroidism
   b) myxoedema
   c) hyperthyroidism
   d) cretinism

5. _____ is associated with hypothyroidism.
   a) Cushing's disease
   b) myxoedema
   c) Graves' disease
   d) gigantism

6. The term _____ indicates a worsening of symptoms.
   a) regression
   b) suppression
   c) remission
   d) exacerbation

7. Oversecretion of the pituitary growth hormone in an adult produces the condition _____.
   a) gigantism
   b) acromegaly
   c) myxoedema
   d) tetany

8. _____ is a condition of excessive potassium concentration in the circulating blood.
   a) hyponatraemia
   b) hypernatraemia
   c) hyperkalaemia
   d) hypokalaemia

9. _____ is a syndrome caused by the hyperproduction of cortisone and hydrocortisone by the adrenal cortex.
   a) Cushing's disease
   b) Addison's disease
   c) Crohn's disease
   d) Graves' disease

10. Hyposecretion of insulin from the pancreas results in _____.
    a) diabetes insipidus
    b) diabetes mellitus
    c) hyperinsulinism
    d) pancreatitis

11. The term _____ means overeating.
    a) anorexia nervosa
    b) polyphasia
    c) polyphagia
    d) bulimia

12. Hyposecretion of the antidiuretic hormone from the pituitary gland results in _____.
    a) diabetes mellitus
    b) diabetes insipidus
    c) dwarfism
    d) ketosis

13. A decrease in levels of thyroid hormones in the blood resulting in lethargy, non-pitting oedema, weakness and slow speech is known as _____.
    a) hypoparathyroidism
    b) myxoedema
    c) goitre
    d) euthyroidism

14. _____ is an abnormal protrusion of the eyeball.
    a) ectropion
    b) entropion
    c) exophthalmos
    d) exophthalmometer

15. A state of general ill health, malnutrition, weakness and emaciation is termed _____.
    a) cachexia
    b) moribund
    c) tetany
    d) goitre

EXERCISE 8.7: MATCH TESTS, PROCEDURES AND MEANINGS

Match the test or procedure in Column A with its meaning from Column B.

Column A	Answer	Column B
1. GTT		A. tests the level of the hormone that controls TSH secretion
2. beta hCG		B. radioactive iodine is given, then the thyroid gland is imaged
3. orchidectomy		C. assesses adrenal medulla function
4. serum cortisol test		D. excision of, or radiation to, the pituitary gland
5. thyroid scan		E. excision of the testes
6. FBS		F. urine test to diagnose Cushing's disease or Addison's disease
7. hypophysectomy		G. measures fasting blood glucose levels
8. TRH test		H. measures the body's response to the administration of a concentrated glucose drink
9. radioimmunoassay		I. a pregnancy test
10. catecholamine analysis		J. nuclear medicine procedure to detect hormones in the blood

EXERCISE 8.8: PRONUNCIATION AND COMPREHENSION

Read the following paragraphs aloud to practise your pronunciation. Using your textbook and a medical dictionary, find the meanings of the underlined medical terms.

Mr Franklin is a 65-year-old man who has had <u>type 2 diabetes mellitus</u> for 3 years. He was referred by his GP to the diabetes clinic at University Hospital for annual review. On presentation, Mr Franklin gave a recent history of weight gain, <u>uncontrolled blood glucose levels</u> (as tested by his GP) and pain in his feet. He had recently stopped taking his <u>oral hypoglycaemic medication</u> because of dizziness, <u>diaphoresis</u> and <u>anxiety</u>. He was taking Lipitor for <u>hypercholesterolaemia</u>. He confessed to never testing his blood glucose levels at home. His healthcare record showed that, despite a referral, he had not seen a <u>diabetic educator</u> so had not been instructed on the correct process for self-monitoring blood glucose nor seen a <u>dietitian</u> for information about a diabetic diet. On examination, he was found to be <u>hypertensive</u> and <u>tachycardic</u>, with <u>diminished peripheral pulses</u> indicating probable <u>peripheral neuropathy</u>.

Because of his obvious poor understanding of his diabetes, it was decided to admit Mr Franklin to hospital for urgent diabetic education and control of his type 2 diabetes mellitus.

EXERCISE 8.9: CROSSWORD PUZZLE

Complete the puzzle by providing the medical term for each of the clues below.

ACROSS

1. Abnormally large extremities (10)
3. Aids digestion through the release of enzymes into the duodenum and produces insulin (8)
4. Advanced hypothyroidism in adults (9)
6. An accumulation of material in the thyroid gland, leading to hypertrophy of the gland (7, 6)
10. Abnormal overgrowth of the body resulting from excess secretion of growth hormone before puberty (9)

DOWN

2. Extreme form of hypothyroidism in infancy and childhood (10, 14)
5. Chemical messengers that transfer instructions from one set of body cells to another to stimulate a response (7)
7. Controls levels of blood sugar (7)
8. Congenital hyposecretion of growth hormone resulting in small and underdeveloped bones (8)
9. Hormones that regulate body activity such as growth, production or energy and other metabolic processes (7)

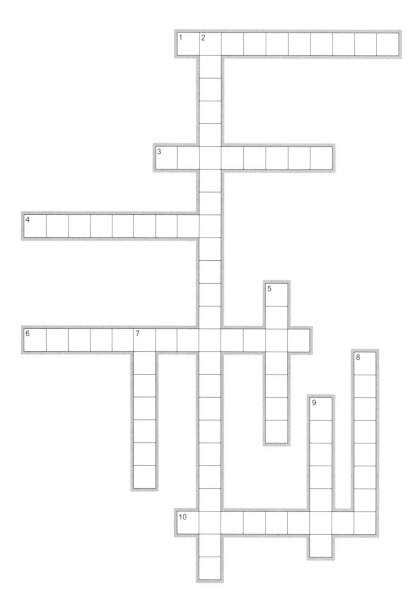

EXERCISE 8.10: ANAGRAMS

Work out each medical term from the jumbled letters below. Then, using the letters in brackets, determine the medical term that matches the description given.

1. smigigtna	__ __ __ __ __ (__) __ __ __	results from a hypersecretion of growth hormone in childhood
2. gemaracoyl	__ __ __ __ __ __ __ __ __ (__)	results from a hypersecretion of growth hormone in an adult
3. tismshiur	(__) __ __ __ __ __ __ __ __	excessive hairiness in a female
4. ycuiosargl	__ __ __ __ __ __ __ (__) __ __	sugar in urine
5. niisuln	(__) __ __ __ __ __ __	hormone secreted by the pancreas
6. trigoe	__ (__) __ __ __ __	an enlarged gland in the neck
7. lopiayipsd	__ __ __ __ (__) __ __ __ __	excessive thirst

Rearrange the letters in brackets to form a word that means 'a gland in the neck that controls body metabolism'.

— — — — — — —

EXERCISE 8.11: DISCHARGE SUMMARY ANALYSIS

Read the discharge summary below and answer the questions.

UNIVERSITY HOSPITAL DISCHARGE SUMMARY	**UR number:** 010204 **Name:** Linda Scott **Address:** 50 Bayview Drive, Hill End **Date of birth:** 12/2/1960 **Sex:** F **Nominated primary healthcare provider:** Dr Michaela Swan
Episode details **Consultant:** Dr Jason Keith **Registrar:** Dr Morton **Unit:** Endocrinology **Admission source:** Elective **Date of admission:** 11/3/2020	**Discharge details** **Status:** Home **Date of discharge:** 17/3/2020

Reason for admission / Presenting problems:
This was a routine admission of a 60-year-old woman with a thyroid goitre. She had noticed neck enlargement since late last year. She had also complained of some mild dysphagia. There were no obvious thyroid symptoms.
Principal diagnosis: Hashimoto's thyroiditis
Comorbidities:
Previous medical history:

Clinical synopsis:

On examination, Ms Scott seemed to have diffuse thyroid enlargement, with the right lobe larger than the left. An ultrasound scan was consistent with a multinodular goitre. Chest x-ray was clear. She had no tracheal compression. A fine-needle aspiration was performed under LA. This showed no signs of malignancy and was consistent with either a multinodular goitre or possibly Hashimoto's thyroiditis. Antithyroid antibodies were not performed preoperatively. A right hemithyroidectomy was performed under GA (ASA = 1NE), where a diffusely enlarged gland was found with associated lymphadenopathy.

Complications:

Her postoperative course was complicated by an early haematoma in her operative wound forming on the evening following surgery. This required a return to the OR and exploration and drainage under GA. Following this, she recovered well.

Clinical interventions:

Fine-needle aspiration

Hemithyroidectomy

Drainage of haematoma

Diagnostic interventions:

Ultrasound

Chest x-ray

FS confirmed Hashimoto's thyroiditis

Final histology was consistent with Hashimoto's thyroiditis

Medications at discharge:

She was placed on 100 ug of thyroxine daily.

Ceased medications:

Allergies:

Alerts:

Arranged services:

Recommendations:

She was discharged home with plans for surgical outpatient review.

Information to patient/relevant parties:

Authorising clinician:

Document recipients:

Patient and LMO

1. **Expand the following abbreviations as found in the discharge summary above.**

   LA

   GA

   OR

   ug

   FS

2. **Is the dysphagia that Ms Scott had on presentation to hospital a known symptom of Hashimoto's thyroiditis?**

3. Why was a chest x-ray performed for Ms Scott?

4. The clinical synopsis states that during surgery a 'diffusely enlarged gland was found with associated lymphadenopathy'. What does this mean?

5. It is noted that Ms Scott had an 'early haematoma in her operative wound forming' after her procedure. Describe what is meant by this and why she had to 'return to the OR and exploration and drainage'.

CHAPTER 9

Cardiovascular System

Contents

OBJECTIVES   180

INTRODUCTION   181

NEW WORD ELEMENTS   181
    Combining forms   181
    Prefixes   182
    Suffixes   182

VOCABULARY   183

ABBREVIATIONS   184

FUNCTIONS AND STRUCTURE OF
THE CARDIOVASCULAR SYSTEM   185
    Heart   185
    Arteries, veins and capillaries   186

PATHOLOGY AND DISEASES   189
    Pathological conditions of the
    heart   189
    Pathological conditions of
    blood vessels   193

TESTS AND PROCEDURES   197

EXERCISES   202

Objectives

After completing this chapter you should be able to:

1. state the meanings of the word elements related to the cardiovascular system

2. build words using the word elements associated with the cardiovascular system

3. recognise, pronounce and effectively use medical terms associated with the cardiovascular system

4. expand abbreviations related to the cardiovascular system

5. describe the structure and functions of the cardiovascular system including the heart and blood vessels

6. describe common pathological conditions associated with the cardiovascular system

7. describe common laboratory tests and diagnostic and surgical procedures associated with the cardiovascular system

8. apply what you have learned by interpreting medical terminology in practice.

Demonstrate your knowledge of the cardiovascular system by completing the exercises at the end of this chapter.

INTRODUCTION

The cardiovascular system (also called the circulatory system) can be thought of as the transport system of the body. It is a closed system that consists of the heart and a network of vessels that carry blood to the body tissues. With each heartbeat, blood is sent through the body, moving oxygen and nutrients to all the cells. Blood is not discussed in this chapter. It is discussed in the haematology chapter, Chapter 6.

Cardi/o comes from the Greek word *kardia*, meaning heart, and vascular comes from the Latin word *vasculum*, meaning small vessel.

The functions of the cardiovascular system are very closely linked with the functions of many other body systems such as the respiratory system. A healthy cardiovascular system is essential for maintaining homeostasis and general good health. If this important system ceases its work, the body will fail.

NEW WORD ELEMENTS

Here are some word elements related to the cardiovascular system. To reinforce your learning, write the meanings of the medical terms in the spaces provided. Use the Glossary of medical terms on page 561 to help you work out the meanings. You may also need to check the meaning in a medical dictionary, but make an attempt yourself first.

Combining forms

Combining Form	Meaning	Medical Term	Meaning of Medical Term
aneurysm/o	aneurysm	aneurysmectomy	
angi/o	vessel	angiospasm	
aort/o	aorta	aortic	
arter/o	artery	endarterectomy	
arteri/o		arteriorrhexis	
arteriol/o	arteriole	arteriolitis	
ather/o	fatty plaque	atherosclerosis	
atri/o	atrium	atrioventricular	
brachi/o	arm	brachial	
cardi/o	heart	cardiomyopathy	
cholesterol/o	cholesterol	hypercholesterolaemia	
coron/o	heart	coronary	
cyan/o	blue	cyanosis	
embol/o	embolism, plug	embolectomy	
haemangi/o	blood vessel	haemangiectasis	
isch/o	deficiency, blockage, hold back	ischaemic	
man/o	pressure	manometer	
my/o	muscle	myocarditis	
myos/o		myositis	
necr/o	death, dead	necrosis	
ox/o	oxygen	hypoxic	
pector/o	chest	pectoralgia	
phleb/o	vein	phlebotomist	
pulm/o	lungs	pulmogram	
pulmon/o		pulmonary	
scler/o	sclera, hardening	atherosclerosis	
sept/o	septum	atrioseptoplasty	
sphygm/o	pulse	sphygmomanometer	
steth/o	chest	stethoscope	
thromb/o	clot	thrombocyte	

Table continued

Combining Form	Meaning	Medical Term	Meaning of Medical Term
valv/o	valve	valvectomy	
valvul/o		valvuloplasty	
varic/o	swollen, twisted vein	varicosis	
vas/o	vessel, vas deferens, duct	vasoconstriction	
vascul/o	vessel	vasculitis	
ven/i	vein	venipuncture	
ven/o		venovenostomy	
ventricul/o	ventricle	atrioventricular	

Prefixes

Prefix	Meaning	Medical Term	Meaning of Medical Term
a-	no, not, without, absence of	arrhythmia	
an-		anaerobic	
brady-	slow	bradycardia	
de-	lack of, less, removal of	deoxygenate	
dys-	bad, painful, difficult	dyslipidaemia	
echo-	reflected, repeated sound	echocardiogram	
endo-	within, inside, inner	endocardium	
extra-	outside	extravascular	
hyper-	above, excessive	hypertension	
hypo-	below, under, deficient, less than normal	hypotensive	
inter-	between	interventricular	
peri-	around, surrounding	pericardium	
tachy-	rapid, fast	tachycardia	
tetra-	four	tetralogy	
trans-	across, through, over	transmural	
tri-	three	tricuspid	

Suffixes

Suffix	Meaning	Medical Term	Meaning of Medical Term
-centesis	surgical puncture to remove fluid	pericardiocentesis	
-constriction	narrowing	vasoconstriction	
-dilation	widening, stretching	vasodilation	
-gram	record, writing	electrocardiogram	
-graph	instrument for recording	electrocardiograph	
-graphy	process of recording	electrocardiography	
-meter	instrument used to measure, measurement	anaesthesiometer	
-plasty	plastic, surgical repair	angioplasty	
-plegia	condition of paralysis	cardioplegia	
-sclerosis	hardening	atherosclerosis	
-stenosis	narrowing, stricture	arteriostenosis	

VOCABULARY

The following list provides many of the medical terms used for the first time in this chapter. Pronunciations are provided with each term. As you read the rest of the chapter, make sure you identify each of these terms and understand their meanings.

Term	Pronunciation
aneurysm	AN-yoo-riz-im
angina pectoris	an-JY-nah pek-TOR-is
angiography	an-jee-OG-raf-ee
aorta	ay-AW-ta
arteriole	ar-TEER-ee-ol
arteriosclerosis	ar-TEER-ee-oh-skler-OH-sis
artery	AH-ter-ee
atherosclerosis	ATH-er-oh-skler-OH-sis
atrioventricular valve	ay-tree-oh-ven-TRIK-yoo-lah valv
blood pressure	blud PRESH-a
capillary	ka-PIL-a-ree
cardiac cycle	KAH-dee-ak sy-kil
cardiac MRI	KAH-dee-ak em-ah-eye
cardiac tamponade	KAH-dee-ak TAM-pon-ahd
cardiomyopathy	KAH-dee-oh-my-OP-a-thee
cardiopulmonary bypass	KAH-dee-oh-pull-mon-ah-ree BY-pahs
cardioversion	KAH-dee-oh-VER-shun
congestive cardiac failure	kon-JES-tiv KAH-dee-ak FAYL-ya
coronary angiography	KO-ron-ah-ree an-jee-OG-raf-ee
coronary artery bypass graft	KO-ron-ah-ree AH-te-ree BY-pahs grahft
coronary artery disease	KO-ron-ah-ree AH-te-ree diz-eez
coronary catheterisation	KO-ron-ah-ree kath-et-er-eye-ZAY-shun
deep vein	deep vayn
deoxygenation	dee-OK-see-jen-AY-shun
diastolic	dy-a-STOL-ik
digital subtraction angiography	DIJ-et-al sub-TRAK-shun an-jee-OG-raf-ee
Doppler ultrasound	DOP-la UL-tra-sownd
echocardiography	ek-o-KAH-dee-OG-raf-ee
electrocardiograph	ee-LEK-troh-KAH-dee-oh-graf
electrophysiological study	e-LEK-troh-fizz-ee-o-LOJ-ik-al STUD-ee

Table continued

Term	Pronunciation
endocarditis	en-doh-kah-DY-tis
heart	hart
Holter monitoring	HOL-ta MON-i-tor-ing
hypertension	hy-per-TEN-shun
hypertensive heart disease	hy-per-TEN-siv hart diz-eez
left atrium	left AY-tree-um
left ventricle	left VEN-tri-kul
ligation and stripping	ly-GAY-shun and strip-ing
lipid tests	LIP-id tests
mitral valve prolapse	MY-tral valv PROH-laps
myocardial infarction	my-oh-KAH-dee-al in-FARK-shun
oxygen	OK-se-jen
oxygenation	OK-se-jen-AY-shun
pacemaker insertion	pays-may-ker in-SIR-shun
percutaneous transluminal coronary angioplasty	per-kyoo-TAY-nee-us tranz-LOO-min-al KO-ron-ah-ree AN-jee-oh-plas-tee
peripheral vascular disease	per-IF-er-al VAS-kyoo-lah diz-eez
positron emission tomography scan	POZ-ee-tron e-MISH-en to-MOG-raf-ee skan
pulmonary artery	PUL-mon-ah-ree AH-ter-ee
pulmonary vein	PUL-mon-ah-ree vayn
pulse	puls
right atrium	rite AY-tree-um
right ventricle	rite VEN-tri-kul
sinoatrial node	sy-noh-AY-tree-al node
sinus rhythm	SY-nus rith-em
stress echocardiogram	stres ek-o-KAH-dee-oh-gram
stress exercise test	stres eks-er-syz test
superficial vein	soop-er-FISH-al vayn
systemic artery	sis-TEM-ik AH-ter-ee
systemic vein	sis-TEM-ik vayn
systolic	sis-TOL-ik
technetium (tc)-99m sestambi scan	tek-NET-ee-um 99-em ses-TAM-bee skan
thrombolytic therapy	throm-boh-LIT-ik ther-a-pee
vein	vayn
ventriculography	ven-trik-yoo-LOG-raf-ee
venule	VEN-yool

ABBREVIATIONS

The following abbreviations are commonly used in the Australian healthcare environment. Because some abbreviations can have more than one meaning, check the context in which the abbreviation is used before assigning a meaning to it.

Abbreviation	Definition
^{99m}Tc	technetium 99m
AAA	abdominal aortic aneurysm
ACE inhibitors	angiotensin-converting enzyme inhibitors
ACS	acute coronary syndrome
AF	atrial fibrillation
AI	aortic insufficiency
AMI	acute myocardial infarction
AR	aortic regurgitation
AS	aortic stenosis
ASD	atrial septal defect
AV, A-V	atrioventricular
BBB	bundle branch block
BP	blood pressure
bpm	beats per minute
CABG	coronary artery bypass graft
CAD	coronary artery disease
CAT	computed axial tomography
CCF	congestive cardiac failure
CCU	coronary care unit
CHD	congenital heart disease, congestive heart disease
CHF	congestive heart failure
CoA	coarctation of aorta
CT	computed tomography
cTn1	cardiac troponin 1
CVA	cerebrovascular accident
CVD	cardiovascular disease, cerebrovascular disease
CVP	central venous pressure
DSA	digital subtraction angiography
DVT	deep venous thrombosis
ECC	extracorporeal circulation, external cardiac compression
ECG	electrocardiogram
Echo	echocardiography
EF	ejection fraction
ETT	exercise tolerance test
HDL	high-density lipoproteins

Table continued

Abbreviation	Definition
HR	heart rate
HTN, H/T	hypertension
ICD	implantable cardioverter defibrillator
LA	left atrium
LBBB	left bundle branch block
LDL	low-density lipoproteins
LFTs	liver function tests
LMWH	low-molecular-weight heparin
LV	left ventricle
LVAD	left ventricular assist device
LVH	left ventricular hypertrophy
MI	myocardial infarction
MIDCAB	minimally invasive direct coronary artery bypass
mmHg	millimetres of mercury
MR	mitral regurgitation
MRI	magnetic resonance imaging
MUGA	multiple gated acquisition scan
MVP	mitral valve prolapse, mean venous pressure
NSR	normal sinus rhythm
NSTEMI	non-ST-segment elevation myocardial infarction
PAC	premature atrial contraction
PCI	percutaneous coronary intervention
PDA	patent ductus arteriosus
PET	positron emission tomography
PTCA	percutaneous transluminal coronary angioplasty
PVC	premature ventricular contraction
PVD	peripheral vascular disease
RA	right atrium
RBBB	right bundle branch block
RFA	radiofrequency ablation
RV	right ventricle
SA, S-A	sinoatrial
SOB	shortness of breath
SPECT	single-photon emission computed tomography
STEMI	ST elevation myocardial infarction
TIA	transient ischaemic attack
TMR	transmyocardial revascularisation
TOE	trans-oesophageal echocardiography
tPA, TPA	tissue plasminogen activator

Table continued

Abbreviation	Definition
UA	unstable angina
VF	ventricular fibrillation
VSD	ventricular septal defect
VT	ventricular tachycardia
VV	varicose vein

FUNCTIONS AND STRUCTURE OF THE CARDIOVASCULAR SYSTEM

The cardiovascular system is also known as the circulatory system and consists of the heart and blood vessels: veins, venules, arteries, arterioles and capillaries. This system plays a vital role in moving blood around the body to ensure every cell, organ and muscle receives oxygen and nutrients and that waste products are removed. Although the blood is intricately involved in the work of the cardiovascular system, it is considered separately in this textbook in Chapter 6 Haematology.

Heart
The heart is made up of cardiac muscle. Approximately the size of a closed adult fist, it is located within the thoracic cavity between the lungs and behind the sternum. It sits in a space called the pericardial cavity surrounded by the ribs and the muscular diaphragm. The main function of the heart is to act as the pump that forces blood to circulate throughout the body. The heart has three layers:
- a smooth inner lining, known as the endocardium
- a muscular middle layer, called the myocardium
- the outer layer, called the epicardium.

The epicardium protects the inner heart layers and also produces pericardial fluid, which fills the double-walled pericardium. The pericardium is also known as the pericardial sac and is the protective and insulating cover in which the heart sits. The pericardial fluid prevents friction during beating of the heart.

Within the heart are two upper chambers known as the right and left atria, and two lower chambers called the right and left ventricles (Fig. 9.1). It is important to remember that when talking about right and left in relation to the heart that the person is considered to be in the anatomical position. Refer back to Chapter 3 The Human Body to define this concept. Separating the right and left sides of the heart is a thick muscle known as the septum.

Figure 9.1 **The pathway of blood flow through the heart**
(© Alila/Fotolia.com)

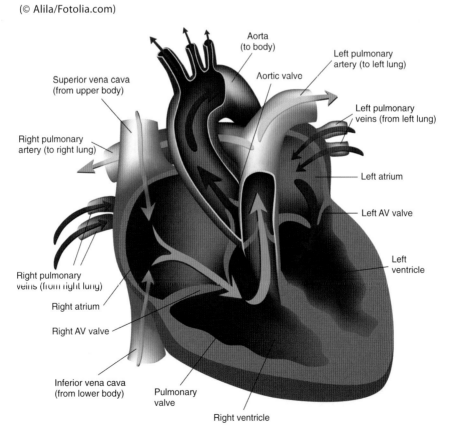

The right atrium receives deoxygenated blood returned from the upper part of the body through the superior vena cava and from the lower body through the inferior vena cava. In addition, blood from the heart itself enters the right atrium through the coronary sinus. The deoxygenated blood then flows into the right ventricle through the right atrioventricular valve (also known as the tricuspid valve because it has three cusps or leaves). The heart valves act to ensure the blood can only flow in one direction. The right ventricle then pumps the blood through the pulmonary valve and into the lungs via the right and left pulmonary arteries. Once in the lungs, the blood is reoxygenated. The pulmonary arteries are unique in that they are the only arteries to carry deoxygenated blood.

The blood, with its new load of oxygen from the lungs, enters the left atrium through the pulmonary veins. These are the only veins in the body to carry oxygenated blood. The left atrium is smaller than the right atrium but has stronger, more muscular walls. Blood then flows through the mitral valve (also known as the left atrioventricular valve or the bicuspid valve because it has two cusps or leaves) into the left ventricle. The left ventricle pumps the blood through the aortic valve into the aorta and then to the rest of the body. The aorta is the largest blood vessel in the body.

The heart beats at an average of 72 times per minute in a resting adult and, with each beat, approximately 30–40 millilitres of blood is released to the body from the left ventricle or returned to the heart and lungs for reoxygenation via the right atrium and then the right ventricle. Thus around 5 litres of blood are pumped by the heart each minute. The amount differs according to body weight and physical fitness. The blood from the left ventricle, being full of oxygen, is pumped to all the cells in the body to ensure they can function optimally. Blood from which the oxygen has been drawn is extracted from the cells and returned to the right atrium and then passed to the right ventricle. This continuous sequence of oxygenation–pumping to body cells–return of deoxygenated blood is known as the cardiac cycle. The cycle includes systole, or contraction, and diastole, or relaxation, of the left and right atria and ventricles. The two atria contract simultaneously. As they relax, the ventricles contract. The ventricles then relax and the atria again contract. This cycle repeats continuously.

As the blood is pumped around the body, it exerts pressure on the walls of the arterial vessels. This is known as blood pressure and is measured as a comparison of systolic (maximum) pressure as the heart contracts and pumps blood, over diastolic (minimum) pressure as the heart relaxes before its next beat. Normal blood pressure is around 120/80 mmHg, although this varies from individual to individual and from time to time in the one person according to the body's requirements.

The rhythmic beating of the heart is controlled by the sinoatrial node located in the right atrium. This node controls the contraction of heart muscle by generating impulses that cause other heart cells to contract in an orderly sequence that forces blood to be pumped around the heart. Normal heart rhythm is known as sinus rhythm. The sympathetic division of the autonomic nervous system can transmit messages to the sinoatrial node, instructing it to increase the heart rate in response to a need for additional oxygen in the body cells, such as during exercise or times of stress. By contrast, the parasympathetic division has the opposite effect, instructing the heart to slow.

The number of times the heart beats in a minute can be felt as contractions in the arteries. This is known as the pulse and is measured by feeling a superficial vessel against a bone, most commonly the radial artery in the wrist. A normal resting heart rate is between 60 and 80 beats per minute, but this is affected by level of fitness, activity or relaxation, body weight and heart health. An abnormally fast heart rate is known as tachycardia and a slower than usual heart rate is called bradycardia.

Arteries, veins and capillaries

There are three types of vessels in the human body, known as arteries, veins and capillaries. **Arteries** are elastic vessels primarily responsible for carrying oxygenated blood away from the heart to the rest of the body. There are two main types of arteries: pulmonary arteries and systemic arteries (Fig. 9.2). The pulmonary arteries are responsible for taking blood from the heart to the lungs to collect oxygen. These are the only arteries in the body to carry deoxygenated blood. The reoxygenated blood is then returned to the heart via the pulmonary veins, the only veins in the body to carry oxygen-rich blood. The systemic arteries, of which the aorta is the largest, transport the blood to the remainder of the body. The aorta originates in the heart but branches out into smaller vessels to supply the head, the heart itself and the lower body. As the arteries branch out, they get smaller and smaller. The smallest branches are called arterioles, and these are involved in circulating the oxygenated blood to the body tissues via the capillaries. Similarly, the venules, which are the smallest branches of the veins, are responsible for circulating deoxygenated blood from the tissues via the capillaries.

There are three main types of **veins**: pulmonary veins, systemic veins and portal veins (Fig. 9.3). As noted above, the pulmonary veins transport the oxygenated blood from the lungs to the left atrium

Figure 9.2 Arteries

(Mosby's Dictionary 2014)

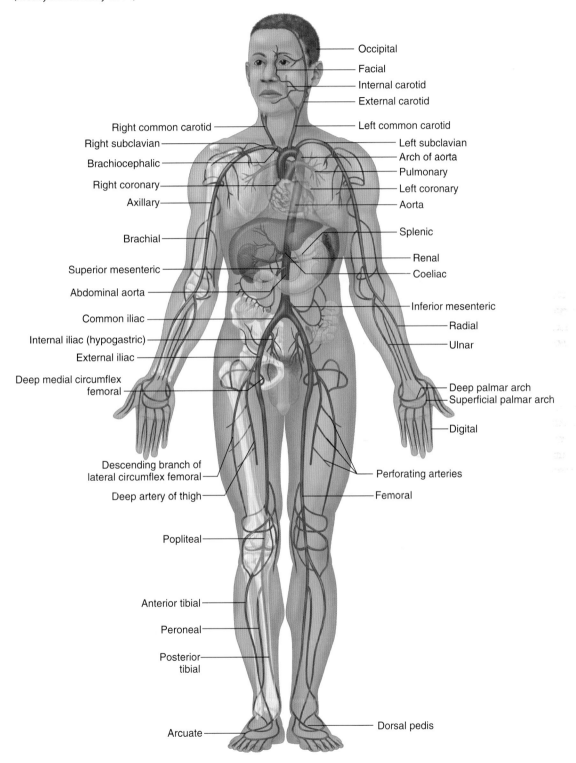

Figure 9.3 Veins

(Mosby's Dictionary 2014)

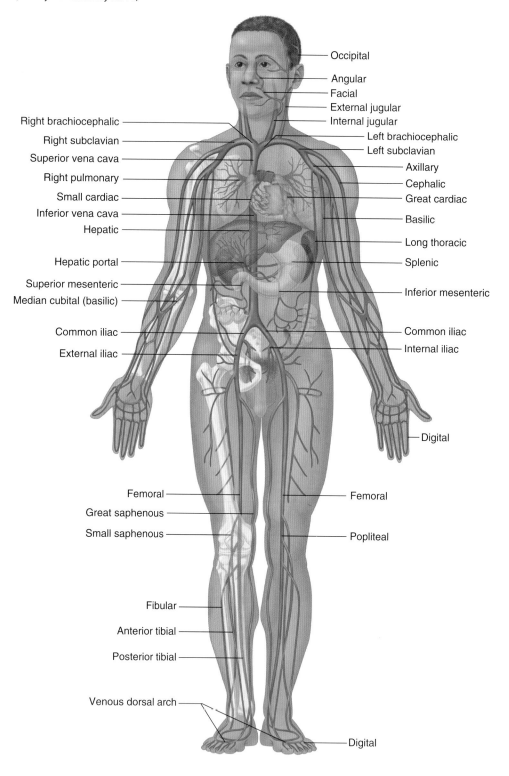

of the heart, while the systemic veins are responsible for returning the deoxygenated blood from the tissues back to the heart. Portal veins drain the gastrointestinal tract carrying blood full of nutrients to the liver. The liver processes these nutrients and is also responsible for filtering the blood of toxic substances such as bacteria before the blood goes back into general circulation around the body. The largest systemic veins are the inferior vena cava and superior vena cava, collectively called the venae cavae. Some veins are located close to the surface of the body and are called superficial veins. Deep veins are those that are found in deep muscle tissue and are usually co-located with a corresponding artery. Within the veins are valves that prevent blood from moving in the wrong direction.

Capillaries are tiny blood vessels that are so small that red blood cells can only pass through them in single file. The capillaries exist in a network like a web that connects the arteries and veins. Oxygen, carbon dioxide, nutrients and wastes pass through the thin walls of capillaries. Capillaries also have a role in regulating temperature within the body. When body temperature rises, the temperature of blood also rises. The heated blood travels in the capillaries to the body tissues where the heat is released. This causes, for example, a flushed look on the faces of people who are feeling hot.

PATHOLOGY AND DISEASES

The following section provides a list of common diseases and pathological conditions relevant to the cardiovascular system.

Pathological conditions of the heart

Term	Pronunciation	Definition
acute coronary syndrome	a-kewt KO-ron-ah-ree SIN-drom	Acute coronary syndrome is an umbrella term referring to ST elevation myocardial infarction (STEMI), non-ST-segment elevation myocardial infarction (NSTEMI) and unstable angina. These are all described in this section. Any condition caused by a sudden reduction in blood flow to the heart is considered part of an acute coronary syndrome.
angina pectoris	an-JY-nah pek-TOR-is	Angina pectoris is the medical term used to describe the temporary chest pain that occurs when the heart is not getting enough blood. It presents as a severe steady pain and a feeling of constriction around the heart, typically radiating from the chest to the left shoulder and down the left arm, creating a feeling of pressure in the chest (Fig. 9.4). The patient will often be very pale or ashen, will experience dyspnoea and have a variable raised blood pressure. An attack of angina pectoris will last a few seconds to a few minutes. It is relieved by removing the stressor and/or taking sublingual nitroglycerin either as a spray or tablet.
		Unstable angina is the term used when the chest pain caused by angina occurs at irregular intervals.

Table continued

Term	Pronunciation	Definition

Figure 9.4 Common sites of pain in angina pectoris

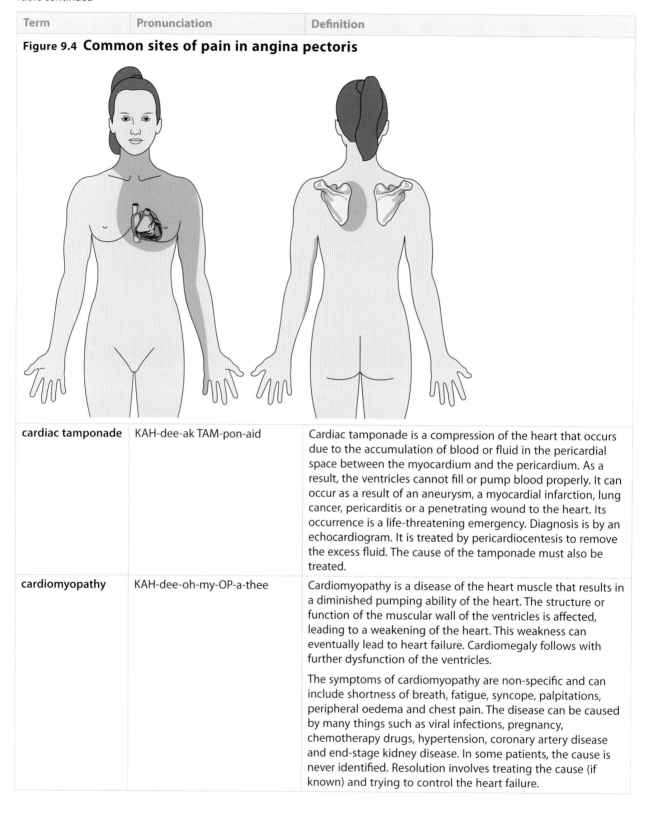

cardiac tamponade	KAH-dee-ak TAM-pon-aid	Cardiac tamponade is a compression of the heart that occurs due to the accumulation of blood or fluid in the pericardial space between the myocardium and the pericardium. As a result, the ventricles cannot fill or pump blood properly. It can occur as a result of an aneurysm, a myocardial infarction, lung cancer, pericarditis or a penetrating wound to the heart. Its occurrence is a life-threatening emergency. Diagnosis is by an echocardiogram. It is treated by pericardiocentesis to remove the excess fluid. The cause of the tamponade must also be treated.
cardiomyopathy	KAH-dee-oh-my-OP-a-thee	Cardiomyopathy is a disease of the heart muscle that results in a diminished pumping ability of the heart. The structure or function of the muscular wall of the ventricles is affected, leading to a weakening of the heart. This weakness can eventually lead to heart failure. Cardiomegaly follows with further dysfunction of the ventricles.
		The symptoms of cardiomyopathy are non-specific and can include shortness of breath, fatigue, syncope, palpitations, peripheral oedema and chest pain. The disease can be caused by many things such as viral infections, pregnancy, chemotherapy drugs, hypertension, coronary artery disease and end-stage kidney disease. In some patients, the cause is never identified. Resolution involves treating the cause (if known) and trying to control the heart failure.

Table continued

Term	Pronunciation	Definition
congestive cardiac failure	kon-JES-tiv KAH-dee-ak FAYL-ya	Congestive cardiac failure is a condition in which the heart cannot pump enough blood and, consequently, enough oxygen around the body. It can result from coronary artery disease such as stenosis, scarring from a previous myocardial infarction, hypertension, damaged heart valves, cardiomyopathy or an infection such as endocarditis.
		The failing heart keeps working but not as efficiently as it should. People with congestive cardiac failure cannot exert themselves because they become fatigued and short of breath very easily. As blood flow out of the heart slows, blood returning to the heart through the veins backs up. Peripheral oedema occurs due to this venous stasis. Sometimes fluid collects in the lungs and interferes with breathing, causing shortness of breath, especially when a person is lying down. Diagnosis is by clinical examination, electrocardiogram, echocardiogram and blood tests. Treatment includes reducing salt and fluid intake, medications such as diuretics, and a cocktail of cardiac-specific medications.
coronary artery disease (CAD)	KO-ron-ah-ree AH-ter-ee diz-eez	CAD occurs when the arteries that supply blood to the heart muscle (the coronary arteries) become hardened and narrowed. This is due to atherosclerosis, which is the build-up of cholesterol-rich plaque on the inner walls of the vessels. Over time, this plaque hardens and may rupture. Hardened plaque narrows the coronary arteries and reduces the flow of oxygen-rich blood to the heart. This reduced blood supply to the heart muscle is called ischaemia. When the heart muscle does not get enough blood, chest pain known as angina may occur. Angina is the most common symptom of CAD. As the disease progresses, CAD can lead to ischaemic heart disease. CAD may also result in myocardial infarction, which is discussed elsewhere in this section.
endocarditis	en-doh-kah-DY-tis	Endocarditis is a bacterial infection of the endocardium on the inner surface of the heart that may result in damage to the heart valves. It most commonly occurs in susceptible patients whose circulatory system has been breached in some way such as through insertion of a central venous line, recent dental work, drug injections or previous cardiac surgery. Long-term intravenous antibiotics are required and heart valve replacement may be necessary.
hypertensive heart disease	hy-per-TEN-siv hart diz-eez	Hypertensive heart disease occurs as a result of long-term hypertension. This causes cardiomegaly as the heart tries to compensate for the increased resistance due to increased arterial pressure.

Table continued

Term	Pronunciation	Definition
mitral valve prolapse	MY-tral valv PROH-laps	A mitral valve prolapse occurs when there is a drooping of one or both cusps of the mitral valve into the left atrium during ventricular systole. This results in incomplete closure of the valve and mitral insufficiency. This may cause regurgitation or backflow of the blood.
myocardial infarction	my-oh-KAH-dee-al in-FARK-shun	A myocardial infarction is commonly known as a heart attack. It occurs when an artery that supplies blood to the heart muscle becomes completely blocked and the heart does not get enough blood or oxygen (Fig. 9.5). Most myocardial infarctions are due to blood clots, which are in turn caused by atherosclerosis. The occlusion can lead to prolonged ischaemia and necrosis of cardiac tissue distal to the occlusion. The two common types of myocardial infarction are **ST elevation myocardial infarction** (STEMI) and **non-ST-segment elevation myocardial infarction** (NSTEMI). Each of these is diagnosed by review of characteristic patterns in the ST segment seen on an electrocardiogram. A STEMI is the more common of the two, causing approximately 70% of all myocardial infarctions. In a STEMI, there is complete or almost complete blockage of a major coronary artery, causing significant heart damage. Although the symptoms of a NSTEMI are similar to a STEMI, the damage to the heart is less because the blockage either occurs in a minor coronary artery or because the obstruction does not cause complete blockage of a major vessel. A myocardial infarction is a life-threatening emergency and needs urgent medical treatment. It may lead to impairment of systolic or diastolic function and to increased predisposition to arrhythmias and other long-term complications. Symptoms include chest pain (which may radiate to the jaw, neck, back or left arm), cardiac arrhythmia, shortness of breath, sweating, nausea, vomiting and a sense of foreboding. Diagnosis is by an electrocardiogram and blood tests to check cardiac enzymes. Treatment may include drug therapy, insertion of a stent, angioplasty or surgery such as a coronary artery bypass graft.

Table continued

Term	Pronunciation	Definition

Figure 9.5 **Myocardial infarction**

The area shadowed in purple indicates affected tissue distal to the blockage after myocardial infarction.

(© Alila/Fotolia.com)

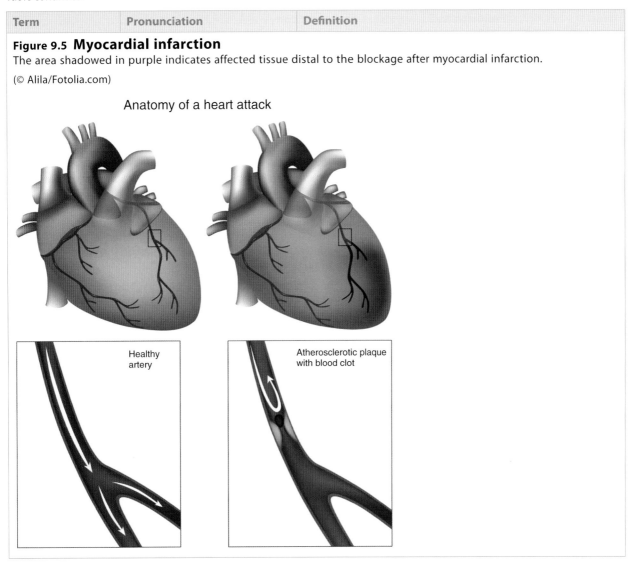

Anatomy of a heart attack

Healthy artery

Atherosclerotic plaque with blood clot

Pathological conditions of blood vessels

Term	Pronunciation	Definition
aneurysm	AN-yoo-riz-im	An aneurysm is a localised dilation or ballooning of an arterial wall due to weakness in the wall of the blood vessel. The aorta, cerebral arteries and mesenteric arteries supplying the intestines are most commonly affected. If the aneurysm ruptures it becomes a life-threatening emergency. Surgery may be performed to repair or clip the defect or may be minimally invasive treatment that involves placing coils or stents, which are introduced through other arteries of the body or neck and guided into the affected vessel. These act to close the aneurysm and preserve normal blood flow through the vessel.
arteriosclerosis	ah-TEE-ree-oh-skler-OH-sis	Arteriosclerosis is a general term for a hardening and thickening of arterial walls with a subsequent loss of elasticity and diminished blood flow to the heart, extremities and cerebrum. It is commonly referred to as hardening of the arteries. Arteriosclerosis may be present in any artery of the body, but the disease is most concerning when it attacks the coronary arteries and threatens to cause a myocardial infarction.

Table continued

Term	Pronunciation	Definition
atherosclerosis	ATH-er-oh-skler-OH-sis	Atherosclerosis is the most common variant of arteriosclerosis. It is a chronic inflammatory disease of large arteries that progresses with age. It is caused by fatty plaques (atheromas) building up in the walls of the arteries (Fig. 9.6). Over time the plaque causes thickening of the walls of the artery with stiffness and a loss of elasticity resulting.
		It is important to note that sometimes the terms arteriosclerosis and atherosclerosis are used interchangeably. However, they are different conditions. Arteriosclerosis is the general term referring to a hardening or stiffening of the vessels, whereas atherosclerosis describes the cause of that problem. To clarify, a patient with arteriosclerosis may not have atherosclerosis (plaque), but a patient with atherosclerosis does have arteriosclerosis. Patients will often have both conditions, which can cause a decrease in the blood flow through the affected vessel.
		In coronary atherosclerosis, atheromas form on the inner lining of the coronary arteries. This leads to a narrowing of the vascular lumen, a reduced volume of blood flow to the heart muscle and eventually myocardial ischaemia. Atherosclerosis can also occur in cerebral and peripheral arteries. There are multiple potential risk factors involved in developing the disease. These include hyperlipidaemia, smoking, sedentary lifestyle, obesity, hypertension, family history, injury to the endothelium of an artery, genetic or acquired abnormality and possibly cancer-producing viruses or carcinogens.
		The presence of atherosclerosis may only be recognised when an ischaemic event such as angina or a myocardial infarction occurs. Various diagnostic tests may be performed if the disease is suspected. These tests include arteriography (which demonstrates type, location and degree of occlusion); CT and MRI scans (imaging for detection and evaluation of pathology); electrocardiography (graphic demonstration of the cardiac cycle); digital subtraction angiography (images taken of vessels using a contrast medium, followed by computerised modification of the image allowing the contrast in the vessels to be seen more clearly); Doppler ultrasound (sound waves used to evaluate blood flow through the heart); echocardiography and an exercise stress test.
		Treatment for atherosclerosis includes: reducing risk factors for atheroma formation such as decreasing fat intake, regular exercise, reduction in weight, control of salt intake, cessation of smoking, reduction in stress levels; taking medications such as anticoagulants, beta blockers, antihypertensives and antidysrhythmic drugs; and surgical interventions such as angioplasty, endarterectomy, cardiac catheterisation (diagnostic and therapeutic), coronary artery bypass graft and possibly amputation if peripheral arterial reconstruction fails or if gangrene, uncontrollable infection or intractable pain develop.

Table continued

Term	Pronunciation	Definition
		Figure 9.6 Atherosclerosis (Shiland 2006) 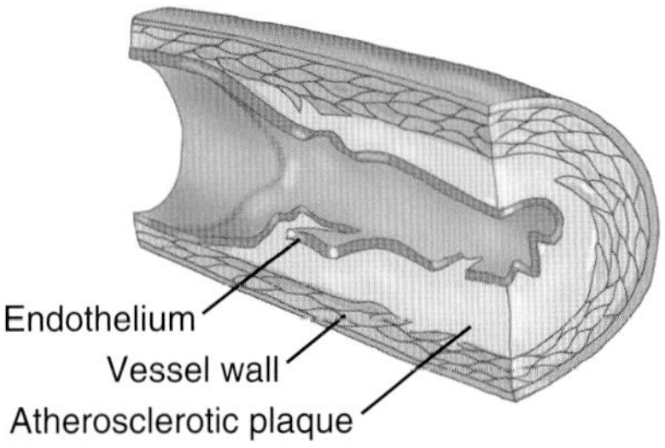 Endothelium Vessel wall Atherosclerotic plaque (Damjanov & Linder 2000) 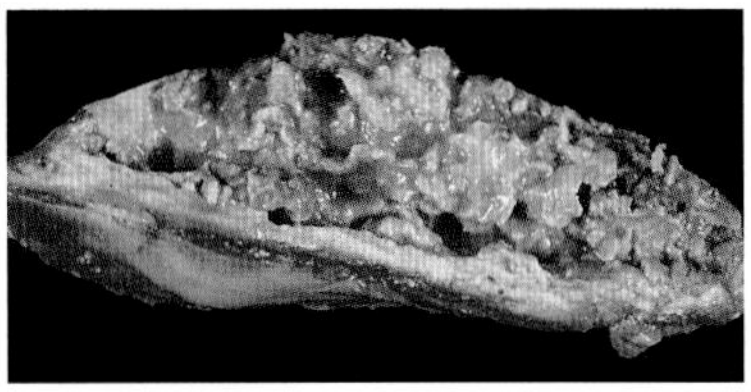
hypertension	hy-per-TEN-shun	Hypertension is more commonly known as high blood pressure. There are two main types of hypertension. Essential (also called primary) hypertension accounts for about 90% of all cases. There is no known cause, but risk factors include hypercholesterolaemia, hypernatraemia, obesity and family history. The other type is secondary hypertension, which occurs when the patient has another disease such as a complication of pregnancy or kidney disease, which causes the hypertension. Treatment of the original condition will often reduce the hypertension to normal levels. Malignant (or accelerated) hypertension is a very serious form of hypertension that is rapidly progressive and severe. It occurs when the diastolic pressure rises above 120 mmHg. Without urgent treatment it can lead to a cerebrovascular accident, uraemia or myocardial infarction.
peripheral vascular disease	pe-RIF-er-al VAS-kyoo-lah diz-eez	Peripheral vascular disease is a condition of the blood vessels that leads to narrowing and hardening of the arteries that supply the legs and feet. Atherosclerosis causes obstruction of the vessels in the peripheries. The narrowing of the blood vessels leads to decreased blood flow, which can damage nerves and other tissues. As a result, when the leg muscles are under strain during exercise or walking, they cannot get enough blood and oxygen. Eventually, there may not be enough blood and oxygen, even when the muscles are at rest. Drug therapy and reduction of risk factors for atherosclerosis are the preferred treatments.
varicose veins	VAR-i-kohs vaynz	Varicose veins are enlarged, twisted veins that are often dark in colour (Fig. 9.7). They have a ropey appearance and are usually thick and enlarged. While any vein can be affected, the veins in the lower legs and thighs have a greater tendency to varicose. This is due to leaking valves in the leg veins that allow blood to flow backwards, resulting in poor venous return to the heart. Over time this causes veins to varicose, becoming dilated and swollen.

Table continued

Term	Pronunciation	Definition
		Varicose veins can be aggravated by many other conditions such as long periods of standing, obesity, pregnancy, advanced age and chronic constipation causing straining. As well as being a causative factor for varicose veins, straining to pass a bowel motion can, over time, result in anorectal varicose veins, more commonly known as haemorrhoids. Haemorrhoids are discussed in detail in Chapter 11, Digestive system.
		Varicose veins are usually harmless but can cause pain and a feeling of heaviness in the legs. On rare occasions they can haemorrhage or cause a thrombus, which can travel to the heart or lungs where it can cause a fatal outcome. Many sufferers choose to have their varicose veins treated for cosmetic reasons (Fig. 9.8). Treatments include sclerotherapy (most effective in treating smaller spider veins), ligation and stripping of the vein, endovascular laser therapy or radiofrequency ablation. It is common for varicose veins to recur due to the defective valves in the veins.

Figure 9.7 Varicose veins

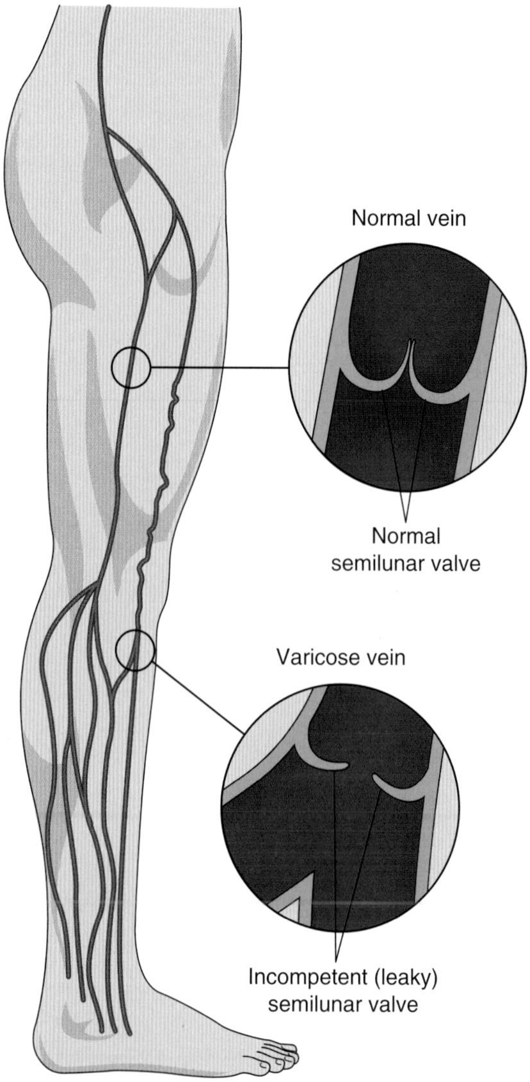

Normal vein

Normal semilunar valve

Varicose vein

Incompetent (leaky) semilunar valve

Table continued

Term	Pronunciation	Definition

Figure 9.8 Varicose veins before and after treatment

A. Posterior aspect of varicose veins before treatment. **B.** Medial aspect of varicose veins before treatment. **C.** Posterior aspect of varicose veins 2 years after initial treatment. **D.** Medial aspect of varicose veins 2 years after initial treatment. **E and F.** Development of new varicose veins after initial treatment and resolution. The saphenofemoral junction is now incompetent bilaterally.

(Golman et al 2011)

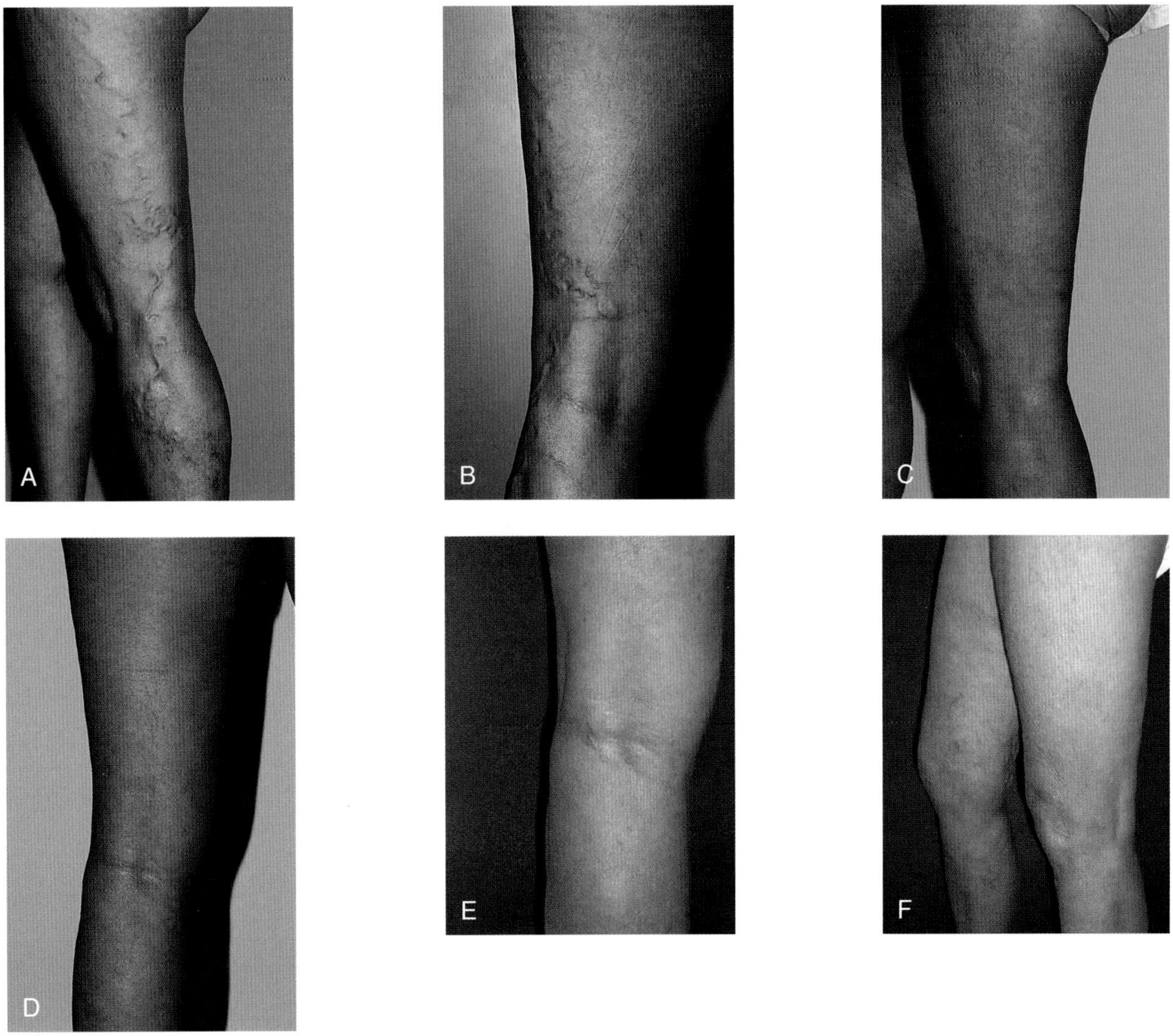

TESTS AND PROCEDURES

The following section provides a list of common diagnostic tests and procedures and clinical interventions and surgical procedures that are undertaken for the cardiovascular system.

Test/Procedure	Pronunciation	Definition
angiography	an-jee-OG-raf-ee	Angiography involves an injection of a contrast medium into blood vessels to enable x-ray imaging of the vessels.
cardiac magnetic resonance imaging (MRI)	KAH-dee-ak mag-NET-ik REZ-on-ans im-a-jing (em-ah-eye)	A cardiac MRI is a diagnostic test that creates images of cardiac tissue using radio waves and a magnetic field to identify aneurysms, patency of coronary arteries and determine cardiac output.

Table continued

Test/Procedure	Pronunciation	Definition
cardiopulmonary bypass	KAH-dee-oh-pull-mon-a-ree BY-pahs	A cardiopulmonary bypass is a technique used in heart surgery, where a machine temporarily takes over the functions of the heart and lungs to maintain the circulation of blood and oxygen. It is commonly used in surgeries performed on the chambers of the heart.
cardioversion	KAH-dee-oh-VER-shun	Cardioversion is a procedure that uses drugs or electricity to convert a fast heart rate or cardiac dysrhythmia or arrhythmia to normal rhythm.
coronary angiography	KOR-on-ah-ree an-jee-OG-raf-ee	Coronary angiography uses radio-opaque contrast to record x-ray images of the coronary arteries to identify issues that affect the circulation of the blood through the arteries. The contrast medium is usually injected into the arteries via cardiac catheterisation.
coronary artery bypass graft	KOR-on-ah-ree AH-ter-ee BY-pahs grahft	A coronary artery bypass graft is a surgical procedure that involves the grafting of vessels from elsewhere in the body to coronary arteries to bypass around blockages (Fig. 9.9). Graft vessels are harvested endoscopically from internal mammary arteries, radial arteries or the saphenous veins. The procedure can be performed as an open procedure involving a sternotomy to open the chest or as a minimally invasive procedure using smaller incisions.

Figure 9.9 Coronary artery bypass graft

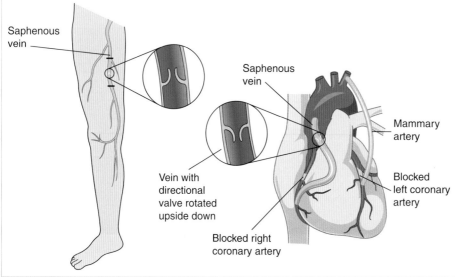

| coronary catheterisation | KOR-on-ah-ree kath-et-er-eye-ZAY-shun | Coronary (or cardiac) catheterisation involves inserting a catheter into the coronary arteries for diagnostic or therapeutic purposes. The catheter is generally inserted via an artery or vein in the arm, groin or neck and threaded through the vessels to the heart. It is often used to deliver contrast medium to the vessels for an angiography. |
| digital subtraction angiography | DIJ-e-tal sub-TRAK-shun an-jee-OG-raf-ee | Digital subtraction angiography is a technique using fluoroscopy to gain an image of blood vessels in a bony or soft tissue environment (Fig. 9.10). Images are obtained by injecting a contrast medium and using a computer to subtract a pre-contrast image from later images with contrast, leaving a clearer image. |

Table continued

Test/Procedure	Pronunciation	Definition

Figure 9.10 **Digital subtraction angiography**

A. Digital subtraction angiography in the anteroposterior projection of the right common femoral artery. CFA, common femoral artery; PFA, profunda femoral artery; SFA, superficial femoral artery. B. Infrapopliteal digital subtraction angiography in the anteroposterior projection. AT, anterior tibial artery; TPT, tibial-peroneal trunk; PT, posterior tibial artery; PA, peroneal artery

(Sellke et al 2009)

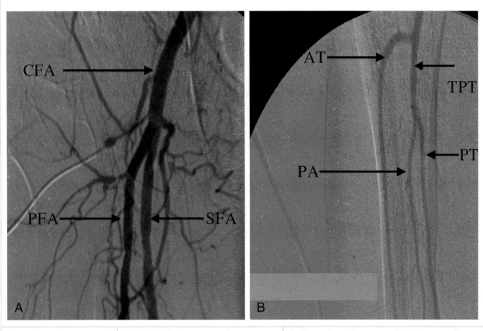

Test/Procedure	Pronunciation	Definition
Doppler ultrasound	DOP-la UL-tra-sownd	A Doppler ultrasound test uses ultrasound technology to analyse the progress of blood flowing through vessels by using a transducer to send, receive and measure echoes of sound waves bouncing off blood cells.
electrocardiograph (ECG)	ee-LEK-troh-KAH-dee-oh-graf	An ECG is a diagnostic test that measures and records the electrical activity of the heart. Electrodes are placed on specific points of the thorax and extremities and electrical activity is recorded. Interpretation of these results allows diagnosis of a wide range of cardiac conditions.
echocardiography	ek-oh-KAH-dee-OG-raf-ee	Echocardiography uses ultrasound or sound wave technology to obtain images of the heart to show the structure and movement of the heart.
electrophysiological study	e-LEK-troh-fizz-ee-oh-loj-ik-al STUD-ee	An electrophysiological study is an invasive procedure that tests the electrical system of the heart to assess rhythm disturbances. The procedure is performed by inserting a catheter into a vein in the groin and advancing it through the veins to the heart, viewed by fluoroscopy. Electrical signals are then sent to the heart via the catheter to evaluate the electrical conduction system.
Holter monitoring	HOL-ta MON-i-tor-ing	Holter monitoring involves a patient wearing a portable ECG machine for 24 hours to identify cardiac arrhythmias.

Table continued

Test/Procedure	Pronunciation	Definition
implantable cardioverter defibrillator (ICD) insertion	im-PLAN-ta-bel kah-dee-o-VER-ta dee-FIB-ril-ay-tor in-SUR-shun	An ICD is a device that uses electrical signals to manage seriously abnormal heart rhythms. ICD insertion involves implanting a defibrillator and leads, which sit subcutaneously under the chest wall to continuously monitor the heart rhythm. When it identifies a life-threatening cardiac dysrhythmia such as ventricular fibrillation, the ICD can deliver either low-level or high-level electrical pulses that are designed to shock the heart back to a normal rhythm. The process of delivering the shock is called defibrillation.
ligation and stripping	ly-GAY-shun and strip-ing	Ligation and stripping is a procedure used to treat varicose veins. For varicose veins in the lower limbs, it involves making a small incision in the groin to expose the diseased great saphenous vein, which is tied off. A series of incisions are then made along the leg and a specialised stripping tool is inserted and threaded through the incisions to strip out the diseased vein.
lipid tests	LIP-id tests	Lipid tests measure the cholesterol and triglyceride levels in blood.
pacemaker insertion	pays-mayk-a in-SIR-shun	Inserting a pacemaker involves placing an artificial device that uses low-level electrical impulses to regulate heartbeat. They are particularly useful for patients who experience bradycardia.
percutaneous transluminal coronary angioplasty (PTCA)	per-kyoo-TAY-nee-us tranz-LOO-min-al KO-ron-ah-ree AN-jee-oh-plas-tee	A PTCA is performed to treat vessel narrowing. A wire is inserted into the femoral or radial artery and progressed through and beyond the point of narrowing in the affected artery. A balloon-tipped catheter is then advanced over the wire to the section that needs to be treated. The balloon is inflated, compressing the plaque that has caused the narrowing and improving the blood flow (Fig. 9.11).

Figure 9.11 Percutaneous transluminal coronary angioplasty

(A: LaFleur Brooks 2005; B: Ballinger & Frank 2003)

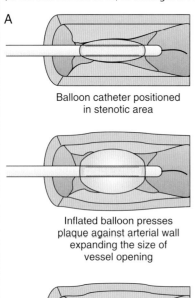

A

Balloon catheter positioned in stenotic area

Inflated balloon presses plaque against arterial wall expanding the size of vessel opening

Balloon is deflated and blood flow reestablished

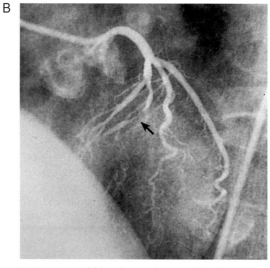

B

B: A narrowed blood vessel caused by the presence of plaque

Table continued

Test/Procedure	Pronunciation	Definition
positron emission tomography (PET) scan	POZ-ee-tron e-MISH-en to-MOG-ra-fee skan	A PET scan is a non-invasive nuclear medicine imaging technique that produces three-dimensional images of the heart using a radioactive tracer. It can also be used for other body sites to identify abnormalities. A camera detects emissions coming from the injected tracer and a computer creates two- and three-dimensional images of the area where the pharmaceutical has travelled. In the heart, this demonstrates blood flow and potential blockages in the cardiac vessels.
stent insertion (stenting)	stent in-SIR-shun	A stent is a mesh tube that is inserted into a coronary artery that is narrowed or blocked due to plaque build-up. Usually a balloon angioplasty is performed first to widen the lumen of the artery (see PTCA above). Then the stent is inserted to act as a scaffold to keep the vessel open to maintain the improved blood flow. Drug-eluting stents are coated with slow-release drugs to prevent the formation of scar tissue to avoid the re-narrowing of the artery.
stress echocardiogram	stres ek-o-KAH-dee-o-gram	A stress echocardiogram provides more specific information than the usual stress exercise test. In addition to a resting ultrasound of the heart taken for baseline monitoring and a stress exercise test monitoring process, a further ultrasound using a transducer is taken immediately after an exercise test on the treadmill while the heart is still beating fast. This provides the opportunity to identify valvular disease and gather information on pressure in the heart and lung.
stress exercise test	stres EKS-er-syz test	A stress exercise test assesses the response of the heart to physical exertion. A recording on ECG is taken at rest and then at 3-minute stages over a period of 30 minutes on a treadmill. The treadmill is progressively elevated throughout the test. The test is used to diagnose coronary artery disease and to assess left ventricular function.
technetium-99m (^{99m}Tc) sestambi scan	tek-NET-ee-um 99-em ses-TAM-bee skan	A ^{99m}Tc sestambi scan is performed to identify ischaemic and infarcted heart tissue. A radioactive tracer compound is injected intravenously and taken up by normal heart tissue. A scan is then used to identify ischaemic cardiac tissue.
thrombolytic therapy	throm-bo-LIT-ik ther-a-pee	Thrombolytic therapy involves injecting drugs into the bloodstream to dissolve clots in patients with coronary thrombosis. It is done to avoid permanent damage caused by the blockage.
ventriculography	ven-trik-yoo-LOG-raf-ee	Ventriculography involves taking images of the ventricles of the heart using echocardiography, blood pool radionuclide imaging, electron beam CT scan, MRI or contrast x-ray.

Exercises

EXERCISE 9.1: LABEL THE DIAGRAM

Using the information provided in this chapter, label the anatomical parts in Fig. 9.12.

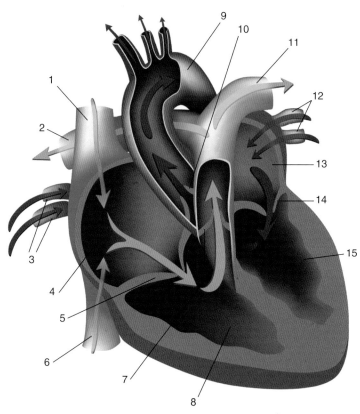

Figure 9.12 The pathway of blood flow through the heart

(© Alila/Fotolia.com)

1 _____

2 _____

3 _____

4 _____

5 _____

6 _____

7 _____

8 _____

9 _____

10 _____

11 _____

12 _____

13 _____

14 _____

15 _____

EXERCISE 9.2: MATCH WORD ELEMENTS AND MEANINGS

Match the prefix, suffix or combining form in Column A with its meaning from Column B.

Column A	Answer	Column B
1. angi/o		A. atrium
2. tachy-		B. vein
3. scler/o		C. plug, embolism
4. arteri/o		D. pulse
5. cyan/o		E. narrowing, stricture
6. echo-		F. slow
7. pector/o		G. hardening, sclera
8. brachi/o		H. surgical puncture to remove fluid
9. -stenosis		I. chest
10. man/o		J. across or through
11. -meter		K. vessel
12. phleb/o		L. rapid, fast
13. -centesis		M. heart
14. atri/o		N. pressure
15. trans-		O. death, dead
16. sphygm/o		P. artery
17. coron/o		Q. instrument to measure, measurement
18. embol/o		R. arm
19. necr/o		S. reflected, repeated sound
20. brady-		T. blue

EXERCISE 9.3: WORD ANALYSIS AND MEANING

Break up the medical terms below into their component parts (prefixes, suffixes, word roots, combining vowels). Provide the meaning for each word element and each term as a whole.

Example:

erythrocyte

erythr/o = red

-cyte = cell

Meaning = cell that is red (red blood cell)

1. vasoconstriction _____

_____

_____

2. hypovolaemia _____

_____

3. angioplasty _____

_____

_____

4. ventriculography _____

_____

_____

5. pancytopenia _____

_____

_____

6. septicaemia _____

_____

_____

7. phlebotomy _____

_____

_____

8. hypochromic microcytic anaemia _____

_____

_____

9. aneurysmorrhaphy _____

_____

10. sphygmomanometer _____

_____

_____

EXERCISE 9.4: VOCABULARY BUILDING

Provide the medical term for each of the definitions below.

1. Condition in which the normal rhythm of the heart is absent:

_____

2. Enlarged heart:

_____

3. A ballooning in the walls of an artery:

_____

4. A form of arteriosclerosis in which there are fatty plaque deposits in the lining of an artery:

_____

5. A recording of heart sounds:

_____

6. Excision of the inner lining of an artery:

_____

7. A bursting forth of blood (usually due to trauma to a blood vessel):

_____

8. Condition in which there is a decrease in the level of oxygen in the blood:

_____

9. Inflammation of the membrane covering the heart:

_____

10. Abnormal condition of bluish discolouration usually of fingertips and lips:

_____

EXERCISE 9.5: EXPAND THE ABBREVIATIONS

Expand the abbreviations to form correct medical terms.

Abbreviation	Expanded Abbreviation
AF	
AMI	
BBB	
BP	
CABG	
CAD	
CCF	
CCU	

Abbreviation	Expanded Abbreviation
CHD	
CVP	
DVT	
HDL	
LDL	
LV	
NSTEMI	
PDA	
PTCA	
SOB	
TOE	
VSD	

EXERCISE 9.6: APPLYING MEDICAL TERMINOLOGY

The combining form cardi/o, meaning heart, is the foundation for most medical terms relating to the heart. Complete the following sentences using the correct prefix, suffix or word root.

1. A doctor who specialises in treating heart-related conditions is a cardio _____.

2. A patient with _____ cardia has a fast heart rate.

3. A condition where the heart is found on the right side of the body is _____ cardia.

4. An enlarged heart is cardio _____.

5. A general term for disease of the heart muscle is cardio _____.

6. An _____ cardio _____ is a graphic record of electrical conduction within the heart.

7. The inner lining of the heart is called the _____ cardium.

8. Cardio _____ is a rupture of the heart usually resulting in immediate death.

9. A procedure to view the pericardium is a _____ cardi _____.

10. Cardio _____ is paralysis of the heart muscle.

EXERCISE 9.7: MATCH DRUG TYPE WITH USE

Match the type of drug in Column A with its use from Column B.

Column A	Answer	Column B
1. anticoagulant		A. increases the formation of urine
2. antihyperlipidaemic		B. controls hypertension and angina pectoris
3. antiarrhythmic		C. prevents blood clotting
4. thrombolytic		D. narrows blood vessels
5. beta blocker		E. widens blood vessels
6. vasodilator		F. lowers blood cholesterol
7. diuretic		G. prevents abnormal heart rhythm
8. vasoconstrictor		H. dissolves blood clots

EXERCISE 9.8: APPLYING MEDICAL TERMINOLOGY

Fill in the missing medical terms to identify the pathway of blood through the heart and lungs.

Deoxygenated blood enters the right (1) _____ from the superior vena cava and the (2) _____. It then passes through the (3)_____ valve into the right ventricle. Blood then leaves this chamber via the (4) _____ valve and flows to the lungs via the right and left (5) _____ arteries. These are the only arteries in the body that carry (6) _____ blood. The blood is reoxygenated in the lungs and is returned to the left (7) _____ via the right and left (8) _____ veins. These are the only veins in the body to carry (9) _____ blood. Blood then enters the left (10) _____ through the (11) _____ valve. Blood leaves the heart through the (12) _____ valve and flows into the (13) _____, which is the largest artery in the body.

EXERCISE 9.9: PRONUNCIATION AND COMPREHENSION

Read the following paragraphs aloud to practise your pronunciation. Using your textbook and a medical dictionary, find the meanings of the underlined medical terms.

A 65-year-old man was admitted to hospital with a prolonged episode of central chest pain that had been present for 11 hours without any significant ECG change or cardiac enzyme rise. The pain had begun while he was having a glass of beer in the afternoon, but there were no gastrointestinal features. The pain was described as a central heaviness that radiated to the right hand. It was atypical in nature with pleuritic and positional elements and also exacerbation with change in posture and use of his arms. There was no associated diaphoresis, nausea or syncope. There was no ongoing exertional chest pain or dyspnoea. Exercise tolerance was normally limited by intermittent leg claudication.

Risk factors for ischaemic heart disease included hypertension, gout and a past history of smoking. He also admitted to heavy alcohol consumption.

On examination he had sinus tachycardia of 110/min and hypertension of 150/100. Pulses were symmetric and blood pressure equal in both upper arms. Heart sounds were dual, chest was clear, carotids were decreased in volume, but there were no associated bruits. Femoral pulses were also decreased in volume. There were well-maintained peripheral pulses. Abdomen was soft to palpation. There was marked chest wall tenderness that reproduced some of the pain.

EXERCISE 9.10: CROSSWORD PUZZLE

Complete the puzzle by providing the medical term for each of the clues below.

ACROSS

3. Controls the rhythmic beating of the heart (10, 4)
4. Takes blood from the heart to the lungs to collect oxygen (9, 6)
5. Receives deoxygenated blood returned from the upper part of the body through the superior vena cava and from the lower body through the inferior vena cava (5, 6)
7. Drooping of one or both cusps of the mitral valve into the left atrium (6, 5, 8)
8. The largest vessel in the body (5)
9. Netlike structure that connects the arteries and veins (9)

DOWN

1. A localised dilatation or ballooning of an arterial wall (8)
2. Carries deoxygenated blood from tissues to the heart (4)
3. A vessel that moves the blood from the heart to the remainder of the body (8, 6)
6. Acts as the pump to circulate blood throughout the body (5)

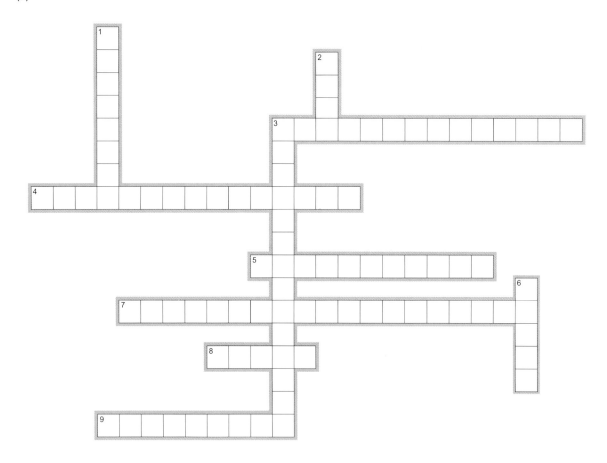

EXERCISE 9.11: ANAGRAMS

Work out each medical term from the jumbled letters below. Then, using the letters in brackets, determine the medical term that matches the description given.

1. ivne	__ __ __ (__)	vessel that takes blood to the heart
2. traoa	(__) __ __ __ __	the large artery that takes blood away from the heart
3. nnfartocii	__ (__) __ __ __ __ __ __ __ __	death of tissue due to a lack of oxygen
4. gbac	__ __ __ (__)	abbreviation for coronary artery bypass graft
5. yoacrmmiud	__ __ __ __ __ __ __ (__) __ __	the middle layer of the heart muscle
6. iiaaechms	__ __ __ __ __ __ __ __ (__)	lack of blood to a part of the heart

Rearrange the letters in brackets to form a word that means 'crushing chest pain'.

__ __ __ __ __ __

EXERCISE 9.12: DISCHARGE SUMMARY ANALYSIS

Read the discharge summary below and answer the questions.

UNIVERSITY HOSPITAL DISCHARGE SUMMARY	**UR number:** 141516
	Name: Barry Fredricks
	Address: 9 First Street, Downey Island
	Date of birth: 5/5/1942
	Sex: M
	Nominated primary healthcare provider: Dr Brian Lowerson

Episode details	**Discharge details**
Consultant: Dr Greyson	**Status:** Home
Registrar: Dr Clark	**Date of discharge:** 8/12/2020
Unit: Cardiac	
Admission source: Emergency department	
Date of admission: 29/11/2020	

Reason for admission / Presenting problems:
Palpitations, dyspnoea, continuing chest pain and breathlessness
Principal diagnosis: Ischaemic cardiomyopathy

Comorbidities:
Continuing angina
Left ventricular failure
Previous medical history:
Clinical synopsis:
Examination demonstrated a tendency towards hypotension, mildly elevated venous pressure, grossly displaced apex beat and pansystolic murmur consistent with mitral regurgitation. Third heart sound was present on auscultation. There was mild pitting oedema involving both ankles. Peripheries were cold on palpation.
During the patient's admission he was worked up with a further transthoracic echocardiogram. The doctor's opinion was that the patient had a severe ischaemic cardiomyopathy with an ejection fraction of less than 30% on formal testing. In view of the patient's continuing symptoms of severe cardiac failure together with his atrial fibrillation we have electively anticoagulated him. We have also introduced a low dose of diuretic.
Complications: Nil reported
Clinical interventions: Nil reported
Diagnostic interventions: Transthoracic echocardiogram
Medications at discharge:
Pepcidine 40 mg nocte
Pulmicort metered aerosol 200 ug 2 puffs b.d.
Digoxin PG 3 tablets mane
Aspirin 100 mg daily
Enalapril 50 mg b.d.
Transiderm patch 50 mg on 8 am off 10 pm
Isordil 5 mg q.i.d.
Diltiazem 60 mg t.d.s.
Lasix 40 mg q.d.
Warfarin 4 mg
Ceased medications: Nil reported
Allergies: Nil reported
Alerts: Nil reported
Arranged services: Nil reported
Recommendations: Patient is a candidate for ongoing medical management. Surgical re-vascularisation should not be considered in this patient.
Information to patient/relevant parties: To see GP for INR in 5 days. For review in cardiac outpatients in 6 weeks.
Authorising clinician: Dr Clark
Document recipients:
Patient and LMO: Dr Brian Lowerson

1. **Expand the following abbreviations as found in the discharge summary above.**

   40 mg nocte

   b.d.

   q.d.

   q.i.d.

   t.d.s.

2. **Under Recommendations it states that the 'patient is a candidate for ongoing medical management'. What does this mean?**

3. Mr Fredricks' principal diagnosis is ischaemic cardiomyopathy. What is this condition?

4. The summary states that Mr Fredricks was anticoagulated. What does this mean and why would it have been done?

5. Under the Clinical synopsis section, there is a statement that Mr Fredricks had a third heart sound present on auscultation. What is auscultation and what is a third heart sound?

CHAPTER 10

Respiratory System

Contents

OBJECTIVES   212

INTRODUCTION   213

NEW WORD ELEMENTS   213
  Combining forms   213
  Prefixes   214
  Suffixes   214

VOCABULARY   215

ABBREVIATIONS   216

FUNCTIONS AND STRUCTURE
OF THE RESPIRATORY SYSTEM   217
  Nose   217
  Pharynx   217
  Larynx   219
  Trachea   219
  Lungs   219
  Bronchi   219
  Alveoli   219

PATHOLOGY AND DISEASES   219

TESTS AND PROCEDURES   226

EXERCISES   231

Objectives

After completing this chapter you should be able to:

1. state the meanings of the word elements related to the respiratory system

2. build words using the word elements associated with the respiratory system

3. recognise, pronounce and effectively use medical terms associated with the respiratory system

4. expand abbreviations related to the respiratory system

5. describe the structure and functions of the respiratory system including the lungs, associated structures and the respiratory process

6. describe common pathological conditions associated with the respiratory system

7. describe common laboratory tests, diagnostic and surgical procedures associated with the respiratory system

8. apply what you have learned by interpreting medical terminology in practice.

Demonstrate your knowledge of the respiratory system by completing the exercises at the end of this chapter.

INTRODUCTION

The system that involves inspiration (also called inhalation or breathing in), expiration (also called exhalation or breathing out), exchange of gases in the lungs and the transport of gases between the lungs and body tissues is known as the respiratory system. Respiration (also known as ventilation) is the process of breathing in and out through this system.

All body cells require oxygen. Without it, they cannot survive. How does the body get oxygen? It is obtained from breathing in air, which the blood circulates to all parts of the body. The goal of breathing is to deliver oxygen to the cells of the body and to take away carbon dioxide and other waste gases. This exchange of gases is vital to life.

Functions of the respiratory system are very closely associated with the functions of many other body systems such as the cardiovascular system. This chapter will look at the medical terminology associated with the respiratory system.

NEW WORD ELEMENTS

To reinforce your learning, write the meanings of the medical terms in the spaces provided. Use the Glossary of medical terms on page 561 to help you work out the meanings. You may also need to check the meaning in a medical dictionary, but make an attempt yourself first.

Combining forms

Combining Form	Meaning	Medical Term	Meaning of Medical Term
adenoid/o	adenoids	adenoiditis	
alveol/o	alveolus, air sac	alveolar	
anthrac/o	black, coal	anthracosis	
bronch/i	bronchus	bronchiectasis	
bronch/o		bronchoscopy	
bronchiol/o	bronchiole	bronchiolitis	
capn/o	carbon dioxide	hypocapnia	
coni/o	dust	pneumoconiosis	
cost/o	rib	costochondritis	
cyan/o	blue	cyanosis	
epiglott/o	epiglottis	epiglottitis	
laryng/o	larynx, voice box	laryngectomy	
lob/o	lobe	lobectomy	
mediastin/o	mediastinum	mediastinitis	
nas/o	nose	nasal	
or/o	mouth	oropharyngeal	
orth/o	straight, upright	orthopnoea	
ox/i	oxygen	oximetry	
ox/o		hypoxaemia	
palat/o	palate	palatoplasty	
pector/o	chest	pectoralgia	
pharyng/o	pharynx, throat	pharyngitis	
phon/o	voice, sound	aphonia	
phren/o	diaphragm, mind	phrenoplegia	
pleur/o	pleura	pleuritic	
pneum/o	lungs, respiration, air, gas	pneumothorax	
pneumat/o		pneumatocoele	
pneumon/o		pneumonia	

Table continued

Combining Form	Meaning	Medical Term	Meaning of Medical Term
pulm/o	lungs	pulmography	
pulmon/o	—	pulmonary	
rhin/o	nose	rhinorrhoea	
sept/o	septum	septoplasty	
sinus/o	sinus, cavity	sinusitis	
spir/o	breathe	spirograph	
steth/o	chest	stethoscope	
tel/o	distant, end, far, complete	telemetry	
thorac/o	thorax, chest	thoracotomy	
tonsill/o *(Note: the word tonsil has one 'l', but the combining form tonsill/o has two)*	tonsils	tonsillitis	
trache/o	trachea	tracheostomy	
uvul/o	uvula, little grape	uvulectomy	

Prefixes

Prefix	Meaning	Medical Term	Meaning of Medical Term
a- an- *(used when the combining form starts with a vowel)*	no, not, without, absence of	apnoea anoxic	
brady-	slow	bradypnoea	
dys-	bad, painful, difficult	dysphonia	
em- *(used when the combining form starts with b, m or p)* en-	in	empyema encapsulate	
endo-	within, inside, inner	endotracheal	
inter-	between	intercostal	
tachy-	rapid, fast	tachypnoea	
tele-	distant, end, far, complete	telehealth	

Suffixes

Suffix	Meaning	Medical Term	Meaning of Medical Term
-capnia	condition of carbon dioxide	hypocapnia	
-centesis	surgical puncture to remove fluid	thoracocentesis	
-eal	pertaining to	pharyngeal	
-ectasia -ectasis	expansion, dilatation, stretching out	pharyngectasia bronchiectasis	
-ema	condition	erythema	
-osmia	condition of sense of smell	dysosmia	
-oxia	condition of oxygen	hypoxia	

Table continued

Suffix	Meaning	Medical Term	Meaning of Medical Term
-pnoea	breathing	dyspnoea	
-ptysis	spitting	haemoptysis	
-scope	instrument to view	bronchoscope	
-scopy	process of viewing	laryngoscopy	
-spasm	involuntary contraction	bronchospasm	
-thorax	pleural cavity, chest	haemopneumothorax	

VOCABULARY

The following list provides many of the medical terms used for the first time in this chapter. Pronunciations are provided with each term. As you read the rest of the chapter, make sure you identify each of these terms and understand their meanings.

Term	Pronunciation
allergic rhinitis	a-LER-jik ry-NY-tis
alveoli	al-vee-OL-eye
asthma	ASS-ma
auscultation	os-kul-TAY-shun
bronchioles	BRON-kee-olz
bronchitis	bron-KY-tis
bronchoscopy	bron-KOS-kop-ee
bronchus (bronchi)	BRON-kus (BRON-ky)
carbon dioxide	KAH-bon dy-OK-syd
chest x-ray	chest EKS-ray
chronic obstructive pulmonary disease	KRON-ik ob-STRUK-tiv PULL-mon-ah-ree diz-eez
computed tomography scan of the chest	kom-PYOO-ted to-MOG-ra-fee skan of the chest
continuous positive airway pressure	kon-TIN-yoo-us POZ-it-iv air-way PRESH-a
coryza	kor-EYE-za
cystic fibrosis	SIS-tik fy-BROH-sis
diaphragm	DY-a-fram
emphysema	em-fa-SEE-ma
endotracheal intubation	en-doh-trak-EE-al in-tyoo-BAY-shun
epiglottis	ep-ee-GLOT-is
exhalation	ex-ha-LAY-shun
influenza	in-floo-EN-za
inhalation	in-ha-LAY-shun
laryngitis	lar-in-JY-tis
laryngoscopy	la-ring-GOS-kop-ee

Table continued

Term	Pronunciation
larynx	LA-rinks
lobectomy	loh-BEK-tom-ee
lower respiratory tract	lo-wa res-PEER-at-or-ee trakt
lung	lung
lung biopsy	lung BY-op-see
lung cancer	lung KAN-sa
lung transplant	lung TRANS-plant
magnetic resonance imaging	mag-NET-ik rez-on-ans IM-a-jing
mediastinoscopy	mee-dee-AS-tin-OS-kop-ee
nose	noze
oxygen	OK-see-jen
parietal pleura	pa-RY-et-al PLOO-ra
percussion	per-KUSH-en
pharynx	FA-rinks
pleura	PLOO-ra
pleural cavity	PLOO-ral KAV-it-ee
pleural effusion	PLOO-ral ef-YOO-shun
pneumoconiosis	NYOO-moh-kon-ee-OH-sis
pneumonectomy	nyoo-mon-EK-tom-ee
pneumonia	NYOO-moh-nee-a
pneumothorax	NYOO-moh-THOR-aks
positron emission tomography	POZ-i-tron e-MISH-en to-MOG-raf-ee
pulmonary angiography	PULL-mon-ah-ree an-jee-OG-raf-ee
pulmonary function tests	PULL-mon-ah-ree FUNK-shun tests
pulmonary oedema	PULL-mon-ah-ree e-DEE-ma
respiration	res-pir-AY-shun
thoracocentesis	thor-a-koh-sen-TEE-sis
thoracoscopy	thor-a-KOS-kop-ee
thoracotomy	thor-a-KOT-om-ee

Table continued

Term	Pronunciation
tonsils	TON-silz
trachea	tra-KEE-a
tracheostomy	tra-kee-OS-tom-ee
tube thoracostomy	tyoob thor-a-KOS-tom-ee
tuberculin test	too-BERK-yoo-lin test
tuberculosis	too-BERK-yoo-LOH-sis
upper respiratory tract infection	up-pa res-PEER-at-or-ee trakt in-fek-shun
upper respiratory tract	up-pa res-PEER-at-or-ee trakt
ventilation perfusion scan	ven-til-AY-shun per-FYOO-shun skan
visceral pleura	VISS-er-al PLOO-ra

ABBREVIATIONS

The following abbreviations are commonly used in the Australian healthcare environment. Because some abbreviations can have more than one meaning, check the context in which the abbreviation is used before assigning a meaning to it.

Abbreviation	Definition
ABGs	arterial blood gases
AFB	acid fast bacilli
ARDS	acute/adult respiratory distress syndrome
ARF	acute respiratory failure
BiPAP	bilevel positive airway pressure
BS	breath sounds
CAL	chronic airways limitation
COAD	chronic obstructive airways disease
COLD	chronic obstructive lung disease
COPD	chronic obstructive pulmonary disease
COVID-19	coronavirus disease
CF	cystic fibrosis
CNPV	continuous negative pressure ventilation
CO_2	carbon dioxide
CPAP	continuous positive airways pressure
CPR	cardiopulmonary resuscitation

Table continued

Abbreviation	Definition
CT	computed tomography
CVS	continuous ventilatory support
CXR	chest x-ray
DOE	dyspnoea on exertion
ENT	ear nose and throat
ETT	endotracheal tube
FEV_1	forced expiratory volume in 1 second
FNA	fine needle aspiration
FVC	forced vital capacity
ICC	intercostal catheter
IMV	intermittent mandatory ventilation
IPPB	intermittent positive-pressure breathing
IPPV	intermittent positive-pressure ventilation
JVP	jugular venous pressure
LLL	left lower lobe (of lung)
LUL	left upper lobe (of lung)
MERS-CoV	Middle East respiratory syndrome coronavirus
MRI	magnetic resonance imaging
N	nitrogen
NIMV	non-invasive mask ventilation
NIPV	non-invasive pressure ventilation
NIV	non-invasive ventilation
O_2	oxygen
PCP	*Pneumocystis carinii* pneumonia
PE	pulmonary embolism
PET	positron emission tomography
PFR	peak flow rate
PND	paroxysmal nocturnal dyspnoea
RDS	respiratory distress syndrome
RLL	right lower lobe (of lung)
RR	respiratory rate
RUL	right upper lobe (of lung)
SARS	severe acute respiratory syndrome
SIMV	synchronised intermittent mandatory ventilation

Table continued

Abbreviation	Definition
SOB	shortness of breath
SOBOE	shortness of breath on exertion
T&A	tonsils and adenoids
TB	tuberculosis
URTI	upper respiratory tract infection
V/Q scan	ventilation perfusion scan

FUNCTIONS AND STRUCTURE OF THE RESPIRATORY SYSTEM

The major function of the respiratory system is respiration, or the exchange of gases between the external environment and the circulatory system. Erythrocytes are responsible for transporting haemoglobin, which carries oxygen to the body cells.

Around one-sixth of the air in the lungs is exchanged for new air with every breath. This exchange, known as external respiration, provides oxygenation of the blood and therefore the body cells, with an associated removal of carbon dioxide and other gaseous metabolic wastes from the cells. Within the brain, the respiratory centre controls the process of respiration. The exchange of gases occurs at the level of the alveoli, the smallest branches of the respiratory system. The walls of the alveoli are almost transparent (approximately 0.2 micrometres thick) and are located adjacent to the tiny capillaries of the cardiovascular system. The gas–blood membrane between the alveolar space and the pulmonary capillaries is extremely thin, allowing for the exchange of gases by diffusion in the presence of pressure differences. Molecules of carbon dioxide move from the erythrocytes in the capillaries through the membrane into the alveoli. At the same time the oxygen molecules pass through the membrane from the inhaled air into the erythrocytes. When the atmospheric pressure is low outside, the air from the lungs flows out. When the air pressure is low inside, then the opposite phenomenon occurs. As gas exchange occurs, the acid–base balance of the body is maintained through the process of homeostasis. The diaphragm, a sheet of muscles positioned across the base of the thoracic cavity, and the intercostal muscles between the ribs contract and relax, pulling air into the lungs and pumping waste products out.

Haemoglobin in the erythrocytes moves around the bloodstream carrying oxygen to the cells of the body. In the cells, there is another respiratory process known as internal or cellular respiration. This occurs when oxygen is released from the blood to tissues or cells and carbon dioxide is absorbed by the blood. Once inside the cells, the oxygen is metabolised to produce energy.

The upper respiratory tract, which includes the nose, pharynx, larynx and trachea, is the passageway for oxygen and carbon dioxide during inhalation and exhalation. The actual gas exchange process takes place in the lower respiratory tract, consisting of the bronchi, lungs and alveolar sacs.

Oxygen enters the respiratory system through the mouth and the nose and then passes through the larynx and the trachea. The larynx is responsible for producing sound and also protects the upper part of the trachea. The larynx is located just below the part of the pharynx which splits into the trachea (which carries air to the lower respiratory tract) and the oesophagus (which carries food and fluid to the digestive tract). A flap of cartilage known as the epiglottis closes over the glottal folds of the larynx during the process of swallowing, preventing food from entering the trachea, which would cause choking. The folds of vocal cords in the larynx are funnel-shaped and have cartilaginous walls and a sophisticated muscle system that allows us to produce various sounds. The upper respiratory tract has an important function in moistening and warming air before it reaches the lungs.

The structures of the respiratory system are as follows (see also Figs 10.1 and 10.2).

Nose

The nose is responsible for the process of olfaction or the sense of smell. In addition to this, it filters the air that is inhaled through it, removing dust, pathogens and irritants by trapping them in the cilia or soft hairs on the inside of the nostrils. It also helps to warm and moisten the air to prevent the remainder of the respiratory tract from drying out. Sneezing is usually caused by foreign particles irritating the nasal mucosa.

Pharynx

The pharynx is divided into three parts known as the nasopharynx, oropharynx and laryngopharynx. The nasopharynx lies behind the nose and above the soft palate. Within the nasopharynx is the pendulous uvula.

The mouth leads into the oropharynx. The walls of the oropharynx are lined with mucous membrane that has adapted to handling food as well as air. It is here that the two types of tonsils are located. The human palatine tonsils and the nasopharyngeal tonsils (also known as the adenoids) are both made up of lymphoepithelial tissues and are believed to have a role in defending the body against inhaled or swallowed pathogens. This process is currently poorly understood.

The laryngopharynx is the common pathway for both air and food and connects to the oesophagus.

Figure 10.1 Structures of the respiratory system

(Mosby's Dictionary 2014)

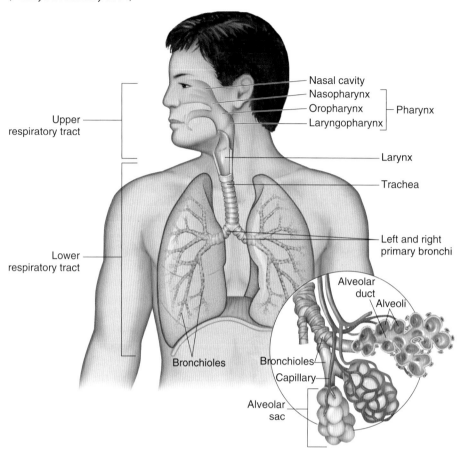

Figure 10.2 Upper respiratory system

(Mosby's Dictionary 2014)

NASAL PASSAGES AND THROAT

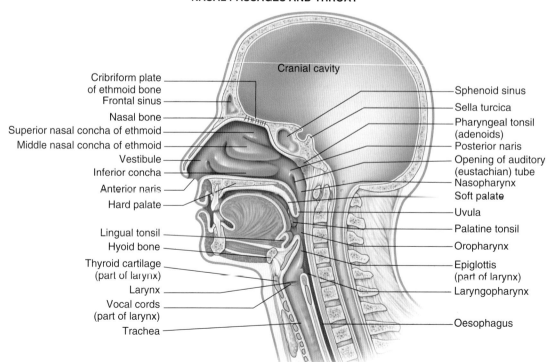

Larynx

As noted above, the larynx contains the vocal cords and the epiglottis (which acts to protect the trachea from inhaled and swallowed food, foreign objects and particles). The larynx also includes rings of cartilage called thyroid, arytenoid and cricoid cartilage. The laryngeal prominence of the thyroid cartilage is more prominent in males. It is commonly called the Adam's apple.

Trachea

The trachea in an adult is approximately 10 centimetres in length and 2.5 centimetres in diameter. It comprises C-shaped cartilage linked by ligaments extending from the larynx to the bronchi at approximately the level of the 4th or 5th thoracic vertebrae.

Lungs

The lungs take up most of the thoracic cavity and are protected by 12 ribs on either side of the cavity. Although they are similar in appearance, the lungs are not identical. Both are separated into lobes, with three lobes in the right lung and two in the left. These five lobes are further divided into segments and then into lobules. Together, the lungs contain approximately 2400 kilometres of airways and around 600 million alveoli surrounded by capillaries. The reason for the left lung having two and not three lobes is so that there is enough space in the left of the thoracic cavity for the heart.

The thoracic cavity includes the mediastinum and pleural cavity. The heart and major vessels are located in the mediastinum. On either side of the mediastinum is the specific part of the thoracic cavity where the lungs are located, known as the pleural cavity. There is a membrane that covers the thoracic cavity known as the parietal pleura and another covering the lungs called the visceral pleura. A small amount of fluid normally fills the gap between the parietal and visceral pleural layers. This fluid lubricates the surface of the layers to prevent friction when the lungs move within the thoracic cavity.

Bronchi

The trachea splits into two similarly structured tubes, known as the right and the left bronchi, at a position known as the carina. The bronchi are made up of rings of hyaline membrane, which become irregular and also become smaller until the tubes are approximately 1 millimetre in diameter, when the cartilage disappears. Smooth muscle covers the length of the bronchi. This muscle becomes thicker when the hyaline membrane stops at the level of the bronchioles. The bronchioles branch into smaller and smaller passageways until they terminate in tiny air sacs called alveoli.

Alveoli

The alveoli are the final branches of the respiratory tract and act as the primary gas exchange units of the lungs. They are shaped like bunches of grapes.

PATHOLOGY AND DISEASES

The following section provides a list of some of the most common diseases and pathological conditions relevant to the respiratory system.

Term	Pronunciation	Definition
allergic rhinitis	a-LER-jik ry-NY-tis	Allergic rhinitis is better known as hay fever. It is a condition in which the nasal mucous membranes and the eyes become itchy and inflamed after exposure to allergens such as animal dander, dust mites, mould spores, pollens, certain foods and tobacco smoke. It is best to avoid exposure to the allergens to prevent the rhinitis from occurring. Medication such as antihistamines may be given to treat individual symptoms and lessen the allergic response.
asthma	ASS-ma	Asthma is a chronic inflammatory condition of the airways characterised by airway obstruction (Fig 10.3). Asthma causes bronchoconstriction, shortness of breath, wheezing and chest tightness and increased mucus production and coughing. Similar to allergic rhinitis, asthma symptoms can be triggered by inhaling allergens such as animal dander, dust mites, mould spores, pollens, certain chemicals and tobacco smoke. Other factors such as cold weather, exercise, stressful situations and respiratory infections can also trigger an attack of asthma. During an asthma attack a person may experience cyanosis, tachycardia, difficulty breathing and severe anxiety.

Table continued

Term	Pronunciation	Definition
		Patients should try to avoid exposure to allergens or factors that can trigger an attack. There are two types of treatment for asthma: drugs such as corticosteroids to prevent an attack and quick-relief drugs such as bronchodilators for use during an attack.
		The complications of poorly controlled and/or inadequately treated asthma can be severe. Patients may experience a persistent cough, inability to exercise or perform activities of daily living, permanent lung damage and even death.
		Figure 10.3 Asthma (Thibodeau & Patton 2007) ![Asthma diagram] Oedema of respiratory mucosa and excessive mucus production obstruct airways. Smooth muscle constriction Mucus Mucus plug Hyperinflation of alveoli
bronchitis	bron-KY-tis	Bronchitis is an inflammation of the bronchi. There are two main types of bronchitis: acute and chronic. **Acute bronchitis** is caused by a bacterial infection or, more commonly, a viral infection. Exposure to tobacco smoke, air pollution, dust and fumes can also cause acute bronchitis. Symptoms include a productive cough, shortness of breath, wheezing, and chest tightness due to obstruction of the bronchi. Acute bronchitis is usually self-limiting, with most people recovering within a few days. Treatments such as rest, fluids and a bronchodilator can help relieve symptoms. Antibiotics are only effective for bacterial infections.
		Chronic bronchitis is the chronic inflammation of the bronchi. It is defined as a persistent productive cough that occurs for at least 3 months per year for 2 consecutive years. It is one of the components of chronic obstructive pulmonary disease (COPD). Symptoms, treatment and prognosis are the same as for COPD.
chronic obstructive pulmonary disease (COPD)	KRON-ik ob-STRUK-tiv PULL-mon-ah-ree diz-eez	COPD is also known as chronic obstructive airways disease (COAD), chronic obstructive lung disease (COLD) and chronic airways limitation (CAL). COPD usually refers to combinations of chronic bronchitis, asthma and emphysema resulting in destruction of the lung tissues. Tobacco smoking or inhalation of industrial pollutants are the usual causes.
		Symptoms of COPD are the same as for emphysema: dyspnoea, wheezing, a productive cough, recurrent chest infections, hypoxia and cyanosis due to poor oxygenation. Heart failure often occurs because the heart has to pump harder to circulate blood to the lungs.

Table continued

Term	Pronunciation	Definition
		While COPD is irreversible, there are several treatment strategies that can be implemented to improve quality of life. Because emphysema is a major component of COPD, the treatments are very similar. It is essential that patients cease smoking. Medications such as bronchodilators, antibiotics and anti-inflammatory drugs are given to improve the symptoms. Pulmonary rehabilitation to assist with maximising a person's remaining lung function is often given. Oxygen therapy is frequently required.
cystic fibrosis (CF)	SIS-tik fy-BROH-sis	Technically, CF is an endocrine disorder, but because the manifestation of progressive lung disease is the predominant cause of illness and death, it is included in this text in the respiratory chapter. CF also affects exocrine glands (sweat glands, pancreas). In CF, thick mucus secretions clog the bronchi in the lungs and ducts from the pancreas and intestines. CF is a recessive genetic condition affecting chromosome 7. The causes of associated problems include chronic bacterial infections (*Pseudomonas aeruginosa* is a common infective agent) and inflammation, resulting in repeated exacerbations and episodes of intense breathing problems. Recurrent infections and blockages can result in irreversible lung damage (Fig. 10.4) and death. Additionally, sweat glands in CF sufferers are unable to absorb salt back into the blood, leaving more than usual amounts of salt in the sweat. Because the level of salt in the blood is not elevated, the patient does not feel thirsty and therefore does not increase their fluid consumption to compensate. This leads to increased risk of dehydration. Signs and symptoms vary depending on the severity and degree of infection but include: a productive cough; a barrel-shaped chest; recurrent respiratory, gastrointestinal and nutritional problems; and extreme weakness due to salt loss. **Figure 10.4 Damaged lung due to cystic fibrosis** (Kumar et al 2005)

Table continued

Term	Pronunciation	Definition
		In Australia, all babies are screened at birth for this genetic disorder. This allows for early treatment, which leads to a better long-term prognosis. Treatment has also improved greatly over the past few decades. Patients now have access to new and improved antibiotics, inhaled bronchodilators, other medications such as steroids and pancreatic enzymes, advanced techniques in chest physiotherapy to dislodge lung secretions, a better understanding of nutritional requirements (high-fat and high-kilojoule intake) and, more recently, single/double/triple heart-lung-liver transplantation. These treatments have resulted in a much-improved life expectancy for CF sufferers. With advances in gene therapy, it is hoped that, in the future, CF may become preventable.
emphysema	em-fa-SEE-ma	Emphysema is a chronic obstructive disease affecting the lungs and bronchi. It is characterised by an abnormal permanent enlargement of the alveoli with a resulting loss of elasticity in the alveolar walls. This affects gaseous exchange, resulting in severe shortness of breath. Tobacco smoking is the most important risk factor in developing the disease. Almost all patients have a long history of smoking or, in some cases, inhalation of industrial pollutants. Symptoms of emphysema include shortness of breath, frequent chest infections, productive cough, generalised fatigue and cyanosis due to a lack of oxygen. Complications of emphysema can include pneumonia, a collapsed lung and heart problems. A multi-focused treatment plan is required. It is essential that patients stop smoking. Medications such as bronchodilators, antibiotics and anti-inflammatory drugs are given. Exercise to improve overall fitness and lung capacity is encouraged. In advanced cases, oxygen therapy may be required. Emphysema often occurs with chronic bronchitis and asthma as part of COPD.
influenza	in-floo-ENZ-a	Influenza, commonly known as 'the flu', is a contagious viral infection of the respiratory tract. It is passed from person to person by droplets produced by sneezing or coughing. Influenza tends to occur mostly in the colder months. Symptoms include a high fever, myalgia, headache and severe malaise. Some patients will have a non-productive cough, pharyngitis and rhinitis. Influenza tends to be self-limiting, with most patients recovering within 1–2 weeks without medical treatment. In susceptible people such as babies, the elderly or those with underlying medical conditions, complications such as pneumonia and even death can occur. Each year, different strains of influenza appear. Vaccinations are developed for each strain.
laryngitis	lar-in-JY-tis	Laryngitis is a swelling and inflammation of the larynx, usually associated with dysphonia or aphonia. It is a type of URTI. Acute laryngitis is usually caused by a cold or other virus and resolves quickly without any treatment except rest. Because laryngitis is usually caused by a virus, antibiotics have no effect. Chronic laryngitis can be caused by recurrent allergic rhinitis, asthma, sinusitis, heavy smoking, excessive use of the voice, or GORD (gastro-oesophageal reflux disease) caused when gastric acid flows back into the oesophagus. Treatment of the underlying cause will help the laryngitis to resolve.

Table continued

Term	Pronunciation	Definition
lung cancer	lung KAN-sa	Lung cancer is also called bronchogenic carcinoma. It is a common cancer in both males and females in Australia and there are four main histological types. Small cell carcinoma (20% of all lung cancers) is the most aggressive and rapidly growing of all lung cancers. Squamous cell carcinoma (50%), adenocarcinoma (20%) and large cell anaplastic carcinoma (10%) are the other main types. Tobacco smoking is the most common cause of lung cancer, particularly small cell carcinoma, but other factors such as inhaling irritants such as asbestos or the presence of other lung diseases such as COPD or tuberculosis also contribute to the incidence of this disease. Signs and symptoms include a persistent cough, haemoptysis, dyspnoea and weight loss. Diagnosis is normally by chest x-ray, CT scan, MRI, bronchoscopy, sputum culture and lung biopsy. Treatment may involve a combination of surgery, radiation therapy and chemotherapy. Lung cancers can be very difficult to treat because they tend to metastasise early. The most common sites for metastatic spread include the liver, brain, bone and adrenal glands. The lung is also a common site for metastases from tumours originating in other sites.
pleural effusion	PLOO-ral ef-YOO-shun	A pleural effusion is the presence of excess fluid between the two layers of the pleura surrounding the lungs. Normally the pleural space contains about 20 millilitres of fluid that acts as a lubricant between the two layers of membranes. Any significant increase in the quantity of pleural fluid is a pleural effusion. Congestive cardiac failure and lung diseases such as cancer, pneumonia, tuberculosis and drug reactions are the most common causes of pleural effusion. Patients may experience chest pain and dyspnoea. However, many pleural effusions cause no symptoms and are discovered as an incidental finding on a chest x-ray. Treatment may include thoracocentesis to drain the excess fluid. The cause of the effusion also needs to be treated. For example, diuretics may be given to treat congestive cardiac failure or antibiotics given for an infection.
pneumoconiosis	NYOO-moh-kon-ee-oh-sis	Pneumoconiosis is a generic term used to describe any lung disease caused by inhaling dust or chemical irritants over a prolonged period of time. This inhalation usually occurs in the workplace when appropriate protective clothing or equipment is not worn. The most common of these diseases is asbestosis. Exposure to asbestos dust most commonly occurs in the mining, building and shipbuilding industries. It takes many years for the symptoms of asbestosis to develop. The disease is caused by an accumulation of asbestos in the lungs, resulting in interstitial fibrosis and scarring of the lungs. Mesothelioma is a malignant tumour arising most commonly in the pleura and is associated with asbestos exposure. Another common disease caused by inhaling dust fibres is silicosis. This type of pneumoconiosis occurs in people exposed to silica in industries such as mining, quarrying, sand blasting, stone cutting and pottery. Silicosis leads to fibrosis of the lungs, which eventually impairs the functioning of the lungs. It is further exacerbated by tobacco smoking. Pneumoconiosis is a fully preventable disease if adequate safety measures are followed in the relevant industries.

Table continued

Term	Pronunciation	Definition
pneumonia	NYOO-moh-nee-a	Pneumonia is an acute inflammation of the lungs affecting one or both sides of the chest, often occurring as a result of an infection (Fig. 10.5). The infection can be caused by several different microorganisms such as bacteria (pneumococci, staphylococci), viruses (e.g. respiratory syncytial virus), fungi (e.g. histoplasmosis) and parasites or by inhaling chemicals, smoke or dust. Aspiration pneumonia is caused by foreign matter such as food stuffs or vomitus entering the respiratory tract. Lobar pneumonia involves one or more entire lobes; bronchopneumonia involves patchy consolidation in the lung parenchyma. Diagnosis of pneumonia is by chest x-ray and sputum culture. Treatment includes antibiotics, oxygen and physiotherapy.

Figure 10.5 Pneumonia
A. Normal PA chest x-ray; **B.** X-ray of lung with pneumonia

(Adam et al 2007)

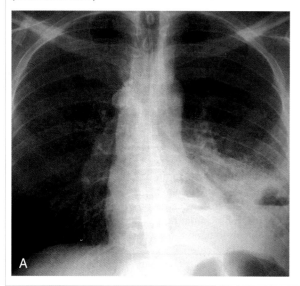 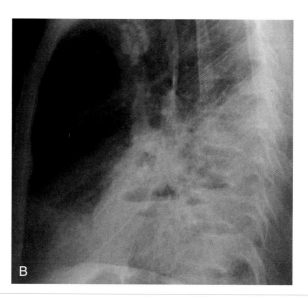

Term	Pronunciation	Definition
pneumothorax	NYOO-moh-thor-aks	A pneumothorax (also called a collapsed lung) is a collection of air or gas in the pleural space. This puts pressure on the lung, preventing it from expanding properly. It can be spontaneous or traumatic. A spontaneous pneumothorax can occur as a result of an existing lung disease (secondary pneumothorax) or due to the rupture of a bulla (an air-filled sac in the lungs). A traumatic pneumothorax occurs as a result of a puncture wound – such as a stabbing, rib fracture or blunt force injury – that causes the lung to collapse. Occasionally it can also be a complication of a medical procedure. A pneumothorax may be treated conservatively to see if it resolves on its own, but in many cases the patient will require an intercostal catheter to drain the air to help the lung re-inflate. A pneumothorax should not be confused with a **haemothorax** (Fig. 10.6), which is the collection of blood and fluid in the pleural cavity between the parietal and visceral pleura. This is usually the result of trauma.

Table continued

Term	Pronunciation	Definition
Figure 10.6 Haemothorax and pneumothorax		

Term	Pronunciation	Definition
pulmonary oedema	PULL-mon-ah-ree e-DEE-ma	Pulmonary oedema occurs when the alveoli fill with fluid instead of air, preventing oxygen from being absorbed into the bloodstream. It is usually due to left ventricular failure or congestive cardiac failure when the left ventricle cannot pump out all the blood it receives from the lungs, meaning that pressure builds up in the left atrium, then in the veins and finally in the capillaries. This causes fluid to be forced through the capillary walls into the alveoli. It is characterised by tachypnoea, dyspnoea, cyanosis, hypertension, tachycardia and peripheral oedema. Pulmonary oedema is potentially a life-threatening condition. The cause needs to be urgently identified and treated.
tuberculosis (TB)	too-BERK-yoo-LOH-sis	TB is a highly contagious infection caused by a bacterium called *Mycobacterium tuberculosis*, transmitted by inhaling airborne droplets. It is most prevalent in areas that are overcrowded and where inhabitants have poor health care and poor nutrition, such as among the homeless, in refugee camps and prisons. It is also common in patients with HIV/AIDS.
		In the early stages there are very few symptoms. As the disease progresses, patients may experience a productive cough, haemoptysis, fatigue, fever, weight loss, swollen lymph nodes and night sweats. Treatment must be thorough because the disease can recur. It normally involves a combination of several drugs continuing for several months.
		If treatment is not adequate, TB can disseminate throughout the body into the bones, the central nervous system, the gastrointestinal system, genitourinary tract and the kidneys causing secondary infections and functional abnormalities. Adequate public health measures need to be introduced to eliminate TB in the population. These include education on preventative strategies, screening of susceptible groups, vaccination against TB and appropriate treatment of infected individuals, including through the internationally recommended Directly Observed Treatment Short course (DOTS) strategy.

Table continued

Term	Pronunciation	Definition
upper respiratory tract infection (URTI)	up-pa res-PEER-at-or-ee trakt in-fek-shun	URTI is a generalised term used to describe any acute infection of the nose, paranasal sinuses, pharynx, larynx or trachea. The most frequently occurring URTI is the common cold or coryza. Other infections include rhinitis, pharyngitis, sinusitis, epiglottitis, laryngitis and tracheitis. Doctors often just use the term URTI to include any, or all, of these infections. Most URTIs are due to a viral infection.

TESTS AND PROCEDURES

The following section provides a list of common diagnostic tests and procedures, clinical interventions and surgical procedures that are undertaken for the respiratory system.

Test/procedure	Pronunciation	Definition
auscultation	os-kul-TAY-shun	Auscultation is the process of listening to the sounds within the body using a stethoscope. It is used to diagnose conditions of the respiratory, cardiovascular and digestive systems as well as assessing a fetus during pregnancy.
bronchoscopy	bron-KOS-kop-ee	Bronchoscopy is a procedure that allows for visual examination of the bronchi and for the sampling of tissue via biopsy. The bronchoscope (either rigid or flexible) is inserted into the bronchi via the pharynx, larynx and trachea (Fig. 10.7).

Figure 10.7 Bronchoscopy

(Elkin et al 2007)

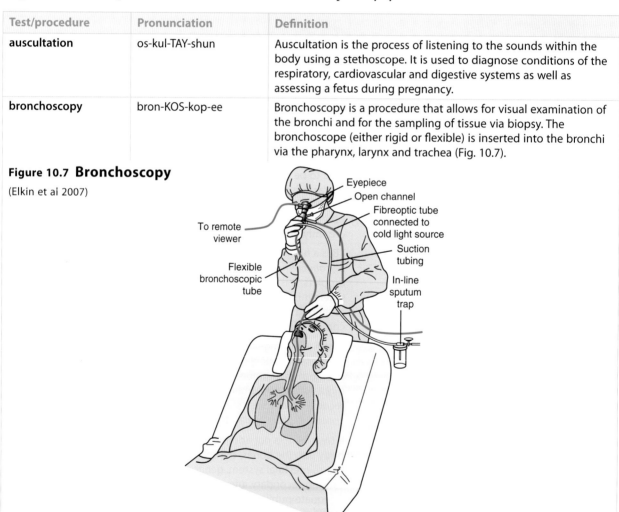

Table continued

Test/procedure	Pronunciation	Definition
chest x-ray	chest EKS-ray	A chest x-ray involves taking radiographic images of the thoracic cavity by passing small amounts of ionising radiation through the body and recording the resultant images on a computer or film. The two most common views of the thorax are taken in the coronal plane (images taken from the anterior–posterior view or posterior–anterior view) and those taken in the sagittal plane (taking a lateral view).
computed tomography (CT) of the chest	kom-PYOO-ted to-MOG-ra-fee	A CT is a diagnostic test to identify disorders of the thoracic structures. Cross-sectional images are taken using a digital computer in conjunction with x-ray beams.
endotracheal intubation	en-doh-trak-EE-al in-tyoo-BAY-shun	Endotracheal intubation involves placing a tube into the trachea to ensure an open airway in patients who are unconscious or unable to breathe on their own. Anaesthetics, or other gaseous medications, can be delivered through the tube. It also provides the opportunity to place the patient on a ventilator if necessary.
laryngoscopy	la-rin-GOS-kop-ee	A laryngoscopy is a procedure that allows the larynx to be examined using a lighted scope called a laryngoscope.
lobectomy	loh-BEK-tom-ee	This is the process of removing a lobe of a lung (Fig. 10.8).
lung biopsy	lung BY-op-see	A lung biopsy involves collecting tissue from the lung for microscopic examination. It is usually done to identify the cause of an abnormality identified on x-ray or scans.
lung transplant	lung TRANZ-plant	A lung transplant is a surgical procedure that involves removing a diseased lung and replacing it with a donor lung. The transplant may involve one or both lungs and can also be done in conjunction with a heart transplant.
magnetic resonance imaging (MRI)	mag-NET-ik REZ-on-ans IM-a-jing	An MRI is a diagnostic test that creates images of the interior of the body using radio waves and a magnetic field. An MRI of the thoracic cavity helps identify lesions in soft tissues, such as the lungs, that cannot be easily noted on a chest x-ray.
mediastinoscopy	mee-dee-AS-tin-OS-kop-ee	A mediastinoscopy is a surgical procedure performed by making an incision into the neck, just above the sternum, and inserting a thin scope to examine the inside of the mediastinum, which is the middle section of the chest cavity that contains all of the thoracic organs other than the lungs.
percussion	per-KUSH-en	Percussion is a technique used in clinical examinations to determine the density of underlying structures of the chest and abdomen. It is done by tapping on the surface of the chest or abdomen to listen to the resonance or feel the vibrations from the underlying structures.

Table continued

Test/procedure	Pronunciation	Definition
pneumonectomy	nyoo-mo-NEK-to-mee	A pneumonectomy is a surgical procedure that involves resecting a lung, which may also include removing mediastinal nodes (Fig. 10.8). **Figure 10.8 Pneumonectomy and lobectomy** (Shiland 2006) 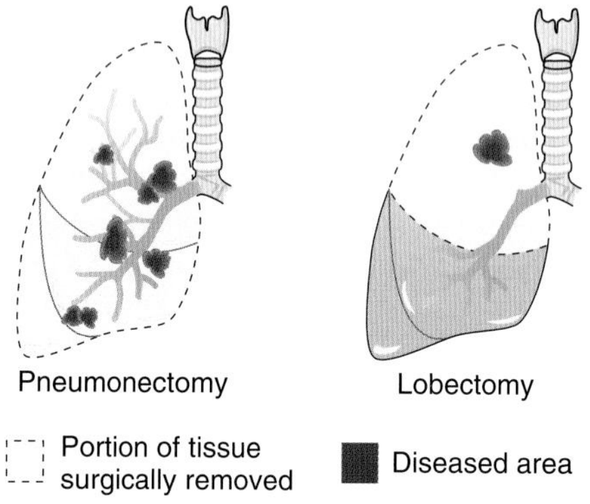 Pneumonectomy Lobectomy Portion of tissue surgically removed Diseased area
positron emission tomography (PET)	POZ-i-tron e-MISH-en to-MOG-raf-ee	A PET scan is a non-invasive nuclear medicine imaging technique that produces three-dimensional images of the chest.
pulmonary angiography	PULL-mon-ah-ree an-jee-OG-raf-ee	Pulmonary angiography uses radio-opaque contrast material to record x-ray images of pulmonary circulation to identify obstructions or pathological conditions, including pulmonary emboli.
pulmonary function tests	PULL-mon-ah-ree FUNK-shun tests	Pulmonary function tests are a group of tests used to measure how well the lungs take in and release air and how well they move gases such as oxygen from the atmosphere into the body's circulation. They are undertaken to: diagnose certain types of lung disease such as asthma, bronchitis and emphysema; identify the cause of shortness of breath; and measure whether contaminants have affected lung function.
thoracocentesis	thor-a-koh-sen-TEE-sis	A thoracocentesis is a surgical procedure that involves removing fluid from the pleural cavity following incision. It can be performed as a method of diagnosis or to drain fluid from a pleural effusion.
thoracoscopy	thor-a-KOS-kop-ee	A thoracoscopy is a procedure that allows a visual examination of the pleural and thoracic cavities via a thoracoscope. It is used to obtain biopsies or for the resection of lesions.
thoracotomy	thor-a-KOT-om-ee	A thoracotomy is a surgical procedure involving an incision into the chest to allow access to the thoracic organs. It is the method of entry for procedures such as lung resections.

Table continued

Test/procedure	Pronunciation	Definition
tracheostomy	trak-ee-OS-tom-ee	A tracheostomy involves making an incision into the trachea to insert a tube, creating an artificial airway (Fig. 10.9).

Figure 10.9 Tracheostomy

(Blamb/Shutterstock)

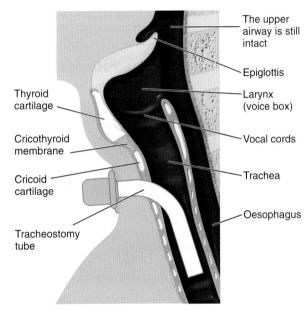

The upper airway is still intact

Epiglottis

Thyroid cartilage

Larynx (voice box)

Cricothyroid membrane

Vocal cords

Cricoid cartilage

Trachea

Tracheostomy tube

Oesophagus

Test/procedure	Pronunciation	Definition
tube thoracostomy	tyoob thor-a-KOS-tom-ee	A tube thoracostomy is a procedure that involves inserting an intercostal catheter into the pleural space following an incision into the chest wall. The tube acts as a mechanism for draining a pleural effusion.
tuberculin test	too-BERK-yoo-lin test	A tuberculin test is also known as a Mantoux test. It is done to identify infection (either old or current) by tuberculosis. It is performed by injecting a tuberculin intradermally and measuring the skin response at 48 hours and 72 hours.
ventilation–perfusion (V/Q) scan	ven-til-AY-shun-per-FYOO-shun skan	A V/Q scan is used to measure the flow of air (ventilation) and the flow of blood (perfusion) into the lung by using inhaled and injected radioactive material. This form of scan is generally performed to identify blockages in the vessels such as those caused by a pulmonary embolism.
ventilatory support (mechanical ventilation)	ven-til-AY-tor-ee suh-port (meh-KAN-i-kal ven-til-AY-shun)	Ventilatory support (mechanical ventilation) is administered via invasive or noninvasive devices to assist or replace a patient's own respiratory efforts. **Continuous ventilatory support** (CVS) refers to ventilation provided after inserting an invasive artificial airway such as an endotracheal or tracheostomy tube.

Table continued

Test/procedure	Pronunciation	Definition
		Continuous positive airway pressure (CPAP) is a type of ventilation therapy that allows air to be delivered into the upper airways through a nasal mask or pillow to deliver pressurised air to ensure that the airways remain open. CPAP is used to treat patients with breathing problems such as sleep apnoea or infants with respiratory distress syndrome or bronchopulmonary dysplasia. It is also used as a weaning stage for patients coming off mechanical ventilation. CPAP can be delivered invasively or noninvasively. **Figure 10.10 Patient sleeping with CPAP machine** (Amy Walters/Fotolia.com) **Bilevel positive airway pressure** (BiPAP) is a noninvasive ventilation therapy using a machine that has one pressure level for inhalation and a lower pressure for exhalation. Increased pressure is applied when the patient inhales to keep the airways from closing during sleep and provides a lower pressure during exhalation that continues to maintain an open airway. BiPAP has been designed to be administered noninvasively via mask ventilators but can also be administered invasively. **Intermittent positive pressure breathing** (IPB), **intermittent positive pressure ventilation** (IPPV), **noninvasive mask ventilation** (NIMV) and **noninvasive pressure ventilation** (NIPV) are all forms of noninvasive ventilatory support used to deliver aerosol medications or to augment lung expansion. **Controlled mechanical ventilation**, **intermittent mandatory ventilation** (IMV) and **synchronised intermittent mandatory ventilation** (SIMV) are all forms of ventilatory support that record a patient's breathing rate and synchronise the patient's own respiration rate with the volume of air provided by the ventilator. This type of ventilation is always administered using an endotracheal or tracheostomy tube and therefore is always invasive. **Continuous negative pressure ventilation** (CNPV) is a form of ventilation not commonly used and is administered by applying negative pressure on the outside of the patient's chest, expanding the lungs to facilitate airflow.

Exercises

EXERCISE 10.1: LABEL THE DIAGRAM

Using the information provided in this chapter, label the anatomical parts in Fig. 10.11.

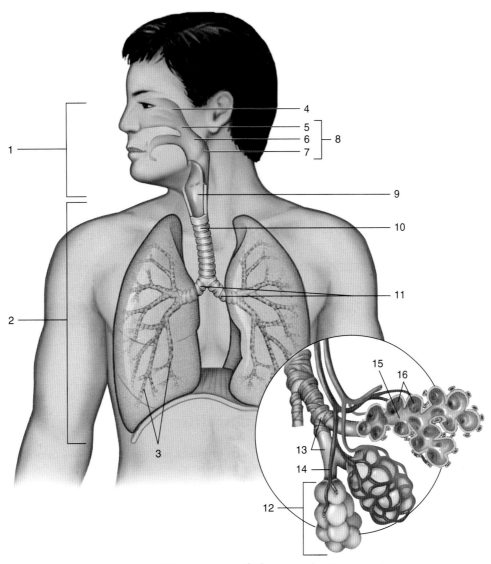

Figure 10.11 Structures of the respiratory system

(Mosby's Dictionary 2014)

1 _____

2 _____

3 _____

4 _____

5 _____

6 _____

7 _____

8 _____

9 _____

10 _____

11 _____

12 _____

13 _____

14 _____

15 _____

16 _____

EXERCISE 10.2: MATCH WORD ELEMENTS AND MEANINGS

Match the prefix, suffix or combining form in Column A with its meaning from Column B.

Column A	Answer	Column B
1. -capnia		A. diaphragm, mind
2. pneumat/o		B. black, coal
3. -oxia		C. nose
4. phren/o		D. carbon dioxide
5. steth/o		E. bad, painful, difficult
6. spir/o		F. expansion, dilatation, stretching out
7. -osmia		G. blue
8. anthrac/o		H. air, respiration, lung
9. pharyng/o		I. lobe
10. coni/o		J. oxygen
11. orth/o		K. septum
12. dys-		L. spitting
13. rhin/o		M. straight, upright
14. -ectasis		N. voice
15. -ptysis		O. distant, end, far, complete
16. tele-		P. breathe
17. cyan/o		Q. pharynx
18. sept/o		R. dust
19. phon/o		S. chest
20. lob/o		T. sense of smell

EXERCISE 10.3: WORD ANALYSIS AND MEANING

Break up the medical terms below into their component parts (prefixes, suffixes, word roots, combining vowels).
Provide the meaning for each word element and each term as a whole.

Example:
rhinorrhoea

rhin/o = nose

-rrhoea = discharge, flow

Meaning = discharge from nose

1. laryngeal _____

_____

_____

2. dysosmia _____

_____

_____

3. intercostal _____

_____

_____

4. apnoea _____

_____

_____

5. thoracoscopy _____

_____

_____

6. tracheotomy _____

_____

_____

7. pneumothorax _____

_____

_____

8. pleuritis _____

_____

_____

9. hypocapnia _____

_____

_____

10. pleural empyema _____

_____

_____

EXERCISE 10.4: VOCABULARY BUILDING

Provide the medical term for each of the definitions below.

1. Surgical repair of the chest: _____

2. Difficulty breathing: _____

3. Surgical removal of the tonsils and adenoids: _____

4. Condition of deficiency of oxygen in the blood: _____

5. Inflammation of the voice box: _____

6. A blood clot in the lungs: _____

7. Prolapse of the diaphragm: _____

8. Surgical repair of the uvula, palate and pharynx: _____

9. Condition of excessive carbon dioxide: _____

10. Involuntary contraction of the bronchus: _____

EXERCISE 10.5: EXPAND THE ABBREVIATIONS

Abbreviation	Expanded Abbreviation
ABGs	
ARF	
BiPAP	
BS	
COAD	
CPAP	
CXR	
CVS	
DOE	
ETT	
FEV$_1$	
LUL	
O$_2$	

Abbreviation	Expanded Abbreviation
PCP	
PE	
RDS	
RLL	
SARS	
SOBOE	
T&A	
TB	
URTI	

EXERCISE 10.6: MATCH MEDICAL TERMS WITH MEANINGS

Match the medical term in Column A with its meaning in Column B.

Column A	Answer	Column B
1. dysphonia		A. absence of the sense of smell
2. bronchiectasis		B. thin, watery discharge from nose
3. status asthmaticus		C. nasal stone
4. laryngostomy		D. inflammation of all the sinuses
5. sinus actinomycosis		E. fungus infection in sinus
6. pleural effusion		F. permanent opening through the neck into the larynx
7. hyperventilation		G. hoarseness
8. rhinolith		H. dilatation of a bronchus or bronchi
9. anosmia		I. lung disease due to prolonged inhalation of coal dust
10. anthracosis		J. removal of a pulmonary lobe
11. pyopneumothorax		K. coughing up and spitting out material from the lungs
12. bradypnoea		L. excess of CO_2 in the circulating blood
13. hypercapnia		M. slow breathing
14. expectoration		N. pus and air in the pleural cavity
15. lobectomy		O. abnormal accumulation of fluid in the pleural space
16. pansinusitis		P. prolonged state of severe asthma
17. rhinorrhoea		Q. spitting of blood
18. haemoptysis		R. excessive movement of air in and out of lungs
19. thoracocentesis		S. irregular breathing
20. Cheyne-Stokes respiration		T. tapping of pleural cavity to remove fluid

EXERCISE 10.7: APPLYING MEDICAL TERMINOLOGY

Fill in the blank or select the correct answer.

1. A/an _____ is an x-ray of the blood vessels of the lungs after injection of a contrast material.
   a) MRI
   b) CT of the thorax
   c) pulmonary angiogram
   d) chest x-ray

2. In total, there are _____ lung lobes.
   a) two
   b) three
   c) four
   d) five

3. Which of the following filters air as it enters the respiratory tract?
   a) lungs
   b) nose
   c) trachea
   d) diaphragm

4. The ability to breathe only in an upright position is _____.
   a) bradypnoea
   b) orthopnoea
   c) anopnoea
   d) hypopnoea

5. Cyanosis means what kind of discolouration of the skin?
   a) reddish
   b) yellowish
   c) bluish
   d) brownish

EXERCISE 10.8: PRONUNCIATION AND COMPREHENSION

Read the following paragraphs aloud to practise your pronunciation. Using your textbook and a medical dictionary, find the meanings of the underlined medical terms.

This 34-year-old male with a history of heavy smoking was admitted for investigation of haemoptysis. He noted that he has lost > 20 kg of weight in the past 6 months for no apparent reason with a current weight of 65 kg. Clinical examination was unremarkable, and spirometry was 4.4/5.7.

A bronchoscopy under IV sedation (ASA 2NE) was performed. Posterior nasal space revealed some tissue swelling but no bleeding. Cords and trachea were normal. There was no airway endobronchial lesion and no source of haemoptysis was seen. The mucosa, however, was slightly bronchitic. There was no growth from washings from the right lower lobe. No malignancy was seen, and smears for AFB were negative. Because of the significant weight loss, thoracic and abdominal computed tomography (CT) scans were performed to check for any evidence of lymphoma. There were no abnormalities found on these scans. Investigations showed a normal coagulation profile; FBC (full blood count) within normal limits; ESR (erythrocyte sedimentation rate) 3 mm/hr; and serum electrolytes (urea, creatinine, glucose, calcium and liver function tests) were all within normal limits. He was discharged into the care of his wife to be reviewed in the outpatients department, with a follow-up chest x-ray.

EXERCISE 10.9: CROSSWORD PUZZLE

Complete the puzzle by providing the medical term for each of the clues below.

ACROSS

2. The process where gaseous waste products are expelled from the body (10)

5. Build-up of extravascular fluid from capillaries of the lung in the alveoli (9, 6)

7. A chronic obstructive disease affecting the lungs and bronchi, characterised by an abnormal permanent enlargement of the alveoli (9)

8. An endocrine disorder that has a respiratory manifestation (6, 8)

10. Filters inhaled air removing respiratory contaminants (4)

DOWN

1. Lung diseases caused by the inhalation of dust or chemical irritants (14)

3. The smallest branches of the respiratory system (7)

4. An opening into the trachea for an indwelling tube to be inserted (12)

6. The inner membrane of the pleura (8, 6)

9. Inflammation of the bronchi (10)

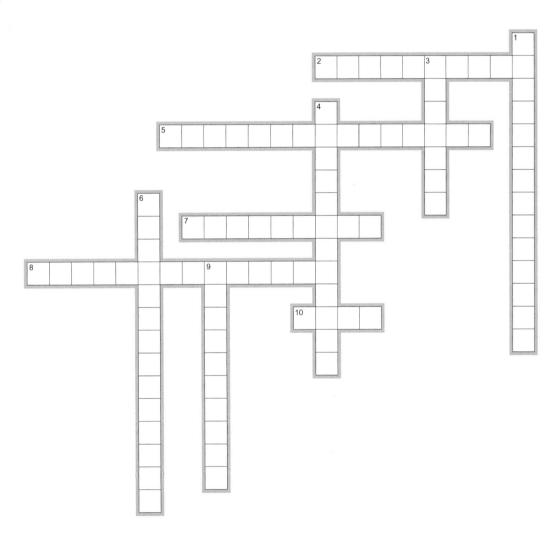

EXERCISE 10.10: ANAGRAMS

Work out each medical term from the jumbled letters below. Then, using the letters in brackets, determine the medical term that matches the description given.

1. doac	__ __ (__) __	abbreviation for a chronic obstruction of the lung
2. chinrob	__ (__) __ __ __ __ __	branches of the trachea that lead into the lungs
3. xprynah	__ __ __ __ __ __ (__)	the throat
4. gunl	__ __ (__) __	major organ of respiration
5. llaeiov	__ (__)__ __ __ __ __	the air sacs of the lung
6. rulepisy	__ __ __ __ __ __ __ (__)	inflammation of the pleura

Rearrange the letters in brackets to form a word that means 'the voice box'.

— — — — — —

EXERCISE 10.11: DISCHARGE SUMMARY ANALYSIS

Read the discharge summary below and answer the questions.

UNIVERSITY HOSPITAL DISCHARGE SUMMARY	**UR number:** 171819 **Name:** Elizabeth Fox **Address:** 55 Brownley Road, Closter **Date of birth:** 15/1/1942 **Sex:** F **Nominated primary healthcare provider:** Dr Phillip Newsome
Episode details **Consultant:** Dr Franklin **Registrar:** Dr Richards **Unit:** Respiratory **Admission source:** Emergency department **Date of admission:** 17/3/2020	**Discharge details** **Status:** Home **Date of discharge:** 25/3/2020
Reason for admission / Presenting problems: Productive cough and SOB	
Principal diagnosis: Bronchitis due to *Haemophilus*	

Comorbidities:

Asthma

Ischaemic heart disease

Cardiac failure

T2DM

Controlled atrial fibrillation

Recently diagnosed non-Hodgkin lymphoma

SCCs of the legs

Previous medical history:

Trigeminal neuralgia 2002

Clinical synopsis:

This well-known patient presented with a 5-day history of cough productive of brown sputum and increasing shortness of breath. She had experienced no fevers or rigors. She was seen by her local doctor, who gave her a course of amoxicillin, but this had made no improvement. On the day of admission, she was worse than usual, complaining of marked shortness of breath and wheeze. She had not taken her Lasix for the 3 days prior to admission. She also needed to sleep on two pillows as opposed to her normal one and the oedema in her legs had increased. When seen she was afebrile with a pulse of 72 in atrial fibrillation, her JVP was +5 cm and Kussmaul's sign negative. She had oedema to her knees. She had a grade 3/6 pansystolic murmur at the apex with no right ventricular heave or increase in her pulmonary 2nd sound. Her breath sounds were decreased bilaterally, with occasional basal wheezes and crackles. She had a soft abdomen. CXR showed an increase in her cardiothoracic ratio, with marked increase in markings, left pleural effusion and pulmonary vascular redistribution. Her ECG showed atrial fibrillation with widespread T wave inversion and T wave flattening.

She was admitted with a provisional diagnosis of infective exacerbation of COAD secondary to penicillinase resistant *Haemophilus*, also for control of her cardiac failure. She was admitted to the ward and given oral Augmentin, started on Captopril and her Lasix was reintroduced. She settled rapidly over the next few days and her JVP fell and her ankle oedema disappeared. Her chest still had occasional wheezes and crackles. She remained afebrile and her sputum greatly cleared.

When seen by her doctor, he re-examined her legs and found there were several areas consistent with recurrent SCCs. She was referred to the dermatologist she has seen previously for excision of these lesions.

Complications:

Clinical interventions:

Diagnostic interventions:

CXR

ECG

Medications at discharge:

Oral Augmentin

Captopril

Lasix

Ceased medications: Nil reported

Allergies: Nil reported

Alerts: Nil reported

Arranged services: Nil reported

Recommendations:

Discharged home to the care of her husband to see her local doctor privately in 2 weeks and to see the dermatologist in outpatients on 25-5-20 regarding removal of her skin lesions.

Information to patient/relevant parties:

Maintain discharge medications and review in respiratory OPD in 6 weeks.

Authorising clinician: Dr Richards

Document recipients:

Patient and LMO: Dr Phillip Newsome

1. **Expand the following abbreviations as found in the discharge summary above.**

   COAD

   CXR

   ECG

   JVP

   T2DM

   OPD

   SCC

   SOB

2. **What is Kussmaul's sign?**

3. **What is Lasix and why did not taking it cause problems for Mrs Fox?**

4. **Mrs Fox's principal diagnosis was bronchitis due to *Haemophilus*. What is *Haemophilus*?**

5. **Mrs Fox's ECG showed atrial fibrillation. What is AF and how is it treated?**

CHAPTER 11

Digestive System

Contents

OBJECTIVES 241

INTRODUCTION 242

NEW WORD ELEMENTS 242

    Combining forms 242

    Prefixes 243

    Suffixes 244

VOCABULARY 244

ABBREVIATIONS 245

FUNCTIONS AND STRUCTURE OF THE DIGESTIVE SYSTEM 246

    Mouth (buccal cavity) 246

    Pharynx and oesophagus 246

    Stomach 246

    Small intestine 247

    Large intestine 248

    Anus 248

    Liver 249

    Pancreas 249

    Gallbladder 249

PATHOLOGY AND DISEASES 249

    Diseases of the oral cavity 249

    Diseases of the salivary glands 250

    Diseases of the oesophagus 250

    Diseases of the stomach 250

    Diseases of the small intestine and associated organs 252

    Diseases of the large intestine 255

    Diseases of the rectum and anus 258

TESTS AND PROCEDURES 259

EXERCISES 264

Objectives

After completing this chapter you should be able to:

1. state the meanings of the word elements related to the digestive system

2. build words using the word elements associated with the digestive system

3. recognise, pronounce and effectively use medical terms associated with the digestive system

4. expand abbreviations related to the digestive system

5. describe the structure and functions of the digestive system including the stomach, liver, gallbladder, small and large intestines and the digestive process

6. describe common pathological conditions associated with the digestive system

7. describe common laboratory tests and diagnostic and surgical procedures associated with the digestive system

8. apply what you have learned by interpreting medical terminology in practice.

Demonstrate your knowledge of the digestive system by completing the exercises at the end of this chapter.

INTRODUCTION

The digestive system (also called the alimentary or gastrointestinal system) consists of a series of hollow organs joined in a tube-like tract starting at the mouth and ending at the anus. So that they can be used as body fuel, the food and fluids we consume must be broken down both physically and chemically into nutrients. They can then be absorbed into the blood and carried to the body cells. The body also has to excrete waste. The organs of the digestive system collectively perform these activities.

A properly functioning digestive system is essential for the effective interactions of almost all other body systems. A problem in the digestive system can cause conditions in other body systems and vice versa. This is why a healthy, well-balanced diet is important.

NEW WORD ELEMENTS

Here are some word elements related to the digestive system. To reinforce your learning, write the meanings of the medical terms in the spaces provided. Use the Glossary of medical terms on page 561 to help you work out the meanings. You may also need to check the meaning in a medical dictionary, but make an attempt yourself first.

Combining forms

Combining Form	Meaning	Medical Term	Meaning of Medical Term
abdomin/o	abdomen	abdominocentesis	
adhesi/o	adhesion	adhesiolysis	
amyl/o	starch	amylase	
an/o	anus	anal	
appendic/o	appendix	appendicitis	
bil/i	gall, bile	biliary	
bilirubin/o	bile pigment	bilirubinuria	
bucc/o	cheek	buccal	
caec/o	caecum	caecopexy	
cheil/o	lip	cheiloplasty	
chol/e	gall, bile	cholesteatoma	
cholangi/o	bile duct	cholangiogram	
cholecyst/o	gallbladder	cholecystectomy	
choledoch/o	common bile duct	choledocholithiasis	
cib/o	meal	cibophobia	
cirrh/o	orange, yellow	hepatic	
coel/o	cavity	coeliac	
col/o	colon, large intestine	colorectal	
colon/o		colonoscopy	
cyst/o	bladder, cyst, sac	cholecystitis	
dent/i	teeth	dentibuccal	
dent/o		dentogingival	
diverticul/o	diverticulum, blind pouch	diverticulosis	
duoden/o	duodenum	duodenoscopy	
enter/o	small intestine	enteropathy	
faci/o	face	facial	
gastr/o	stomach	gastroenterology	
gingiv/o	gums	gingivoplasty	
gloss/o	tongue	glossorrhaphy	

Table continued

Combining Form	Meaning	Medical Term	Meaning of Medical Term
gluc/o	glucose, sugar, sweet(ness)	glucose	
glyc/o		glycolysis	
glycogen/o	glucose, animal starch	glycogenesis	
hepat/o	liver	hepatitis	
herni/o	hernia	herniorrhaphy	
ile/o	ileum, small intestine	jejunoileitis	
inguin/o	groin	inguinal	
jejun/o	jejunum	jejunostomy	
labi/o	lip	labiodental	
lapar/o	abdomen	laparotomy	
lingu/o	tongue	sublingual	
lip/o	fat	lipolytic	
lith/o	stone, calculus	cholecystolithiasis	
mandibul/o	lower jaw, mandible	mandibulofacial	
odont/o	teeth	endodontology	
oesophag/o	oesophagus	oesophagogastrostomy	
or/o	mouth	oral	
palat/o	palate	palatomaxillary	
pancreat/o	pancreas	pancreatoma	
pept/o	digestion	peptic	
peritone/o	peritoneum	peritonitis	
phag/o	eating, swallowing	dysphagia	
pharyng/o	pharynx, throat	pharyngitis	
proct/o	anus, rectum	proctodynia	
prote/o	protein	protease	
pylor/o	pylorus, pyloric sphincter	pyloric stenosis	
rect/o	rectum	rectocele	
sial/o	saliva, salivary	sialolithiasis	
sigmoid/o	sigmoid colon	rectosigmoidoscopy	
splen/o *(Note: the word spleen has two 'e's but the combining form splen/o has one 'e')*	spleen	splenomegaly	
steat/o	fat	steatolysis	
stomat/o	mouth	stomatopathy	

Prefixes

Prefix	Meaning	Medical Term	Meaning of Medical Term
dia-	through, across	diarrhoea	
hemi-	half	hemigastrectomy	
hyper-	above, excessive	hyperemesis	
post-	after, behind	postprandial	
sub-	under, below	subgastric	

Suffixes

Suffix	Meaning	Medical Term	Meaning of Medical Term
-ase	enzyme	lipase	
-chezia	defecation, elimination of waste products	dyschezia	
-emesis	vomiting	haematemesis	
-iasis	abnormal condition or state	cholelithiasis	
-pepsia	condition of digestion	dyspepsia	
-prandial	meal	preprandial	

VOCABULARY

The following list provides many of the medical terms used for the first time in this chapter. Pronunciations are provided with each term. As you read the rest of the chapter, make sure you identify each of these terms and understand their meanings.

Term	Pronunciation
abdominal ultrasonography	ab-DOM-in-al ul-tra-son-OG-ra-fee
absorption	ab-SAWP-shun
adhesiolysis	add-heez-ee-o-LY-sis
alimentary canal	ayl-i-MEN-tree can-al
anal fissure	AY-nal FISH-a
anus	AY-nus
appendicitis	ah-pen-de-SY-tis
appendix	a-PEN-diks
Barrett's oesophagus	BA-rets e-SOF-a-gus
bile	byl
bolus	BO-lus
caecum	SEE-kum
capsule endoscopy	KAPS-yool en-DOS-kop-ee
chemical digestion	KEM-i-kal dy-JES-jun
cholangiography	kol-an-jee-OG-ra-fee
cholecystectomy	kol-EE-sis-TEK-tom-ee
cholecystitis	kol-ee-sist-EYE-tis
cholelithiasis	kol-ee-lith-EYE-a-sis
chyme	kyme
cirrhosis	si-ROH-sis
coeliac disease	SEE-lee-ak diz-eez
colon	KOH-lon
colonic polyp	koh-LON-ik POL-ip
colorectal cancer	koh-loh-REK-tal KAN-sa
computed tomography	kom-PYOO-ted tom-OG-ra-fee

Table continued

Term	Pronunciation
Crohn's disease	KROHNs diz-eez
defecation	dee-fa-KAY-shun
dental caries	DEN-tal KAIR-eez
diarrhoea	dy-a-REE-a
digestion	dy-JES-jun
diverticular disease	dy-ver-TIK-yoo-la diz-eez
diverticulum	DY-ver-TIK-yoo-lum
duodenal ulcer	dyoo-oh-DEE-nal UL-sa
duodenum	dyoo-oh-DEE-num
elimination	e-lim-in-AY-shun
endoscopy	en-DOS-kop-ee
enterostomy	en-ter-OS-to-mee
eructation	e-ruk-TAY-shun
faeces culture	FEE-seez KUL-cha
flatulence	FLAT-yoo-lens
fundoplication	fun-doh-pli-KAY-shun
gallbladder	GAWL-blad-a
gastric banding	GAS-trik BAN-ding
gastric carcinoma	GAS-trik kar-sin-OH-ma
gastric ulcer	GAS-trik UL-sa
gastritis	gas-TRY-tis
gastroenteritis	GAS-troh-en-tah-RY-tus
gastrointestinal endoscopy	gas-troh-in-TES-tin-al en-DOS-kop-ee
gastro-oesophageal reflux disease	GAS-troh-e-sof-a-JEE-al REE-fluks diz-eez
gastro-oesophageal sphincter	GAS-troh-e-sof-a-JEE-al SFINK-ta
guaiac faecal occult blood test (or haemoccult test)	GWY-ak FEE-kal OK-ult blud test (heem-OK-ult test)
haemorrhoidectomy	HEM-a-royd-EK-to-mee
haemorrhoids	HEM-a-roydz

Table continued

Term	Pronunciation
hepatitis	hep-a-TY-tis
hernia	HER-nee-a
herniorrhaphy	her-nee-O-raf-ee
ileum	IL-ee-um
ingestion	in-JES-jun
irritable bowel syndrome	i-rit-a-bel BOW-el SIN-drohm
jejunum	jay-JOO-num
laparoscopy	lap-ahr-OS-ko-pee
large intestine	larj in-TES-tyn
liver	LIV-a
liver biopsy	LIV-a BY-op-see
liver function tests	LIV-a FUNK-shun tests
liver scan	LIV-a skan
lower gastrointestinal series	LOW-a gas-troh-in-TES-tin-al SEE-reez
magnetic resonance imaging	mag-NET-ik REZ-on-ans IM-a-jing
mechanical digestion	mek-AN-i-kal dy-JEST-jun
mouth	mowth
nasogastric intubation	NAY-zo-GAS-trik in-tyoo-BAY-shun
non-alcoholic steatohepatitis	non al-ko-HOL-ik stee-at-o-hep-a-TY-tis
oesophageal varices	e-sof-a-JEE-al VAR-is-eez
pancreas	PAN-kree-as
paracentesis (abdominocentesis)	par-a-sen-TEE-sis (ab-dom-in-o-sen-TEE-sis)
parotitis	par-o-TY-tis
percutaneous endoscopic gastrostomy tube	per-kyoo-TAYN-ee-us en-dos-KOP-ik gas-TROS-tom-ee tyoob
percutaneous endoscopic jejunostomy tube	per-kyoo-TAYN-ee-us en-dos-KOP-ik je-joon-OS-tom-ee tyoob
peristalsis	per-ee-STAL-sis
pharynx	FA-rinks
propulsion	pro-PUL-shun
rectum	REK-tum
saliva	sa-LY-va
salivary gland	sa-LY-va-ree gland
secretion	se-KREE-shun
small intestine	small in-TES-tyn
stomach	STUM-ak
stomatitis	stoh-ma-TY-tus

Table continued

Term	Pronunciation
teeth	teeth
tongue	tung
ulcerative colitis	UL-ser-a-tiv kol-EYE-tis
upper gastrointestinal series	UP-pa gas-troh-in-TES-tin-al SEE-reez

ABBREVIATIONS

The following abbreviations are commonly used in the Australian healthcare environment. Because some abbreviations can have more than one meaning, check the context in which the abbreviation is used before assigning a meaning to it.

Abbreviation	Definition
Ba	barium
BMI	body mass index
ERCP	endoscopic retrograde cholangiopancreatography
FIT	faecal immunochemical test
GI(T)	gastrointestinal (tract)
GORD	gastro-oesophageal reflux disease
IBD	inflammatory bowel disease
IBS	irritable bowel syndrome
iFOBT	immunochemical faecal occult blood test
LFTs	liver function tests
NASH	non-alcoholic steatohepatitis
N&V	nausea and vomiting
NG	nasogastric
NPO, NBM	*nil per os*, nil by mouth
NSAID(s)	non-steroidal anti-inflammatory drug(s)
OGD	oesophagogastroduodenoscopy
PEG tube	percutaneous endoscopic gastrostomy tube
PEJ tube	percutaneous endoscopic jejunostomy tube
PR	per rectum, by way of the rectum
PTHC	percutaneous transhepatic cholangiography
PUD	peptic ulcer disease
TPN	total parenteral nutrition

FUNCTIONS AND STRUCTURE OF THE DIGESTIVE SYSTEM

The digestive system consists of a series of organs and glands that work together to process and digest food and to excrete wastes. Controlled by the enteric nervous system, digestion is a complex process of motility, secretion and absorption. Most of the digestive system is made up of a long cylindrical tube (most commonly known as the digestive tract, but can also be called the alimentary canal or gastrointestinal tract) that moves the food from the mouth to the anus, plus accessory organs that assist with the chemical and mechanical breakdown of food. The digestive tract is 9–10 metres in length, and food takes between 12 and 48 hours to move from one end to the other. There are seven basic processes that occur in the digestive system:

Ingestion is the process of eating and drinking.

Propulsion moves the food along the digestive tract by a process called peristalsis, which is the rhythmic contraction and relaxation of the smooth muscle that lines the walls of the digestive organs. These muscular waves force the food down the digestive tract.

Secretion of enzymes helps to process the food into liquid by adjusting the pH of the food and chemically breaking it down.

Mechanical digestion occurs when the food is physically broken down into smaller and smaller pieces. This process begins in the mouth as food is chewed to make it small enough to swallow and continues in the stomach and small intestine through muscular action.

Chemical digestion takes place as enzymes in the stomach and small intestine break down food into simpler molecules.

Absorption occurs when these molecules move from the digestive tract to adjacent blood and lymphatic vessels for transport around the body.

Elimination occurs when undigested waste products are defecated from the body through the anus.

The digestive organs are the:

- Mouth, salivary glands, tongue and teeth
- Pharynx
- Stomach
} upper digestive tract

- Small and large intestines
- Rectum
- Anus
} lower digestive tract

- Liver
- Pancreas
- Gallbladder
} accessory organs

The organs of the digestive system are shown in Fig. 11.1 and the pathway of food through the gastrointestinal tract is shown in Fig. 11.2.

Mouth (buccal cavity)

The digestive process begins before food is placed in the mouth, as the senses (such as smell) identify the presence of food and alert the other digestive organs to produce various gastric juices in preparation for digestion. The salivary glands in the mouth produce saliva, which mixes with the food, acting as a lubricant and also killing some of the microorganisms present. The major salivary glands are the parotid, submandibular and sublingual glands. Saliva contains amylase, an enzyme that begins the chemical process to break starches down into sugars. The teeth have a mechanical function, crushing, grinding and tearing the food into a size and consistency suitable for swallowing. There are two types of teeth – incisors at the front of the mouth, which cut and tear food, and the molars, located in the middle and back of the mouth, which act to crush and grind the food. The tongue, which is a band of muscle, is covered with mucous membrane and contains papillae. In between these papillae are the taste buds, which identify sweet, sour, salty, savoury (umami) and bitter tastes.

The decision to swallow starts as a voluntary movement, but once swallowing begins, the process becomes involuntary and is controlled by the nervous system. The ball of food, once swallowed, is known as a bolus.

Pharynx and oesophagus

The pharynx is the part of the throat that lies directly behind the mouth. As discussed in Chapter 10 Respiratory System, the pharynx contains openings to both the trachea and the oesophagus. The bolus of food is directed by the pharynx into the oesophagus where waves of peristalsis move it down to the stomach. The entrance to the stomach is guarded by the gastro-oesophageal sphincter (also called the cardiac sphincter), a ring-like valve that detects the approach of the bolus, relaxes and opens to allow it into the stomach. The sphincter then closes, helping to ensure the food only moves in one direction.

Stomach

The stomach undertakes three mechanical processes – it stores the food and liquid in its upper part or fundus, mixes them up with various digestive juices through the muscular action of the middle-lower stomach or corpus, and moves the resultant partially digested mixture into the small intestine through the antrum and pylorus. In addition to these mechanical actions, the stomach also has chemical digestive processes that are triggered by the release of gastrin, a hormone, in

Figure 11.1 Organs of the digestive system

(Mosby's Dictionary 2014)

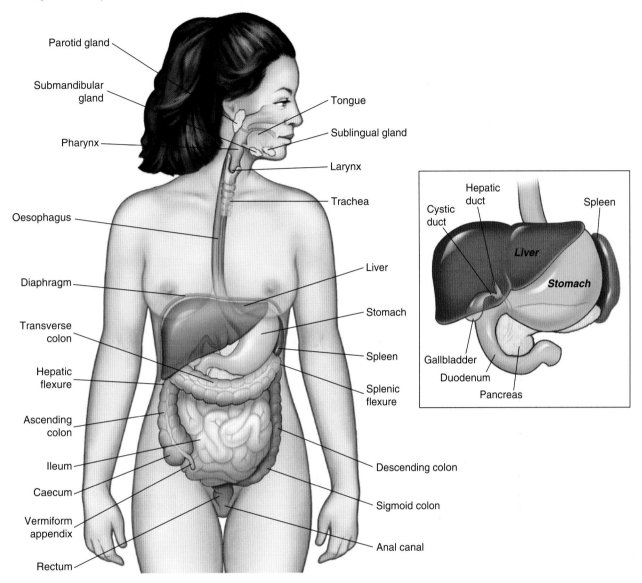

the blood. Various types of gastric juices are produced by the stomach – proteases (such as pepsin), mucus and hydrochloric acid. In humans, gastric juices are very acidic and help the process of breaking down the food into chyme, a liquid. The high acidity level also helps with killing microorganisms.

An empty adult stomach has a volume of about 45 millilitres but can expand to hold as much as 3 litres, although a normally full stomach is about 1 litre in volume.

Small intestine

The small intestine, consisting of the duodenum, jejunum and ileum, is the longest part of the intestinal tract, being around 6 metres in length. As the chyme moves through the pyloric sphincter, it enters the first part of the small intestine, the duodenum. This is where alkalis neutralise the acids from the stomach. Bile from the gallbladder and enzymes from the pancreas enter the duodenum through ducts and mix with mucus to coat the chyme. The majority of proteins, carbohydrates and fats are absorbed into the bloodstream in the duodenum.

The second part of the small intestine is the jejunum. Through its villi (finger-like projections), it absorbs more carbohydrates and proteins, which then enter the bloodstream. The jejunum directs the remainder of the material into the distal part of the small intestine, known as the ileum. The ileum absorbs vitamin B_{12} and bile salts as well as any remaining nutrients. Peristaltic waves then move remaining products through the ileocaecal valve into the large intestine.

Figure 11.2 Pathway of food through the gastrointestinal tract

(Mosby's Dictionary 2014)

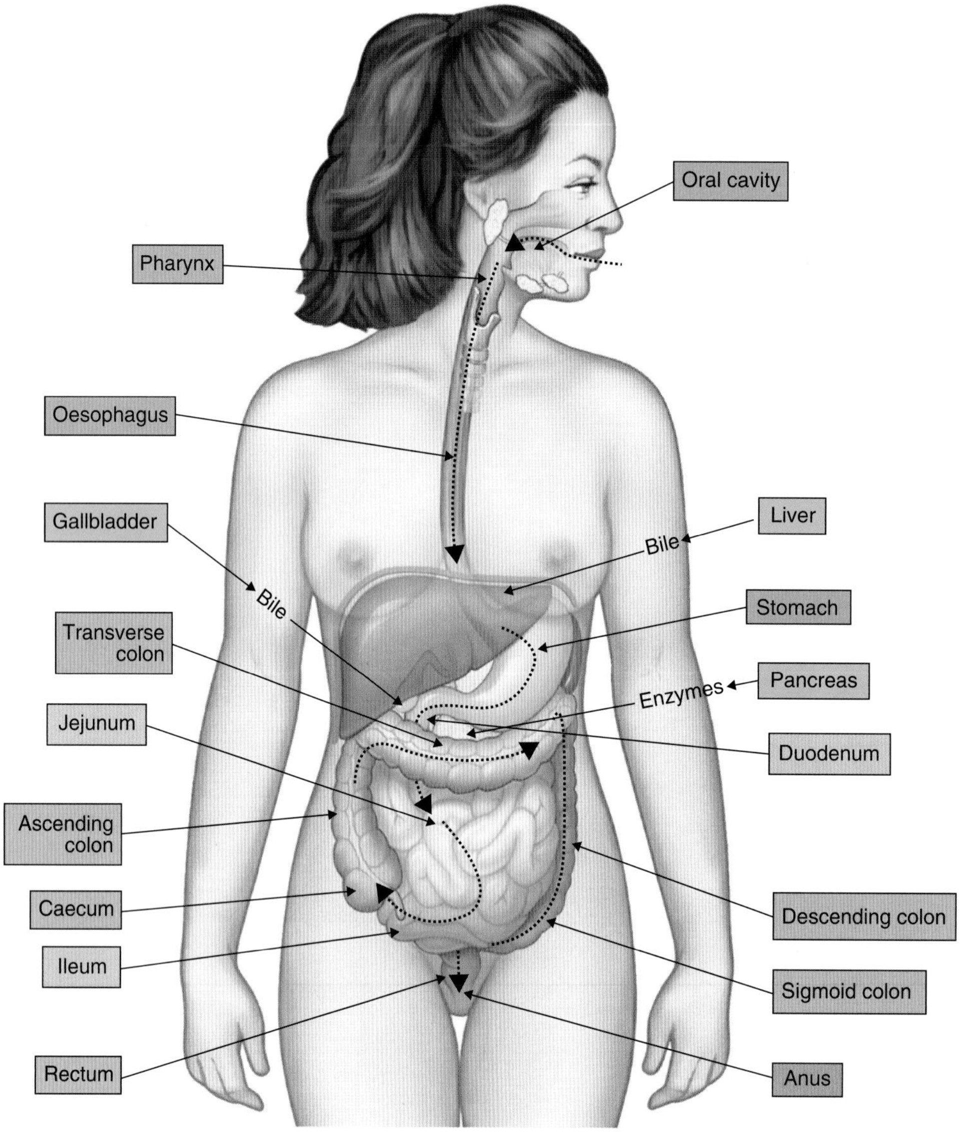

Large intestine

The large intestine consists of the caecum, colon and rectum (Fig. 11.3). Altogether, the large intestine is only about 1 metre in length but is 4 centimetres wide, the width giving it the name large intestine. The caecum is a pouch-like structure at the junction between the small intestine and the remainder of the large intestine. It is also attached to the appendix, a blind-ended structure the principal purpose of which is unknown. It has been suggested that the appendix previously had a role in the immune system but that natural selection has changed its purpose.

The middle portion of the large intestine is called the colon and has four parts – the ascending, transverse, descending and sigmoid colon. As it moves through these parts, salts, residual vitamins, minerals and water are extracted from the remainder of the ingested materials. What is left is now considered waste product. This product mixes with mucus and bacteria to become faeces. In the sigmoid colon, the walls retract, forcing the faeces into the rectum where it is stored.

Anus

The anus is a sphincter that relaxes to allow the faeces stored in the rectum to be released to the external environment. This process is known as defecation.

Figure 11.3 Large intestine

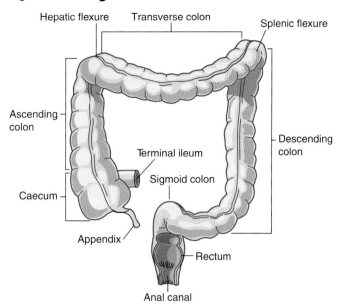

Liver

The liver has a vital role in helping the body to remove toxins, process nutrients and regulate metabolism. It is located on the upper right-hand side of the abdominal cavity and is the second largest organ in the body after the skin. All blood, containing nutrients obtained in the digestive process, is filtered through the liver prior to being transported around the rest of the body. The liver detoxifies chemicals and noxious materials and further breaks down nutrients into more manageable products. The liver produces bile, which is then stored in the gallbladder before being used to break down fats in the duodenum as part of the digestive process. Vitamin B$_{12}$, iron and copper are also stored in the liver, and cholesterol and other fats are produced there.

Glucose is made by the liver and stored as glycogen until it is needed by the body. When it is required, glycogen is converted back into glucose and used by the body for energy.

Pancreas

The pancreas is a small glandular organ located behind the stomach and attached to the duodenum via the pancreatic duct. It has two major functions and is considered both an exocrine and endocrine gland. Its exocrine function is to produce digestive enzymes that pass through the pancreatic duct into the small intestine to help in the breakdown of fats, carbohydrates and proteins and to neutralise stomach acids. The important endocrine function of the pancreas is to produce insulin, which regulates the levels of sugars in the blood. Insulin is produced by the islets of Langerhans, a small clump of cells in the pancreas. The pancreas also produces glucagon, which helps with blood sugar regulation.

Gallbladder

The gallbladder is a pear-shaped organ connected to the liver and duodenum via the hepatic duct and the common bile duct. Its primary function is to store the bile created by the liver and make it more concentrated. Bile is used by the small intestine to emulsify fats and to neutralise some acids so they are easier to digest.

PATHOLOGY AND DISEASES

The following section provides a list of some of the most common diseases and pathological conditions relevant to the digestive system.

Diseases of the oral cavity

Term	Pronunciation	Definition
dental caries	DEN-tal KAIR-eez	Dental caries is the medical term for the common condition of tooth decay. Bacteria in the mouth cause a film on the teeth called plaque. This in turn converts starches in food to acid. The acid erodes the enamel of the teeth, causing caries. A high standard of oral hygiene is the best preventative measure.

Table continued

Term	Pronunciation	Definition
stomatitis	stoh-mat-TY-tus	Stomatitis is an inflammation of the mucous membrane lining of the mouth including the cheeks, gums, lips, tongue and palate. It can be caused by injury such as burns from hot food or drinks, poorly fitting oral appliances, cheek biting, mouth breathing and poor oral hygiene.

Diseases of the salivary glands

Term	Pronunciation	Definition
parotitis	pa-ro-TY-tis	Parotitis is an inflammation of one or both parotid glands. **Acute bacterial parotitis** results from a bacterial infection commonly occurring after radiation therapy or in immunocompromised patients. **Chronic parotitis** is recurrent bouts of infection in patients with a blocked or narrowed salivary duct. **Viral parotitis**, commonly called mumps, is caused by the paramyxovirus and causes a severe swelling of the parotid glands.

Diseases of the oesophagus

Term	Pronunciation	Definition
Barrett's oesophagus	BA-rets e-SOF-a-gus	Barrett's oesophagus is a pre-malignant condition in which the tissue lining the oesophagus is replaced by tissue that is similar to the lining of the stomach and intestine. The Barrett's lining always begins at the bottom of the oesophagus and extends upward towards the mouth for varying distances. It is commonly found in people with gastro-oesophageal reflux disease (GORD). It can progress to adenocarcinoma of the oesophagus.
oesophageal varices (singular: varix)	e-SOF-a-JEE-al VAR-is-eez	Oesophageal varices are dilated (varicosed) veins in the lower part of the oesophagus or in the upper part of the stomach. They are associated with the increased venous pressure that occurs in liver diseases such as cirrhosis. Oesophageal varices can rupture and cause extreme bleeding, which may be life threatening.

Diseases of the stomach

Term	Pronunciation	Definition
eructation	e-ruk-TAY-shun	Eructation, better known as belching or burping, is the act of expelling gas from the stomach out through the mouth. The usual cause of this is a distended stomach caused by swallowed air. The distension of the stomach causes abdominal discomfort, and the belching expels the air and relieves the discomfort.
gastric carcinoma	GAS-trik kah-sin-OH-ma	Gastric carcinoma is also called stomach cancer. Most gastric cancers are adenocarcinomas. The risk factors for developing stomach cancer are *Helicobacter pylori* (*H. pylori*) infection, cigarette smoking, excessive consumption of alcohol and a diet that is high in foods and beverages that contain nitrates and nitrites such as smoked and salted fish/meats and pickled vegetables. Symptoms may include anorexia, dysphagia, indigestion, bloating, nausea and haematemesis. Treatment for gastric cancer includes surgery, radiotherapy and chemotherapy.

Table continued

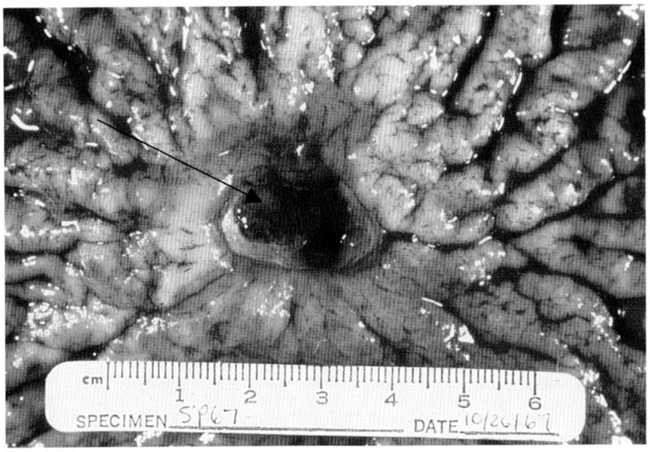

Term	Pronunciation	Definition
gastric ulcer, duodenal ulcer	GAS-trik UL-sa, dyoo-o-DEEN-al UL-sa	Gastric ulcers and duodenal ulcers are also known as peptic ulcers. They are erosions in the lining of the stomach or intestinal tract (Fig. 11.4). Most peptic ulcers are caused by the bacterium *H. pylori*. Long-term use of non-steroidal anti-inflammatory agents (NSAIDs), such as aspirin and ibuprofen, is another common cause. Lifestyle factors, stress and diet used to be thought to cause ulcers, but recent research has shown that while these factors can worsen ulcers and prevent healing, they do not cause them. Peptic ulcers result in a burning pain in the stomach and duodenum. The pain may be temporarily relieved by eating food, drinking milk or by taking antacids. A combination of antibiotics and acid-reducing medication is the most effective treatment for *H. pylori*-induced peptic ulcers.
	Figure 11.4 Gastric ulcer (Patton & Thibodeau 2010)	
gastritis	gas-TRY-tis	Gastritis is a condition in which there is an abnormal inflammation of the mucous lining of the stomach. Symptoms may include dyspepsia, nausea or vomiting. There are many causes of gastritis. One of the most common causes is infection by the bacteria *H. pylori*. Treating *H. pylori* infection is important because it may lead to gastric ulcer disease or cancer. Other causes of gastritis include prolonged use of alcohol, NSAIDs such as aspirin, iron supplements and chemotherapy.
gastroenteritis	GAS-troh-en-ter-EYE-tus	Gastroenteritis is the inflammation of the lining of the stomach and intestines resulting in diarrhoea, abdominal cramps, nausea and vomiting. It is usually caused by a virus such as norovirus but can also have a bacterial aetiology. These types of gastroenteritis are highly contagious. Other types of gastroenteritis are non-infectious and can be the result of medications or food allergies. Dehydration is the most common complication of gastroenteritis. Adequately replacing fluids can avoid this. Most cases of gastroenteritis resolve over time without specific treatment.

Table continued

Term	Pronunciation	Definition
gastro-oesophageal reflux disease (GORD)	GAS-troh-e-sof-a-JEE-al REE-fluks diz-EEZ	GORD is a form of chronic heartburn caused by the backflow (reflux) of acidic stomach contents into the oesophagus (Fig. 11.5). This is often due to incompetence of the cardiac sphincter between the stomach and oesophagus. It results in a severe burning pain in the oesophagus and can lead to oesophagitis or ulceration.

Figure 11.5 Gastro-oesophageal reflux disease

Oesophagus lining becomes irritated

Acid backs up into oesophagus

Lower oesophageal sphincter

Stomach acid

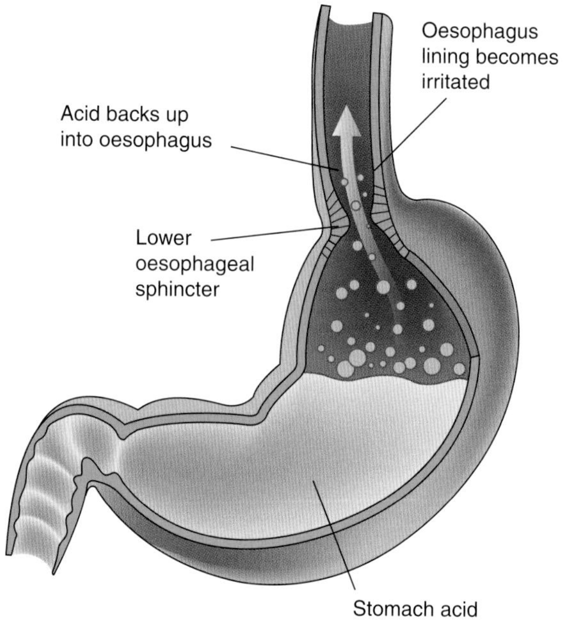

Diseases of the small intestine and associated organs
Appendix

Term	Pronunciation	Definition
appendicitis	a-pen-de-SY-tis	Appendicitis occurs when the lumen of the appendix becomes obstructed by faeces, lymphatic tissue or other materials, resulting in a painful swelling and infection of the appendix. The severe pain of appendicitis is usually sudden, begins near the umbilical region and then moves to the lower right quadrant. It progressively worsens over a few hours. Other symptoms of appendicitis may include anorexia, nausea, vomiting, a low-grade fever and raised white cell count that indicates an infection.
		Appendicitis is diagnosed by a physical examination that often demonstrates guarding and rebound tenderness when the area is palpated. Appendicitis can be confirmed by CT scan or ultrasound. If appendicitis is suspected, surgery will often be performed without conducting extensive diagnostic testing (Fig. 11.6). Prompt surgery decreases the likelihood the inflamed appendix will burst. If the appendix does burst, infection can spread throughout the abdominal cavity, resulting in a potentially dangerous condition called peritonitis.
		Sometimes a mass forms around a burst appendix, resulting in a condition called an appendiceal abscess. This pus-filled abscess will either be drained before surgery or removed as part of the appendicectomy procedure.

Table continued

Term	Pronunciation	Definition
Figure 11.6 Laparoscopic view of an appendix being removed (Sudhakaran & Ade-Ajayi 2010)		

Gallbladder

Term	Pronunciation	Definition
cholecystitis	kol-ee-sist-EYE-tis	Cholecystitis is inflammation of the gallbladder. This can be either acute or chronic. **Acute cholecystitis** occurs when a calculus, or gallstone, becomes lodged in the cystic duct, trapping bile in the gallbladder. This results in sudden severe pain usually in the right upper quadrant. **Chronic cholecystitis** occurs as a result of long-term irritation of the gallbladder, usually after recurrent attacks of acute cholecystitis. Because the function of the gallbladder to emulsify fats is adversely affected, consuming a fatty meal will often bring on an attack.
cholelithiasis	kol-ee-lith-EYE-a-sis	Cholelithiasis is the presence of calculi or stones in the gallbladder (Fig. 11.7). It may occur in conjunction with cholecystitis. Gallstones form when bile hardens in the gallbladder. It tends to be more common among adults over 40 years of age, especially: females; those with a family history of gallstones; people who are overweight or undergo rapid weight loss; and those taking cholesterol-lowering drugs. Symptoms include eructation, pain or discomfort in the right upper quadrant radiating to the back and intolerance to foods with a high fat content. Gallstones can cause serious problems if they become trapped in the bile ducts. A laparoscopic choledocholithotomy or cholecystectomy are the most common forms of treatment.
	Figure 11.7 Cholelithiasis (Kumar et al 2009)	

Liver

Term	Pronunciation	Definition
cirrhosis	si-ROH-sis	Cirrhosis is a chronic disease in which the liver slowly deteriorates, with scar tissue replacing healthy liver tissue and partially blocking the flow of blood through the liver (Fig. 11.8). This reduced blood flow affects the way the liver performs its functions. Excessive alcohol consumption and chronic hepatitis B and C are the most common causes of cirrhosis. Other conditions such as fatty liver disease associated with obesity, blocked bile ducts and haemochromatosis also cause cirrhosis. Cirrhosis cannot be cured, so treatment aims to prevent the disease from progressing. Treatment includes avoiding alcohol and other drugs, nutrition therapy and medications to treat specific complications or causes of the disease. If the cirrhosis progresses and the liver fails, a liver transplant may be required.

Figure 11.8 Liver with alcoholic cirrhosis
Gross and microscopic images of a normal and cirrhotic liver. A. Gross image of a normal liver with a smooth surface and homogeneous texture; B. Microscopically, liver sinusoids are organised, and vascular structures are normally distributed; C. Gross image of a cirrhotic liver. The liver has an orange-tawny colour with an irregular surface and a nodular texture; D. Microscopically, the architecture is disorganised, and there are regenerative nodules surrounded by fibrous tissue.

(Goldman & Schafer 2011)

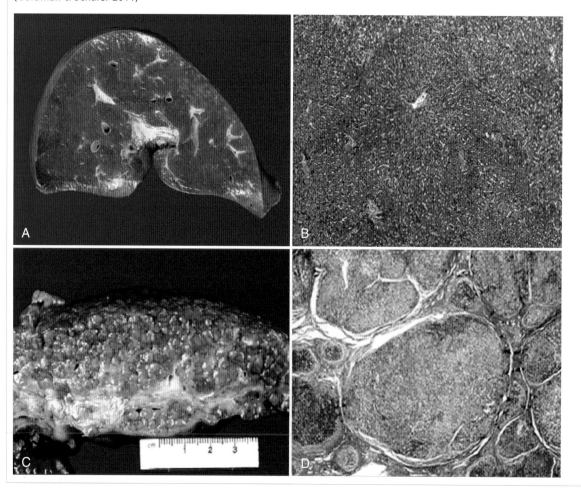

Table continued

Term	Pronunciation	Definition
hepatitis	hep-a-TY-tis	Hepatitis is an inflammation of the liver that can result in damage to the cells in the liver. It can lead to cirrhosis or cancer of the liver and, in some cases, death. Patients with hepatitis will have symptoms that include hepatomegaly, jaundice, clay-coloured faeces, dark urine, abnormal liver function tests and generalised malaise. There are at least five viruses that cause different types of hepatitis – these are hepatitis A, B, C, D and E. They all result in similar symptoms but differ in prognosis and the way in which they are transmitted.
		Hepatitis A is transmitted by ingesting food or water that has been contaminated with the faeces of an infected person. **Hepatitis B** is transmitted by infected body fluids such as blood or semen. It is potentially fatal. **Hepatitis C** is transmitted by infected blood and blood products. It can also be associated with unsafe injection practices and poorly sterilised medical equipment. It can now be successfully treated using antiviral medications. **Hepatitis D** is also transmitted by infected body fluids such as blood or semen but only occurs in people who already have hepatitis B. **Hepatitis E** is also contracted by ingesting contaminated food or water. It is usually a comparatively mild form of hepatitis, with patients recovering in a few weeks.
non-alcoholic steatohepatitis (NASH)	non al-ko-HOL-ik stee-at-o-hep-a-TY-tis	NASH is caused by a build-up of fat in the liver leading to liver inflammation and damage. It is an advanced form of non-alcoholic fatty liver disease. NASH can be difficult to diagnose because many people do not display any symptoms or the symptoms are non-specific to the disease, leading to diagnosis at a late stage of the disease. The condition can cause scarring of the liver, which leads to cirrhosis. NASH is most common in people who are overweight or obese, with other risk factors including diabetes and hypercholesterolaemia.

Small intestine

Term	Pronunciation	Definition
coeliac disease	SEE-lee-ak diz-eez	Coeliac disease is a disorder that damages the small intestine and interferes with absorption of nutrients from food. It is caused by intolerance to gluten, a protein found in wheat, rye and barley. A person with coeliac disease may be asymptomatic or may experience abdominal pain and bloating, diarrhoea or constipation, failure to thrive (in children), and a general feeling of being unwell. Diagnosis involves blood tests and biopsy of the small intestine. Family members should also be tested because coeliac disease is hereditary. Coeliac disease is treated by eliminating all gluten from the diet. The gluten-free diet may be a lifetime requirement.

Diseases of the large intestine

Term	Pronunciation	Definition
colonic polyp	ko-LON-ik POL-ip	A colonic polyp is a growth on the internal surface of the colon. Some colonic polyps are benign, but others may be malignant. Flat polyps are more likely to be cancerous than raised polyps. Most colonic polyps are asymptomatic. Polyps are usually diagnosed during a colonoscopy. If found, they are removed and sent for biopsy. Patients are more likely to develop colonic polyps if they are over 50 years of age, are overweight, a smoker, eat a high-fat, low-fibre diet, or have a personal or family history of colonic polyps or colon cancer. Polyps can also occur in other body sites.

Table continued

Term	Pronunciation	Definition
colorectal cancer	koh-loh-REK-tal KAN-sa	Colorectal cancer (also called bowel cancer) refers to a malignant tumour found in the colon and/or rectum. It is one of the most commonly occurring cancers in Australia. Almost all colorectal cancers begin as benign polyps, which slowly develop into cancer.
		Symptoms of colorectal cancer include changes in bowel habits, rectal bleeding, abdominal pain, weight loss, unexplained anaemia and tiredness. A colonoscopy and biopsy are performed for diagnosis. A CT scan or PET scan can identify any metastatic disease. On diagnosis, colorectal cancers are staged to show the extent of the disease.
		Treatment includes surgery to remove part or all of the colon (colectomy) and associated lymph nodes and chemotherapy. The stage at diagnosis will determine a person's prognosis. If diagnosed early, colorectal cancer is often curable.
Crohn's disease	KROHNs diz-eez	Crohn's disease is an autoimmune disease in which the body's immune system attacks the digestive tract, causing inflammation. It is a type of chronic inflammatory bowel disease. Crohn's disease can affect any area of the digestive tract, from the mouth to the anus, but it most commonly affects the ileum. Consequently, Crohn's disease may also be called ileitis or regional enteritis. Crohn's disease causes changes in the bowel wall, which can range from mild inflammation to severe inflammation, with thickening and ulceration affecting all the layers of the bowel wall. There can be healthy patches of bowel tissue between diseased areas.
		The symptoms of Crohn's disease include abdominal pain, diarrhoea, rectal bleeding causing anaemia, weight loss and fever. Because the symptoms of Crohn's disease are similar to other digestive disorders, it can be difficult to diagnose.
		Diagnosis is by colonoscopy with biopsy. Treatment may include drugs such as anti-inflammatories, steroids, antibiotics and nutrition supplements. In severe cases, surgery such as a colectomy with ileostomy may be required. Often, a combination of treatments is necessary.
diarrhoea	dy-a-REE-a	Diarrhoea is loose, watery faeces or an increase in the frequency of passing faeces. Diarrhoea can be symptomatic of a bacterial or viral infection, or it can be related to a functional disorder, reaction to medication or intestinal disease. Diarrhoea lasting more than a few days may be a sign of a more serious condition. As diarrhoea may result in dehydration, it should be closely monitored and, if required, fluids given to maintain hydration.
diverticular disease	dy-ver-TIK-yoo-la diz-eez	A **diverticulum** (plural: diverticula) is an abnormal side pocket or pouch in the wall of the colon usually related to a lack of fibre in the diet. Diverticular disease, also called diverticulosis, is the presence of diverticula in the colon (Fig. 11.9). **Diverticulitis** is an inflammation or infection in the pouches caused by the collection of faecal material. This may lead to an abscess forming and the wall of the colon perforating. Fever, raised white cell count and pain in the left lower quadrant are common symptoms. Antibiotics and a fluid diet may alleviate symptoms, but often surgery is required to remove the affected section of the colon.

Table continued

Term	Pronunciation	Definition

Figure 11.9 A. Diverticular disease. B. Colonoscopic view of sigmoid diverticulosis.

(A: Waugh et al 2010; B: Sleisenger and Fordtran 2016.)

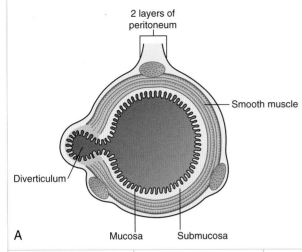 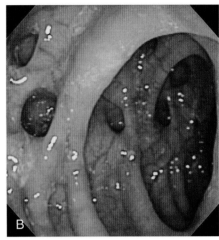

flatulence	FLAT-yoo-lens	Flatulence is the presence of gas in the digestive tract. The gas enters the tract through swallowing air during eating or the air is produced by bacteria that normally inhabit the colon. Air is propelled along the tract by peristalsis. The gurgling noise made by this movement of gas is called borborygmos. The average person produces around 1 litre of gas a day and passes it as flatus through the anus about 20 times each day.
hernia	HER-nee-a	A hernia is an abnormal protrusion of part of an organ or tissue through the structure that normally contains it – usually the abdominal wall or diaphragm. A hernia may be present at birth or develop later in life. There are many types of hernia, which are categorised by their location or cause: umbilical, inguinal, femoral, abdominal, diaphragmatic, hiatal and incisional. Potential complications of a hernia include strangulation and obstruction of the protruding tissue, which can lead to gangrene and ultimately death if urgent surgery is not performed. Treatment options will vary depending on the site but include manual reduction, herniorrhaphy and hernioplasty. Mesh is often used to reinforce the area of weakness to reduce the likelihood of recurrence of the hernia. Common hernia sites are shown in Fig. 11.10.

Figure 11.10 Common sites of hernias

(Leonard 2005)

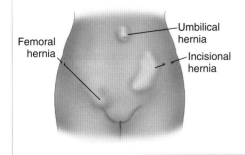 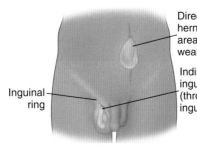

Table continued

Term	Pronunciation	Definition
irritable bowel syndrome (IBS)	i-rit-a-bel BOW-el SIN-drohm	IBS is a non-specific intestinal disorder that causes crampy abdominal pain, bloating and alternating constipation and diarrhoea. People with IBS are more sensitive to factors such as stress, large meals, flatulence, certain medications, certain foods, caffeine and alcohol. IBS is a disease of exclusion – it is diagnosed by its signs and symptoms in the absence of other diseases. It can be controlled by taking medication to relieve specific symptoms such as laxatives, antidiarrhoeals, antispasmodics or antidepressants. Reducing stress and dietary changes are also prescribed.
ulcerative colitis	UL-sa-rat-iv kol-EYE-tis	Ulcerative colitis is a type of chronic inflammatory bowel disease. It causes irritation, ulceration and abscesses in the top layer of the lining of the rectum and colon.
		The most common symptoms of ulcerative colitis are severe abdominal pain and bloody diarrhoea. Other symptoms include anaemia, fevers, weight loss, anorexia, fatigue and rectal bleeding.
		Ulcerative colitis can be difficult to diagnose because its symptoms are similar to other intestinal disorders such as Crohn's disease. A detailed medical history is required, and blood tests to check for anaemia, which could indicate bleeding in the colon or rectum, or high white blood cell count, which is a sign of inflammation – are done. A faecal sample is tested for infection and bleeding. A colonoscopy with biopsy is the most accurate test to diagnose ulcerative colitis.
		Treatment needs to be tailored for individual patients depending on their specific symptoms. Medications include anti-inflammatory agents, corticosteroids and immunomodulators. If symptoms are not controlled by medication, surgery may be necessary to improve quality of life. Surgery for ulcerative colitis includes proctocolectomy or total colectomy with ileostomy or ileoanal anastomosis.

Diseases of the rectum and anus

Term	Pronunciation	Definition
anal fissure	AY-nal FISH-ya	An anal fissure is a tear or split in the lining of the anal canal due to minor trauma such as from passing hard faeces or from childbirth. Recurrent diarrhoea can also result in an anal fissure. Pain and bleeding after defecation are common symptoms. An anal fissure may be treated conservatively with anaesthetic medication and creams supplemented by use of laxatives but may require surgical intervention with an anal sphincterotomy. More recently, injections of Botox to relax the anal sphincter while the fissure heals naturally have been successful.

Table continued

Term	Pronunciation	Definition
haemorrhoids	HEM-a-roydz	Haemorrhoids are swollen, inflamed veins found in the anus or in the lower part of the rectum. External haemorrhoids are located under the skin surrounding the anus. They can cause itching, pain and bleeding with a bowel motion. It is quite common for external haemorrhoids to become thrombosed. Internal haemorrhoids develop in the inside lining of the lower rectum. They are usually painless but may protrude, or prolapse, through the anus and cause bleeding during a bowel motion. Severely prolapsed haemorrhoids may protrude permanently and require treatment.
		Haemorrhoids are caused by several factors, including chronic constipation, straining during bowel movements and a lack of fibre in the diet. Pregnancy can also cause haemorrhoids because of increasing pressure in the abdomen, which may enlarge the veins in the lower rectum and anus. For most women, haemorrhoids caused by pregnancy disappear after childbirth.
		Treatment of haemorrhoids may be conservative (changes to diet to include more fibre and fluids, warm baths, regular exercise and topical creams to reduce pain and inflammation) or surgical (including ligation, sclerotherapy or haemorrhoidectomy).

TESTS AND PROCEDURES

The following section provides a list of common diagnostic tests and procedures and clinical interventions and surgical procedures that are undertaken for the digestive system.

Test/Procedure	Pronunciation	Definition
abdominal ultrasonography (ultrasound or sonography)	ab-DOM-in-al ul-tra-son-OG-ra-fee (UL-tra-sownd or son-OG-ra-fee)	Abdominal ultrasonography is performed using high-frequency sound waves to produce two-dimensional images of the abdominal cavity and its structures. It can be used as a diagnostic tool or as a method of guidance in other treatment procedures such as biopsies.
adhesiolysis	ad-heez-ee-o-LY-sis	Adhesiolysis is a procedure performed to separate or divide adhesions or scar tissue that may be causing an intestinal obstruction.
bariatric therapies	BA-ree-at-rik ther-a-pees	Bariatric medicine is a field of medicine focusing on the control and treatment of obesity and the diseases associated with obesity. Obesity can be treated in several ways. Diet, exercise or oral medications can be successful in some patients. However, in other patients, especially those who are morbidly obese, surgical interventions are required for weight reduction.
		Vagal-blocking therapy delivers electrical impulses from a neuroregulator, via electrodes, to the vagus nerves, blocking the actions of the nerves. This results in a slower emptying of the stomach and an earlier feeling of fullness.
		Intragastric balloon insertion is a reversible procedure in which a soft, expandable silicone balloon is inserted into the stomach via endoscopy. The balloon is inflated using a sterile saline solution to create a feeling of fullness. The balloon is left in place for a period of up to 6 months.
		Gastric banding involves the laparoscopic placement of a band around the top of the stomach, thus reducing the amount of food that can enter the stomach.
		Gastric plication is a laparoscopic procedure that involves suturing one or more large folds in the stomach, reducing the stomach volume to approximately 70%. The procedure may be reversed or lead to other bariatric procedures.

Table continued

Test/Procedure	Pronunciation	Definition
		Sleeve gastrectomy is a non-reversible laparoscopic procedure. The outer part of the stomach is removed, resulting in the creation of a tube-like section in the upper part of the stomach. With only a small portion of the stomach remaining, food intake capacity is reduced along with food absorption.
		Gastric bypass surgery (Roux-en-Y gastric bypass) is a non-reversible procedure, commonly performed via laparoscope. The stomach is divided into two sections, the upper and lower parts of the stomach. The upper section is then connected directly to the lower section of the small intestine, resulting in reduced absorption.
		Biliopancreatic division is generally only performed on people with a body mass index of 50+ who have not been able to lose weight through other means. Up to 70% of the stomach is removed and the remaining portion is connected to the lower portion of the small intestine. A less involved version of this procedure is the biliopancreatic diversion with switch, which involves connecting the stomach to the duodenum and not the lower part of the small intestine.
capsule endoscopy	KAPS-yool en-DOS-kop-ee	This form of endoscopic examination of the digestive tract uses a camera the size of a pill. The patient swallows the camera and images are taken throughout the gastrointestinal tract, with the images being transferred to a computer via bluetooth technology. The capsule endoscopy is particularly useful for diagnosing diseases of the small intestine, which are often difficult to identify through other endoscopic procedures.
cholangiography	kol-an-jee-OG-ra-fee	A cholangiography is a diagnostic procedure that involves radiographic imaging of the bile ducts with contrast medium administered orally or injected intravenously or percutaneously.
cholecystectomy	kol-EE-sis-TEK-tom-ee	A cholecystectomy is a surgical procedure to remove the gallbladder (Fig. 11.11). The majority of cholecystectomies are now undertaken via laparoscopy. **Figure 11.11 Laparoscopic cholecystectomy** (Lau et al 2013) 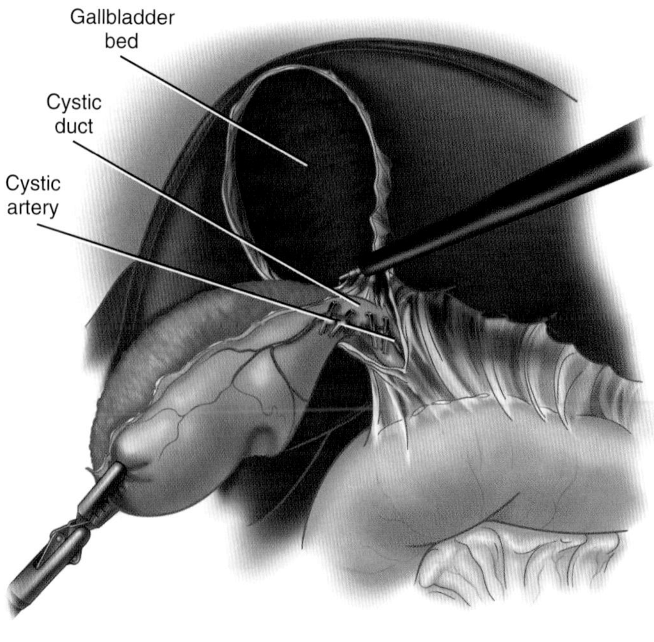

Table continued

Test/Procedure	Pronunciation	Definition
computed tomography (CT) scan (of the) abdomen	kom-PYOO-ted to-MOG-raf-ee skan ab-doh-MEN	A CT scan of the abdomen is a diagnostic test to identify disorders of the digestive tract. Cross-sectional images are taken using a computer in conjunction with x-ray beams.
enterostomy (colostomy, ileostomy, duodenostomy)	en-te-ROS-tom-ee (co-LOS-tom-ee, il-ee-OS-tom-ee, dyoo-o-den-OS-tom-ee)	An enterostomy is a procedure that involves incising the small or large intestine to insert a tube to make an artificial opening (stoma) for drainage or feeding purposes (Fig. 11.12). The stoma can be temporary or permanent. Enterostomies are named according to the part of the intestine where the stoma has been created (e.g. ileostomy, colostomy and duodenostomy).

Figure 11.12 Ileostomy construction

(Copyright 1991, Mayo Clinic, Rochester, Minn.)

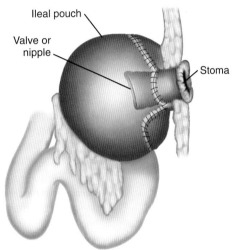

Ileal pouch

Valve or nipple

Stoma

faecal occult blood test (guaiac, haemoccult or immunochemical test)	fee-kal OK-ult blud test (GWY-ik, heem-OK-ult or im-YOON-o-kem-ee-kal test)	A faecal occult blood test is used to detect blood in faeces that is not visibly apparent, otherwise known as faecal occult (hidden) blood. A guaiac test involves applying a faeces sample to a thick piece of paper coated with a film of guaiac (a wood resin from a guiaicum tree), which reacts to the presence of blood. A FIT (faecal immunochemical test), sometimes called an iFOBT (immunochemical faecal occult blood test), is an increasingly common form of faecal occult blood test that gives improved results.
faeces culture	FEE-seez KUL-cha	This test is also known as a stool culture and tests for parasites or microorganisms in faeces. The test is undertaken when a patient has had diarrhoea for several days or if they have blood or mucus in their faeces.
fundoplication	fun-doh-pli-KAY-shun	Fundoplication is a surgical procedure that is undertaken to treat GORD or hiatus hernia. It involves wrapping (folding) the gastric fundus (upper part) of the stomach around the lower end of the oesophagus and stitching it in place, reinforcing the closing function of the lower oesophageal sphincter.
gastrointestinal endoscopy	gas-tro-in-TES-tin-al en-DOS-kop-ee	This procedure involves using an endoscope to view the digestive tract. The entry point for the endoscope can be either the mouth or the anus. The types of endoscopies are named for the site of the digestive tract being viewed, including gastroscopy, colonoscopy, sigmoidoscopy (Fig. 11.13), proctoscopy, oesophagoscopy, and oesophagogastroduodenoscopy. These procedures are either diagnostic or allow access to parts of the digestive tract for biopsy or to remove lesions.

Table continued

Test/Procedure	Pronunciation	Definition
Figure 11.13 Colonoscopy with sigmoidoscopy (Ballinger & Frank 2003)		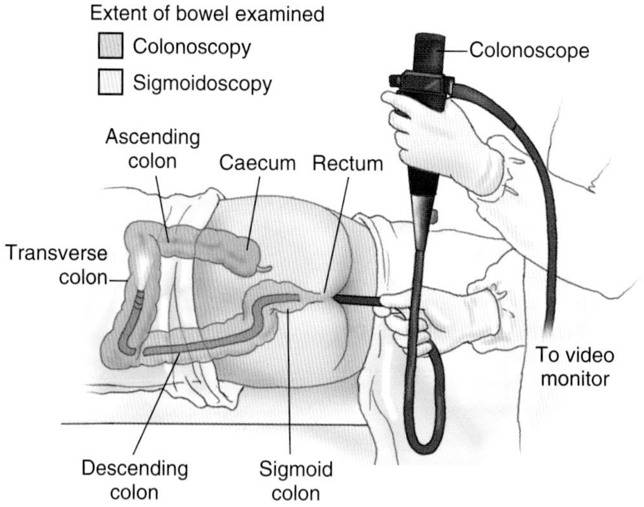 Extent of bowel examined ☐ Colonoscopy ☐ Sigmoidoscopy
haemorrhoidectomy	HEM-a-royd-EK-tom-ee	A haemorrhoidectomy is a surgical procedure to repair swollen, varicose veins in the rectal region by removing the haemorrhoids using a scalpel, laser or staple gun. The membranes lining the rectum and anus are then sutured to the underlying muscle.
herniorrhaphy	HER-nee-O-raf-ee	A herniorrhaphy is a surgical procedure involving opening the hernial sac, placing the contents in their normal location, removing the sac and suturing the surgical wound. Mesh may be used to reinforce the area of weakness to reduce the likelihood of recurrence of the hernia.
laparoscopy	lap-ah-ROS-kop-ee	A laparoscopy is a procedure that allows for the visual examination of the abdominal and pelvic cavities for diagnostic purposes via a small incision into the abdominal cavity and insertion of a lighted scope. It can also be used as a method for entry to the abdominal cavity for surgical treatment, with the addition of further small incisions to introduce a laser and other equipment.
liver biopsy	LIV-a BY-op-see	A liver biopsy is a diagnostic procedure that involves removing a small amount of liver tissue for microscopic examination. The most common biopsy method is a percutaneous liver biopsy, involving the use of a hollow needle inserted through the skin of the abdomen for removing a small sample of tissue. Other methods include laparoscopic, transvenous and intraoperative.

Table continued

Test/Procedure	Pronunciation	Definition
liver function tests (LFTs)	LIV-a FUNK-shun tests	LFTs are a series of tests measuring the enzymes and bilirubin in serum to identify liver disease, the severity of the disease and for monitoring treatment of the disease. The tests that are undertaken include tests for the following:
		Alanine aminotransferase (ALT) is an enzyme that has a role in metabolism. High levels of ALT are an indication of damage to liver cells, particularly in acute hepatitis.
		Alkaline phosphatase (ALP) is an enzyme found in the liver, bones, intestines, kidneys and other organs. Elevated levels can be an indication of viral infections, liver diseases or blocked bile ducts.
		Aspartate aminotransferase (AST) is an enzyme that has a role in processing protein, with elevated levels indicating that the liver is damaged or inflamed.
		Total bilirubin and direct bilirubin. Bilirubin results from the normal breakdown of red blood cells. The normal process is for the bilirubin to pass through the liver and be excreted. However, if this does not happen the skin can take on a yellow discolouration from the rise in bilirubin levels. Bilirubin tests can be total (a measure of the level of all bilirubin in the body) or direct (a measure of only the bilirubin that has been processed by the liver and attached to other chemicals).
liver scan	LIV-a skan	A liver scan is a diagnostic nuclear radiology procedure that uses a radioactive substance to diagnose various conditions such as tumours, abscesses, haematomas, organ enlargement or cysts.
lower gastrointestinal series	LOW-a gas-troh-in-TES-tin-al SEE-reez	A lower gastrointestinal series is a diagnostic tool using x-rays to identify problems of the large intestine. The patient is given a barium enema, which coats the lining of the large intestine to highlight abnormalities more clearly on x-ray.
magnetic resonance imaging (MRI)	mag-NET-ik REZ-on-ans IM-a-jing	An MRI is a diagnostic test that creates images of the abdominal cavity using radio waves and a magnetic field to identify lesions that cannot be easily noted on x-ray.
nasogastric intubation	NAY-zo-GAS-trik in-tyoo-BAY-shun	Nasogastric intubation involves inserting a tube through the nose into the stomach. The purpose is to: relieve gastric distension by removing gas, gastric secretions or food; administer medication, food or fluids; or obtain a specimen for laboratory analysis.
paracentesis (abdominocentesis)	pa-ra-sen-TEE-sis (ab-dom-in-o-sen-TEE-sis)	Paracentesis is a procedure to drain accumulated fluid (ascites) from the peritoneal cavity using a long, thin needle.
percutaneous endoscopic gastrostomy (PEG) tube	per-KYOO-tayn-ee-us en-do-SKOP-ik gas-TROS-tom-ee tyoob	A PEG is also known as a feeding tube. The tube is placed by passing an endoscope through the mouth into the stomach. Using the light from the endoscope as a guide, a small incision is made in the abdominal wall for inserting the feeding tube. PEG feeding tubes are generally inserted for long-term enteral nutrition where the patient cannot maintain adequate oral nutritional intake.
percutaneous endoscopic jejunostomy (PEJ) tube	per-KYOO-tayn-ee-us en-DO-SKOP-ik je-JYOON-os-tom-ee tube	A PEJ is a surgical procedure for placing the feeding tube into the jejunum, similar to a PEG.
upper gastrointestinal series	UP-pa gas-troh-in-TEST-in-al SEE-reez	An upper gastrointestinal series is a diagnostic technique using x-rays to identify problems of the oesophagus, stomach and duodenum. The patient is given a carbonated drink to expand the stomach by creating gas, followed by a barium medication that coats the lining of the stomach to highlight abnormalities more clearly on x-ray.

Exercises

EXERCISE 11.1: LABEL THE DIAGRAM

Using the information provided in this chapter, label the anatomical parts in Figs 11.14a and b.

1 _____

2 _____

3 _____

4 _____

5 _____

6 _____

7 _____

8 _____

9 _____

10 _____

11 _____

12 _____

13 _____

14 _____

15 _____

16 _____

17 _____

18 _____

19 _____

20 _____

21 _____

22 _____

23 _____

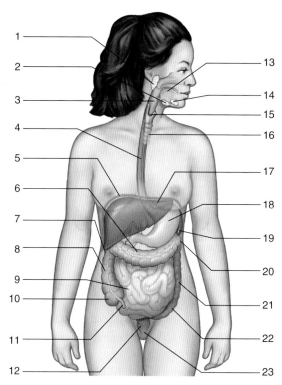

Figure 11.14a Organs of the digestive system

(Mosby's Dictionary 2014)

1 _____

2 _____

3 _____

4 _____

5 _____

6 _____

7 _____

8 _____

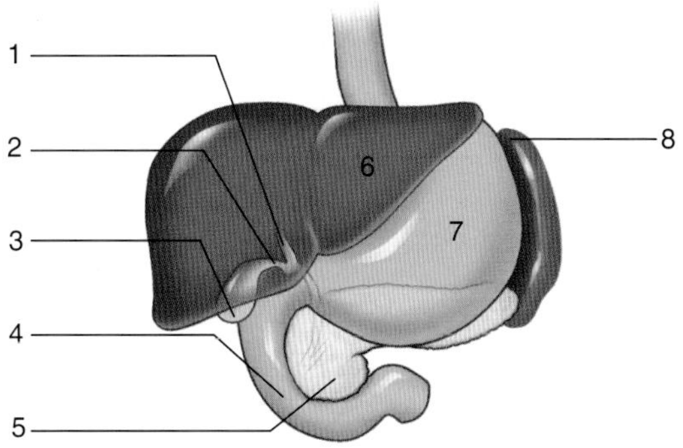

Figure 11.14b **The liver and stomach**

(Mosby's Dictionary 2014)

EXERCISE 11.2: WORD ELEMENT MEANINGS AND WORD BUILDING

Insert the missing word elements, then use each element correctly in a medical term.

Meaning	Word Element	Medical Term
anus		
bile duct		
bile pigment		
bladder, cyst, sac		
cheek		
defecation, elimination of waste products		
digestion		
eat, swallow		
enzyme		
gall		
bile		
gallbladder		
ileum		
lip		
meal		
orange/yellow		
small intestine		
starch		
through, across		
vomiting		

EXERCISE 11.3: MATCH MEDICAL TERMS AND MEANINGS

Match the medical term in Column A with its meaning in Column B.

Column A	Answer	Column B
1. cholecystectomy		A. breaking down of fat
2. sublingual		B. suture of a hernia
3. steatolysis		C. pertaining to the colon and rectum
4. jejunoileitis		D. fixation of the caecum
5. proctodynia		E. difficulty swallowing
6. dyspepsia		F. surgical removal of the gallbladder
7. cheiloplasty		G. protein enzyme
8. splenomegaly		H. pain in the rectum
9. pharyngoscope		I. drainage of fluid from the abdomen
10. stomatitis		J. excessive vomiting
11. enterostomy		K. pertaining to the teeth and gums
12. herniorrhaphy		L. viewing of the stomach
13. colorectal		M. artificial opening of the intestine
14. dysphagia		N. pertaining to under the tongue
15. dentogingival		O. difficult digestion
16. gastroscopy		P. instrument to view the pharynx
17. protease		Q. inflammation of the jejunum and ileum
18. abdominocentesis		R. repair of the lip
19. caecopexy		S. enlarged spleen
20. hyperemesis		T. inflammation of the mucous membrane of the mouth

EXERCISE 11.4: CIRCLE THE CORRECT SPELLING

Circle the correctly spelled medical term from the options provided.

diarhea	diarhoea	diorrhea	diarrhoea
haemorhoid	haemorrhoid	hemorhoid	heemorhoid
cholecystitis	cholicystitis	colecystitis	colicystitis
intassusception	intersusception	intussusception	intususception
paroditis	parotitis	parottitis	parrotitis
polidipsia	polidypsia	polydipsia	polydypsia
esophagescopy	esophogoscopy	oesophagoscopy	oesophogoscopy
disentery	disentry	dysentery	dysentry
cirhosis	cirrhosis	serosis	serrhosis
gluecose	glucoze	glucose	glukose

EXERCISE 11.5: EXPAND THE ABBREVIATIONS

Expand the abbreviations to form correct medical terms.

Abbreviation	Expanded Abbreviation
Ba	
b.i.d.	
BMI	
ERCP	
GORD	
IBD	
IBS	
LFTs	
N&V	
NG	
OGD	
PEJ tube	
PTHC	
PUD	
TPN	

EXERCISE 11.6: VOCABULARY BUILDING

Provide the medical term for each of the definitions below.

1. Food that has been broken down into a liquid: _____

2. An abnormal side pocket or pouch in the wall of the colon, usually related to a lack of fibre in the diet: _____

_____

3. A tear or split in the lining of the anal canal due to minor trauma: _____

4. Rhythmic contraction and relaxation of the smooth muscle that lines the walls of the digestive organs: _____

_____

5. Gas in the digestive tract: _____

6. Dilated veins in the lower part of the oesophagus or in the upper part of the stomach: _____

_____

7. A growth on the internal surface of the colon: _____

8. Movement of food along the digestive tract through a process called peristalsis: _____

9. Mixes with food to lubricate and to also kill microorganisms: _____

10. Release of faeces into the external environment: _____

EXERCISE 11.7: PRONUNCIATION AND COMPREHENSION

Read the following paragraphs aloud to practise your pronunciation. Using your textbook and a medical dictionary, find the meanings of the underlined medical terms.

This was a routine admission of a 49-year-old woman for <u>open cholecystectomy</u>. She had a 12-month history of <u>epigastric</u> pain associated with nausea and sweating. She was admitted in the previous December with probable <u>gallstone pancreatitis</u>. At this time she had an <u>amylase</u> rise of 550. An ultrasound scan at this time revealed gallstones. The common bile duct was not dilated.

Open cholecystectomy was performed under general <u>anaesthetic</u> (ASA = 1NE) on 21.1.20 via a <u>Kocher's</u> incision. An operative <u>cholangiogram</u> at this time revealed filling defects with an obstructed flow into the <u>duodenum</u>. Subsequently the common bile duct was explored and multiple stones were removed. Following this a T-tube was inserted.

<u>Postoperatively</u> she suffered some pain at the site of her T-tube. She also had some transient fevers. This was not thought to be <u>cholangitis</u> and the pain was attributed to irritation of the T-tube in the abdominal wall. A T-tube cholangiogram performed on day 7 showed <u>choledocholithiasis</u> but with flow into the duodenum. At this stage the patient was <u>asymptomatic</u> and not <u>jaundiced</u>. A decision to perform an <u>endoscopic retrograde cholangeopancreatography</u> (ERCP) was made and carried out. A T-tube cholangiogram following this procedure showed good flow into the duodenum, with no further stones apparent. The T-tube was then removed without any further problems. The patient was discharged home with review in surgical outpatients planned.

EXERCISE 11.8: CROSSWORD PUZZLE

Complete the puzzle by providing the medical term for each of the clues below.

ACROSS

3. Ball of food (5)

6. A weight reduction procedure used to treat morbidly obese patients (7, 7)

8. Breaking down food into smaller components to allow for absorption in the digestive tract (9)

11. Inflammation of the liver that can result in damage to the cells in the liver (9)

DOWN

1. Surgical removal of the gallbladder (15)

2. A series of tests measuring the enzymes and bilirubin in serum to identify liver disease (5, 8, 5)

4. The part of the large intestine between the caecum and the rectum (5)

5. The passage of digested food molecules through the intestinal cells into the bloodstream (10)

7. Inflammation of parotid gland(s) (9)

9. A band of muscle in the mouth (6)

10. Mixes with food to lubricate and to also kill microorganisms (6)

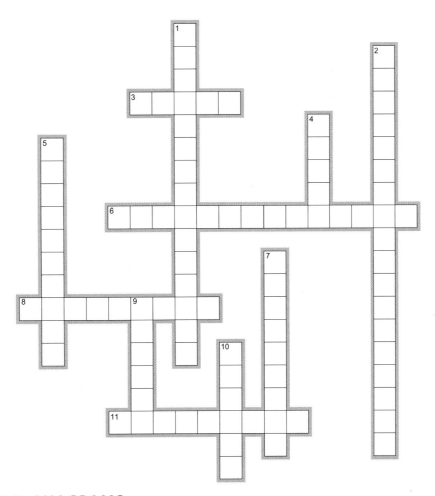

EXERCISE 11.9: ANAGRAMS

Work out each medical term from the jumbled letters below. Then, using the letters in brackets, determine the medical term that matches the description given.

1.	evirl	__ __ __ (__) __	large organ located in the right upper quadrant
2.	suproly	__ (__) __ __ __ __ __	opening between the stomach and duodenum
3.	melui	__ __ __ __ (__)	third part of the small intestine
4.	gadyphias	__ __ __ __ (__) __ __ __ __	difficulty in swallowing
5.	muccea	(__) __ __ __ __ __	first part of the large intestine

Rearrange the letters in brackets to form a word that means 'the semi-fluid contents of the stomach'.

__ __ __ __ __

EXERCISE 11.10: DISCHARGE SUMMARY ANALYSIS

Read the discharge summary below and answer the questions.

UNIVERSITY HOSPITAL DISCHARGE SUMMARY	**UR number:** 202122
	Name: Karen Green
	Address: 55 Alexander Street, Woodley
	Date of birth: 23/10/1943
	Sex: F
	Nominated primary healthcare provider: Dr Kerry Trackson

Episode details	**Discharge details**
Consultant: Dr Morrison	**Status:** Home
Registrar: Dr Pringle	**Date of discharge:** 11/4/2020
Unit: Gastroenterology	
Admission source: ED	
Date of admission: 6/4/2020	

Reason for admission / Presenting problems:

RUQ pain of sudden onset, N&V for 24 hours

Principal diagnosis: Gastric ulcer

Comorbidities:

Smoker – 20 cigarettes a day

Hx of light alcohol intake

Rheumatoid arthritis – using NSAIDs regularly for many years

Previous medical history:

Clinical synopsis:

On examination, Ms Green had an acute abdomen with tenderness and guarding on the right side, absent bowel sounds and gas under the diaphragm shown on erect chest x-ray. LFTs and amylase were normal. Her WCC was 14. She was taken to theatre that day for an urgent laparotomy where a 5 mm perforation in the anterior stomach was oversewn with an omental patch under GA. ASA = 1NE. Postoperatively, she improved rapidly.

Complications: Nil reported

Clinical interventions:

Oversew of perforated gastric ulcer

Diagnostic interventions:

Chest x-ray

LFTs and amylase were normal

Medications at discharge:

Zantac

Ceased medications: Nil reported

Allergies: Nil reported

Alerts: Nil reported

Arranged services: Nil reported

Recommendations: For review in 6 weeks in surgical outpatients

Information to patient/relevant parties:

For review in 6 weeks in surgical outpatients

Authorising clinician: Dr Pringle

Document recipients:

Patient and LMO: Dr Kerry Trackson

1. **Expand the following abbreviations as found in the discharge summary above.**

   ED

   Hx

   LFTs

   LMO

   N&V

   NSAIDs

   RUQ

   WCC

2. **It is stated that Ms Green had an 'acute abdomen'. What does this mean?**

3. **Ms Green has been taking aspirin for many years for her rheumatoid arthritis. Does research show a link between long-term ingestion of aspirin and gastric ulcers?**

4. **What does perforation of a gastric ulcer mean and why is it a serious condition?**

5. **Why was Ms Green discharged on Zantac medication?**

CHAPTER 12

Nervous System

Contents

OBJECTIVES   272

INTRODUCTION   273

NEW WORD ELEMENTS   273
   Combining forms   273
   Prefixes   274
   Suffixes   274

VOCABULARY   275

ABBREVIATIONS   276

FUNCTIONS AND STRUCTURE
OF THE NERVOUS SYSTEM   276
   Central nervous system   278
   Brain   278
   Spinal cord   279
   Peripheral nervous system   280
   Neurons   281

PATHOLOGY AND DISEASES   282
   Degenerative and motor
   disorders   282
   Episodic neurological disorders 284
   Inflammatory and infectious
   diseases   284
   Neoplasms   285
   Disorders of nerves   285
   Disorders due to trauma   285
   Paralysis   286
   Vascular disorders   287
   Miscellaneous conditions   288

TESTS AND PROCEDURES   288

EXERCISES   291

Objectives

After completing this chapter you should be able to:

1. state the meanings of the word elements related to the nervous system

2. build words using the word elements associated with the nervous system

3. recognise, pronounce and effectively use medical terms associated with the nervous system

4. expand abbreviations related to the nervous system

5. describe the structure and functions of the nervous system including the brain, spinal cord and nerves

6. describe common pathological conditions associated with the nervous system

7. describe common laboratory tests, diagnostic and surgical procedures associated with the nervous system

8. apply what you have learned by interpreting medical terminology in practice.

Demonstrate your knowledge of the nervous system by completing the exercises at the end of this chapter.

INTRODUCTION

The nervous system is arguably the most complex system in the body. It facilitates internal communication within the body by integrating and controlling the various functions of the body. Sense organs provide the nervous system with information about the external environment by means of such senses as sight, hearing, smell, taste and touch. The nervous system is then responsible for sending, receiving and processing nerve impulses to react to the various stimuli in the environment that the senses have identified.

The activities that keep the body operating such as respiration, digestion, heart pumping, movement, the senses, and the unique processes that make us human such as thinking, dreaming, laughing and memory are not possible without a properly functioning nervous system. The nervous system is discussed in this chapter, while the sense organs are discussed in Chapter 13.

NEW WORD ELEMENTS

Here are some word elements related to the nervous system. To reinforce your learning, write the meanings of the medical terms in the spaces provided. Use the Glossary of medical terms on page 561 to help you work out the meanings. You may also need to check the meaning in a medical dictionary, but make an attempt yourself first.

Combining forms

Combining Form	Meaning	Medical Term	Meaning of Medical Term
aesthesi/o	sensation, feeling	anaesthesiology	
astr/o	star	astrocyte	
caus/o	burn, burning	causalgia	
cephal/o	head	cephalic	
cerebell/o	cerebellum	cerebellar	
cerebr/o	cerebrum, brain	cerebral	
comat/o	coma	comatose	
crani/o	skull, cranium	cranial	
dendr/o	tree, branches	oligodendria	
dur/o	dura mater	extradural	
encephal/o	brain	encephalopathy	
gangli/o	ganglion, knot	gangliocytoma	
gli/o	glue	glioneuroma	
gnos/o	knowledge	prognosis	
hydr/o	water	hydrocephalus	
hypn/o	sleep	hypnosis	
kinesi/o	movement, motion	kinesiology	
kinet/o		akinetic	
lex/o	word, phrase	dyslexia	
mening/o	meninges	meningoencephalitis	
meningi/o		meningioma	
myel/o	spinal cord, bone marrow	myelomalacia	
narc/o	stupor, sleep	narcolepsy	
neur/o	nerve	neurogenic	
phas/o	speech	dysphasic	
plex/o	network (of nerves)	plexopathy	
psych/o	mind	psychotic	
rachi/o	spine	rachiocentesis	
radic/o	nerve root	radicotomy	
radicul/o		radiculopathy	
somat/o	body	somatosensory	

Table continued

Combining Form	Meaning	Medical Term	Meaning of Medical Term
somn/i	sleep	insomnia	
somn/o		somnolence	
spin/o	spine, thorn	cerebrospinal	
spondyl/o	vertebra	spondylosis	
syncop/o	cut short	syncopal	
tax/o	order, coordination	ataxic	
thalam/o	thalamus	hypothalamus	
thec/o	sheath	intrathecal	
ventricul/o	ventricle	ventriculotomy	
vertebr/o	vertebra, spine	vertebrocostal	

Prefixes

Prefix	Meaning	Medical Term	Meaning of Medical Term
bi-	two, twice, double	bilateral	
echo-	repeated, reflected sound	echoencephalogram	
electro-	electricity, electrical activity	electroencephalograph	
hemi-	half	hemiplegia	
para-	beside, near, alongside	paraesthesia	
polio-	grey matter	poliomyelitis	
poly-	many, much	polyneuritis	
quadri-	four	quadriplegia	
tetra-	four	tetraplegia	
uni-	one	unilateral	

Suffixes

Suffix	Meaning	Medical Term	Meaning of Medical Term
-aesthesia	condition of sensation, feeling	anaesthesia	
-al	pertaining to, drug action	neural	
-algesia	condition of pain	analgesia	
-algia	condition of pain	cephalgia	
-asthenia	condition of weakness, debility	myasthenia	
-cele	hernia, protrusion	myelocele	
-form	having the form of	somatoform	
-kinesia	condition of movement, motion	hyperkinesia	
-lepsy	seizure	epilepsy	
-oma	tumour, collection, mass, swelling	neuroma	
-paresis	slight or incomplete paralysis	hemiparesis	
-phasia	speech	dysphasia	
-plegia	condition of paralysis	paraplegia	
-praxia	achieve, to do	hypopraxia	

Table continued

Suffix	Meaning	Medical Term	Meaning of Medical Term
-rrhage	bursting forth, excessive discharge or flow	haemorrhage	
-us	thing, structure	macrocephalus	

VOCABULARY

The following list provides many of the medical terms used for the first time in this chapter. Pronunciations are provided with each term. As you read the rest of the chapter, make sure you identify each of these terms and understand their meanings.

Term	Pronunciation
Alzheimer's disease (dementia)	ALZ-hy-mers diz-eez (de-MENT-cha)
amygdala	a-MIG-dal-a
arachnoid membrane	a-RAK-noyd membrayn
autonomic nervous system	aw-ton-om-ik NER-vus sis-tem
axon	AK-son
brainstem	BRAYN-stem
carpal tunnel syndrome	KAR-pul TUN-el SIN-drohm
cell body	SEL bod-ee
central nervous system	SEN-tral NER-vus sis-tem
cerebellum	SE-re-BEL-um
cerebral angiography	SE-re-bral an-jee-OG-ra-fee
cerebral concussion	SE-re-bral kon-KUSH-un
cerebral contusion	SE-re-bral kon-TOO-shun
cerebral palsy	SE-re-bral PAWL-zee
cerebral tumour	SE-re-bral TYOO-ma
cerebrospinal fluid	SE-re-broh-SPY-nal FLOO-id
cerebrospinal fluid analysis	SE-re-broh-SPY-nal FLOO-id a-NAL-e-sis
cerebrovascular accident	SE-re-broh-VAS-kyoo-la AK-se-dent
cerebrum	SE-re-brum
computed tomography	kom-PYOO-ted to-MOG-ra-fee
dendrite	DEN-dryt
Doppler ultrasound studies	DOP-la UL-tra-sownd stud-eez
dura mater	dyoo-ra MAH-ta
electroencephalography	ee-LEK-tro-en-kef-a-LOG-ra-fee
encephalitis	en-kef-a-LY-tus
epilepsy	EP-il-ep-see
forebrain	FOR-brayn

Table continued

Term	Pronunciation
frontal lobe	FRUN-tal lohb
hindbrain	HYND-brayn
hippocampus	hip oh KAM pus
hydrocephalus	hy-droh-KEF-a-lus
hypothalamus	hy-poh-THAL-a-mus
interneuron	in-ta-NYOO-ron
intracranial haemorrhage	in-tra-KRAYN-ee-al HEM-ah-raj
limbic system	LIM-bik SIS-tem
lumbar (spinal) puncture	LUM-bah (spy-nal) PUNK-cha
magnetic resonance imaging	mag-NET-ik REZ-on-ans IM-a-jing
medulla oblongata	me-DUL-a ob-long-GAH-ta
meninges	men-IN-jeez
meningitis	men-in-JY-tus
midbrain	MID-brayn
migraine	MY-grayn
motor neuron disease	MOH-ta NYOO-ron diz-eez
multiple sclerosis	MUL-tip-el skler-OH-sis
myelography	my-el-OG-ra-fee
neuron	NYOO-ron
neurotransmitter	nyoo-roh-tranz-MIT-a
occipital lobe	ok-SIP-it-al lohb
parietal lobe	par-EYE-e-tal lohb
Parkinson's disease	PAH-kin-sonz diz-eez
peripheral nervous system	pe-RIF-er-al NER-vus SIS-tem
pia mater	pee-a MAH-ta
poliomyelitis	POL-ee-o-my-a-LY-tus
pons	ponz
positron emission tomography	POZ-i-tron e-MISH-en to-MOG-ra-fee
receptor	ree-SEP-ta
sciatica	sy-AT-ik-a
sensory neuron	SEN-sor-ee NYOO-ron
sleep apnoea	sleep AP-nee-ah
somatic nervous system	soh-MAT-ik NER-vus sis-tem
spinal cord	SPY-nal kord

Table continued

Term	Pronunciation
stereotactic radiosurgery	STE-ree-oh-TAK-tik RAY-dee-oh-ser-jer-ee
synapse	SY-naps
tectum	TEK-tum
tegmentum	teg-MEN-tum
temporal lobe	TEM-por-al lohb
thalamus	THAL-a-mus
transient ischaemic attack	TRANZ-ee-ent is-KEE-mik a-TAK

ABBREVIATIONS

The following abbreviations are commonly used in the Australian healthcare environment. Because some abbreviations can have more than one meaning, check the context in which the abbreviation is used before assigning a meaning to it.

Abbreviation	Definition
ANS	autonomic nervous system
CNS	central nervous system
CSF	cerebrospinal fluid
CT	computed tomography
CAT	computerised axial tomography
CTS	carpal tunnel syndrome
CVA	cerebrovascular accident
ECT	electroconvulsive therapy
EEG	electroencephalogram
GCS	Glasgow Coma Scale/Score
ICP	intracranial pressure
LOC	loss of consciousness

Table continued

Abbreviation	Definition
LP	lumbar puncture
MRI	magnetic resonance imaging
MS	multiple sclerosis
NSAID(s)	non-steroidal anti-inflammatory drug(s)
PET	positron emission tomography
PNS	peripheral nervous system
REM	rapid eye movement
TBI	traumatic brain injury
TENS	transcutaneous electrical nerve stimulation
TIA	transient ischaemic attack

FUNCTIONS AND STRUCTURE OF THE NERVOUS SYSTEM

The nervous system plays an important role in coordinating and regulating body functions and communicating within and between the brain, spinal cord and all other parts of the body. Another important function is to interpret stimuli from the external environment so the body can respond accordingly. Working in association with the endocrine system, the nervous system acts to maintain homeostasis, the body's ability to maintain a constant internal state even in changing external environments. The nervous system consists of a network of specialised cells called neurons. Signals move between the brain and body via these neural networks. The nervous system has two divisions: the central nervous system, which includes the brain and spinal cord, and the peripheral nervous system, which is composed of nerves and neural networks throughout the rest of the body (Figs 12.1 and 12.2).

Figure 12.1 Structure of the nervous system

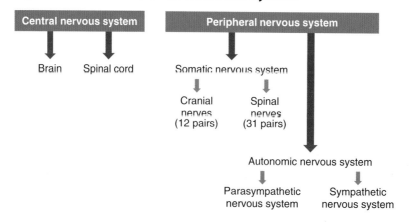

Figure 12.2 **The nervous system**

A. Simplified view of the nervous system; B. Cranial nerves.

(Thibodeau & Patton 2003)

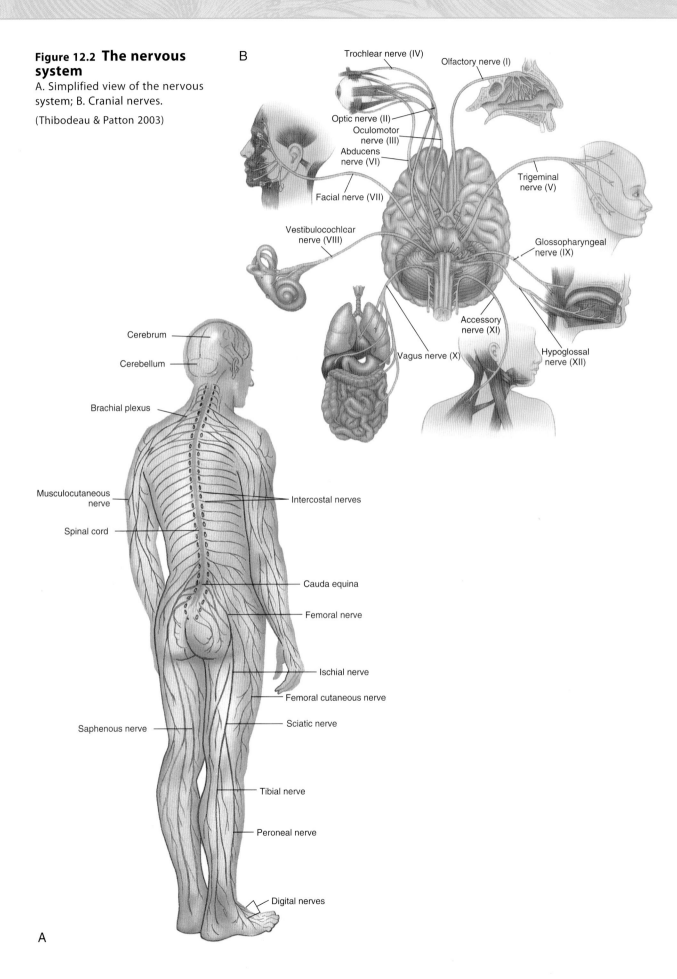

B

Trochlear nerve (IV)

Olfactory nerve (I)

Optic nerve (II)

Oculomotor nerve (III)

Abducens nerve (VI)

Facial nerve (VII)

Trigeminal nerve (V)

Vestibulocochlear nerve (VIII)

Glossopharyngeal nerve (IX)

Accessory nerve (XI)

Vagus nerve (X)

Hypoglossal nerve (XII)

Cerebrum

Cerebellum

Brachial plexus

Musculocutaneous nerve

Intercostal nerves

Spinal cord

Cauda equina

Femoral nerve

Ischial nerve

Femoral cutaneous nerve

Saphenous nerve

Sciatic nerve

Tibial nerve

Peroneal nerve

Digital nerves

A

Central nervous system

The central nervous system (CNS) consists of the brain and spinal cord. These structures serve as the main processing centres for the rest of the nervous system, controlling the operations of the body. All nerve impulses either originate or terminate in the CNS. The CNS is responsible for processing sensations and thoughts using information gathered from sensory receptors throughout the body. The CNS also sends messages to the rest of the body to control movement, actions and responses to the environment. The main form of communication in the CNS occurs through the neurons.

The CNS consists of two types of tissue: grey matter and white matter. In the brain, the grey matter is primarily found on the surface although some is located deep in the cerebellum. It is primarily made up of neuronal cell bodies and axons which do not have a myelin sheath coating and it is mainly responsible for processing information in the brain. Also in the grey matter are glial cells which carry nutrients and energy to the neurons. White matter is mainly found deep in the cerebral cortex of the brain although some is also found in the optic nerves and the brainstem. It is made up of axons covered with myelin, which provides them with a protective covering, insulation and support for the transmission of neuronal signals. The myelin gives the tissue its characteristic white colouring. In the spinal cord, the location of the grey and white matter is the opposite to the brain – the grey matter is found deep inside the spinal cord and the white matter twists around the outside of the cord.

Protection for the central nervous system

Because of their delicacy and importance, the body has protective barriers surrounding the organs of the CNS, including the skull and bones of the spine and membranous tissues called meninges.

There are three layers of meninges (Fig. 12.3). The outermost and toughest layer is the **dura mater**, which lines the skull and covers the brain and spinal cord. The middle layer is the **arachnoid mater** (sometimes called **arachnoid membrane**). It is a delicate, web-like membrane attached to the inside of the dura and surrounds the brain and spinal cord. The innermost layer is the **pia mater**, which is richly supplied with blood vessels. It is attached firmly to the brain. The space between the dura mater and the arachnoid mater is called the **subdural space**. The region between the arachnoid mater and pia mater is the **subarachnoid space** and is filled with cerebrospinal fluid (CSF). The spinal cord is also surrounded by meninges and by CSF.

Brain

The brain performs the main regulatory and coordination functions in the body. The brain is made up of three main parts: the forebrain, midbrain and hindbrain, each part controlling different activities. The forebrain includes the cerebrum, thalamus and hypothalamus. The midbrain consists of the tectum and tegmentum and the hindbrain includes the cerebellum, pons and medulla oblongata. Together the midbrain, pons and medulla are referred to as the brainstem.

The brain contains a network of interconnected spaces called ventricles. There are four ventricles: the right and left lateral ventricles, the third ventricle and the fourth ventricle. They are filled with cerebrospinal fluid (CSF), which is a clear fluid created in the ventricles which flows through the ventricular system and into the subarachnoid space. CSF is designed to act as support, lubrication and cushioning between the brain and spinal cord and the surrounding bones. It also removes waste products from the tissues of the CNS and is eventually absorbed into the venous circulation.

- The **cerebrum** is the largest, uppermost part of the brain, associated with higher brain functions such as thought and action. The cerebrum is divided into right and left hemispheres, connected by a mass of nerve fibres called the corpus callosum, which allows communication between the two hemispheres. The right hemisphere controls and processes signals from the left side of the body, while the left hemisphere controls and processes signals from the right side of the body. The surface of the cerebrum consists of a series of ridges called gyri and fissures called sulci. This structure gives the cerebrum a greater surface area. The outer layer of the cerebrum is called the cerebral cortex. It has four divisions in each hemisphere: the frontal lobe, parietal lobe, occipital lobe and temporal lobe, each named for the overlying cranial bone (Fig. 12.4). The frontal lobe is responsible for reasoning, planning, some speech, movement, emotion and problem solving. The parietal lobe is associated with perception of stimuli, movement, orientation and recognition. The occipital lobe has a role in visual processing, and the temporal lobe in perception, olfaction and recognition of sounds, memory and speech.
- The **limbic system** is located within the cerebrum and is responsible for controlling emotions, motivation, memories and behavioural responses. It contains the thalamus (sensory perception (except olfaction) and regulation of motor functions), hypothalamus (homeostasis, emotion, thirst, hunger, circadian rhythms, control of the autonomic nervous system and the pituitary

Figure 12.3 **The layers of the meninges**

A. Superior coronal view; B. Continuity with the spinal meninges.

(Drake et al 2009)

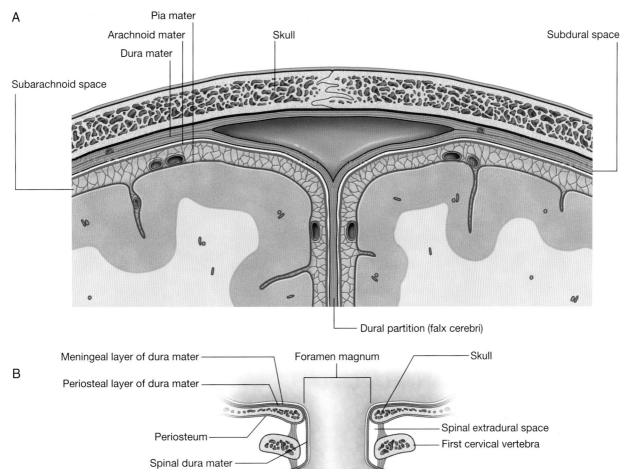

A

Pia mater

Arachnoid mater

Dura mater

Skull

Subdural space

Subarachnoid space

Dural partition (falx cerebri)

B

Meningeal layer of dura mater

Foramen magnum

Skull

Periosteal layer of dura mater

Periosteum

Spinal extradural space

First cervical vertebra

Spinal dura mater

gland), amygdala (memory, emotion, fear) and hippocampus (learning and memory).

- The **cerebellum** is the second largest part of the brain. It is associated with controlling and coordinating movement, posture and balance. It also consists of two hemispheres.
- The **brainstem** is located beneath the limbic system. It is a pathway for nerve impulses between the brain and the spinal cord. The brainstem directs functions vital to life. It is made up of three parts. The **midbrain** is involved in functions such as vision, hearing, eye movement and body movement. The **pons** maintains motor control and has a role in analysing information from the sense organs. It acts as a bridge between

the cerebrum and other parts of the nervous system. The **medulla oblongata** is responsible for maintaining vital body functions, such as breathing, blood pressure and heart rate. It connects with the spinal cord (Fig. 12.5).

- The human brain receives nerve impulses from the spinal cord and 12 pairs of cranial nerves.

Spinal cord

The spinal cord is an extension of the medulla oblongata in the brainstem and continues to the level of the first or second lumbar vertebra. It is a long, narrow collection of nervous tissues protected by the vertebral column and the meninges. The spinal cord has two main functions: transmission of nerve impulses to and from

Figure 12.4 Lobes of the brain

(Nicol & Walker 2007)

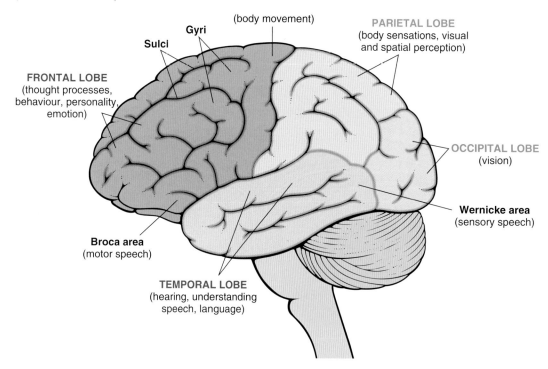

Figure 12.5 Major structures of the brain

(Monahan et al 2007)

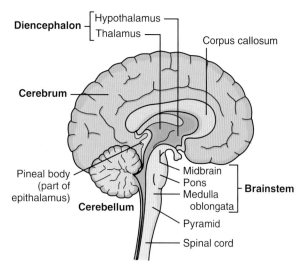

the brain and coordination of some simple reflexes. An example of a reflex action is the withdrawal of the hand from a hot object to avoid a burn.

Peripheral nervous system

The main role of the peripheral nervous system (PNS) is to act as a communication channel between the CNS and the body's organs, glands and muscles and to sensory receptors in the limbs and the skin. The PNS can be divided into the somatic nervous system and the autonomic nervous system.

- **Somatic nervous system:** The somatic nervous system transmits communications relating to the senses and is responsible for managing voluntary body movements. The somatic nervous system consists of 31 pairs of spinal nerves and 12 pairs of cranial nerves. The spinal nerves carry sensory impulses into, and motor impulses out of, the spinal cord. They are named according to the vertebrae they are associated with. There are 8 pairs of cervical nerves, 12 pairs of thoracic nerves, 5 pairs of lumbar nerves, 5 pairs of sacral nerves and 1 pair of coccygeal nerves. These nerves branch off from the spinal cord into the thorax, abdomen and extremities. Cranial nerves carry impulses into and out of the cerebrum or brainstem. They are named according to their function or structure and are designated by the Roman numerals I–XII. Fig. 12.2 B gives the names of all the cranial nerves. They include nerves associated with the senses of smell, sight, hearing and taste, movement of eye muscles and tongue and the muscles that control facial expression and chewing.

- **Autonomic nervous system:** The autonomic nervous system (ANS) directs involuntary body functions such as respiration, digestion, urine production, heartbeat and blood pressure, and has a role in creating emotional responses such as sweating and crying. The ANS is also responsible for the way that the body reacts automatically to certain stimuli without any conscious thought about the movement or responses required. These reactions are called reflexes. In some instances, the reflexes cause a reaction to a stimulus without a message being sent to the brain as local nerves process information from the stimulus and react to it automatically. For example, moving the body away from a hot object or blinking in a dusty environment. Reflexes are one of the body's automatic defence mechanisms. Another example of the body's reflexes is the patellar reflex, the knee jerk reaction that happens when an area just below the patella is struck during a medical examination. The ANS also monitors internal bodily functions; the information gained is integrated in the brain and then in response, the ANS sends commands to involuntary smooth muscle in organs, glands and blood vessels. The autonomic system has two subsystems called the sympathetic and parasympathetic nervous systems.
- The **sympathetic nervous system** manages the body's reaction to stress and emergencies. When this system is activated, the heart and breathing rates increase, digestion slows or stops, pupils dilate and the body begins to sweat. This is called the fight-or-flight response and works to prepare the body to either fight danger or flee from it.
- The **parasympathetic nervous system** counteracts the functions of the sympathetic nervous system by helping to calm the body after the danger has passed. Heart and breathing rates return to normal, digestion resumes, pupils contract and sweating stops.

Neurons

Neurons are the specialised nerve cells which are responsible for communicating information in both chemical and electrical forms. Neurons vary in size, shape and characteristics depending on their function and role. Neurons have three parts (Fig. 12.6):

- cell body, containing the nucleus
- dendrites which are hair-like structures that surround the cell body and which manage and direct incoming signals
- axon or nerve fibre, which guides the outgoing signals from the neuron. Axons are covered in a fatty sheath called myelin, which acts to insulate

Figure 12.6 A neuron

(Hall 2010)

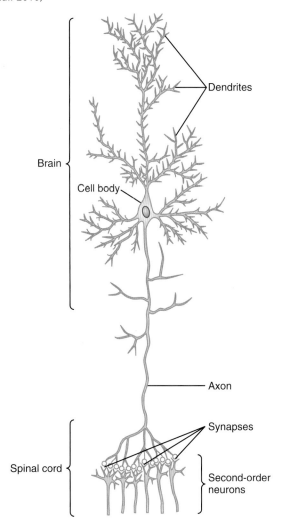

the axon and facilitates the transmission of impulses.

Neurons communicate by transmitting information both within the neuron and from one neuron to the next. The neuron's dendrites receive the information from sensory receptors or other neurons. This information is transferred to the cell body and then travels down the length of the axon in the form of an electrical signal known as an action potential. The point at which the message passes between two nerve cells is called a synapse. The synapse is a small gap across which chemical neurotransmitters diffuse or electrical impulses connect to pass instructions to the dendrites of other neurons or to activate specialised sites called receptors on a target cell. The target cell may be a specialised part of a muscle cell or a gland. In some cases, the electrical signal can almost instantaneously connect across the space between the neurons and continue along its path. In other cases, the chemical messenger (neurotransmitter) diffuses across the synapse to reach the receptor sites of other neurons in a process that is slower than the electrical signal. There are around one hundred known types of neurotransmitters. Common types include:

- **Acetylcholine** (a-se-TIL-koh-leen): this neurotransmitter works with memory, muscle contractions and learning. A lack of acetylcholine in the brain is correlated with a diagnosis of Alzheimer's disease.
- **Endorphins** (en-DOR-finz): are connected with emotions and the perception of pain, fear and trauma. They reduce pain.
- **Dopamine** (DOPE-a-meen): neurotransmitter related to thought and feelings of pleasure. Deficits in dopamine are related to Parkinson's disease; excessive amounts are thought to be linked to schizophrenia.

There are three classes of neurons, each with a unique role:

- **Sensory neurons** receive information from the body's internal and external sensory receptors and convert the messages received into electrical impulses for transfer to the central nervous system. The external sensory receptors react as we look, listen, smell, taste, touch and feel, while the internal receptors report on the condition of the internal organs, such as the state of the bladder, the digestive system, blood pressure and osmolality. Other receptors respond to the position of the body and its movements.
- **Interneurons** transfer messages and impulses to and from the sensory neurons and to and from other interneurons. Branching from the end of the interneurons are dendrites, which receive information by means of signals sent from the axon of another neuron. Interneurons can only transmit information in one direction.
- **Motor neurons** send messages from the central nervous system to the muscles and glands to initiate an action or carry out a response. Most motor neurons are stimulated by interneurons, but some receive direct stimulation from sensory neurons.

PATHOLOGY AND DISEASES

The following section provides a list of common diseases and pathological conditions relevant to the nervous system.

Degenerative and motor disorders

Term	Pronunciation	Definition
Alzheimer's disease (dementia)	ALZ-hy-mers diz-eez (de-MENT-cha)	Alzheimer's disease, also known as Alzheimer's dementia, is an irreversible, progressive brain disorder of deteriorating mental capacity. It is characterised by confusion, memory loss, other cognitive defects and eventually even the inability to carry out the simplest tasks or activities of daily living. The Alzheimer's brain is characterised by the deposit of amyloid (protein) plaques and atrophy. Alzheimer's disease is the most common cause of dementia among older people.

Table continued

Term	Pronunciation	Definition
cerebral palsy	SE-re-bral PAWL-zee	Cerebral palsy refers to a variety of neurological conditions that manifest as disorders of movement or posture. Body movement and muscle coordination are permanently affected. While it may appear to be a muscular disorder, cerebral palsy is actually due to damage to the part of the brain that controls muscle movements. Damage may be due to a developmental abnormality or a brain injury prior to or shortly after birth. This may include cerebral haemorrhage, hypoxia and hypoglycaemia. Occasionally cerebral palsy can develop in early childhood as a result of brain damage after a head injury or infection such as bacterial meningitis or viral encephalitis.
		Patients with cerebral palsy will have varying degrees of ataxia, the loss of control over voluntary muscle functions. Also symptomatic of the disease are stiff or tight muscles (spasticity), hypertonic or hypotonic muscles causing uncontrolled or uncoordinated movements as well as gait abnormalities. Cerebral palsy severity and symptoms differ from individual to individual. For some, the condition may be relatively minor (e.g., affecting one hand and causing minor disability) whereas for others it may be severely disabling, with the requirement for total care for the affected individual. While there is no cure, physiotherapy and rehabilitation can improve muscle control. Botox injections have recently been used as a means of controlling palsy.
multiple sclerosis	MUL-tip-el skle-ROH-sis	Multiple sclerosis (MS) is a progressive degenerative neurological disease with scattered patches of demyelination of nerve fibres of the brain and spinal cord. These fibres are replaced by scar tissue with a resulting loss of neural function and conduction. Patients may experience almost any neurological symptoms. Common symptoms include: tingling, numbness, muscle weakness or spasm, ataxia, dysarthria, dysphagia, visual problems (such as diplopia), fatigue, pain and bladder and bowel incontinence. MS is a progressive disease but in some patients it may be episodic, with long periods of remission in between attacks.
Parkinson's disease	PAH-kin-sons diz-eez	Parkinson's disease is a slowly progressive, degenerative neurologic disorder. Nerve cells in the brain deteriorate causing a deficiency of the neurotransmitter dopamine. Dopamine plays a part in many brain functions, including motor coordination and memory, by promoting communication between the brain cells. Parkinson's disease is characterised by rhythmic fine tremors or trembling in the hands, arms, legs, jaw and face; stiffness of the limbs and joints; bradykinesia; and impaired balance and coordination. It causes weakness and stiffness of the muscles and interferes with speech, walking and daily tasks. There is no cure for Parkinson's disease, therefore treatment is aimed at improving the symptoms.

Episodic neurological disorders

Term	Pronunciation	Definition
epilepsy	EP-il-ep-see	Epilepsy is an episodic neurological disorder characterised by recurrent, transient abnormal electrical activity in the brain. The normal pattern of neuronal activity becomes disturbed, causing a variety of symptoms including periods of confusion, sensory disturbances, staring spells, convulsions, muscle spasms and loss of consciousness. Epilepsy has many possible causes, including illness, an imbalance of neurotransmitters, brain injury and abnormal brain development. In many cases, the cause is unknown. Epilepsy is classified by the part of the brain where the seizure starts (partial/focal or generalised), if the person is aware during the seizure or not and whether movement is involved in the seizure. In partial seizures, there is no loss of consciousness; rather the patient may appear to be daydreaming with only mild symptoms. Generalised seizures include a loss of consciousness with possible muscle spasm. Epilepsy can usually be controlled by anticonvulsant medications.
sleep apnoea	sleep AP-nee-a	Sleep apnoea is a common disorder in which breathing repeatedly stops and starts during sleep. Pauses can last from a few seconds to minutes and occur from 5 to 30 times or more per hour. This results in poor sleep quality and excessive daytime sleepiness, slow reflexes, poor concentration and an increased risk of accidents. In obstructive sleep apnoea, the soft tissue in the throat relaxes during sleep causing a blockage of the airway. Air that squeezes past the blockage can cause loud snoring. It is more common in people who are overweight, but it can affect anyone including children with enlarged tonsils. Lifestyle changes, mouth splints, surgery and/or the use of a continuous positive airway pressure (CPAP) device can successfully treat sleep apnoea in many people.

Inflammatory and infectious diseases

Term	Pronunciation	Definition
encephalitis	en-kef-a-LY-tus	Encephalitis is an inflammation of the brain secondary to another infection (usually viral) such as influenza, measles or herpes virus. It is more common in the very young or old. It results in cerebral oedema and sometimes intracerebral haemorrhage. It is characterised by fever, headache, photophobia, vomiting and disorientation. Diagnosis is by CT scan of the head, a brain MRI and a lumbar puncture to withdraw cerebrospinal fluid for examination. Treatment includes antiviral and antiseizure medications as well as rest and fluids.
meningitis	men-in-JY-tus	Meningitis is an inflammation in the meninges. Most cases are due to a bacterial or viral infection. Meningitis usually has a sudden onset and is characterised by a severe headache, neck stiffness, irritability, fever, nausea, vomiting and delirium. A particular type of meningitis, meningococcal meningitis, is also characterised by a rapidly spreading rash. Meningitis can be life threatening because of the proximity to the brain and spinal cord, therefore the condition is classified as a medical emergency. A lumbar puncture is performed to diagnose the condition. Treatment is with specific antibiotics.
poliomyelitis	POL-ee-oh-my-a-LY-tus	Poliomyelitis is an acute viral infection of the grey matter of the brain/spinal cord, often resulting in spinal or muscle deformity and paralysis. In most countries the incidence has decreased due to immunisation but poliomyelitis is still endemic in a few highly populated and developing countries.

Neoplasms

Term	Pronunciation	Definition
cerebral tumours	SE-re-bral TYOO-maz	Cerebral tumours are better known as brain tumours. There are many different types of brain tumours that are named according to their location or histology. Examples include: gliomas, meningiomas, astrocytomas, Schwannomas. They can cause CNS changes by invading and destroying tissues. Depending on the site, they can also have secondary effects such as blindness. An increase in intracranial pressure from the tumour can threaten life through brain herniation, coma, respiratory arrest or cardiac arrest.
		There are many theories as to the cause of cerebral tumours. For example: genetic mutation, exposure to chemicals such as vinyl chloride and pesticides, a virus or heredity.
		Diagnosis is by physical examination, skull x-ray, CT scan, MRI scan, cerebral angiography, biopsy of lesion (to determine histology and grading) or a lumbar puncture. Treatment will vary depending on the histologic type, radiosensitivity of the tumour and location, but may include: surgery, radiotherapy, chemotherapy, decompression of intracranial pressure and palliative measures such as steroids for cerebral oedema, and anticonvulsants to prevent seizures.

Disorders of nerves

Term	Pronunciation	Definition
carpal tunnel syndrome	KAR-pul TUN-el SIN-drohm	Carpal tunnel syndrome (CTS) is the entrapment of the median nerve in the wrist. Compression of the nerve causes loss of movement and sensation in the wrist, hand and fingers. Symptoms include weakness, pain, burning, numbness or paraesthesia in the hand.
		CTS is more common in people who perform repetitive tasks such as meatworkers, hairdressers, data entry workers or workers using vibrating equipment. Oedema-producing conditions such as diabetes and pregnancy or pre-existing hypothyroidism are all risk factors for CTS. Treatment depends on the severity and presence of any underlying condition. In milder cases conservative treatment such as splinting the wrist, corticosteroid injections or oral NSAIDs can be effective. In more severe cases, surgical decompression of the nerve may be required.
sciatica	sy-AT-ik-a	Sciatica is an inflammation of the sciatic nerve resulting in pain in the buttock, thigh and leg. It results from compression of the nerve often due to osteoarthritis of the lumbosacral spine or a ruptured intervertebral disc.

Disorders due to trauma

Term	Pronunciation	Definition
cerebral concussion	SE-re-bral kon-KUSH-un	A cerebral concussion is a transient neurogenic dysfunction caused by a force to the brain. It is the most common form of head injury. It results in a change in mental status, with headache, confusion, disorientation and retrograde amnesia, with or without a brief loss of consciousness. A concussion occurs when the head hits or is hit by an object, or when the brain is jarred against the skull, as can happen in a motor vehicle accident, a fall or in collision/contact sports.

Table continued

Term	Pronunciation	Definition
cerebral contusion	SE-re-bral kon-TOO-shun	Cerebral contusions are scattered areas of bleeding on the surface of the brain resulting in bruising of the brain tissue and cerebral oedema. They occur when the brain rebounds against the skull in a serious head injury. The signs and symptoms of a contusion include severe headache, dizziness, vomiting, increased size of one pupil and sudden weakness in an arm or leg. The person may seem restless, agitated or irritable with a loss of memory. As the cerebral oedema progresses, the person may feel increasingly drowsy or confused. A cerebral contusion is diagnosed by a CT brain scan. If pressure on the brain increases significantly or if there is a large blood clot, a craniotomy may be required to remove the cerebral contusion.

Paralysis

Term	Pronunciation	Definition
paralysis	pah-RAL-a-sis	Paralysis is loss of the ability to move one or more muscles. It may be associated with loss of feeling and other bodily functions. Paralysis may be partial or complete, and temporary or permanent. It is not usually caused by problems with the muscles, but by problems with the spinal cord or nerves that control muscles. A person with paralysis will usually have some form of nerve damage. Most paralysis results from cerebrovascular accidents and spinal cord injuries. Other causes of paralysis include Bell's palsy, multiple sclerosis and Guillain-Barré syndrome.
– flaccid paralysis	FLAS-id pah-RAL-a-sis	Flaccid paralysis is a condition in which there is weakened or absent muscle tone. It is caused by disease or by injury to the nerves associated with the involved muscles.
– spastic paralysis	SPAS-tik pah-RAL-a-sis	In spastic paralysis, muscles are affected by persistent spasms and involuntary contractions. It is usually caused by a central nervous system disorder such as cerebral palsy. Tendon reflexes are also exaggerated.
– monoplegia	mon-oh-PLEE-jee-a	In monoplegia, only one limb is paralysed.
– hemiplegia	hem-ee-PLEE-jee-a	A person with hemiplegia will experience paralysis of one side of the body, affecting the arm and leg and sometimes part of the trunk on the same side of the body. It often occurs as the result of a cerebrovascular accident.
– paraplegia	para-PLEE-jee-a	A person with paraplegia will have paralysis of the trunk and lower limbs. The degree of paralysis will depend on the level of the spinal cord injury. The paralysis can result from a spinal cord injury or conditions such as a tumour or multiple sclerosis.
– quadriplegia, tetraplegia	KWAD-ra-PLEE-jee-a, tet-ra-PLEE-jee-a	Quadriplegia or tetraplegia result in paralysis of all four extremities (and often the trunk). It generally results from an injury to the spinal cord at the level of the cervical vertebrae. The severity of the condition is linked to the level of the spinal cord injury.

Vascular disorders

Term	Pronunciation	Definition
cerebrovascular accident (CVA)	SE-re-broh-VAS-kyoo-la AK-se-dent	A cerebrovascular accident is more commonly known as a stroke. It is a general term to indicate disruption of blood supply to a part of the brain causing cells to die. The part of the body that is affected by a CVA is dependent on which brain cells are damaged or die (Fig. 12.7). It is caused by a blockage to a cerebral artery or by atherosclerosis in the carotid or cerebral arteries. The vessels can become occluded by a thrombus or an embolus resulting in ischaemia. This is called an ischaemic stroke. A CVA can also be due to a ruptured cerebral artery or aneurysm causing a haemorrhage. This is called a haemorrhagic stroke. A cerebral haemorrhage is usually due to uncontrolled hypertension or a weakening of a cerebral blood vessel.

Figure 12.7 Cerebrovascular accident
A. Events causing stroke; **B.** MRI showing haemorrhagic stroke in left cerebrum; **C.** Areas of the body affected by CVA.

(Black et al 2005)

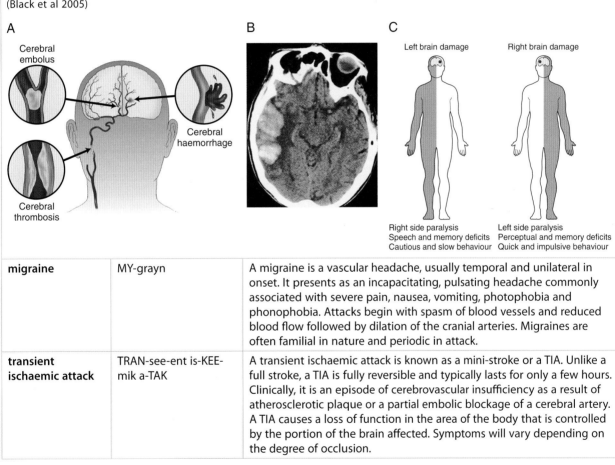

Term	Pronunciation	Definition
migraine	MY-grayn	A migraine is a vascular headache, usually temporal and unilateral in onset. It presents as an incapacitating, pulsating headache commonly associated with severe pain, nausea, vomiting, photophobia and phonophobia. Attacks begin with spasm of blood vessels and reduced blood flow followed by dilation of the cranial arteries. Migraines are often familial in nature and periodic in attack.
transient ischaemic attack	TRAN-see-ent is-KEE-mik a-TAK	A transient ischaemic attack is known as a mini-stroke or a TIA. Unlike a full stroke, a TIA is fully reversible and typically lasts for only a few hours. Clinically, it is an episode of cerebrovascular insufficiency as a result of atherosclerotic plaque or a partial embolic blockage of a cerebral artery. A TIA causes a loss of function in the area of the body that is controlled by the portion of the brain affected. Symptoms will vary depending on the degree of occlusion.

Miscellaneous conditions

Term	Pronunciation	Definition
hydrocephalus	hy-droh-KEF-a-lus	Hydrocephalus results from an increased amount of cerebrospinal fluid (CSF) within the ventricles of the brain. It causes an abnormal widening of the ventricles. This widening creates a potentially harmful increase in pressure on the cerebral tissues. Hydrocephalus is either congenital or acquired. It may also be either communicating, where the CSF can still flow around the ventricles, or obstructive, where the CSF cannot flow between the ventricles. Treatment most commonly involves the insertion of a shunt to drain the CSF from the ventricles into the peritoneal cavity where it is reabsorbed by the body.
intracranial haemorrhage	in-tra-KRAYN-ee-al HEM-ah-raj	An intracranial haemorrhage is a bleed inside the head. It can be caused by a trauma, hypertension or vascular diseases such as an aneurysm. The haemorrhage is named for its location: extradural, subdural, subarachnoid, intracerebral. It is a medical emergency because the accumulation of blood can result in increased intracranial pressure and the potential for permanent brain damage.

TESTS AND PROCEDURES

The following section provides a list of common diagnostic tests and procedures, clinical interventions and surgical procedures that are undertaken for the nervous system.

Test/Procedure	Pronunciation	Definition
cerebral angiography	SE-re-bral an-jee-OG-ra-fee	Cerebral angiography is a procedure which uses radio-opaque contrast to record x-ray images of the blood vessels in the brain to identify conditions such as aneurysms, occlusion and haemorrhage in the brain.

Figure 12.8 Cerebral angiography
A. Insertion of dye through a catheter in the common carotid artery outlines the vessels of the brain; B. Internal carotid artery injection, lateral projection, arterial phase. The arteries are primarily opacified during this phase.

(A: Shiland 2006; B: Sattenberg et al 2016)

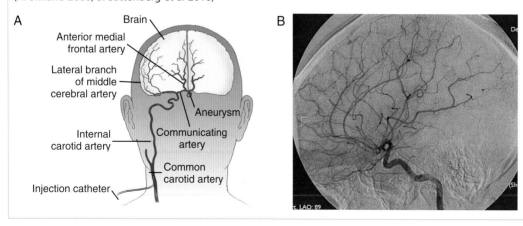

Table continued

Test/Procedure	Pronunciation	Definition
cerebrospinal fluid analysis	SE-re-broh-SPY-nel FLOO-id a-NAL-e-sis	Cerebrospinal fluid (CSF) analysis is a test that is undertaken to diagnose a range of diseases and conditions affecting the CNS. A sample of CSF is collected for the analysis from the lower back by a lumbar puncture or spinal tap. The analysis tests for conditions such as infectious diseases (meningitis and encephalitis), haemorrhage from the brain and tumours within the CNS.
computed tomography (CT)	kom-PYOO-ted to-MOG-ra-fee	A CT is a diagnostic test that can be used to identify disorders of the brain and spinal cord. Cross-sectional images are created using computerised digital technology in conjunction with x-ray beams.
Doppler ultrasound study	DOP-la UL-tra-sownd stud-ee	A Doppler ultrasound study is a test using ultrasound technology to analyse the speed of blood flow in the major arteries and veins, such as the carotid and intracranial arteries. It is performed using a handheld scanner connected to a computer to measure echoes from the blood vessels.
electroencephalography (EEG)	ee-LEK-troh-en-kef-a-LOG-ra-fee	An EEG is a test that measures the electrical activity of the brain using electrodes attached to the scalp. It is most commonly used to identify the type and location of activity in the brain during seizures but can also be used to identify tumours and other lesions in the brain.
lumbar (spinal) puncture (LP)	LUM-bah PUNK-cha	A LP is a procedure that involves the insertion of a needle into the cerebrospinal fluid surrounding the spinal nerve roots in the lower back to remove CSF for analysis. The LP may also be done to measure the pressure of the circulating CSF or as a method for injecting contrast material for a myelography.

Figure 12.9 Lumbar puncture procedure and positioning of the needle during a lumbar puncture

The procedure involves introducing a needle or its respective introducer at the superior aspect of the inferior spinal process into the subarachnoid space of the lumbar sac, at the L4/L5 level or other level safely (L3/L4) below the spinal cord.

(Engelborghs et al 2017)

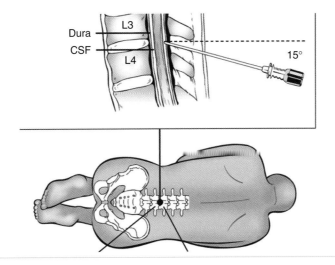

Table continued

Test/Procedure	Pronunciation	Definition
magnetic resonance imaging (MRI)	mag-NET-ik REZ-on-ans IM-a-jing	MRI is a process of diagnostic testing using a magnetic field and radio waves to take images of internal organs, muscles and soft tissues which do not show up well on x-rays.
myelography	my-el-OG-ra-fee	Myelography is the process of testing using fluoroscopy, a real time x-ray examination of the structures within the spinal column, following injection of a contrast medium into the subarachnoid space around the spinal cord and nerve roots. The images identify conditions such as spinal tumours, spinal cord swelling and herniated (slipped) discs.
positron emission tomography (PET)	POZ-i-tron e-MISH-en to-MOG-ra-fee	A PET scan is a non-invasive nuclear medicine imaging technique which produces two- and three-dimensional images of organs, in particular the brain. It involves injection of a radiopharmaceutical which travels to the organ being investigated where it lodges and releases emissions, allowing images to be captured using a PET scanner.
stereotactic radiosurgery	STE-ree-oh-TAK-tik RAY-dee-oh-ser-jer-ee	Stereotactic radiosurgery is the delivery of radiation using three-dimensional coordinates to a precise targeted area of the brain, while avoiding damage to healthy tissue in surrounding areas. A head frame is fixed to the skull and is used as a guide to ensure the radiation is delivered to the correct location.

Exercises

EXERCISE 12.1: LABEL THE DIAGRAMS

Using the information provided in this chapter, label the anatomical parts in Figs 12.10 and 12.11.

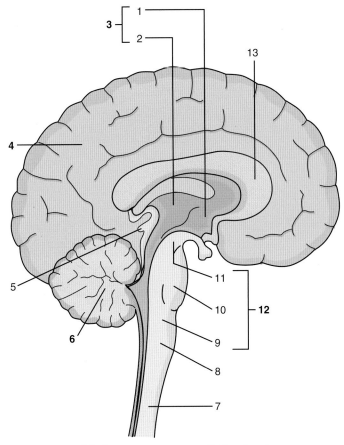

Figure 12.10 Major structures of the brain

(Monahan et al 2007)

1 _____	8 _____	
2 _____	9 _____	
3 _____	10 _____	
4 _____	11 _____	
5 _____	12 _____	
6 _____	13 _____	
7 _____		

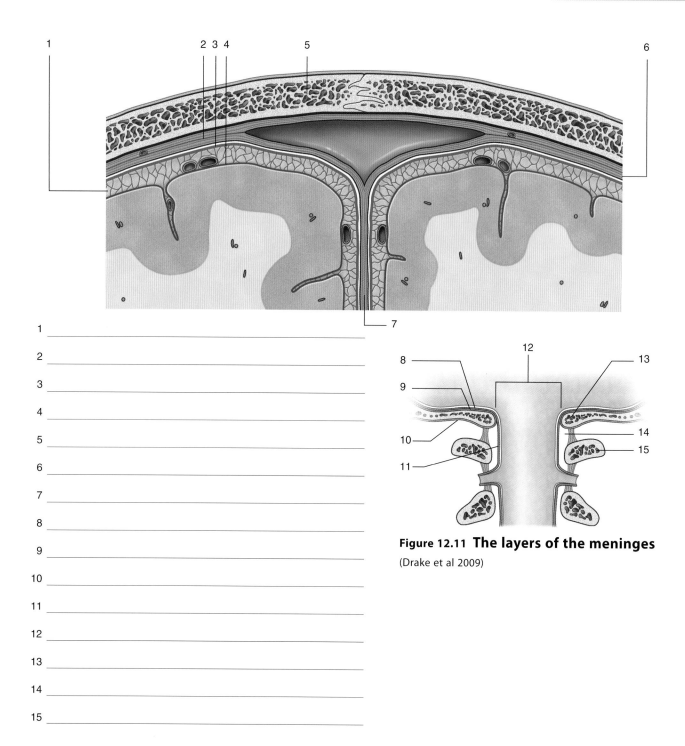

Figure 12.11 The layers of the meninges
(Drake et al 2009)

1 _____

2 _____

3 _____

4 _____

5 _____

6 _____

7 _____

8 _____

9 _____

10 _____

11 _____

12 _____

13 _____

14 _____

15 _____

EXERCISE 12.2: PROVIDE THE WORD ELEMENTS

Provide the correct word element for each of the terms below.

Meaning	Word Element
burning	
cut short	
electrical	
glue	
head	
knowledge	
nerve	
sound	
star	
water	

EXERCISE 12.3: WORD ELEMENT MEANINGS AND WORD BUILDING

Provide the meaning for each of the word elements below, then use each element correctly in a medical term and provide the meaning of each term.

Word Element	Meaning	Medical Term	Meaning of Medical Term
ment/o			
-praxia			
som/o			
pont/o			
radicul/o			
-lepsy			
-plegia			
thec/o			
atel/o			
gli/o			

EXERCISE 12.4: WORD ANALYSIS AND MEANING

Break up the medical terms below into their component parts (prefixes, suffixes, word roots, combining vowels). Provide the meaning for each word element and each term as a whole.

Example:

dysphasia

dys = bad, difficult

-phasia = speech

Meaning = difficult speech

1. anencephaly _____

_____

_____

2. craniotomy _____

_____

_____

3. polioencephalomeningomyelitis _____

_____

_____

4. hemiplegia _____

_____

_____

5. astrocytoma _____

_____

_____

6. radiculitis _____

_____

_____

7. bradykinesia _____

_____

_____

8. glioblastoma _____

_____

_____

9. hyperaesthesia _____

_____

_____

10. psychosomatic _____

_____

EXERCISE 12.5: EXPAND THE ABBREVIATIONS

Expand the abbreviations to form correct medical terms.

Abbreviation	Expanded Abbreviation
CNS	
CSF	
CVA	
ECT	
EEG	
GCS	
ICP	
LP	
MS	
PET	
PNS	
REM	
TBI	
TENS	
TIA	

EXERCISE 12.6: MATCH MEDICAL TERMS AND MEANINGS

Match the medical term in Column A with its meaning in Column B.

Column A	Answer	Column B
1. meningitis		A. uncontrollable sleepiness
2. ataxia		B. dizziness
3. dementia		C. tumour composed of astrocytes
4. vertigo		D. paralysis
5. aphasia		E. loss of speech function
6. astrocytoma		F. inflammation of meninges
7. apraxia		G. loss of muscular coordination
8. syncope		H. fainting
9. narcolepsy		I. inability to perform purposeful actions
10. palsy		J. mental decline

EXERCISE 12.7: PRONUNCIATION AND COMPREHENSION

Read the following paragraphs aloud to practise your pronunciation. Using your textbook and a medical dictionary, find the meanings of the underlined medical terms.

This 39-year-old lady was admitted for investigation of a headache. She had a sudden onset of <u>bifrontal</u> headache followed by collapse and, according to her husband, possible right <u>focal fitting</u>. There was no associated <u>incontinence</u>. She was noted to be confused afterwards. She proceeded to her local doctor. At the local doctor's surgery she was noted to be <u>hypertensive</u>, with a blood pressure of 180/120 on arrival at hospital. There was no associated fever, cough, nausea, vomiting, <u>diplopia</u> or focal weakness. There was no past history of migraine or other headache. She had had a head injury at the age of 18 when she had been admitted to hospital but there had been no problems since then.

On examination she was very obese and <u>hirsute</u>. She was noted to have a blood pressure of 150/105 in both arms, although this was labile, pulse of 90/min and regular. She was <u>afebrile</u>. <u>Auscultation</u> of her heart sounds was normal and chest was clear. Abdominal examination was unremarkable. <u>Cranial</u> nerves were normal. Power and tone in the upper and lower limbs were normal. There were no <u>cerebellar</u> signs. Sensation was normal and there was no <u>meningism</u>. Her <u>Kernig's</u> was negative. Due to the suspicion of a <u>subarachnoid haemorrhage</u>, contrast <u>CT head scan</u> was performed. This was entirely normal. She then proceeded to a <u>lumbar puncture</u>, which was also normal, showing one red cell, two white cells and normal biochemistry. Full blood count did show some <u>neutrophilia</u>, with a white cell count of 18.53, predominantly neutrophils, normal coagulation profile and normal SMA. ECG was normal.

She was admitted to the ward where she was observed. Headache resolved and there was no further evidence of fitting. <u>Neurological</u> signs returned to normal. Blood pressure continued to be erratic, ranging from 140/100 to 170/110. It was elected to commence Adalat 20 mg b.d. Further investigations for an underlying cause for her hypertension were undertaken. <u>Microurine</u> was negative. She was very keen to return home. Outstanding investigations include renal ultrasound, urinary analyses and EEG. She has also been referred to the dietitian for weight loss.

EXERCISE 12.8: CROSSWORD PUZZLE

Complete the puzzle by providing the medical term for each of the clues below.

ACROSS

5. Controls and coordinates movement, posture and balance (10)
6. Nerve fibre (4)
7. Maintains motor control and analyses information from the sense organs (4)
8. Commonly known as a stroke (15, 8)
9. A neurological disorder characterised by recurrent, transient abnormal electrical activity in the brain (8)

DOWN

1. Responsible for homeostasis, emotion, thirst, hunger, circadian rhythms and control of the autonomic nervous system and pituitary gland (12)
2. Controls motor function (9)
3. Middle layer of the meninges (9, 8)
4. A vascular headache, usually temporal and unilateral in onset (8)

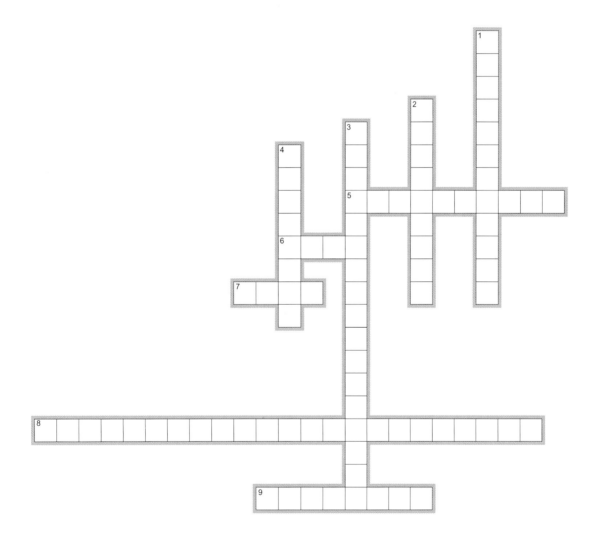

EXERCISE 12.9: ANAGRAMS

Work out each medical term from the jumbled letters below. Then, using the letters in brackets, determine the medical term that matches the description given.

1.　magloi	__ __ __ (__) __ __	a type of brain tumour
2.　posceny	__ __ __ __ __ __ (__)	fainting
3.　spno	__ __ (__) __	part of the midbrain
4.　nirab	__ (__) __ __ __	the combining form encephal/o refers to this organ
5.　lionggna	__ __ (__) __ __ __ __ __	a knot of nerves
6.　rubercem	__ __ __ __ __ __ (__) __	the largest part of the brain

Rearrange the letters in brackets to form a word that means 'a nerve cell'.

— — — — — —

EXERCISE 12.10: DISCHARGE SUMMARY ANALYSIS

Read the discharge summary below and answer the questions.

UNIVERSITY HOSPITAL DISCHARGE SUMMARY	**UR number:** 242526 **Name:** Joanne Lyons **Address:** 7/89 Bryans Court, Longlands **Date of birth:** 28/9/1980 **Sex:** F **Nominated primary healthcare provider:** Dr David Dresden
Episode details **Consultant:** Dr Willows **Registrar:** Dr Meakin **Unit:** Neurology **Admission source:** Neurology outpatient **Date of admission:** 30/11/2020	**Discharge details** **Status:** Home **Date of discharge:** 8/12/2020
Reason for admission / Presenting problems: Progressive tremor involving all limbs and neck present for at least 12 months. Ms Lyons complained of weakness and spasticity in the right leg, difficulties with balance, tingling in her extremities, blurred vision and fatigue and malaise. She had experienced multiple episodes of loss of bladder control.	
Principal diagnosis: MS	
Comorbidities: Familial tremor	
Previous medical history: Family history of familial tremor – father and grandfather	

Clinical synopsis:

Examination demonstrated marked cerebellar signs together with increased tone generally, sustainable clonus in the legs and positive Hoffman's sign together with up-going Babinski's. The patient was assessed by the neurologist, who felt that MS was likely to be the major underlying entity. This was further supported by the presence of oligoclonal bands.

Complications: Nil reported

Clinical interventions:

LP investigations demonstrated an unremarkable CSF apart from elevated protein of 0.8. Specific testing for oligoclonal bands on the CSF was positive.

Diagnostic interventions:

TFTs were normal, biochemistry normal. Baseline vitamin assays were normal. RPR was negative. Blood count normal. Contrast CT scanning of the brain demonstrated areas of periventricular lucency.

Medications at discharge: Nil reported

Ceased medications: Nil reported

Allergies: Nil reported

Alerts: Nil reported

Arranged services: She has been put in contact with MS support services.

Recommendations: Follow-up MRI scan as an outpatient.

Information to patient/relevant parties:

Authorising clinician: Dr Meakin

Document recipients: Patient and LMO: Dr David Dresden

1. **Expand the following abbreviations as found in the discharge summary above.**

   MRI

   MS

   RPR

   TFTs

2. **What is a Hoffman's test?**

3. **What is a Babinski's test?**

4. **Identify five of the MS symptoms that Ms Lyons has experienced.**

5. **Why is it important for an MRI to be performed on Ms Lyons?**

CHAPTER 13

The Senses

Contents

OBJECTIVES	301
INTRODUCTION	301
NEW WORD ELEMENTS FOR THE SENSE OF SIGHT	301
Combining forms	301
Prefixes	302
Suffixes	303
ABBREVIATIONS FOR THE SENSE OF SIGHT	303
FUNCTIONS AND STRUCTURE OF THE EYE – THE SENSE OF SIGHT	303
The orbit	304
Eyelids and eyelashes	304
Sclera	304
Conjunctiva	304
Cornea	304
Anterior chamber	305
Iris and pupil	305
Posterior chamber, lens and ciliary body	306
Vitreous cavity	306
Retina, macula and choroid	306
Optic nerve	306
PATHOLOGY AND DISEASES FOR THE SENSE OF SIGHT	306
NEW WORD ELEMENTS FOR THE SENSE OF HEARING	309
Combining forms	309
Prefixes	310
Suffixes	310
ABBREVIATIONS FOR THE SENSE OF HEARING	310
FUNCTIONS AND STRUCTURE OF THE EAR – THE SENSE OF HEARING	311
Outer ear	312
Middle ear	312
Inner ear	312
PATHOLOGY AND DISEASES FOR THE SENSE OF HEARING	312
NEW WORD ELEMENTS FOR THE SENSE OF SMELL	314
Combining forms	315
Prefixes	315
FUNCTIONS AND STRUCTURE OF THE NOSE – THE SENSE OF SMELL	315
NEW WORD ELEMENTS FOR THE SENSE OF TASTE	315
Combining forms	315
FUNCTIONS AND STRUCTURE RELATING TO THE TONGUE – THE SENSE OF TASTE	315
NEW WORD ELEMENTS FOR THE SENSE OF TOUCH	316
Combining forms	316
FUNCTIONS AND STRUCTURE RELATING TO THE SENSE OF TOUCH	316
VOCABULARY FOR THE SENSES	316
TESTS AND PROCEDURES FOR THE SENSES	317
EXERCISES	321

Objectives

After completing this chapter you should be able to:

1. state the meanings of the word elements related to each of the senses

2. build words using the word elements associated with each of the senses

3. recognise, pronounce and effectively use medical terms associated with each of the senses

4. expand abbreviations related to each of the senses

5. describe the structure and functions of the senses including sight, hearing, taste, smell and touch

6. describe common pathological conditions associated with each of the senses

7. describe common laboratory tests and diagnostic and surgical procedures associated with each of the senses

8. apply what you have learned by interpreting medical terminology in practice.

Demonstrate your knowledge of the senses by completing the exercises at the end of this chapter.

INTRODUCTION

In this chapter, the five special senses will be discussed. These are sight, hearing, smell, taste and touch. The senses are based on receptor cells or groups of receptor cells called sense organs. Receptors respond to stimuli in the environment and send nerve impulses along sensory neurons. Everything we see, hear, feel, smell or taste requires billions of these nerve impulses to send messages to the brain. The brain interprets the nerve impulses and thus, we perceive the impulse through one of our senses. Other than the vocabulary and the tests and procedure sections, all topics in this chapter have been divided according to the respective sense.

NEW WORD ELEMENTS FOR THE SENSE OF SIGHT

Here are some word elements related to the sense of sight. To reinforce your learning, write the meanings of the medical terms in the spaces provided. Use the Glossary of medical terms on page 561 to help you work out the meanings. You may also need to check the meaning in a medical dictionary, but make an attempt yourself first.

Combining forms

Combining Form	Meaning	Medical Term	Meaning of Medical Term
ambly/o	dull, dim	amblyopia	
aque/o	water	aqueous	
blephar/o	eyelid	blepharoplasty	
choroid/o	choroid	choroidopathy	
conjunctiv/o	conjunctiva	conjunctivitis	
cor/o	pupil of the eye	leucocoria	
core/o		coreopexy	
corne/o	cornea	corneal	
cycl/o	ciliary body of the eye, circular	cycloplegia	
dacry/o	tears, tear duct, lacrimal sac	dacryocystitis	
dipl/o	double	diplopia	
foc/o	focus	multifocal	
glauc/o	grey	glaucoma	
iri/o	iris	iritis	
irid/o		iridokinesis	

Table continued

Combining Form	Meaning	Medical Term	Meaning of Medical Term
kerat/o	cornea, hard, horny tissue	keratomalacia	
lacrim/o	tears	lacrimotomy	
mi/o	smaller, less	miotic	
mydr/o	widen, enlarge	mydriatic	
nyct/o	night, darkness	nyctalopia	
ocul/o	eye	oculonasal	
ophthalm/o	eye	ophthalmoscope	
opt/i	eye, vision	orthoptic	
opt/o		optometry	
optic/o		optical	
palpebr/o	eyelid	palpebral fissure	
papill/o	nipple-shaped projection (refers to optic disc here)	papilloretinitis	
phac/o	lens of the eye	phacomalacia	
phot/o	light	photophobic	
presby/o	old age	presbyopia	
pupill/o *(Note: pupil has one 'l' but the combining form has two)*	pupil	pupilloplegia	
retin/o	retina	retinoblastoma	
scler/o	sclera, hardening	sclerectasis	
scot/o	darkness	scotopia	
ton/o	tone, pressure, tension	tonometer	
uve/o	uvea, vascular layer of eye	uveal	
vitre/o	glassy	vitreous	
xer/o	dry	xerophthalmia	

Prefixes

Prefix	Meaning	Medical Term	Meaning of Medical Term
aniso-	unequal, asymmetrical, dissimilar	anisocoria	
bi-	two, twice, double	bifocal	
bin-		binocular	
eso-	inward, within	esotropia	
exo-	outward, outside	exophthalmic	
hetero-	different	heteropsia	
hyper-	above, excessive	hyperopia	
iso-	equal, same	isocoria	
mono-	one, single	monocular	

Suffixes

Suffix	Meaning	Medical Term	Meaning of Medical Term
-gyric	pertaining to circular motion	oculogyric	
-metry	process of measuring	pupillometry	
-opia	condition of vision	myopia	
-opsia	condition of vision	achromatopsia	
-phobia	condition of fear	photophobia	
-plasty	surgical, plastic repair	keratoplasty	
-tropia	to turn	exotropia	

ABBREVIATIONS FOR THE SENSE OF SIGHT

The following abbreviations are commonly used in the Australian healthcare environment. Because some abbreviations can have more than one meaning, check the context in which the abbreviation is used before assigning a meaning to it.

Abbreviation	Definition
AC	anterior chamber
acc	accommodation
ACG	angle-closure glaucoma
ARMD	age-related macular degeneration
ASC	anterior subcapsular cataract
CACG	chronic angle-closure glaucoma
CE	cataract extraction
ECCE	extracapsular cataract extraction
EOM	extraocular movements
ICCE	intracapsular cataract extraction
IOFB	intraocular foreign body
IOL	intraocular lens
IOP	intraocular pressure
LASIK	laser-assisted in situ keratomileusis
OD	*oculus dexter* (right eye)
OS	*oculus sinister* (left eye)
OU	*oculus uterque* (both eyes)
PEARL	pupils equal and reactive to light
PEARLA	pupils equal and reactive to light and accommodation
phaco	phacoemulsification
POAG	primary open angle glaucoma
REM	rapid eye movement
ROP	retinopathy of prematurity
SLE	slit lamp examination

Table continued

Abbreviation	Definition
VA	visual acuity
VF	visual field
YAG	yttrium-aluminium-garnet laser

FUNCTIONS AND STRUCTURE OF THE EYE – THE SENSE OF SIGHT

The primary function of the eye is to capture light rays. The light rays are modified into nerve impulses that are transferred to the visual cortex of the brain to be translated and interpreted into images, thereby enabling a person to 'see' in a process that seems instantaneous. Of the five senses, the ability to see is one of the most important to allow us to gather information about the external environment. The eye is a very complex organ and has functions that include light perception, focusing of the light onto the retina, refraction, light accommodation, transmission of messages to the brain and production of tears. The way that the eye operates to allow us to see is as follows.

Light enters the eye by first passing through the cornea, the clear outer portion of the eye (Fig. 13.1). The cornea is curved, focusing the light through the pupil, a round hole located in the centre of the iris. The thin circular iris is responsible for controlling the diameter and size of the pupil and therefore regulating the amount of light that can reach the retina. Muscles attached to the iris expand or contract the pupil depending on how much light is present. The larger the pupil, the more light that can enter. As the light passes through the lens, muscles in the eye cause the shape of the lens to become thicker or thinner to focus the light on the fovea centralis, which is in the middle of the macula on the retina at the back of the eye. This process is known as refraction. The retina converts the light into an electric signal that travels via the optic

Figure 13.1 Cross-section of the eye

(Mosby's Dictionary 2014)

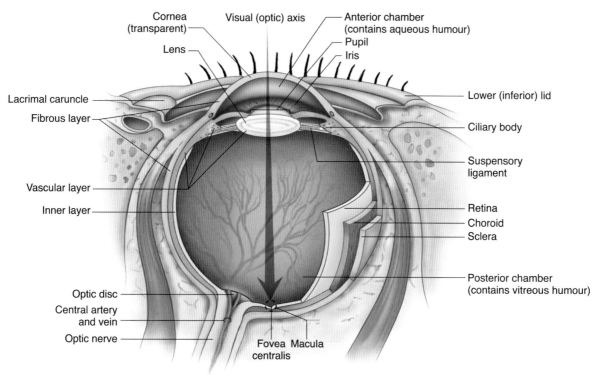

nerve to the brainstem and then to the visual cortex in the occipital lobe, where it is translated into an image. This is the way that a person with perfect eyesight sees. However, sometimes the eye is asymmetrically shaped or the light rays are not focused accurately on the retina. In these cases, the person has a problem with their vision.

The orbit

The orbit is the eye socket, a space adjoined by the bone of the cheek, the forehead, the temporal bone and the side of the nose. Fat pads protect the eye within the orbit. The orbit also contains the lacrimal gland under the outer portion of the upper eyelid. The role of the lacrimal gland is to produce tears to lubricate and moisten the eye and help clear the eye of any foreign matter, such as dust, that enters it. The tears are drained from the eye through the nasolacrimal duct in the inner corner of the eye.

Eyelids and eyelashes

The eye is protected from foreign bodies and bright light by the eyelids – thin folds of skin that cover the eye. The eyelids help keep the eye moist through the operation of blinking, which spreads tears across the eye's surface. Eyelashes also help filter out dust

and debris and prevent sweat from getting into the eye.

Sclera

The sclera is the protective outer wall of the eye and is made up of strong, fibrous tissue that expands from the cornea to the optic nerve. The sclera is what gives the eye its white colour and its shape. The sclera is also attached to the extraocular muscles, which move the eye from side to side, up and down and diagonally.

Conjunctiva

The conjunctiva is a thin, transparent layer of skin that begins at the outer edge of the cornea, covers the outer part of the sclera and coats the inside of the eyelids. The conjunctiva produces a thick clear fluid that lubricates the eye as well as producing some tears, which help keep bacteria and foreign material from getting into the eye. The conjunctiva is made up of microscopic blood vessels. When the eye is irritated, injured or infected, the blood vessels dilate and make the eye look red.

Cornea

The cornea is the clear dome-shaped layer at the front and centre of the eye in front of the iris. Its main role is to help bend or refract light into the lens as it enters the eye. About 70% of the eye's ability to focus comes from the cornea. The cornea also acts as a filter to screen out the most damaging ultraviolet (UV) waves present in sunlight. It contains no blood vessels, but tears and the aqueous humour that fills the chamber behind the cornea provide nourishment and protection from infection.

Anterior chamber

Immediately behind the cornea and the iris is a fluid-filled space known as the anterior chamber. A fluid known as the aqueous humour fills the anterior chamber, providing nourishment for the cornea and the lens.

Iris and pupil

The iris controls the amount of light that enters the eye. The iris is a circular shape with a round opening in the centre known as the pupil (Fig. 13.2). The iris can be coloured green, blue, brown or a mixture of these. A ring of muscles around the iris allows the pupil to contract in bright light and expand in darkness or dim light. The pupil also dilates in response

Figure 13.2 Visible surface of the eye

(Drake et al 2009)

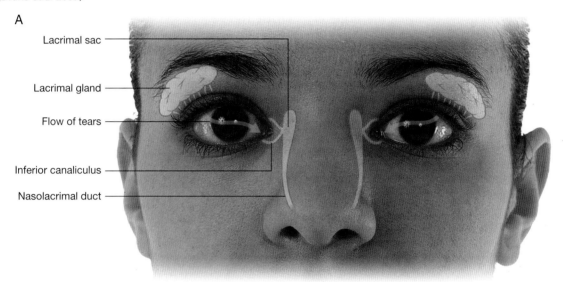

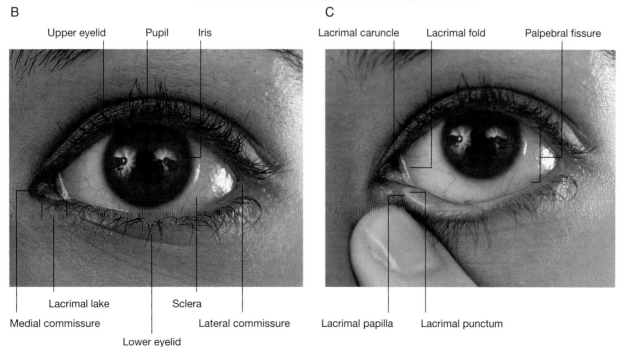

to extreme emotional circumstances such as to fear or pain.

Posterior chamber, lens and ciliary body

The posterior chamber is the fluid-filled space in front of the lens and behind the iris. The lens is a clear, flexible structure that is located just behind the iris and the pupil. The posterior chamber is filled with aqueous humour produced by the ciliary body. The ciliary body is a ring of tissue that is located around the lens. It consists of ciliary muscles and ciliary processes, which contain blood vessels. The aqueous humour moves through the posterior chamber and then forward through the pupil into the anterior chamber. In addition to producing aqueous humour, the muscles of the ciliary body control the eye's ability to accommodate or focus by changing the shape of the lens. When the ciliary body contracts, the lens thickens, increasing the eye's ability to focus up close. When looking at an object at a distance, the ciliary body relaxes and the lens thins out. As we age, the ciliary body muscle and lens gradually lose elasticity.

Vitreous cavity

The vitreous cavity is located behind the lens and in front of the retina and is filled with a jelly-like fluid called the vitreous humour. The role of the vitreous humour is to help maintain the shape of the eyeball.

Retina, macula and choroid

The retina is located at the back of the eye and contains a layer of cells that convert light into nerve signals, which are then transferred via the optic nerve to the brain where the image is processed and we 'see' an object. The retina is made up of two types of cells or photoreceptors known as rods and cones. Rods are more sensitive to light, allowing vision in dim light. Rods do not allow colour to be detected. Cones provide colour sensitivity but need more light.

In the centre of the retina is the macula, which provides sharp vision in an area known as the fovea centralis, where a concentration of cones is located. This area allows the eye to see detail and perform tasks such as reading.

In between the retina and the sclera is the choroid, a layer of tissue mainly made up of blood vessels. The choroid helps nourish the retina.

Optic nerve

The optic nerve is responsible for transmitting visual information from the eye to the visual cortex of the brain for processing into an image. The optic nerve is the second of 12 pairs of cranial nerves.

PATHOLOGY AND DISEASES FOR THE SENSE OF SIGHT

The following section provides a list of common diseases and pathological conditions relevant to the sense of sight.

Term	Pronunciation	Definition
astigmatism	ay-STIG-ma-tiz-em	Astigmatism occurs when the refractive surface of the cornea or lens is abnormally curved. Light rays cannot focus sharply on the retina, causing vision to be out of focus. Astigmatism frequently occurs with other vision conditions such as myopia and hyperopia.
blindness	BLYND-ness	Blindness refers to a partial or complete loss of vision. It may also refer to a loss of vision that cannot be adequately corrected with glasses or contact lenses. Partial blindness means a person has very limited vision. Complete blindness means a person cannot see anything and is also unable to perceive light. The leading causes of blindness among Australians are macular degeneration, glaucoma, cataracts and diabetes.

Table continued

Term	Pronunciation	Definition
cataract	KAT-a-rakt	A cataract is a degenerative eye condition characterised by a clouding or opacity of the lens or the lens capsule (Fig. 13.3). It is a common cause of gradual vision loss. Light shining through the cornea is blocked by the clouded lens – the image cast onto the retina is blurred, therefore the brain interprets a hazy image. There are many different types of cataracts including senile, congenital, traumatic, complicated, toxic and diabetic. Symptoms of cataracts include cloudy or blurry vision, faded colours and sensitivity to glare. A halo may appear around lights. Night vision is poor. Cataracts are usually surgically removed and a replacement lens is inserted.

Figure 13.3 Cataract

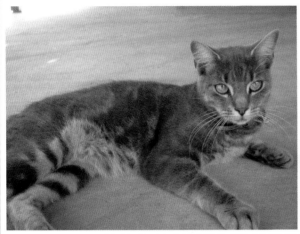 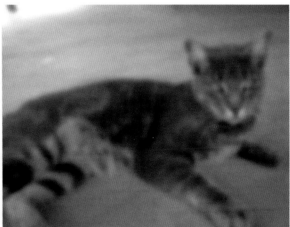

Term	Pronunciation	Definition
glaucoma	glaw-KOH-ma	Glaucoma is an eye disease in which the optic nerve at the back of the eye atrophies (Fig. 13.4). In most people this damage is caused by raised intraocular pressure due to problems with the drainage of the aqueous humour. Chronic (primary open-angle) glaucoma is the most common type. Damage progresses very slowly and destroys vision gradually, starting with peripheral vision. It has no real symptoms until eyesight is lost at a late stage. It can lead to blindness if not treated. Acute (closed-angle) glaucoma occurs when the drainage angle between the iris and cornea is blocked suddenly and the aqueous humour is unable to drain from the anterior chamber.

Figure 13.4 Open angle glaucoma

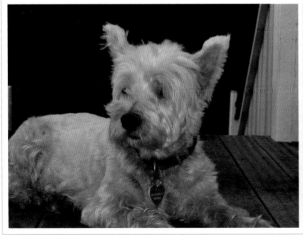 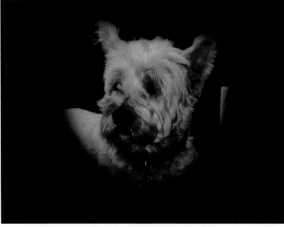

Table continued

Term	Pronunciation	Definition
hyperopia	hy-per-O-pee-a	Hyperopia is diagnosed when a person struggles to see close objects clearly because light is not focused onto the retina. Also called farsightedness, the condition is caused when images are focused behind the retina. This occurs when the eyeball is too short, or where the cornea or lens are odd shapes.
macular degeneration	mak-YOO-lah de-jen-e-RAY-shun	Macular degeneration is a progressive deterioration of the macular tissue of the retina leading to a loss of central vision affecting the ability to see fine detail, drive, read and recognise faces (Fig. 13.5). It tends to be age-related. A spot may appear in the central part of vision or the size of an object may appear different for each eye. It is the visual acuity that is most affected. There are two types of macular degeneration: the dry atrophic form and the wet neovascular form. The dry form results from the slow deterioration of the macula, resulting in a gradual blurring of central vision. Spots called drusen located on the outer retina are the key identifiers for the dry type. Most people with age-related macular degeneration begin with the dry form. In the wet form of macular degeneration, newly created abnormal blood vessels develop in the centre of the retina. These blood vessels can leak and scar the retina, damaging central vision. Vision loss may be rapid in the wet type of macular degeneration.

Figure 13.5 Macular degeneration

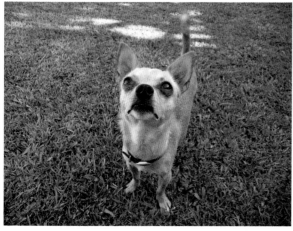 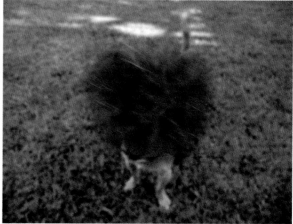

Term	Pronunciation	Definition
myopia	my-O-pee-a	Myopia is a condition that is more commonly known as shortsightedness. It is caused when light is focused in front of the retina, resulting in blurred vision. Shortsighted people can generally see clearly at short distances but have difficulty with seeing distant objects distinctly.
nystagmus	ny-STAG-mus	Nystagmus occurs when there are involuntary rhythmical movements of the eyes, also known as 'dancing eyes'. Nystagmus causes blurred vision because the eyes are always moving. In some people with the condition, head posture is also affected because the eye movements reduce in particular positions. The condition may be unilateral or bilateral and may be congenital or acquired. Often the cause of acquired nystagmus is unknown but may be due to central nervous system or metabolic disorders or alcohol and drug toxicity.
presbyopia	prez-bee-O-pee-a	Presbyopia is a natural condition of ageing that occurs as the muscles around the lens weaken and lose flexibility, causing difficulty in focusing on close objects and print.

Table continued

Term	Pronunciation	Definition
retinal detachment	RET-in-al dee-TACH-ment	Retinal detachment occurs when the retina separates from the supporting layer (the choroid), resulting in loss of vision. Infection, haemorrhage, injury and ageing can cause it. Retinal detachments are often associated with a tear or hole in the retina through which the vitreous humour may leak. If not treated, the detachment can lead to blindness.
retinoblastoma	ret-in-o-blah-STOH-ma	A retinoblastoma is an aggressive malignant tumour arising in the retina. It mostly affects children under 5 years of age. Around two-thirds of cases are unilateral and one-third bilateral, heredity being a factor in some cases. A retinoblastoma will present as a mass of white tissue called leucocoria, which is visible through the pupil. The eye will be inflamed and the eyeball will appear enlarged. Strabismus may be present. Irides may be heterochromic. As it grows, a retinoblastoma can spread to the orbit and along the optic nerve to the central nervous system. It is a potentially fatal condition if not treated. Retinoblastoma is classified by the number of tumours (single or multiple), the size of the tumour and spread (or not) into surrounding tissue.
strabismus	stra-BIZ-mus	Strabismus occurs when the eyes are not able to focus in the same direction at the same time. One eye is misaligned in relation to the other when focusing on an object. It is most commonly due to a weakness of the extraocular muscles. There are four main types: **esotropia** is an inward turning, **exotropia** is an outward turning, **hypertropia** is an upward deviation and **hypotropia** is a downward deviation.
trachoma	tra-KOH-ma	Trachoma is a chronic contagious infection of the conjunctiva caused by the *Chlamydia trachomatis* bacterium. It occurs mostly in settings where standards of hygiene are poor. Trachoma is spread through direct contact with infected eye, nose or throat secretions. Contact with contaminated objects such as towels or clothes can also spread the disease. Symptoms include pain, photophobia, excessive lacrimation and the presence of granulated lesions. If not treated, trachoma can lead to blindness.

NEW WORD ELEMENTS FOR THE SENSE OF HEARING

Here are some word elements related to the sense of hearing. To reinforce your learning, write the meanings of the medical terms in the spaces provided. Use the Glossary of medical terms on page 561 to help you work out the meanings. You may need to check the meaning in a medical dictionary, but attempt it yourself first.

Combining forms

Combining Form	Meaning	Medical Term	Meaning of Medical Term
acous/o	hearing	acoustic	
aer/o	air, gas	aerotitis	
audi/o	hearing	audiology	
audit/o		auditory	

Table continued

Combining Form	Meaning	Medical Term	Meaning of Medical Term
aur/i	ear	auriscope	
aur/o		aural	
auricul/o		auricular	
cerumin/o	wax	ceruminosis	
cochle/o	cochlea	cochleovestibular	
incud/o	incus	incudomalleal	
labyrinth/o	labyrinth, inner ear	labyrinthitis	
malle/o	malleus, hammer	malleotomy	
mastoid/o	mastoid process	mastoidocentesis	
myring/o	eardrum, tympanic membrane	myringotome	
ossicul/o	ossicle	ossiculectomy	
ot/o	ear	otorhinolaryngologist	
salping/o	eustachian (auditory) tube, fallopian tube	salpingoscope	
staped/o	stapes	stapedectomy	
tympan/o	eardrum, tympanic membrane	tympanostomy	
vestibul/o	vestibule	vestibulotomy	

Prefixes

Prefix	Meaning	Medical Term	Meaning of Medical Term
bin-	two, twice, double	binauricular	
electro-	electricity, electrical activity	electrocochleography	
macro-	large	macrotia	
micro-	small	microtia	

Suffixes

Suffix	Meaning	Medical Term	Meaning of Medical Term
-acusis	hearing	anacusis	
-algia	condition of pain	otoneuralgia	
-cusis	hearing	presbycusis	
-otia	ear condition	polyotia	
-rrhoea	discharge, flow	otopyorrhoea	
-scope	instrument to view	auriscope	
-scopy	process of viewing	otoscopy	

ABBREVIATIONS FOR THE SENSE OF HEARING

The following abbreviations are commonly used in the Australian healthcare environment. Because some abbreviations can have more than one meaning, check the context in which the abbreviation is used before assigning a meaning to it.

Abbreviation	Definition
AD	*auris dextra* (right ear)
AL, AS	*auris laeva, auris sinistra* (left ear)
AOM	acute otitis media
AU, a.u.	*aures unitas, auris uterque* (both ears)
aur	*auris* (the ear)

Table continued

Abbreviation	Definition
BAER	brainstem auditory evoked response
BERA	brainstem evoked response audiometry
BSM	bilateral suction myringotomy
EAC	external auditory canal
ENT	ear, nose and throat
ERA	evoked response audiometry
ET	eustachian tube
NIHL	noise-induced hearing loss
OE	otitis externa
OM	otitis media
OME	otitis media with effusion
PE tube	pressure-equalising tube
SNHL	sensorineural hearing loss
SOM	serous otitis media
SSNHL	sudden sensorineural hearing loss
TM	tympanic membrane
TORP	total ossicular replacement prosthesis

FUNCTIONS AND STRUCTURE OF THE EAR – THE SENSE OF HEARING

The auditory system allows mechanical processing and recognition of sounds. The major organ of the auditory system is the ear, which acts as the receiver for sound and also has a major responsibility for maintaining balance and body position (Fig. 13.6). The ear operates with the nerves of the central nervous system to change sound pressure waves and transfer them as electrical impulses to the cerebral cortex in the brain, which processes them and allows us to 'hear'. Sounds are produced when an object vibrates in another substance – this might be something solid such as the earth, a liquid such as water, or a gas such as air. The latter is the most common way that sound is transferred in the environment. When an object vibrates, it moves the air particles around it. The vibrating air particles closest to the object then move the air particles around them, and they move the air particles next to them, and so on – thus the pulse of the vibration travels through the air. The process of hearing occurs as follows:

1. The pinna or external ear captures and directs the sound waves into the ear canal to the eardrum.

Figure 13.6 The ear

(Mosby's dictionary 2014)

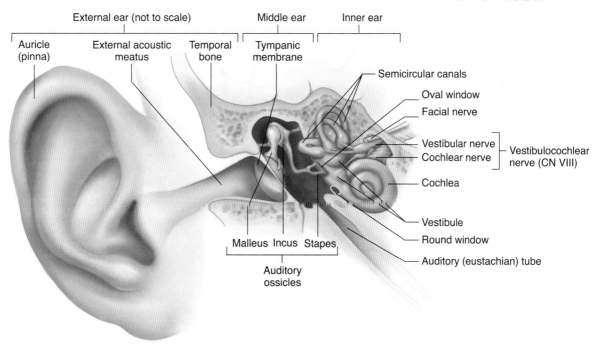

GROSS ANATOMY OF THE EAR

2. The eardrum starts to vibrate, which moves three tiny bones (malleus, incus and stapes) in the middle ear and this causes the fluid in the inner ear or cochlea to also move.

3. The movement of the fluid causes bending of the hair cells in the cochlea. The hair cells change the movement into electrical impulses.

4. The electrical impulses are transmitted via the auditory nerve to the brain, where they are interpreted as sound.

Outer ear

The outer ear is the part of the ear that can be seen. The parts of the outer ear are called the pinna, concha and external auditory meatus. The irregular cartilaginous shape of the pinna (also known as the auricle) helps modify, filter and amplify different sounds. The deepest indent in the pinna is the concha, which is responsible for gathering sound energy and funnelling it to the tympanic membrane, or eardrum. The external auditory ear canal or meatus consists of sweat glands that have adapted to produce cerumen (earwax) in the ear canal. The cerumen is designed to protect, clean and lubricate the ear. If there is an excess of cerumen, this could lead to eardrum damage or block sound transmission.

Middle ear

The external ear canal funnels sound waves to the tympanic membrane, which is similar to a thin, sensitive drum stretched tightly over the entrance to the middle ear. The waves cause the membrane to vibrate, and these vibrations are passed on to the malleus or hammer – one of three tiny bones in the middle ear. The hammer vibrating causes the incus or anvil, another small bone adjacent to the hammer, to also begin vibrating. The anvil transfers the vibrations to the stapes or stirrup, the third small bone in the middle ear. From the stirrup, the vibrations move into the oval window, a connective tissue membrane located between the middle and inner ear.

Inner ear

The inner ear has two roles – one relating to hearing and the other to the sense of balance, known as the vestibular system. It is composed of three structures: the cochlea, three semicircular canals and the vestibule or labyrinth.

The cochlea is a snail-shaped cavity located in the bony labyrinth and contains the nerves that convert the sound vibrations in the fluid of the inner ear (known as perilymph) into nerve impulses, which are transmitted to the brain from the organ of Corti (the body's 'microphone' in the inner ear) via the auditory nerve.

The vestibule (labyrinth) and semicircular canals help maintain balance or equilibrium. To achieve balance, the eyes, ears and the musculoskeletal system need to work together. The brain receives, translates and processes the information from these systems to maintain balance. The semicircular canals in the inner ear contain fluid called endolymph, which helps the brain to identify or detect the extent of body movement and positioning of the head.

PATHOLOGY AND DISEASES FOR THE SENSE OF HEARING

The following section provides a list of common diseases and pathological conditions relevant to the sense of hearing.

Term	Pronunciation	Definition
acoustic neuroma	a-KOO-stik nyoo-ROH-ma	An acoustic neuroma (also called a vestibular Schwannoma) is a benign tumour that arises in the Schwann cells that surround the acoustic nerve (also called the vestibulocochlear nerve or cranial nerve VIII). The tumour can cause symptoms such as tinnitus, vertigo, balance problems and deafness. The tumour grows in the auditory canal and may invade the brainstem and affect other local cranial nerves if not treated.
cholesteatoma	kol-ES-lee-at-OH-ma	A cholesteatoma is a benign cyst-like tumour of the middle ear. It can be either congenital or, more commonly, occurs as a complication of a chronic otitis media. After infections, layers of old skin can build up inside the middle ear resulting in a cholesteatoma. Over time, it can increase in size and erode the bones of the middle ear, resulting in deafness. The initial signs of a cholesteatoma are a recurring discharge from the ear canal and hearing loss. Surgery is often performed to prevent permanent conductive deafness.

Table continued

Term	Pronunciation	Definition
deafness	DEF-nes	Deafness or hearing loss is a partial or complete inability to distinguish or hear sounds. It can be caused by heredity, premature birth, Rh incompatibility, diseases such as rubella and meningitis or damage to ear structures from continual exposure to loud noise. Deafness can be broadly grouped into two main types. Conductive deafness occurs when the sound-conducting abilities of the auditory meatus, the tympanic membrane or the ossicles are affected. Sensorineural deafness occurs as a result of damage to, or disease of, the nerves of the ear, such as in acoustic neuroma.
labyrinthitis	lab-i-rin-THY-tus	Labyrinthitis is an inflammation of the inner ear that occurs as a result of a bacterial or viral infection. It is characterised by vertigo, nausea/vomiting, tinnitus, loss of balance and visual disturbances such as difficulty in focusing the eyes. There is often a loss of hearing in the affected ear.
Ménière's disease	men-ee-YAIRS diz-eez	Ménière's disease is a chronic disease of the inner ear characterised by tinnitus, vertigo, a feeling of fullness or pressure in the ear and fluctuating deafness. Attacks are unpredictable and may occur in clusters. Between attacks, the patient usually exhibits no symptoms of the disease. The cause of Ménière's disease is unknown but may be related to an infection of the inner ear, head injury, migraine or an allergic reaction.
otitis media	oh-TY-tis MEE-dee-a	Otitis media is a general term for an infection or inflammation of the middle ear. Ear infections occur when the eustachian tube becomes blocked with fluid. This causes a build-up of mucus and pus behind the eardrum resulting in pressure and severe pain known as otalgia. The two main types of ear infections are acute otitis media and acute otitis media with effusion. **Acute otitis media (AOM)** is also called suppurative otitis media and is the most common type of ear infection (Fig. 13.7). It most often occurs in young children. Acute otitis media is diagnosed by inflammation in the middle ear and the presence of fluid behind the tympanic membrane. This results in **myringitis**. The tympanic membrane may bulge and perhaps perforate, otalgia will be experienced and there is often drainage of purulent material from the ear canal. AOM is usually of rapid onset and short duration. **Otitis media with effusion (OME)** is also called serous otitis media. It is defined as the presence of inflammation and non-purulent fluid in the middle ear without the signs and symptoms of an acute ear infection. OME may occur after an acute ear infection has resolved but fluid is still trapped behind the tympanic membrane. More commonly OME occurs when the eustachian tube is blocked and does not ventilate the ear normally. As a result, fluid accumulates in the middle ear. If this is not diagnosed and treated, eventually the fluid will become thick and glue-like, resulting in a condition called glue ear. This can lead to conductive deafness. Glue ear is treated by a myringotomy and the insertion of tympanostomy tubes (grommets) to help drain the accumulated fluid (Fig. 13.7).

Table continued

Term	Pronunciation	Definition
Figure 13.7 Disorders of the ear **A.** Acute otitis media – note the red, bulging and thickened tympanic membrane; **B.** Tympanostomy tube or grommet inserted to relieve pressure and permit drainage in otitis media; **C.** Cerumen (earwax) in ear canal (Thibodeau & Patton 2010)		
otosclerosis	ot-oh-skler-O-sis	Otosclerosis is a hereditary condition where the bony tissue of the middle or inner ear hardens. Spongy bone forms around the oval window causing ankylosis (fixation) of the stapes. This prevents transmission of sound energy to the inner ear, resulting in deafness. Other symptoms may include tinnitus and dizziness.
tinnitus	TIN-i-tus	Tinnitus is the presence of a ringing sound in the ears. Tinnitus can arise in any part of the ear (outer, middle or inner ear) or the brain. It can occur as a result of a chronic exposure to loud noise such as music or firearms, deafness or as a symptom of other diseases such as Ménière's disease. While very annoying for the patient, tinnitus does not often require treatment and generally resolves spontaneously.
vertigo	VER-tee-goh	Vertigo is a sensation of moving or spinning that is often symptomatic of inner ear disease. A person with vertigo either feels that they are spinning (**subjective vertigo**) or their surroundings are spinning (**objective vertigo**). Nausea is often present and balance is affected.

NEW WORD ELEMENTS FOR THE SENSE OF SMELL

Here are some word elements related to the sense of smell. To reinforce your learning, write the meanings of the medical terms in the spaces provided. Use the Glossary of medical terms on page 561 to help you work out the meanings. You may need to check the meaning in a medical dictionary, but attempt it yourself first.

Combining forms

Combining Form	Meaning	Medical Term	Meaning of Medical Term
olfactor/o	sense of smell	olfactory	
osm/o	sense of smell	anosmia	
osphresi/o	odour	osphresiology	
oz/o	to smell, odour	ozostomia	
rhin/o	nose	rhinoplasty	

Prefixes

Prefix	Meaning	Medical Term	Meaning of Medical Term
dys-	bad, painful, difficult	dysosmia	
hyper-	above, excessive	hyperosphresia	
hypo-	below, under, deficient, less than normal	hyposmia	

FUNCTIONS AND STRUCTURE OF THE NOSE – THE SENSE OF SMELL

The olfactory system contains the organs and processes that allow us to smell. The system interprets chemical signals – odours – in the brain through the actions of the olfactory epithelium and the olfactory bulb. The olfactory system is a very important part of the body's limbic system, which is involved in memories, emotional responses and behaviour.

The olfactory epithelium is a highly specialised area inside the nose that is responsible for capturing odours and passing them on to the brain via receptors. The exact way that this occurs is not fully understood. The epithelium has many neurons, but the precise means by which they work together to distinguish between different smells is unknown. As we breathe air through the nose, fine hairs and mucus in the nose trap any potentially harmful particles and the remainder of the air flows over the olfactory epithelium. The neurons in the epithelium react to different odours and send signals to the olfactory nerve, which is a part of the peripheral nervous system. The end of the olfactory nerve is the olfactory bulb, which is a part of the central nervous system. The olfactory bulb processes and recognises specific odours by identifying their chemical structures. Mammals also have an accessory olfactory system that principally operates to detect pheromones or chemicals that trigger a sexual or social reaction to other members of the same species.

NEW WORD ELEMENTS FOR THE SENSE OF TASTE

Here are some word elements related to the sense of taste. To reinforce your learning, write the meanings of the medical terms in the spaces provided. Use the Glossary of medical terms on page 561 to help you work out the meanings. You may need to check the meaning in a medical dictionary, but attempt it yourself first.

Combining forms

Combining Form	Meaning	Medical Term	Meaning of Medical Term
geus/o	sense of taste	glycogeusia	
lingu/o	tongue	epilingual	

FUNCTIONS AND STRUCTURE RELATING TO THE TONGUE – THE SENSE OF TASTE

The sense of taste is also called gustation. The sensation of taste can be classified into five basic categories: sweet, bitter, sour, salty and savoury or umami. Taste allows us to identify products as appetitive or aversive, depending upon the effect they have on the body. Appetitive means the instinctive desire to eat specific foods to maintain life, while aversive refers to the body's tendency to reject noxious substances.

The five basic tastes contribute to the sensation and flavour of food in the mouth but are supported by other factors including the sense of smell (as described above) and the texture and temperature of the food. The organ of taste is the taste bud, of which there are approximately 10,000 on the human tongue. Each taste bud has between 50 and 150 receptor cells, each of which responds best to one of the basic tastes. Receptors can respond to the other tastes but respond most strongly to a particular taste. Receptor cells live for only 1–2 weeks and are then replaced by new receptor cells. Taste buds themselves are contained in cup-shaped papillae.

Cranial nerves are necessary for taste: the facial nerve (cranial nerve VII) and the glossopharyngeal nerve (cranial nerve IX). The facial nerve works with the anterior two-thirds of the tongue and the glossopharyngeal nerve works on the posterior part of the tongue. A third cranial nerve (the vagus nerve, X) transmits taste information from the back of the mouth. These nerves convey taste information to a specific part of the brainstem, then to the thalamus and on to the cerebral cortex. In a similar way to the sense of smell, taste is also associated with the limbic system, which is responsible for behavioural and emotional responses.

NEW WORD ELEMENTS FOR THE SENSE OF TOUCH

Here is a word element related to the sense of touch. To reinforce your learning, write the meaning of the medical term in the space provided. Use the Glossary of medical terms on page 561 to help you work out the meanings. You may need to check the meaning in a medical dictionary, but attempt it yourself first.

Combining forms

Combining Form	Meaning	Medical Term	Meaning of Medical Term
palpat/o	touch, feel, stroke	palpatory	

FUNCTIONS AND STRUCTURE RELATING TO THE SENSE OF TOUCH

While the four other human senses (sight, hearing, smell and taste) are located in particular parts of the body, the sense of touch is found throughout the body. Because there are different numbers of nerve endings in various parts of the body, some areas are more sensitive to touch than others. The reason that touch is perceived all over the body is because the sense of touch stems from the dermal skin layer. The human skin acts as the protective barrier between the internal body systems and the external environment. The perception of touch provides the process whereby the skin tells the brain about its surroundings through an arrangement of nerve endings and touch receptors known as the somatosensory system. This system is responsible for sensations such as cold, heat, texture, pressure, irritation, pain and vibration. Within this system, the four types of main receptors are:

1. mechanoreceptors, which react to pressure, vibrations and texture
2. thermoreceptors, which respond to temperature
3. pain receptors, which detect pain or stimuli that could cause damage to the tissues of the body
4. proprioceptors, which act as part of the musculoskeletal system to perceive the position of the different parts of the body in relation to each other and their environment.

The receptors transmit information via sensory nerves in the spinal cord into the brain. The brain processes the message in the parietal lobe of the cerebral cortex and sends a response message back to the body.

VOCABULARY FOR THE SENSES

The following list provides many of the medical terms used for the first time in this chapter. Pronunciations are provided with each term. As you read the rest of the chapter, make sure you identify each of these terms and understand their meanings.

Term	Pronunciation
acoustic neuroma	a-KOO-stik nyoo-ROH-ma
anterior chamber	an-TEE-ree-a CHAYM-ba
astigmatism	ay-STIG-ma-tiz-em
audiometry	aw-dee-OM-e-tree
auditory meatus	AW-di-tor-ee mee-AY-tus
auditory tube	AW-di-tor-ee tyoob

Table continued

Term	Pronunciation
blindness	BLYND-ness
cataract	KAT-a-rakt
cholesteatoma	kol-ES-tee-at-O-ma
choroid	KO-royd
ciliary body	SIL-a-ree BOD-ee
cochlea	KOK-lee-a
cochlear implant	KOK-lee-ar im-plant
concha	KON-ka
conjunctiva	kon-junk-TY-va
cornea	kaw-nee-a
deafness	DEF-ness
ear thermometry	ee-a ther-MOM-e-tree
entropion repair	en-TROH-pee-on ree-pair
enucleation	e-NYOO-klee-AY-shun
fluorescein angiography	FLOO-res-in an-jee-OG-ra-fee
gustation	gus-TAY-shun
glaucoma	glaw-KOH-ma
hyperopia	hy-per-O-pee-a
incus	INK-us
iris	EYE-ris
keratoplasty	ke-RAT-o-plas-tee
labyrinth	LAB-i-rinth
labyrinthitis	lab-i-rinth-EYE-tus
laser photocoagulation	LAY-za foh-to-koh-AG-yoo-LAY-shun
LASIK (laser-assisted in situ keratomileusis)	LAY-sik (LAY-za a-SIS-ted in sy-tyoo ke-RAT-o-my-LOO-sis
lens	lenz
macula	MAK-yoo-la
macular degeneration	MAK-yoo-la de-jen-e-RAY-shun
malleus	MAL-ee-us
Ménière's disease	men-ee-YAIRZ diz-eez
myopia	my-O-pee-a
myringotomy	my-rin-GOT-om-ee
nasendoscopy	naz-en-DOS-kop-ee
nystagmus	ny-STAG-mus
olfactory bulb	ol-FAK-tor-ee bulb
olfactory epithelium	ol-FAK-tor-ee ep-ee-THEEL-ee-um
olfactory nerve	ol-FAK-tor-ee nerv
ophthalmoscopy	off-thal-MOS-kop-ee

Table continued

Term	Pronunciation
optic nerve	OP-tik nerv
otitis media	o-TY-tis MEE-dee-a
otosclerosis	ot-o-skler-O-sis
otoscopy	o-TOS-kop-ee
phacoemulsification	FAY-koh e mul-sif-i-KAY-shun
pinna	PIN-a
presbyopia	prez-bee-O-pee-a
pupil	PYOO-pil
refraction	ree-FRAK-shun
retina	RET-in-a
retinal detachment	RET-in-al dee-TACH-ment
retinoblastoma	ret-in-o-blah-STOH-ma
sclera	SKLEE-ra
scleral buckle	SKLEE-ral buk-el
semicircular canal	sem-ee-SER-kyoo-la kan-AL
septoplasty	SEP-toh-plas-tee
sinusoscopy	syn-us-OS-kop-ee
slit lamp microscopy	slit lamp my-KROS-kop-ee
stapes	STAY-peez
strabismus	stra-BIZ-mus
taste bud	tayst bud
tinnitus	TIN-i-tus
trachoma	trak-O-ma
tuning fork test	TYOO-ning fawk test
turbinectomy	tur-bin-EK-tom-ee
tympanic membrane	tim-PAN-ik MEM-brayn
vertigo	VER-tee-goh
vestibule	VES-tib-yool
visual acuity test	VIZ-yoo-al a-KYOO-i-tee test
visual field test	VIZ-yoo-al FEELD test
vitrectomy	vi-TREK-tom-ee
vitreous cavity	VI-tree-us KAV-i-tee
vitreous humour	VI-tree-us HYOO-ma

TESTS AND PROCEDURES FOR THE SENSES

The following section provides a list of common diagnostic tests and procedures and clinical interventions and surgical procedures that are undertaken for the senses.

Test/Procedure	Pronunciation	Definition
audiometry	aw-dee-OM-e-tree	Audiometry is a test of a person's hearing ability, usually performed using an audiometer and used to determine hearing loss or diseases of the ear. The tests may also involve testing the person's ability to differentiate between sounds.
cochlear implant	KOK-lee-a im-plant	A cochlear implant is a surgical procedure that involves implanting an electrode into the cochlea to allow for a person with sensorineural hearing loss to be able to detect sounds (Fig. 13.8). The electrode is connected to a small computer attached to the external ear. The computer converts the sound waves to electronic impulses, which stimulate nerve fibres. **Figure 13.8 Cochlear implant** (Baker et al 2017) 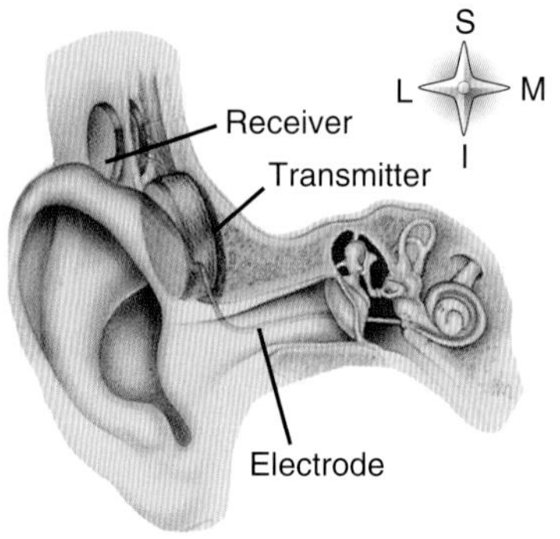
ear thermometry	ee-a ther-MOM-e-tree	Ear thermometry is a test that measures the temperature of the tympanic membrane by detecting infrared radiation from the eardrum.
entropion repair	en-TROH-pee-on ree-pair	Entropion repair involves making an incision in the lateral corner of the eye or an incision just beneath the lower eyelashes and then tightening the muscles to resolve the imbalance.
enucleation	e-NYOO-klee-AY-shun	Enucleation is the surgical removal of an eye and is used to treat tumours of the eye, severe trauma or eyes that are blind and painful. The muscle and other orbital structures are left in place. An artificial eye is generally inserted for cosmetic reasons.
fluorescein angiography	FLOO-res-in an-jee-OG-ra-fee	Fluorescein angiography is the process of imaging the blood vessels of the retina at the back of the eye following the injection of fluorescent dye into the bloodstream. It assists in diagnosing and managing conditions such as diabetic retinopathy and macular degeneration.

Table continued

Test/Procedure	Pronunciation	Definition
keratoplasty	KE-RAT-o-plas-tee	A keratoplasty is a surgical procedure to repair a cornea. It is also known as a corneal transplant. It involves removing a person's damaged cornea and replacing it with a donor cornea.
laser photocoagulation	LAY-za foh-to-koh-ag-yoo-LAY-shun	Laser photocoagulation involves cauterising ocular blood vessels to treat diabetic retinopathy and macular degeneration.
LASIK (laser-assisted in situ keratomileusis)	LAY-sik (LAY-za a-SIS-ted in sy-tyoo ke-RAT-o-my-LOO-sis)	LASIK is a refractive surgery used to correct myopia, hyperopia and astigmatism. The procedure involves creating a flap of corneal tissue, then remodelling the cornea under the flap with a laser and repositioning the flap.
myringotomy	my-rin-GOT-o-mee	A myringotomy is performed to relieve pressure from fluid or pus build-up. It involves making a small incision into the eardrum and can involve inserting a tube to aid ventilation of the middle ear.
nasendoscopy	naz-en-DOS-kop-ee	A nasendoscopy allows for visual examination of the nose and upper airway linings through a small flexible endoscope.
ophthalmoscopy	off-thal-MOS-kop-ee	An ophthalmoscopy is a diagnostic test using an ophthalmoscope to visualise the fundus (back of the eye), usually performed during a routine eye examination.
otoscopy	ot-OS-ko-pee	Otoscopy is an examination of the external auditory canal and eardrum using an otoscope. It is used to identify conditions such as otitis externa, otitis media, excessive wax production, foreign bodies and eczema.
phacoemulsification	FAY-ko-ee-mul-sif-i-KAY-shun	Phacoemulsification is the most common form of treatment for cataracts (Fig. 13.9). It involves removing the lens by breaking it into tiny pieces and suctioning them off the eye. The back of the capsule is left in place and an intraocular lens is implanted as a replacement.

Figure 13.9 Cataract removal by phacoemulsification

(Malavazzi & Nery 2010)

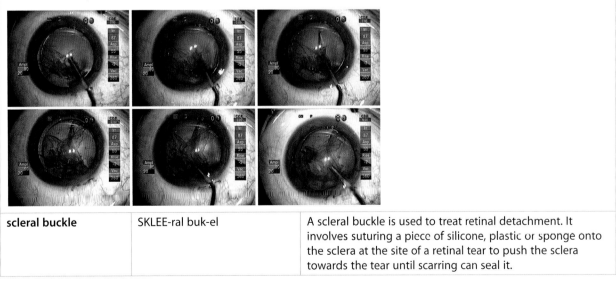

scleral buckle	SKLEE-ral buk-el	A scleral buckle is used to treat retinal detachment. It involves suturing a piece of silicone, plastic or sponge onto the sclera at the site of a retinal tear to push the sclera towards the tear until scarring can seal it.

Table continued

Test/Procedure	Pronunciation	Definition
septoplasty	SEP-toh-plas-tee	A septoplasty is a surgical procedure to repair the nasal septum, performed to correct a deviated nasal septum.
sinusoscopy	syn-us-OS-kop-ee	A sinusoscopy is a procedure that allows for endoscopic visual examination of the maxillary sinus.
slit lamp microscopy	slit lamp my-KROS-kop-ee	A slit lamp microscopy examines the endothelium on the posterior surface of the cornea using a corneal microscope with a special attachment.
tuning fork test	TYOO-ning fawk test	The tuning fork test is a simple diagnostic test for hearing that involves placing a tuning fork in the middle of the forehead, chin or head at equal distance from the person's ears. The person then identifies in which ear the sound is loudest.
turbinectomy	tur-bin-EK-to-mee	A turbinectomy is a surgical procedure that involves removing enlarged inferior turbinates to relieve nasal obstruction.
visual acuity test	VIZ-yoo-al a-KYOO-i-tee test	A visual acuity test is a diagnostic test to determine the smallest letters a person can read on a standard eye chart from a prescribed distance.
visual field test	VIZ-yoo-al FEELD test	Visual field tests are performed to identify any loss of vision. The test is performed by having the person watch a fixed spot on the wall in front of them and identify when a target first appears.
vitrectomy	vit-REK-to-mee	Vitrectomy is a surgical procedure that involves removing some or all of the vitreous humour from the eye. It is used to treat conditions such as vitreous floaters, macular degeneration, retinal detachment and macular pucker.
YAG laser capsulotomy	YAG LAY-zer kap-syul-OT-o-mee	A YAG laser capsulotomy is performed following surgery for a cataract when the lens membrane (or capsule) thickens and becomes cloudy, causing light to fail to reach the back of the eye. The YAG laser creates a tiny hole in the capsule of the lens, allowing light to get through.

Exercises

EXERCISE 13.1: LABEL THE DIAGRAMS

Using the information provided in this chapter, label the anatomical parts in Figs 13.10 and 13.11.

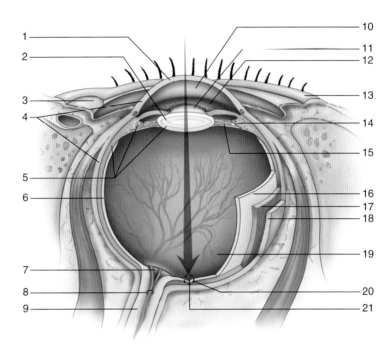

Figure 13.10 The eye

(Mosby's Dictionary 2014)

1 _____	12 _____
2 _____	13 _____
3 _____	14 _____
4 _____	15 _____
5 _____	16 _____
6 _____	17 _____
7 _____	18 _____
8 _____	19 _____
9 _____	20 _____
10 _____	21 _____
11 _____	

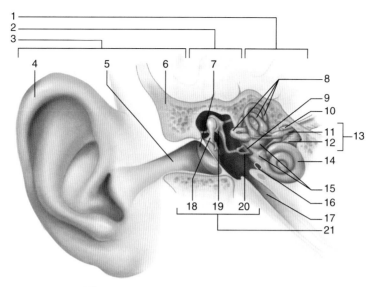

Figure 13.11 The ear

(Mosby's Dictionary 2014)

1 _____

2 _____

3 _____

4 _____

5 _____

6 _____

7 _____

8 _____

9 _____

10 _____

11 _____

12 _____

13 _____

14 _____

15 _____

16 _____

17 _____

18 _____

19 _____

20 _____

21 _____

EXERCISE 13.2: MATCH WORD ELEMENTS AND MEANINGS

Match the prefix, suffix or combining form in Column A with its meaning from Column B.

Column A	Answer	Column B
1. myring/o		A. odour
2. aque/o		B. iris
3. geus/o		C. hearing
4. ambly/o		D. grey
5. malle/o		E. eardrum, tympanic membrane
6. palpat/o		F. the sense of smell
7. dacry/o		G. eyelid
8. acous/o		H. sense of taste
9. xer/o		I. lens of eye
10. corne/o		J. water
11. phac/o		K. darkness
12. glauc/o		L. stapes
13. osphresi/o		M. dull, dim
14. blephar/o		N. cornea
15. mydr/o		O. tears
16. irid/o		P. wax
17. staped/o		Q. touch, feel, stroke
18. osm/o		R. malleus, hammer
19. scot/o		S. widen, enlarge
20. cerumin/o		T. dry

EXERCISE 13.3: WORD ANALYSIS AND MEANING

Break up the medical terms below into their component parts (prefixes, suffixes, word roots, combining vowels). Provide the meaning for each word element and each term as a whole.

Example:
keratoplasty

kerat/o = cornea

-plasty = surgical, plastic repair

Meaning = surgical repair of the cornea

1. ozostomia _____

2.　otosclerosis _____

_____

_____

3.　hyperosphresia _____

_____

_____

4.　vestibulotomy _____

_____

_____

5.　aerotitis _____

_____

_____

6.　dacroadenitis _____

_____

_____

7.　asthenopia _____

_____

_____

8.　ceruminosis _____

_____

_____

9.　anacusis _____

_____

_____

10.　anosmia _____

_____

_____

EXERCISE 13.4: VOCABULARY BUILDING

Provide the medical term for each of the definitions below.

1. Condition of an absence of the lens of the eye: _____

2. Condition of unequal pupils of the eye: _____

3. Inflammation of the eyelid: _____

4. Condition of an outward eye: _____

5. Condition of vision at night: _____

6. Condition of vision without colour: _____

7. One who specialises in the study of the ear, nose and throat: _____

8. Surgical puncture to remove fluid from the mastoid process: _____

9. Discharge, flow of pus from the ear: _____

10. Condition of vision in old age: _____

EXERCISE 13.5: EXPAND THE ABBREVIATIONS

Expand the abbreviations to form correct medical terms.

Abbreviation	Expanded Abbreviation
ACG	
ARMD	
ASC	
BSM	
EAC	
ENT	
IOFB	
IOL	
OM	
PE tube	
POAG	
REM	

Abbreviation	Expanded Abbreviation
ROP	
SLE	
SOM	
SSNHL	
TM	
TORP	
VA	
VF	

EXERCISE 13.6: MATCH MEDICAL TERMS AND MEANINGS

Match the medical term in Column A with its meaning in Column B.

Column A	Answer	Column B
1. retinopathy		A. nearsightedness
2. anosmia		B. savoury taste
3. hypergeusia		C. another term for 'stye'
4. hordeolum		D. excessive sense of taste
5. conjunctivitis		E. loss of hearing associated with age
6. presbycusis		F. absence of a sense of smell
7. blepharoptosis		G. flow of fluid from the ear
8. umami		H. drooping of the eyelid
9. myopia		I. inflammation of the conjunctiva
10. otorrhoea		J. general term for disease of the retina

EXERCISE 13.7: APPLYING MEDICAL TERMINOLOGY

Fill in the blank with the correct medical term.

1. An outward turning of the rim of the eyelid is called
   _____.
   a) entropion
   b) esotropia
   c) strabismus
   d) ectropion

2. The excision of an eyeball is called _____.
   a) blepharectomy
   b) trabeculectomy
   c) enucleation
   d) dacryocystectomy

3. A ringing in the ear is called _____.
   a) otalgia
   b) tinnitus
   c) vertigo
   d) otorrhoea

4. Inflammation of the eardrum is _____.
   a) cerumen impaction
   b) otosclerosis
   c) otitis media
   d) myringitis

5. The term emmetropia means _____.
    a) blindness
    b) shortsighted
    c) longsighted
    d) normal vision

6. The term _____ means snail.
    a) stapes
    b) pinna
    c) cochlea
    d) endolymph

7. A test to measure _____ is known as audiometry.
    a) acuity of hearing
    b) balance
    c) visual acuity
    d) glaucoma

8. A repair of the tympanic membrane is a _____.
    a) membranoplasty
    b) otoplasty
    c) tympanostomy
    d) myringoplasty

9. The medical term to describe double vision is _____.
    a) myopia
    b) presbyopia
    c) exoptropia
    d) diplopia

10. Removal of the vitreous humour is known as _____.
    a) blepharorrhaphy
    b) vitrectomy
    c) iridotomy
    d) coreoplasty

EXERCISE 13.8: PRONUNCIATION AND COMPREHENSION

Read the following paragraphs aloud to practise your pronunciation. Using your textbook and a medical dictionary, find the meanings of the underlined medical terms.

1

A 64-year-old woman was admitted routinely for a left keratoplasty for Fuchs' endothelial dystrophy. This was performed under general anaesthetic (ASA = 1NE). Her postoperative course was uneventful and she was discharged home on 5.3.20 and will be reviewed in the OPD.

2

A 27-year-old woman was admitted with a history of suffering some nasal trauma 4 years prior to admission, with subsequent nasal obstruction since that time. She has a past history of an appendicectomy 10 years ago. Systematic questioning revealed no symptoms of cardiac failure. She smokes 40 cigarettes a day and has a non-productive chronic cough.

On examination she was an obese young woman, pulse 80 and regular, BP 110/70. She had a few cervical nodes in her left anterior triangle and a slight nasal obstruction with the septum deviated to the left. The remainder of the examination was unremarkable.

A septorhinoplasty was performed under a general anaesthetic (ASA = 1NE). During surgery, the cartilage deformity was corrected successfully. She had an uneventful postoperative course and was discharged home.

EXERCISE 13.9: ANAGRAMS

Work out each medical term from the jumbled letters below. Then, using the letters in brackets, determine the medical term that matches the description given.

1. onlneeutaci	__ __ __ __ (__) __ __ __ __ __ __	The surgical removal of an eye
2. easlcr	(__) __ __ __ __ __	The white part of the eye
3. iphmyops	__ __ __ __ __ __ __ (__)	Deficient sense of smell
4. caalmaoklrtea	__ __ __ __ __ __ (__) __ __ __ __ __	Softening of the cornea in the eye

5. ilafca	__ __ __ __ __ (__)	One of the cranial nerves involved in taste
6. dtgaioisuol	__ (__) __ __ __ __ __ __ __ __ __	One who specialises in the study of hearing
7. gnteolaruaio	__ __ __ __ (__) __ __ __ __ __ __	Condition of pain in the nerves of the ear

Rearrange the letters in brackets to form a word that is 'the name of one of the bones in the middle ear that transmits sound waves'.

__ __ __ __ __ __ __

EXERCISE 13.10: CROSSWORD PUZZLE

Complete the puzzle by providing the medical term for each of the clues below.

ACROSS

2. A sensation of moving or spinning that is often symptomatic of inner ear disease (7)

4. A test of a patient's hearing ability (10)

6. Visual examination of the nose and upper airway linings (12)

8. Contains the nerves which convert sound vibrations to nerve impulses (7)

9. Surgical removal of an eye (11)

10. Occurs when the refractive surface of the cornea or lens is abnormally curved (11)

DOWN

1. Changing of the shape of the lens to focus light on the retina (10)

3. Occurs when the eyes are not able to focus in the same direction at the same time (10)

5. Inflammation of the inner ear (13)

7. A partial or complete inability to distinguish or hear sounds (8)

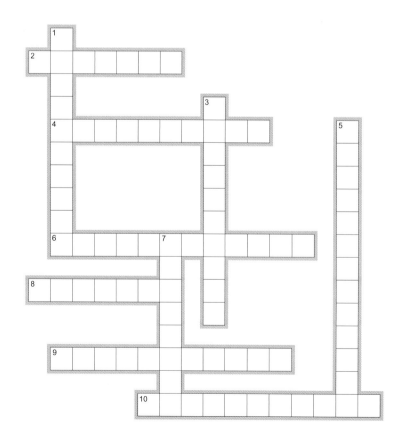

EXERCISE 13.11: DISCHARGE SUMMARY ANALYSIS

Read the discharge summary below and answer the questions.

UNIVERSITY HOSPITAL DISCHARGE SUMMARY	**UR number:** 262728
	Name: Lisa Harris
	Address: 6 Otter Place, Seaview
	Date of birth: 3/8/1937
	Sex: F
	Nominated primary healthcare provider:
	Dr Jason Crighton

Episode details	**Discharge details**
Consultant: Dr White	**Status:** Home
Registrar: Dr Bruce	**Date of discharge:** 5/12/2020
Unit: ENT	
Admission source: Emergency department	
Date of admission: 30/11/2020	

Reason for admission / Presenting problems:

Dizziness, without mention of tinnitus, severe vomiting, hearing deficit, nystagmus or focal neurological signs

Principal diagnosis: Vestibular neuronitis

Comorbidities:

Diverticulosis

Hypertension

Previous medical history:

Partial thyroidectomy for goitre

Left THR

Clinical synopsis:

With a provisional diagnosis of vestibular neuronitis or viral labyrinthitis, Lisa was managed conservatively with IV fluids and Stemetil as required. This was met with a good symptomatic response. Her hypertension was somewhat erratic during her hospitalisation but settled after a change in her medication. She required assistance with mobilisation because of her hip replacement.

Complications:

Clinical interventions:

Diagnostic interventions:

FBC, electrolytes and renal function – all within normal limits. LFTs normal with the exception of a mildly elevated ALT at 53 units/litre (upper limit of normal 45). ECG showed sinus rhythm and chest x-ray was within normal limits.

Medications at discharge:

Tenormin 50 mg daily

Enalapril 2.5 mg daily

Valium 5 mg nocte

Tryptanol 25 mg nocte

Stemetil 5 mg p.r.n.

Panadol ii q.i.d., p.r.n.

Ceased medications:

Allergies: Bee stings

Alerts:

Arranged services:

| **Recommendations:** |
| Lisa was discharged on the above medications and is to be followed up by her local doctor. No follow-up appointment was made for outpatients. |
| **Information to patient/relevant parties:** |
| **Authorising clinician:** Dr Bruce |
| **Document recipients:** |
| Patient and LMO: Dr Jason Crighton |

1. **Expand the following abbreviations as found in the discharge summary above.**

   5 mg p.r.n.

   ALT

   ECG

   ENT

   FBC

   IV

   LFTs

   THR

2. **Ms Harris was said to have a provisional diagnosis of vestibular neuronitis or viral labyrinthitis. What is vestibular neuronitis and is it the same as viral labyrinthitis?**

3. **List five symptoms of vestibular neuronitis.**

4. **Which of these common symptoms did Ms Harris present with?**

5. **Why was Ms Harris prescribed Stemetil?**

CHAPTER 14

Urinary System

Contents

OBJECTIVES   331

INTRODUCTION   332

NEW WORD ELEMENTS   332

    Combining forms   332

    Prefixes   332

    Suffixes   333

VOCABULARY   333

ABBREVIATIONS   334

FUNCTIONS AND STRUCTURE OF THE URINARY SYSTEM   334

    The kidneys   334

    Ureters   336

    Bladder   336

    Urethra   336

    Urinary sphincters   336

PATHOLOGY AND DISEASES   336

    Disorders of the kidneys   338

    Disorders of the bladder   340

    Disorders of the ureter and urethra   342

TESTS AND PROCEDURES   342

    Urinalysis   347

EXERCISES   348

Objectives

After completing this chapter you should be able to:

1. state the meanings of the word elements related to the urinary system

2. build words using the word elements associated with the urinary system

3. recognise, pronounce and effectively use medical terms associated with the urinary system

4. expand abbreviations related to the urinary system

5. describe the structure and functions of the urinary system including the kidneys, bladder and associated structures

6. describe common pathological conditions associated with the urinary system

7. describe common laboratory tests and diagnostic and surgical procedures associated with the urinary system

8. apply what you have learned by interpreting medical terminology in practice.

Demonstrate your knowledge of the urinary system by completing the exercises at the end of this chapter.

INTRODUCTION

The urinary system is the system responsible for producing, storing and excreting urine and for removing metabolic wastes. The urinary system also maintains homeostasis by regulating the concentrations and balance of water, salts, nutrients and nitrogenous wastes in the body. The kidneys work with the lungs, skin and intestines to keep this balance correct.

The urinary system is developmentally and anatomically associated with the male and female reproductive systems. It is sometimes described as the 'genitourinary' system. However, in this textbook the urinary system, male reproductive system and female reproductive system are all discussed in separate chapters.

NEW WORD ELEMENTS

Here are some word elements related to the urinary system. To reinforce your learning, write the meanings of the medical terms in the spaces provided. Use the Glossary of medical terms on page 561 to help you work out the meanings. You may also need to check the meaning in a medical dictionary, but make an attempt yourself first.

Combining forms

Combining Form	Meaning	Medical Term	Meaning of Medical Term
albumin/o	albumin	pseudoalbuminuria	
azot/o	nitrogen, urea	azoturia	
bacteri/o	bacteria	bacteraemia	
cali/o	calyx, cup	pyelocaliectasis	
cyst/o	bladder, cyst, sac	cystoscope	
dips/o	thirst	polydipsia	
glomerul/o	glomerulus	glomerulonephritis	
kal/i	potassium	hypokalaemia	
ket/o	ketone bodies	ketosis	
keton/o		ketonuria	
lith/o	stone, calculus	nephrolithotomy	
meat/o	meatus	meatorrhaphy	
nephr/o	kidney	hydronephrosis	
noct/i	night	nocturia	
olig/o	scanty, deficiency, few	oliguresis	
py/o	pus	pyonephrolithiasis	
pyel/o	renal pelvis	pyelolithotomy	
ren/o	kidney	renal	
trigon/o	trigone (base of the bladder)	trigonitis	
ur/o	urine, urinary tract, urea	urologist	
ureter/o	ureter	ureterocele	
urethr/o	urethra	urethrodynia	
urin/o	urine	urinometer	
vesic/o	urinary bladder, blister	vesicovaginal	

Prefixes

Prefix	Meaning	Medical Term	Meaning of Medical Term
an-	no, not, without, absence of	anuria	
dia-	through, across	dialysis	
dys-	bad, painful, difficult	dysuria	
poly-	many, much	polyuria	
supra-	above, excessive	suprarenal	

Suffixes

Suffix	Meaning	Medical Term	Meaning of Medical Term
-cele	protrusion, hernia	cystocele	
-clysis	irrigating, washing	vesicoclysis	
-gram	record, writing	pyelogram	
-lysis	separation, destruction, breakdown, dissolution	urinalysis	
-poietin	substance that forms	erythropoietin	
-ptosis	downward displacement, prolapse	nephroptosis	
-scope	instrument to view	cystoscope	
-scopy	process of viewing	cystoscopy	
-tripsy	to crush	nephrolithotripsy	
-uresis	excrete in urine, urinate	diuresis	
-uria	urination, urine condition, presence of substance in urine	pyuria	

VOCABULARY

The following list provides many of the medical terms used for the first time in this chapter. Pronunciations are provided with each term. As you read the rest of the chapter, make sure you identify each of these terms and understand their meanings.

Term	Pronunciation
adrenal glands	ad-REE-nal glandz
atonic bladder	a-TOH-nik BLAD-a
bladder cancer	BLAD-a KAN-sa
blood urea nitrogen	BLUD yoo-REE-a NY-tro-jen
calculi	KAL-kyoo-lye
calculus	KAL-kyoo-lus
computed tomography	kom-PYOO-ted to-MOG-ra-fee
creatinine clearance test	kree-AT-in-in KLEE-rans test
cystitis	sis-TY-tus
cystocele	SIS-toh-seel
cystoscopy	sis-TOS-kop-ee
dialysis	dy-AL-e-sis
extracorporeal shock wave lithotripsy	eks-tra-KOR-por-EE-al shok wayv LITH-oh-trip-see
filtration	fil-TRAY-shun
glomerulonephritis	glom-ER-yoo-loh-nef-RY-tus
hydroureter	HY-droh-YOO-ret-a
hypertensive kidney disease	hy-per-TEN-siv kid-nee diz-eez

Table continued

Term	Pronunciation
intravenous pyelogram	in-tra-VEEN-us PY-el-oh-gram
kidney	kid-nee
kidney agenesis	kid-nee a-JEN-a-sis
kidneys, ureters and bladder	kid-neez, YOO-ret-ers and BLAD-a
magnetic resonance imaging	mag-NET-ik REZ-on-ans IM-a-jing
micturition	mic-tyu-RISH-en
nephrolithiasis	nef-roh-lith-EYE-a-sis
nephroptosis	nef-roh-TOH-sis
nephrotic syndrome	nef-ROT-ik SIN-drohm
neurogenic bladder	nyoo-roh-JEN-ik BLAD-a
polycystic kidney disease	pol-ee-SIS-tik kid-nee dis-eez
pyelonephritis	PY-el-oh-nef-RY-tis
radioisotope scan	ray-dee-oh-EYE-so-tope skan
reabsorption	ree-ab-SAWP-shun
renal angiography	REE-nal an-jee-OG-raf-ee
renal angioplasty	REE-nal AN-jee-oh-plas-tee
renal biopsy	REE-nal BY-op-see
renal failure	REE-nal FAYL-ya
renal transplantation	REE-nal trans-plan-TAY-shun
renin	REN-in
retrograde pyelogram	RET-roh-grayd PY-el-oh-gram
tubular necrosis	TU-byoo-lah nek-ROH-sis
ultrasonography	ul-tra-son-OG-ra-fee

Table continued

Term	Pronunciation
urea	yoo-REE-a
ureter	YOO-ret-a
ureteric colic	yoo-ree-TER-ik KOL-ik
ureteric stent	yoo-ree-TER-ik stent
urethritis	yoo-reeth-RY-tus
uric acid	YOO-rik AS-id
urinalysis	yoo-rin-AL-ee-sis
urinary bladder	YOO-rin-ree BLAD-a
urinary catheterisation	YOO-rin-ree kath-e-ter-eye-ZAY-shun
urinary incontinence	YOO-rin-ree in-KON-tin-ens
vesical fistula	VEE-sik-al FIST-yoo-la
vesicoureteral reflux	VEE-sik-oh-yoo-REET-a-ral REE-flux
voiding cystourethrogram	VOYD-ing sis-toh-yoo-REETH-roh-gram

ABBREVIATIONS

The following abbreviations are commonly used in the Australian healthcare environment. Because some abbreviations can have more than one meaning, check the context in which the abbreviation is used before assigning a meaning to it.

Abbreviation	Definition
ADH	antidiuretic hormone
ARF	acute renal failure
ATN	acute tubular necrosis
BNO	bladder neck obstruction
BUN	blood urea nitrogen
C&S	culture and sensitivity
CAPD	continuous ambulatory peritoneal dialysis
CCPD	continuous cycling peritoneal dialysis
CKD	chronic kidney disease
CRF	chronic renal failure
eGFR	estimated glomerular filtration rate
ESKD	end-stage kidney disease
ESRD	end-stage renal disease
ESWL	extracorporeal shock wave lithotripsy
GFR	glomerular filtration rate
IVP	intravenous pyelogram
KUB	kidneys, ureters, bladder
MSU	midstream urine

Table continued

Abbreviation	Definition
PD	peritoneal dialysis
pH	a measure of acidity
PKD	polycystic kidney disease
PKU	phenylketonuria
PUL	percutaneous ultrasonic lithotripsy
RP, RPG	retrograde pyelogram
UA, U/A	urinalysis
UACR	urine albumin/creatinine ratio
UTI	urinary tract infection
VCU(G)	voiding cystourethrogram

FUNCTIONS AND STRUCTURE OF THE URINARY SYSTEM

The urinary system performs several functions. One of the main functions is excretion. Excretion is the process of eliminating the waste products of metabolism and other unusable materials from the body. These metabolic wastes include urea, creatinine, ammonia and uric acid. The process of excretion also ensures the correct concentrations of electrolytes such as sodium, potassium and calcium in the body fluids. Another function is to regulate blood volume and blood pressure by a process called osmoregulation. Blood volume and blood pressure are closely related to salt balance. Osmoregulation maintains the proper balance of water and salts in the blood. The urinary system maintains an appropriate fluid volume in the body by regulating the amount of water that is excreted in the urine. The urinary system also regulates the acid–base balance (or pH level) of the blood. A pH level of around 7.4 is considered optimal. Finally, the urinary system secretes some hormones such as activated vitamin D (which promotes the absorption of calcium), erythropoietin (which stimulates the production of erythrocytes) and renin (which in turn leads to the secretion of aldosterone, which regulates blood pressure).

The urinary system operates through an arrangement of organs, tubes, muscles and nerves to perform these functions. Some of these functions will be examined in more detail as each of the structures of the urinary system is discussed.

The main structures of the urinary system are the right and left kidneys, two ureters, the urinary bladder, two sphincter muscles and the urethra (Fig. 14.1).

The kidneys

The human body has two kidneys, each around the size of a closed fist and located in the retroperitoneal region just below the rib cage on either side of the

Figure 14.1 Urinary system and associated structures

(Mosby's Dictionary 2014)

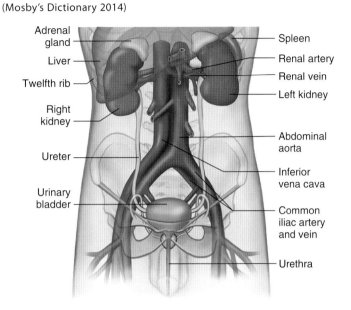

spine. The internal structure of a kidney is quite complex. It consists of three regions (Fig. 14.2). The renal cortex is the outer layer. It is covered by a fibrous sheath called the renal capsule. The renal medulla is the inner layer. It contains cone-shaped structures called renal pyramids, which house the renal tubules. The renal pelvis is the central cavity.

Each kidney is composed of more than a million nephrons, which are the functional units of the kidney. A nephron contains a renal corpuscle, which consists of a glomerulus surrounded by a glomerular capsule (or Bowman capsule). The glomerulus is a cuplike structure containing capillaries that filter the blood as it passes through. This filtrate then passes through a renal tubule consisting of a number of smaller tubules or canals. The tubules of several nephrons connect to one collecting duct.

The main functions of the kidneys are to remove toxic waste products from the blood and to maintain homeostasis in the body by controlling pH levels, the concentration of electrolytes, the volume of extracellular fluid and the regulation of blood pressure. The main waste products managed by the urinary system are urea and uric acid. Accumulation of too much of these in the bloodstream may cause serious illness.

Removing the waste products and maintaining homeostasis is a four-stage process. These stages are filtration, reabsorption, secretion and excretion. These processes, except excretion, are carried out by the nephrons. Clinicians measure the glomerular filtration rate in assessing the functioning of the kidney. Blood from the renal arteries (which branch off the aorta) moves into the kidneys. As it enters each kidney, the blood is filtered by the nephrons, and water and other

small molecules are reabsorbed through capillaries back into the bloodstream. Waste products that are filtered out move into urine. Creatinine is one of the waste products made by the muscles and is usually removed from the blood by the kidneys before passing out in the urine. When the kidneys are not operating effectively, increased amounts of creatinine stay in the blood and can be assessed with the glomerular filtration rate test. The body produces approximately 180 litres of filtered fluid each day, but only around 2 litres end up as urine, with the remaining filtrate being reabsorbed. The functions of the kidney are under the control of the endocrine system through regulating hormones such as antidiuretic hormone, aldosterone and parathyroid hormone.

The kidneys also work to regulate levels of water and salt in the body. Water is absorbed by the gastrointestinal system and passed into the bloodstream, effectively diluting the blood. The kidneys remove excess water and turn it into urine. Similarly, excess amounts of salt in the blood are removed by the kidneys and filtered out into urine. By controlling the amount of water and salt in the blood, the kidneys manage concentrations of these substances.

Another vital function of the kidneys involves regulating blood pressure. The kidneys secrete renin, which is known as a peptide hormone. This specific group includes proteins that are considered both enzymes and hormones. Renin triggers the production of other hormones that control blood pressure and electrolyte balance. If the body's blood pressure drops, the kidneys release renin, which operates to turn blood protein into a hormone called angiotensin. This in turn instructs the adrenal glands, which are located

Figure 14.2 **Internal structure of the kidney**
(Mosby's Dictionary 2014)

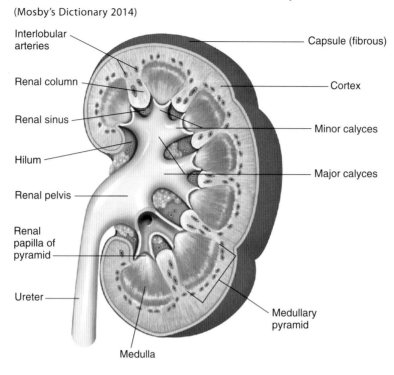

on top of the kidneys, to release another hormone called aldosterone. Aldosterone causes more salt and water to be reabsorbed into the blood in the kidneys, increasing blood volume and therefore blood pressure.

Ureters
A ureter is a hollow tube that moves urine from the renal pelvis in the kidney to the bladder by peristalsis. Usually there is one ureter for each kidney. In an adult, the ureters are usually 25–30 centimetres in length and have a width of about 3 millimetres.

Bladder
The urinary bladder (more commonly referred to as just the bladder) is a hollow muscular organ located in the lower pelvic cavity. It acts as a temporary reservoir for collecting urine prior to micturition. The muscle that controls the bladder is the detrusor muscle, which relaxes to allow the bladder to fill up. At the same time, sphincter muscles located at the base of the bladder and upper urethra contract to keep the urine within the bladder. When urinating, the brain instructs these two muscles to change their functions so that muscles at the base of the bladder relax to let the urine flow through the urethra and the detrusor muscle contracts to force the urine out. The amount of urine that a bladder can hold varies from person to person and decreases with age. When the bladder volume reaches around 300 millilitres (about half full), receptors in the

wall of the bladder send signals along the pelvic nerves to the spinal cord and on to the brain to alert to the need to urinate. This urge can be ignored for a certain amount of time, but eventually the need to urinate becomes urgent as the bladder reaches capacity.

Urethra
The urethra is a tube that carries urine from the bladder to an opening on the exterior of the body called the urethral meatus. In males, the urethra is about 20 centimetres in length and travels through the penis, carrying semen as well as urine (Fig. 14.3). In females, the urethra is only around 4 centimetres in length and emerges above the vaginal opening (Fig. 14.4).

Urinary sphincters
The body has two urinary sphincters, which control the release of urine. The external urethral sphincter is a striated muscle that provides voluntary control over urination. The internal sphincter is a muscle that compresses the internal urethral orifice at the junction of the urethra and the urinary bladder. This is made of smooth muscle, so therefore it is involuntary.

PATHOLOGY AND DISEASES

The following section provides a list of common diseases and pathological conditions relevant to the urinary system.

Figure 14.3 Male urinary system

(Mosby's Dictionary 2014)

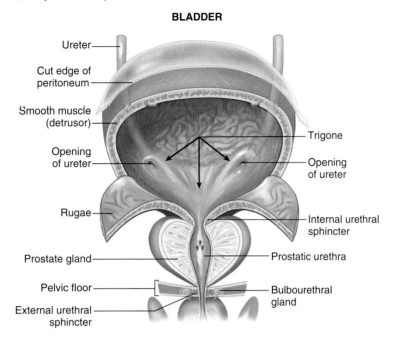

Figure 14.4 Female urinary system

(Nicol and Walker 2007)

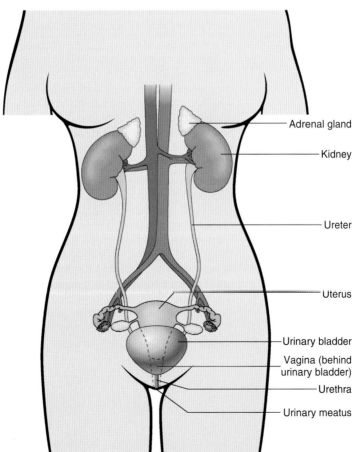

Disorders of the kidneys

Term	Pronunciation	Definition
chronic kidney disease (CKD)	KRON-ik kid-nee diz-eez	CKD is the preferred terminology for chronic renal failure. CKD is diagnosed by blood test for creatinine to determine the patient's glomerular filtration rate. High levels of creatinine means the glomerular filtration rate is falling, which means that the kidney's ability to filter and excrete waste products is inhibited. In the early stages of CKD, creatinine levels may be normal but urinalysis demonstrates a loss of protein or red blood cells into the urine. There are five stages of CKD categorised according to the level of reduced kidney function and evidence of kidney damage, such as blood or protein in the urine. The most severe stage is end-stage kidney disease, also called end-stage renal disease or CKD stage 5. This is diagnosed when kidney function deteriorates to the extent that irreversible kidney failure occurs, requiring kidney dialysis or a kidney transplant.
kidney agenesis	kid-nee a-JEN-a-sis	Kidney (renal) agenesis occurs when the kidneys do not form during fetal development. Renal agenesis can be unilateral, with one kidney present, or bilateral, with no kidneys or very little kidney tissue present (dysgenesis). If the agenesis is unilateral, the other kidney will usually hypertrophy to compensate for the missing kidney. Unilateral agenesis is often asymptomatic and is frequently discovered later in life. Bilateral agenesis is not conducive to life, and the baby will die soon after birth.
glomerulonephritis	glom-ER-yoo-loh nef-RY-tus	Glomerulonephritis is a kidney disease in which the glomeruli – the parts of the kidneys responsible for filtering waste and fluids from the blood – become inflamed. This causes blood and protein to be lost in the urine. Glomerulonephritis may be caused by specific problems with the body's immune system, but often the cause is unknown. Glomerulonephritis can be acute (a sudden attack of inflammation) or chronic (beginning gradually). In some patients there is no history of kidney disease and the disorder first manifests as chronic renal failure.
hypertensive kidney disease	hy-per-TEN-siv kid-nee dis-eez	When high blood pressure causes kidney disease it is called hypertensive kidney disease. This occurs most often in those who have undetected, untreated, or poorly controlled hypertension. High blood pressure makes the heart work harder. In turn, this can damage blood vessels throughout the body. If the blood vessels in the kidneys are damaged, the kidneys can lose their ability to filter blood, allowing a build-up of toxic substances and extra fluid in the body. The extra fluid in the blood vessels may then raise blood pressure even more and the cycle continues.
nephrolithiasis	nef-roh-lith-EYE-a-sis	Nephrolithiasis refers to the presence of calculi in the kidneys. If the calculi are in the urinary tract the condition is called urolithiasis. Renal calculi are small deposits of calcium, phosphate and other components of food that form small crystals and subsequently stones. They are a common cause of haematuria. Renal calculi may form when the urine becomes overly concentrated with certain substances. Calculi tend to be asymptomatic until they begin to move down the ureter, then cause severe pain known as renal colic. If the stone is less than 5 millimetres in diameter, it will most likely pass on urination. If the stone is larger than 5 millimetres, a procedure such as extracorporeal shock wave lithotripsy may be required to crush and destroy the stone.

Table continued

Term	Pronunciation	Definition
nephroptosis	nef-roh-TOH-sis	Nephroptosis is also known as a floating kidney or renal ptosis. It refers to the downward movement of the kidney into the pelvis when the patient stands up. The cause is a congenital or traumatic weakness of the perirenal connective tissue, which is supposed to hold the kidney in place. Nephroptosis is asymptomatic in most patients. However, some patients may experience severe colicky pain in the groin, haematuria, proteinuria, nausea or hypertension. Symptomatic nephroptosis is treated with nephropexy to secure the floating kidney to the retroperitoneum.
nephrotic syndrome	nef-ROT-ik SIN-drohm	Nephrotic syndrome is a general term for a group of diseases affecting the glomeruli. Damage to the kidney's filtration system allows proteins in the blood (such as albumin) to leak into the urine, resulting in proteinuria. Eventually, hypoalbuminaemia and hypercholesterolaemia occurs. Accompanying abnormalities of renal function lead to tissue oedema. Medication is required to improve glomerular function.
polycystic kidney disease	pol-ee-SIS-tik kid-nee dis-eez	Polycystic kidney disease is usually a congenital condition, although it may manifest as an acquired disorder in the presence of other kidney diseases. It causes the kidney to become enlarged with many fluid-filled cysts, which reduce renal function and may lead to kidney failure. Fig. 14.5 shows a nephrectomy specimen from a patient with polycystic kidney disease. **Figure 14.5** **Size, shape and appearance comparison of normal kidney (left) with polycystic kidney (right)** (Salvo, 2009) 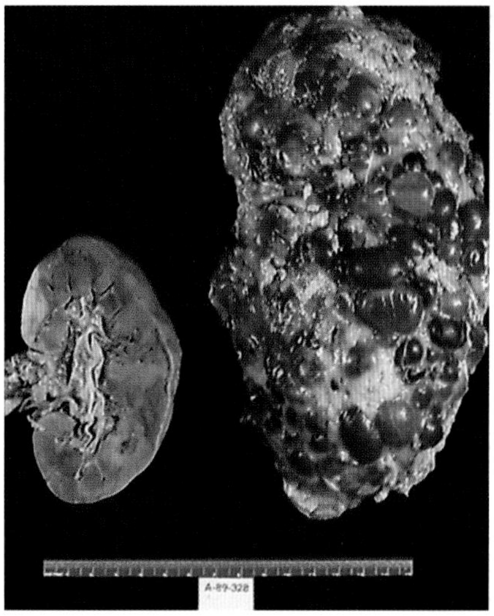
pyelonephritis	PY-el-oh-nef-RY-tis	Pyelonephritis is an infection of the renal pelvis and renal medulla of the kidneys that is usually a result of an infection that has ascended the urinary tract, or from an obstruction in the urinary tract causing urine to backflow into the ureters and kidneys. It is a specific form of the general condition called urinary tract infection.

Table continued

Term	Pronunciation	Definition
renal failure	REE-nal FAYL-ya	Renal failure refers to the inability of the kidneys to maintain proper filtration function, to excrete wastes appropriately and to maintain electrolyte balance. There are three main stages: acute, chronic and end-stage.
		Acute kidney disease (AKD) (also known as acute kidney injury or acute renal failure) is the sudden loss of the ability of the kidneys to remove waste and concentrate urine. It is usually initiated by an underlying cause such as severe dehydration, infection, trauma to the kidney or the chronic use of analgesics. AKD is often reversible with no lasting damage. **End-stage kidney disease** (chronic kidney disease stage 5 or end-stage renal disease) is the complete failure of the kidneys to function, or where chronic kidney disease has worsened to the point at which kidney function is less than 10% of normal. See chronic kidney disease above.
tubular necrosis	TU-byoo-lah nek-ROH-sis	Tubular necrosis is a kidney disorder involving the tubular segment of the nephron. The internal structures of the kidney, particularly the tissues of the kidney tubule, become damaged or destroyed. It is caused by ischaemia of the kidneys. It is a common cause of acute kidney disease and uraemic syndrome.

Disorders of the bladder

Term	Pronunciation	Definition
atonic bladder	a-TOH-nik BLAD-a	Atonic bladder refers to a large dilated urinary bladder that does not empty. It is usually due to disturbance of innervation or to chronic obstruction.
bladder calculus	BLAD-a KAL-kyoo-lus	Bladder calculus is also known as vesical calculus. It refers to the presence of calculi (stones) in the bladder.
bladder cancer	BLAD-a KAN-sa	Bladder cancer is the presence of malignant cells in the urinary bladder. There are several types of bladder cancers. The most common histological type is transitional cell carcinoma, which begins in the cells lining the bladder, kidneys, ureters and urethra. This accounts for about 90% of cases. Squamous cell carcinoma and adenocarcinoma account for the rest. The exact causes of bladder cancer are not known, but there are well-established risk factors for developing the disease such as smoking, occupational exposure to certain chemicals and fumes, chronic bladder infections, family history and gender (male). It is treated by electrocautery for superficial tumours, but more invasive tumours may require cystectomy, chemotherapy and/or radiation therapy.

Table continued

Term	Pronunciation	Definition
cystitis	sis-TY-tus	Cystitis is inflammation of the bladder that may be caused by irritation or infection. A bacterial infection may move up from the urethra. Most infections arise from *Escherichia coli* bacteria, which normally live in the colon. Cystitis is characterised by frequency of micturition, burning and haematuria. It is a specific form of the general condition called a urinary tract infection. It most commonly affects women, possibly due to the shorter length of the urethra, allowing infection to enter the bladder more easily.
cystocele	SIS-toh-seel	A cystocele is a herniation or protrusion of the urinary bladder through the anterior vaginal wall that causes the bladder to prolapse into the vagina. This results in discomfort, incomplete emptying of the bladder and leakage of urine due to stretching of the urethral opening.
neurogenic bladder	nyoo-roh-JEN-ik BLAD-a	Neurogenic bladder refers to dysfunction of the urinary bladder due to a disease of the central nervous system or peripheral nerves involved in the control of micturition. Muscles and nerves in the urinary system work together to retain urine in the bladder then release it at the appropriate time. In a neurogenic bladder, the muscles and nerves do not work properly. This can result in leakage of urine, urine retention and frequent urinary tract infections.
urinary incontinence	YOO-rin-ree in-KON-tin-ens	Urinary incontinence is the loss of ability to control the release of urine, or the inability to hold urine until appropriate to pass it. It is linked to the ageing process, diseases such as benign prostatic hypertrophy, some medications and/or the onset of an illness such as a urinary tract infection. A specific variant of urinary incontinence is called enuresis or bed wetting. This generally occurs in young children and usually resolves by about age five. In rare cases, it can persist into, or develop in, adulthood. The two main types of urinary incontinence are: • urge incontinence – the inability to hold urine long enough to reach a toilet • stress incontinence – the leakage of urine during exercise, coughing, laughing or other body movements that put pressure on the bladder. Treatment may include behavioural techniques such as pelvic muscle exercises and bladder training, medications, surgery and eliminating certain substances such as caffeine and alcohol.
vesical fistula	VEE-sik-al FIST-yoo-la	A vesical fistula is an abnormal opening communicating with the bladder. For example: a vesicovaginal fistula is a channel between the bladder and the vagina.

Disorders of the ureter and urethra

Term	Pronunciation	Definition
hydroureter	HY-droh-YOO-ret-a	A hydroureter is an abnormal distension of the ureter with urine due to obstruction of any cause (Fig. 14.6). Hydroureter secondary to obstruction can lead to hypertension, loss of renal function and sepsis. **Figure 14.6 Hydroureter** (Young & Proctor 2007)
ureteric colic	yoo-ree-TER-ik KOL-ik	Ureteric colic is severe pain caused by an obstruction of the ureter by ureteric calculus.
urethritis	u-reeth-RY-tus	Urethritis is an inflammation of the urethra. Most cases result from an infection by bacteria such as *Escherichia coli* that enter the urethra from the skin around the urethral opening. This is usually due to faecal contamination. Urethritis is also commonly associated with sexually transmitted infections such as gonorrhoea (caused by *Neisseria gonorrhoeae*) or chlamydia (caused by *Chlamydia trachomatis*). The main symptoms of urethritis are urethral discharge, dysuria and frequency of urination. A course of antibiotics is an effective treatment.
vesicoureteral reflux	VEE-sik-oh-u-REET-a-ral REE-fluks	Vesicoureteral reflux occurs when urine in the bladder flows back into the ureters and often back into the kidneys. Ureters normally have a valve system that prevents urine from flowing back up the ureters in the direction of the kidneys. In vesicoureteral reflux, the mechanism that prevents the backflow of urine does not work, allowing urine to flow in both directions. This condition is most frequently diagnosed in infancy. Children with this condition are at risk of developing recurrent kidney infections, which, over time, can result in scarring of the kidneys.

TESTS AND PROCEDURES

The following section provides a list of common diagnostic tests and procedures and clinical interventions and surgical procedures that are undertaken for the urinary system.

Test/Procedure	Pronunciation	Definition
blood urea nitrogen (BUN)	BLUD yoo-REE-a NY-tra-jen	A BUN is a diagnostic test to determine how well the kidneys are functioning to eliminate waste from the body. The test measures the level of nitrogen in urea, with a higher level indicating an issue with kidney function.

Table continued

Test/Procedure	Pronunciation	Definition
computed tomography (CT) scan	kom-PYOO-ted to-MOG-ra-fee skan	A CT is a diagnostic test that can be used to identify disorders of urinary structures. Cross-sectional images are taken using a computer in conjunction with x-ray beams.
creatinine clearance test	kree-AT-in-in KLEER-ans test	A creatinine clearance test compares the levels of creatinine in the blood with that in the urine. The test is performed by collecting urine for 24 hours and then taking a blood sample. Both samples are then measured for the amount of creatinine, along with the amount of urine collected, allowing for a clearance rate to be measured. If there is a greater amount of creatinine in the blood sample than in the urine sample, this is an indication of problems with kidney function.
cystoscopy	sis-TOS-kop-ee	A cystoscopy is a procedure that allows the bladder to be examined using a cystoscope. The procedure is performed by inserting the scope into the urethra and passing it up to the bladder (Fig. 14.7). Inserting a catheter into the scope allows for biopsies of the bladder to be taken for microscopic examination. Figure 14.7 **Male cystoscopy** 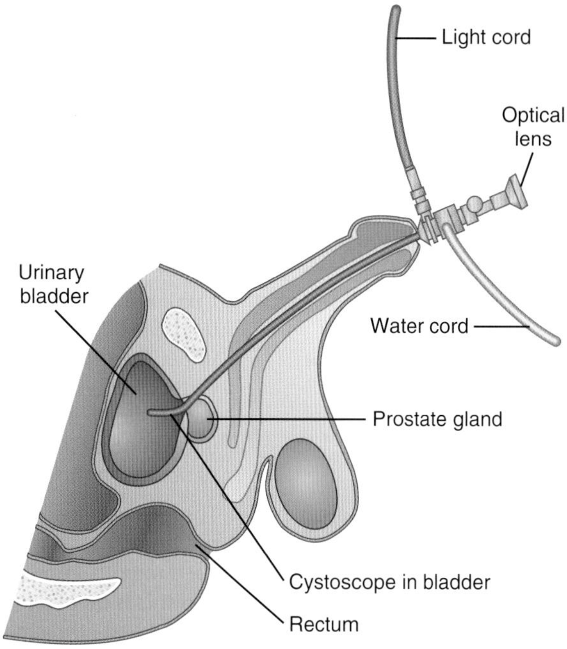
dialysis	dy-AL-e-sis	Dialysis is a procedure that involves removing waste products from the bloodstream when the kidneys can no longer perform this function. There are two types of dialysis available to patients: **Haemodialysis** involves connecting the patient to a dialyser (artificial kidney machine) that contains semi-permeable membranes to allow for the blood to be filtered and then returned to the patient's body (Fig. 14.8). **Peritoneal dialysis** involves introducing a sterile solution (dialysate) containing glucose through a tube (catheter) into the peritoneal cavity, resulting in the peritoneal membrane acting as a semi-permeable membrane. The dialysate absorbs the waste products and is then removed from the body via the catheter.

Figure 14.7 **Male cystoscopy**

Light cord
Optical lens
Urinary bladder
Water cord
Prostate gland
Cystoscope in bladder
Rectum

Table continued

Test/Procedure	Pronunciation	Definition

Figure 14.8 Haemodialysis

(Goldman & Schafer 2011)

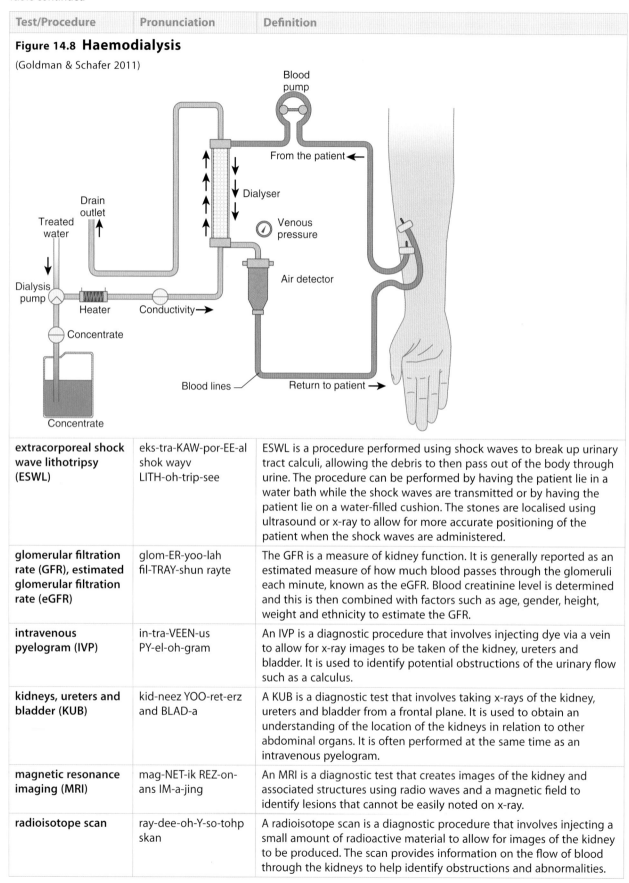

Test/Procedure	Pronunciation	Definition
extracorporeal shock wave lithotripsy (ESWL)	eks-tra-KAW-por-EE-al shok wayv LITH-oh-trip-see	ESWL is a procedure performed using shock waves to break up urinary tract calculi, allowing the debris to then pass out of the body through urine. The procedure can be performed by having the patient lie in a water bath while the shock waves are transmitted or by having the patient lie on a water-filled cushion. The stones are localised using ultrasound or x-ray to allow for more accurate positioning of the patient when the shock waves are administered.
glomerular filtration rate (GFR), estimated glomerular filtration rate (eGFR)	glom-ER-yoo-lah fil-TRAY-shun rayte	The GFR is a measure of kidney function. It is generally reported as an estimated measure of how much blood passes through the glomeruli each minute, known as the eGFR. Blood creatinine level is determined and this is then combined with factors such as age, gender, height, weight and ethnicity to estimate the GFR.
intravenous pyelogram (IVP)	in-tra-VEEN-us PY-el-oh-gram	An IVP is a diagnostic procedure that involves injecting dye via a vein to allow for x-ray images to be taken of the kidney, ureters and bladder. It is used to identify potential obstructions of the urinary flow such as a calculus.
kidneys, ureters and bladder (KUB)	kid-neez YOO-ret-erz and BLAD-a	A KUB is a diagnostic test that involves taking x-rays of the kidney, ureters and bladder from a frontal plane. It is used to obtain an understanding of the location of the kidneys in relation to other abdominal organs. It is often performed at the same time as an intravenous pyelogram.
magnetic resonance imaging (MRI)	mag-NET-ik REZ-on-ans IM-a-jing	An MRI is a diagnostic test that creates images of the kidney and associated structures using radio waves and a magnetic field to identify lesions that cannot be easily noted on x-ray.
radioisotope scan	ray-dee-oh-Y-so-tohp skan	A radioisotope scan is a diagnostic procedure that involves injecting a small amount of radioactive material to allow for images of the kidney to be produced. The scan provides information on the flow of blood through the kidneys to help identify obstructions and abnormalities.

Table continued

Test/Procedure	Pronunciation	Definition
renal angiography	REE-nal an-jee-OG-ra-fee	Renal angiography is a process using radio-opaque contrast to record x-ray images of the vessels of the kidney to identify disorders such as aneurysms, blood clots, renal stenosis and kidney failure.
renal angioplasty	REE-nal AN-jee-oh-plas-tee	A renal angioplasty is a procedure that uses an inflatable balloon to widen renal arteries. A needle is inserted into the artery under x-ray guidance. A guide wire is then inserted and, once positioned correctly, a catheter with the balloon attached is inserted and the balloon inflated. A stent may also need to be inserted to ensure the artery remains open.
renal biopsy	REE-nal BY-op-see	Renal biopsy involves taking a sample of kidney tissue for laboratory examination. It can be performed as an open procedure or percutaneously, using a biopsy needle (generally under ultrasound guidance).
renal transplantation	REE-nal trans-plan-TAY-shun	Renal transplantation is a surgical procedure that involves replacing a diseased kidney with a donor organ (either from a living donor or a cadaver). Living donor kidneys can be either from an identical twin (isograft) or other individual (allograft), preferably from a close relative. The diseased kidney is usually left in situ.
retrograde pyelogram (RP or RPG)	RET-roh-grayd PY-el-oh-gram	An RP is a diagnostic procedure that assists in identifying calculi, obstructions and tumours in the kidneys and ureters. The procedure is performed by injecting contrast medium via a urinary catheter into the ureters. X-ray images can then be taken of the kidneys, ureters and bladder.
ultrasonography	ul-tra-son-OG-raf-ee	An ultrasound is a diagnostic procedure that produces two-dimensional images of the urinary system and its structures. It can be used to identify conditions such as tumours of the kidney and bladder, obstruction of the ureters or bladder and disorders of the kidney such as hydronephrosis and polycystic kidney disease.
ureteric stent	yoo-re-TER-ik stent	A ureteric stent is a flexible plastic tube that is placed in the ureter to temporarily relieve obstruction.
urinary catheterisation	YOO-rin-ree kath-e-ter-eye-ZAY-shun	Urinary catheterisation involves inserting a flexible tube into the bladder either via the urethra or percutaneously from above the symphysis pubis. It is performed to drain urine from the bladder, either as a short-term or long-term measure. Indwelling catheters are those that are inserted via the urethra and are secured in place through using a small inflated balloon that prevents the catheter from sliding out of the body. A Foley catheter is a form of indwelling catheter. Suprapubic catheters are inserted into the bladder percutaneously via a cystotomy and are performed when there is no urethral access, urethral catheterisation has failed, for long-term management or when there is urethral trauma.
urine albumin/ creatine ratio (UACR)	YOO-rin AL-byoo-min kree-AT-in-in ray-she-oh	UACR is used to screen for chronic conditions such as diabetes and hypertension to identify if the kidneys are functioning correctly. The two key indicators for chronic kidney disease are abnormalities in urinary albumin levels and estimated glomerular filtration rate (eGFR). If the kidneys are functioning correctly, then there should only be small amounts of albumin in the urine. The albumin and creatinine are measured in a random urine sample to calculate the albumin/ creatinine ratio.
voiding cystourethrogram (VCUG)	VOY-ding sis-toh-yoo-REETH-roh-gram	A VCUG is a diagnostic test using contrast medium inserted into the bladder to allow for x-ray images to be undertaken while the bladder is emptying (voiding) (Fig. 14.9). The procedure is performed to identify urethral strictures and urinary reflux.

Table continued

Test/Procedure	Pronunciation	Definition

Figure 14.9 Cystogram and voiding cystogram

A. Preliminary kidney, ureter, bladder (KUB) film; B. Film of filled bladder; C. Post-evacuation film comparing posterior extravasation with the preliminary KUB film.

(Marx et al 2009)

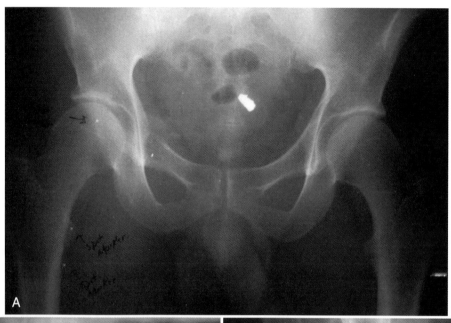

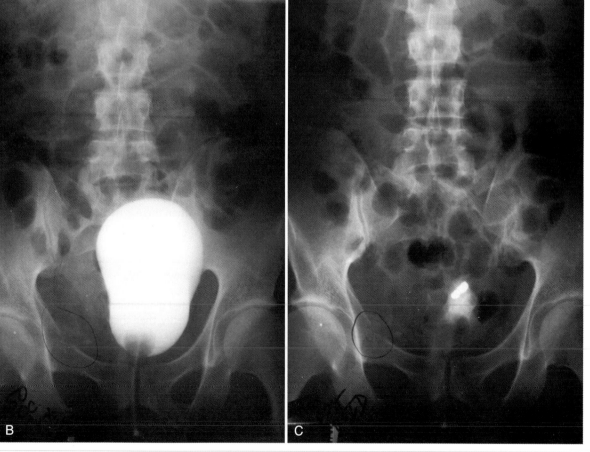

Urinalysis

Urinalysis is a diagnostic or screening tool routinely used to detect microorganisms and physical and chemical abnormalities in the urine. Listed below are a number of tests that can be performed on urine to identify pathological conditions.

Test/Procedure	Pronunciation	Definition
bilirubin	bil-ee-ROO-bin	A bilirubin test measures the amount of bilirubin in the urine. Bilirubin is a pigmented substance found in bile and removed from the blood by the liver. If the liver has difficulty excreting the bilirubin or if there is a blockage of the biliary drainage then bilirubin may appear in urine, giving the urine a darker appearance.
colour	kul-la	The normal colour of urine ranges from straw colour to darker yellow. Urochrome is the colour pigment in urine. Urine that is pale may indicate the presence of an excessive amount of water in the urine. Urine that has a red or brown appearance may contain blood. Caution needs to be observed when looking at the colour of urine because some foods and drugs can alter the colour, with no underlying disease or disorder present.
glucose	GLOO-kohs	A glucose test measures the amount of glucose (sugar) in urine. Its presence is called glycosuria and may be an indication of diabetes mellitus.
ketone bodies	KEE-tohn bod-eez	A ketone test is done to measure the presence or absence of ketone bodies in the urine. Ketones are the result of excessive fatty-acid breakdown. They will appear in urine when the levels in the blood are excessive. The presence of ketones in urine can be an indication of abnormal nutrition (e.g. starving), disorders of increased metabolism, metabolic disorders (e.g. uncontrolled diabetes) and excessive vomiting over a long period of time.
microalbumin test	my-kroh-AL-byoo-min test	A microalbumin test measures small amounts of albumin (protein) in the urine – too small in amount to be detected on dipstick analysis. It usually involves 24-hour, or timed overnight, urine collection. The detection of microalbumin may be an early sign of altered glomerular permeability and, in diabetes, is an indicator of other vascular complications.
microscopy	my-kros-ko-pee	Normal urine is sterile. A microscopy of urine is performed to identify if bacteria (bacteriuria) or other microorganisms are present. The presence of such organisms would indicate an infection.
pH	pee-aych	A urinary pH test is done to identify changes in the body's acid levels, which range between 0 (very acidic) through to 7, which is neutral, and up to 14 (very alkaline). The average pH level of urine is around 6 so is slightly acidic. A high pH level may be an indication of kidney failure, kidney tubular acidosis, urinary tract infection or vomiting. A low pH may be an indication of diabetic ketoacidosis, diarrhoea or starvation.
phenylketonuria (PKU)	fen-el-kee-ton-YOO-ree-a	A PKU test is undertaken on newborns to detect the presence of phenylketones in the urine, a condition known as phenylketonuria. If this genetic condition is present in a newborn, a special milk formula and a low-protein diet that excludes the amino acid phenylalanine is required to prevent permanent intellectual disability, caused by high levels of the phenylalanine that cannot be broken down by the body.
protein test	PROH-teen test	A protein test measures the levels of proteins in the urine. Proteinuria may indicate the presence of a range of conditions such as kidney disease, severe anaemia and heart disease. Albumin is the major protein in blood plasma and when found in urine (albuminuria) is an indication of leakage of albumin through the glomerular membrane into the renal tubules and into the urine.
sediment test	SED-ee-ment test	A sediment test identifies the presence of abnormal substances such as epithelial cells, white blood cells, red blood cells, bacteria, crystals and casts. Normal urine is clear. Urine with sediment will appear cloudy or turbid. The most common cause of turbid urine is a urinary tract infection.
specific gravity test	spe-SIF-ik GRAV-it-ee test	A specific gravity test measures the concentration of all chemical particles in urine. An increase in the concentration of solutes in urine can be an indication of symptoms such as dehydration, diarrhoea, emesis, excessive sweating, glycosuria, renal artery stenosis or hepatorenal syndrome. It is an indication of conditions such as pyelonephritis, renal failure, diabetes insipidus, acute tubular necrosis, interstitial nephritis and excessive fluid intake.

Exercises

EXERCISE 14.1: LABEL THE DIAGRAMS

Using the information provided in this chapter, label the anatomical parts in Figs 14.10 and 14.11.

1 _____

2 _____

3 _____

4 _____

5 _____

6 _____

7 _____

8 _____

9 _____

10 _____

11 _____

12 _____

13 _____

14 _____

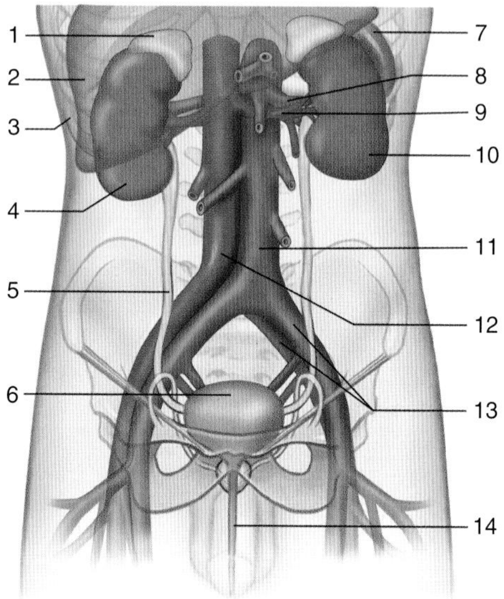

Figure 14.10 Urinary system and associated structures

(Mosby's Dictionary 2014)

1 _____

2 _____

3 _____

4 _____

5 _____

6 _____

7 _____

8 _____

9 _____

10 _____

11 _____

12 _____

13 _____

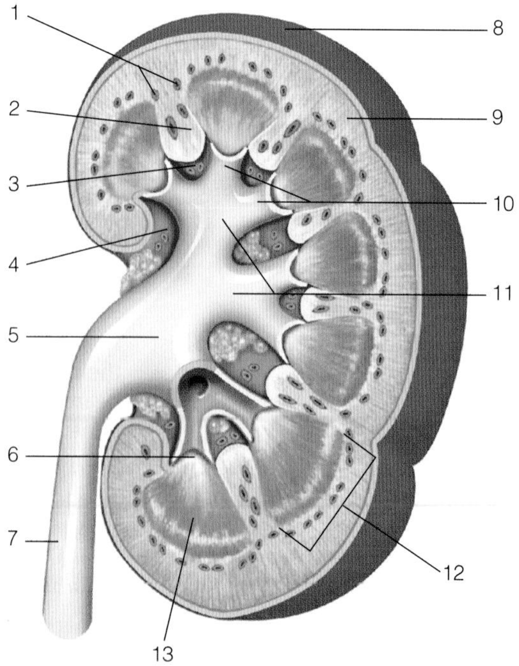

Figure 14.11 Internal structure of the kidney

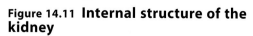

(Mosby's Dictionary 2014)

EXERCISE 14.2: MATCH WORD ELEMENTS AND MEANINGS

Match the prefix, suffix or combining form in Column A with its meaning from Column B.

Column A	Answer	Column B
1. trigon/o		A. urethra
2. pyel/o		B. potassium
3. meat/o		C. thirst
4. -cele		D. substance that forms
5. -clysis		E. trigone (base of the bladder)
6. cali/o		F. stone
7. urethr/o		G. renal pelvis
8. kal/i		H. ketones
9. olig/o		I. kidney
10. dips/o		J. nitrogen, urea
11. ur/o		K. meatus
12. -poietin		L. protrusion, hernia
13. ket/o		M. pus
14. nephr/o		N. irrigation, washing
15. -gram		O. scanty
16. -uresis		P. many, much
17. py/o		Q. calyx
18. lith/o		R. excrete in urine, urinate
19. poly-		S. record, writing
20. azot/o		T. urine, urinary tract, urea

EXERCISE 14.3: WORD ANALYSIS AND MEANING

Break up the medical terms below into their component parts (prefixes, suffixes, word roots, combining vowels). Provide the meaning for each word element and each term as a whole.

Example:
anuria

an = without

ur/o = urine, urinary tract, urea

ia = condition of

Meaning = condition of without urine

1. nephrolithotripsy _____

_____

_____

2. cystectomy _____

_____

_____

3. glomerulonephritis _____

_____

_____

4. ureterocystostomy _____

_____

_____

5. haematuria _____

_____

_____

6. polydipsia _____

_____

_____

7. pyelography _____

_____

_____

8. urology _____

_____

_____

9. erythropoietin _____

_____

_____

10. meatorrhaphy _____

_____

_____

EXERCISE 14.4: VOCABULARY BUILDING

Provide the medical term for each of the definitions below.

1. Hernia or protrusion of the ureter: _____

2. Condition of blood where there is excessive potassium: _____

3. Creation of surgical opening into the ureter and (small) intestine: _____

4. Incision into the urinary bladder: _____

5. Downward displacement of the kidney: _____

6. Abnormal condition of ketone bodies: _____

7. Recording of the urinary bladder: _____

8. Expansion or dilatation of the ureter: _____

9. Pertaining to above the kidney: _____

10. Pain in the urethra: _____

EXERCISE 14.5: MATCH THE ABBREVIATIONS AND MEANINGS

Match each abbreviation in Column A with its meaning in Column B.

Column A	Answer	Column B
1. IVP		A. peritoneal dialysis
2. CRF		B. chronic kidney disease
3. PKD		C. voiding cystourethrogram
4. ESWL		D. end-stage renal disease
5. UTI		E. bladder neck obstruction
6. BUN		F. acute tubular necrosis
7. ARF		G. intravenous pyelogram
8. GFR		H. phenylketonuria
9. BNO		I. chronic renal failure
10. ESRD		J. urinalysis
11. VCU(G)		K. extracorporeal shock wave lithotripsy
12. ATN		L. polycystic kidney disease
13. CKD		M. acute renal failure
14. PKU		N. glomerular filtration rate
15. CAPD		O. antidiuretic hormone
16. UA		P. culture and sensitivity
17. C&S		Q. continuous cycling peritoneal dialysis
18. PD		R. urinary tract infection
19. ADH		S. blood urea nitrogen
20. CCPD		T. continuous ambulatory peritoneal dialysis

EXERCISE 14.6: VOCABULARY BUILDING

Provide the medical term for each of the definitions below.

1. Process of passing urine: _____

2. The main nitrogenous constituent of urine: _____

3. Sugar in the urine: _____

4. An excess of acetone bodies in the urine: _____

5. Abnormally high levels of albumin in the urine: _____

6. Doctor who specialises in diseases of the urinary tract: _____

7. X-ray of the ureter and renal pelvis: _____

8. To introduce a catheter into the urinary bladder: _____

9. Irrigating the bladder (to cleanse it): _____

10. Excessive urination during the night: _____

Now briefly define the following terms.

11. nephroptosis _____

_____

_____

12. ureteral colic _____

_____

_____

13. hydronephrosis _____

_____

_____

14. nephrotic syndrome _____

_____

_____

15. uretovesicoplasty _____

_____

_____

EXERCISE 14.7: APPLYING MEDICAL TERMINOLOGY

Fill in the blank or select the correct medical term.

1. Urethrocystitis is inflammation of the urethra and _____.
   a) kidney
   b) bladder
   c) renal pelvis
   d) renal tubule

2. What is the operative term for the fixation of a displaced kidney?
   a) nephrectomy
   b) nephropexy
   c) nephrotomy
   d) nephrorrhaphy

3. _____ is used for stone retrieval or stent replacement in the urinary tract.
   a) intracorporeal electrohydraulic lithotripsy
   b) urostomy
   c) urologic endoscopic surgery
   d) pyeloplasty

4. Enuresis refers to _____.
   a) an involuntary discharge of urine often while asleep
   b) an inability to urinate
   c) urinating at night
   d) excessive urination

5. Oliguria means _____.
   a) scanty production of urine
   b) excessive production of urine
   c) presence of bacteria in the urine
   d) difficulty in urination

6. Cystitis is an inflammation of the _____.
   a) bladder
   b) kidney
   c) ureter
   d) urethra

7. An excess of urea in the blood as a result of kidney failure is _____.
   a) urethritis
   b) uraemia
   c) haematuria
   d) dysuria

8. The inner part of the kidney is called the _____.
   a) cortex
   b) core
   c) medulla
   d) renal tubule

9. Involuntary discharge of urine is known as _____.
   a) incompetence
   b) impotence
   c) incontinence
   d) intussception

10. Urine passes from the kidney to the bladder via the _____.
    a) urethra
    b) ureter
    c) glomerulus
    d) renal pelvis

EXERCISE 14.8: PRONUNCIATION AND COMPREHENSION

Read the following paragraphs aloud to practise your pronunciation. Using your textbook and a medical dictionary, find the meanings of the underlined medical terms.

A 13-month-old boy was admitted with right <u>vesicoureteric junction obstruction</u> for right <u>ureteral</u> reimplant. He was originally admitted in August last year, with <u>*Klebsiella septicaemia*</u> secondary to a <u>urinary tract infection</u> (UTI) at the age of 7 months. A subsequent <u>ultrasound</u> showed mild <u>dilatation</u> of the right <u>pelvicalyceal</u> system, with the left kidney being normal. An <u>MCU</u> was normal showing no <u>vesicoureteric reflux</u> and a renal scan showed a grossly dilated right <u>pelvicalyceal junction</u> (PUJ), with significant functional obstruction at the PUJ level. In December he was admitted for an <u>antegrade pyelogram</u>, which again showed right vesicoureteric obstruction and a tortuous right ureter.

The right ureteric reimplant was performed under general anaesthetic (ASA = 1NE) without complication. He was subsequently admitted to ICU for <u>epidural analgesia</u>, and his postoperative recovery was uneventful. This child was discharged on a <u>prophylactic</u> dose of <u>trimethoprim</u> and is to be reviewed in outpatients in 6 weeks with the results of a repeat renal ultrasound scan. Arrangements will then be made to remove the <u>ureteral stent</u> that was inserted during the operation.

EXERCISE 14.9: CROSSWORD PUZZLE

Complete the puzzle by providing the medical term for each of the clues below.

ACROSS

1. A floating kidney (12)
5. Occurs when urine in the bladder flows back into the ureters and often back into the kidneys (14, 6)
6. Filtering of blood through the nephrons in the kidney (10)
8. A kidney disorder involving the tubular segment of the nephron, which becomes damaged or destroyed (7, 8)
9. The inability of the kidneys to maintain proper filtration function, excrete wastes or maintain the electrolyte balance (5, 7)

DOWN

2. Abnormal distension of the ureter with urine (11)
3. Occurs when the kidneys do not form during fetal development (6, 8)
4. Infection of the renal pelvis and renal medulla of the kidneys (14)
7. Herniation or protrusion of the urinary bladder through the anterior vaginal wall (9)

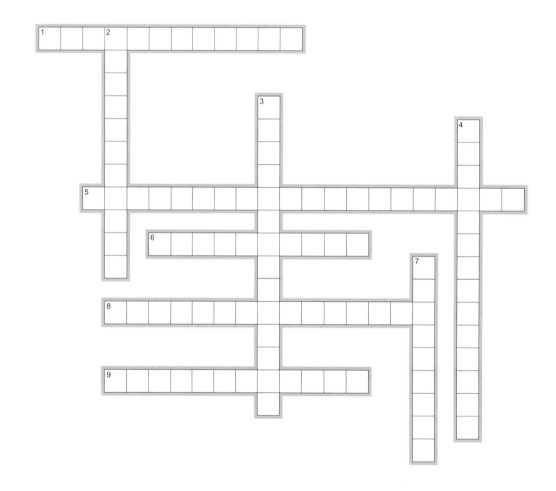

EXERCISE 14.10: ANAGRAMS

Work out each medical term from the jumbled letters below. Then, using the letters in brackets, determine the medical term that matches the description given.

1. iupayr	__ (__) __ __ __ __	pus in the urine
2. turrhea	__ __ (__) __ __ __ __	the tube that carries urine from the bladder to the exterior
3. divgnoi	__ __ __ (__) __ __ __	the process of excreting urine
4. seksito	(__) __ __ __ __ __ __	an abnormal accumulation of ketones in the body
5. cirauton	__ __ __ __ __ __ (__) __	need to pass urine frequently at night
6. pnrhone	__ __ __ __ __ __ (__)	the functional unit of the renal system

Rearrange the letters in brackets to form a word that means a 'retroperitoneal bean-shaped organ'.

__ __ __ __ __ __

EXERCISE 14.11: DISCHARGE SUMMARY ANALYSIS

Read the discharge summary below and answer the questions.

UNIVERSITY HOSPITAL DISCHARGE SUMMARY	**UR number:** 293031 **Name:** Alison Mitchell **Address:** 17 Bluebird Street, Minorton **Date of birth:** 21/7/1948 **Sex:** F **Nominated primary healthcare provider:** Dr Joanna Brown
Episode details **Consultant:** Dr Fells **Registrar:** Dr Hampson **Unit:** Urology **Admission source:** Elective **Date of admission:** 4/9/2020	**Discharge details** **Status:** Home **Date of discharge:** 7/9/2020
Reason for admission / Presenting problems: Five-year history of stress incontinence for which she has had two previous anterior repairs.	
Principal diagnosis: Stress incontinence	
Comorbidities: Mildly elevated BP	

| **Previous medical history:** |
| Two previous anterior repairs for stress incontinence |
| Three vaginal deliveries |
| Cholecystectomy |
| Incisional hernial repair |
| Gut obstruction due to adhesions |
| T&As and vocal cord polyps excised |

Clinical synopsis:

Booked as an elective admission for a urethral suspension. This was performed on 4/9/2020 under general anaesthetic via a Pfannenstiel incision. The procedure was uncomplicated. Following surgery she remained an inpatient for 3 days before discharge. An IDC inserted during surgery was removed on day 2. She was asked to come back to the outpatient clinic about 4 weeks following her surgery.

Prior to discharge, she reported that she could void well, and ultrasonography of her bladder confirmed that her residual urine was minimal. She was therefore discharged home to continue resting for a further fortnight prior to a gradual increase in all activities to normal.

Complications:

Clinical interventions:

Urethral suspension

Diagnostic interventions:

Medications at discharge:

Ceased medications:

Allergies: Bandaids

Alerts:

Arranged services:

Recommendations: Outpatient clinic about 4 weeks following her surgery.

Information to patient/relevant parties:

Continue resting for a further fortnight prior to a gradual increase in all activities to normal.

Authorising clinician: Dr Hampson

Document recipients:

Patient and LMO: Dr Joanna Brown

1. **Expand the following abbreviations as found in the discharge summary above.**

   BP

   IDC

   T&As

2. **Ms Mitchell's principal diagnosis was stress incontinence. What does this mean?**

3. **What is a Pfannenstiel incision and why is it preferred?**

4. It is stated that, post-surgery, Ms Mitchell's residual urine was minimal. What does this mean?

5. List all the procedures that Ms Mitchell had performed during her current admission.

CHAPTER 15

Male Reproductive System

Contents

OBJECTIVES   358

INTRODUCTION   359

NEW WORD ELEMENTS   359
  Combining forms   359
  Prefixes   360
  Suffixes   360

VOCABULARY   360

ABBREVIATIONS   361

FUNCTIONS AND STRUCTURE
OF THE MALE REPRODUCTIVE
SYSTEM   361
  External reproductive
  structures   361
  Internal reproductive
  structures   363

PATHOLOGY AND DISEASES   363

TESTS AND PROCEDURES   367

EXERCISES   368

Objectives

After completing this chapter you should be able to:

1. state the meanings of the word elements related to the male reproductive system

2. build words using the word elements associated with the male reproductive system

3. recognise, pronounce and effectively use medical terms associated with the male reproductive system

4. expand abbreviations related to the male reproductive system

5. describe the structure and functions of the male reproductive system including the penis, testes, seminal vesicles, prostate gland, semen and the reproductive process

6. describe common pathological conditions associated with the male reproductive system

7. describe common laboratory tests and diagnostic and surgical procedures associated with the male reproductive system

8. apply what you have learned by interpreting medical terminology in practice.

Demonstrate your knowledge of the male reproductive system by completing the exercises at the end of this chapter.

INTRODUCTION

The male reproductive system consists of the male sexual organs and is involved in sexuality, fertility and propagation of the species. It is primarily concerned with producing semen and transferring the semen into the female reproductive tract. The male reproductive system also secretes various hormones that maintain secondary sexual characteristics. It has a very close link to the male urinary system because some of the male reproductive organs also have urinary functions.

NEW WORD ELEMENTS

Here are some word elements related to the male reproductive system. To reinforce your learning, write the meanings of the medical terms in the spaces provided. Use the Glossary of medical terms on page 561 to help you work out the meanings. You may also need to check the meaning in a medical dictionary, but make an attempt yourself first.

Combining forms

Combining Form	Meaning	Medical Term	Meaning of Medical Term
andr/o	male	androgenic	
balan/o	glans penis	balanoplasty	
cry/o	cold	cryotherapy	
epididym/o	epididymis	vasoepididymostomy	
fer/o	carry, bear	seminiferous	
gonad/o	gonads, sex glands	gonadoblastoma	
hydr/o	water, fluid	hydrocoele	
oligo-	scanty, deficiency, few	oligospermia	
orch/o	testis, testicle	orchitis	
orchi/o		orchialgia	
orchid/o		orchidoepididymectomy	
pen/i	penis	penile	
perine/o	perineum	perineotomy	
phall/o	penis	phallorrhoea	
phim/o	muzzle	phimosis	
posth/o	prepuce, foreskin	balanoposthitis	
prostat/o	prostate gland	prostatomegaly	
scrot/o	scrotum, bag, pouch	scrotitis	
semin/i	semen, seed	seminoma	
sperm/i	spermatozoa, sperm	spermicidal	
sperm/o		spermopathy	
spermat/o		spermatolysis	
terat/o	monster, malformed	teratospermia	
test/i	testis, testicle	testitis	
test/o		testosterone	
testicul/o		testicular	
urethr/o	urethra	urethroplasty	
varic/o	varicose veins	varicosis	
vas/o	ductus (vas) deferens, vessel, duct	vasectomy	
vesicul/o	seminal vesicle	vesiculography	
zo/o	animal life	azoospermia	

Prefixes

Prefix	Meaning	Medical Term	Meaning of Medical Term
a-	no, not, without, absence of	aspermatogenesis	
an-	no, not, without, absence of	anorchia	
circum-	around, about	circumcise	
crypto-	hidden	cryptorchidism	
para-	near, beside, alongside	paraphimosis	
trans-	across, through, over	transurethral	

Suffixes

Suffix	Meaning	Medical Term	Meaning of Medical Term
-cele	hernia, protrusion	rectocele	
-cision	cutting	circumcision	
-coele	cavity	hydrocoele	
-genesis	pertaining to formation, producing	spermatogenesis	
-ism	state of	anorchism	
-one	hormone	testosterone	
-pexy	fixation, put in place	orchidopexy	
-stomy	create surgical opening	vasovasostomy	

VOCABULARY

The following list provides many of the medical terms used for the first time in this chapter. Pronunciations are provided with each term. As you read the rest of the chapter, make sure you identify each of these terms and understand their meanings.

Term	Pronunciation
anorchism	an-ORK-iz-em
aspermatogenesis	ay-SPER-mat-oh-JEN-e-sis
aspermia	ay-SPER-mee-ah
azoospermia	ay-zoo-oh-SPER-mee-ah
bacterial prostatitis	bak-tee-ree-al pros-tat-EYE-tis
balanitis	bal-an-EYE-tis
benign prostatic hypertrophy	bee-nyn pros-TAT-ik hy-PER-troh-fee
bulbourethral gland	bul-boh-yoo-REETH-ral gland
circumcision	SER-kum-SI-shun
cryptorchidism	kript-OR-kid-iz-em
digital rectal examination	DIJ-e-tal REK-tal ek-ZAM-in-AY-shun

Table continued

Term	Pronunciation
ductus (vas) deferens	DUKT-us (vas) DEF-er-enz
ejaculatory duct	e-jak-yoo-LAY-tor-ee dukt
epididymis	ep-ee-DID-e-mis
epididymitis	ep-ee-did-e-MY-tis
epispadias	ep-ee-SPAY-dee-as
erectile dysfunction	ee-REK-tyl dis-FUNK-shun
gynaecomastia	GY-nee-koh-MAS-tee-ah
hydrocoele	HY-droh-seel
hypospadias	hy-poh-SPAY-dee-as
orchitis	or-KY-tis
paraphimosis	pa-ra-fy-MOH-sis
penile cancer	PEE-nyl KAN-sa
penis	PEE-nis
phimosis	fy-MOH-sis
priapism	PREE-ah-piz-em
prostate biopsy	PROS-tayt BY-op-see
prostate cancer	PROS-tayt KAN-sa
prostate gland	PROS-tayt gland
PSA test	pee-ess-ay test

Table continued

Term	Pronunciation
scrotum	SKROH-tum
semen analysis	SEE-men a-NAL-e-sis
seminal vesicle	SEM-in-al VEE-sik-el
spermatocele	sper-MAT-oh-seel
spermatogenesis	sper-mat-oh-JEN-e-sys
spermatozoa	sper-mat-oh-ZOH-a
testicular cancer	tes-TIK-yoo-lah KAN-sa
testis (testes)	TES-tis (TES-teez)
testosterone	tes-TOS-ter-ohn
transurethral resection of the prostate	tranz-yoo-REETH-ral ree-SEK-shun of the PROS-tayt
urethra	yoo-REETH-ra
varicocele	VA-ree-koh-seel
vasectomy	va-SEK-tom-ee

ABBREVIATIONS

The following abbreviations are commonly used in the Australian healthcare environment. Because some abbreviations can have more than one meaning, check the context in which the abbreviation is used before assigning a meaning to it.

Abbreviation	Definition
BPH	benign prostatic hypertrophy
DRE	digital rectal examination
ED	erectile dysfunction
FSH	follicle-stimulating hormone
HPV	human papillomavirus
HSV	herpes simplex virus
LH	luteinising hormone
NGU	non-gonococcal urethritis
NSU	non-specific urethritis
PSA	prostate-specific antigen
RPR	rapid plasma reagin (test for syphilis)
STD	sexually transmitted disease
STI	sexually transmitted infection
TRUS	transrectal ultrasound
TULIP	transurethral ultrasound-guided laser-induced prostatectomy
TUNA	transurethral needle ablation
TURP	transurethral resection of the prostate
VD	venereal disease

FUNCTIONS AND STRUCTURE OF THE MALE REPRODUCTIVE SYSTEM

The reproductive system in the male consists of hormones that work in combination with the pelvic organs and structures to play a part in the process of reproduction through fertilisation of a female egg. Within the testes (testicles), spermatozoa (or sperm) are produced and stored until sexual intercourse. Spermatozoa are the male gametes, or sex cells. At the time of intercourse, the sperm mix with a protective liquid called semen in the epididymis. This is then ejaculated through the ductus deferens out of the penis via the urethra.

The main hormones involved in the functioning of the male reproductive system are follicle-stimulating hormone (FSH), luteinising hormone (LH) and the main androgen (male sex hormone) called testosterone.

FSH and LH are manufactured by the pituitary gland in the brain. FSH is responsible for producing sperm in a process called spermatogenesis. LH initiates the production of testosterone, which also supports spermatogenesis. In addition, testosterone is responsible for the development of the secondary male sexual characteristics, including distinctive male muscle dimensions and strength, fat distribution, bone mass, deepening of the voice, growth of facial and body hair, the development of the Adam's apple and sex drive.

The male reproductive system has both internal and external organs (Fig. 15.1).

External reproductive structures
Penis – the human penis consists of three parts: the root, which is connected to the abdominal wall; the shaft or body of the penis; and the glans penis. The glans penis is the round, sensitive end of the penis. The foreskin is a loose layer of skin covering the glans. The opening of the urethra, the tube that transports semen and urine, is at the head of the glans. The penis has many sensitive nerve endings.

The body of the penis is shaped like a cylinder and has three internal chambers made up of spongy erectile tissue. This tissue contains thousands of large spaces that fill with blood when a male is sexually aroused. As the penis fills with blood, it becomes rigid and erect, which allows penetration to occur during sexual intercourse. The skin of the penis is loose and elastic to allow it to change size during an erection.

Testicles – the testicles or testes (singular: testis) are two oval-shaped organs located behind the penis in an external sac called the scrotum. Sperm are produced in the testes in a process known as spermatogenesis. The testes also produce male

Figure 15.1 Male reproductive organs and associated structures

(Mosby's Dictionary 2014)

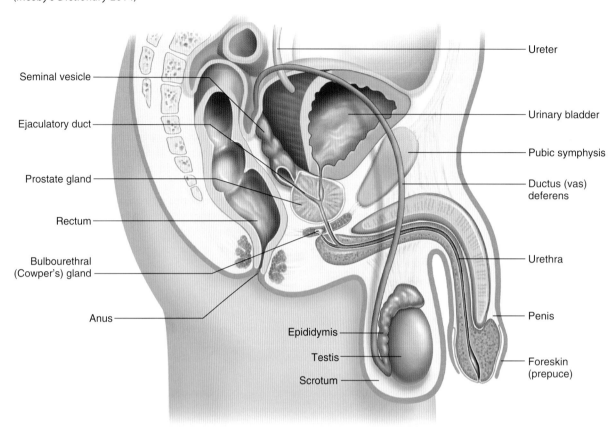

EXTERNAL GENITALS OF THE MALE

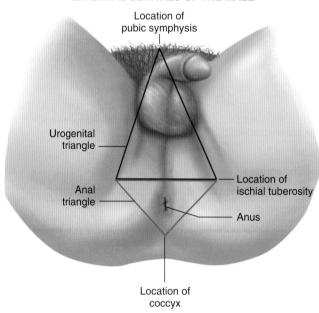

hormones, such as testosterone, which are responsible for the development of the typical male characteristics. The anterior pituitary gland in the brain releases two types of gonadotrophins that affect the testes. These are LH, which causes the release of testosterone from the testes and FSH, which maintains spermatogenesis.

Scrotum – the scrotum consists of a sac of skin and muscle divided by a septum, in which the two testes are contained. By allowing the testes to hang outside the body and by the action of loosening and tightening the scrotal muscle that moves the testes closer to or away from the abdomen, the testes are kept at a slightly cooler temperature than the rest of the body, thus maintaining the viability of the sperm, which are highly sensitive to fluctuations in temperature. Sperm is optimally produced when the testicles are 2–4° Celsius below body temperature.

Epididymis – there are two epididymides (singular: epididymis) in the male, formed of a series of small coiled tubes located at the back of the testes. The epididymis collects and stores sperm prior to the seminal fluid being ejaculated via the ductus deferens.

Internal reproductive structures

Ductus deferens – the ductus deferens (plural: ductus deferentes or ductus deferentia) is a long muscular tube (duct) that transports sperm via peristalsis from each epididymis to the ejaculatory ducts and ultimately to the urethra. There are a pair of these ducts, with each also known as a vas deferens. Along the way, semen is formed from the secretions from other male sex glands such as the seminal vesicles, prostate and the bulbourethral gland, and these mix with the sperm before ejaculation.

Ejaculatory ducts – the two ejaculatory ducts are formed where each ductus deferens connects with the seminal vesicles to pass through the prostate and into the urethra. Semen travels along this path before it exits the body through the penis during ejaculation.

Seminal vesicles – there are two seminal vesicles, which are tubular glands located in close proximity to the prostate. The main role of the seminal vesicles is to produce a fluid that makes up most of the semen.

Prostate – the prostate is a small muscular gland surrounding the urethra just below the bladder. Its function is to secrete some of the seminal fluid that protects and enriches the sperm as it is transported out of the body. The prostate is enclosed in the muscles of the pelvic floor, which contract during the ejaculatory process and also assist with penile erection. Prostate-specific antigen (PSA) is an enzyme called a protease that breaks protein secretions into smaller molecules, thus making the semen liquid.

Bulbourethral glands – these glands are also called Cowper's glands. During sexual arousal each of the bulbourethral glands produces a clear, sticky fluid known as pre-ejaculate. The pre-ejaculate helps to lubricate the urethra for the sperm to pass through and plays a role in neutralising acids from urine that are in the urethra from earlier urination.

Urethra – the urethra is the tube that connects the bladder to the penis for removing fluids from the body. In males, the urethra carries semen as well as urine and hence has a role in the urinary system as well as the male reproductive system.

PATHOLOGY AND DISEASES

The following section provides a list of common diseases and pathological conditions relevant to the male reproductive system.

Term	Pronunciation	Definition
anorchism	an-ORK-iz-em	Anorchism is a congenital absence of one or both testes.
aspermatogenesis	ay-SPER-mat-oh-JEN-a-sis	Aspermatogenesis is the failure to produce mature functional spermatozoa.
aspermia	ay-SPER-mee-ah	Also called aspermatism, aspermia refers to the failure to produce or ejaculate semen.
azoospermia	ay-zo-o-SPER-mee-ah	Azoospermia refers to semen without a measurable number of living spermatozoa. It is linked to infertility.
bacterial prostatitis	bak-TEER-ee-al pros-tat-EYE-tis	Bacterial prostatitis is an infection of the prostate gland caused by bacteria. It often occurs in conjunction with urethritis or an infection of the lower urinary tract. It is characterised by fever, chills, dysuria, urethral discharge and a tender prostate.

Table continued

Term	Pronunciation	Definition
balanitis	bal-an-EYE-tis	Balanitis is an inflammation of the glans penis and foreskin often associated with poor hygiene in uncircumcised men. It results in a painful penis and foreskin and a foul-smelling urethral discharge. Chronic balanitis can result in phimosis.
benign prostatic hypertrophy (BPH)	bee-nyn pros-TAT-ik hy-PER-troh-fee	BPH is also called benign prostatic hyperplasia or prostatomegaly. It is the enlargement of the prostate gland. It is common in males over 50 years of age. Because BPH can result in bladder neck obstruction, it can cause urinary symptoms such as an irritable bladder, urgency and frequency of micturition, hesitancy, nocturia and urinary incontinence.
cryptorchidism	kript-OR-kid-iz-em	Cryptorchidism (also called cryptorchism) is a failure of one or both testicles to descend into the scrotum before birth (Fig. 15.2). It is more common in premature babies than in full-term infants. The undescended testicle will often descend spontaneously by 1 year of age. If not, surgical intervention such as an orchiopexy may be performed.

Figure 15.2 Inguinal orchiopexy for cryptorchidism

(Wein et al 2016)

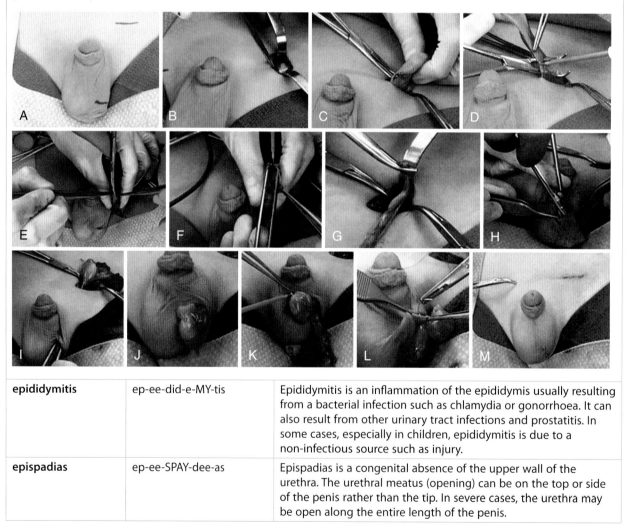

epididymitis	ep-ee-did-e-MY-tis	Epididymitis is an inflammation of the epididymis usually resulting from a bacterial infection such as chlamydia or gonorrhoea. It can also result from other urinary tract infections and prostatitis. In some cases, especially in children, epididymitis is due to a non-infectious source such as injury.
epispadias	ep-ee-SPAY-dee-as	Epispadias is a congenital absence of the upper wall of the urethra. The urethral meatus (opening) can be on the top or side of the penis rather than the tip. In severe cases, the urethra may be open along the entire length of the penis.

Table continued

Term	Pronunciation	Definition
erectile dysfunction	ee-REK-tyl dis-FUNK-shun	Erectile dysfunction is also called impotence. It refers to the inability of the male to achieve or maintain a penile erection during sexual intercourse. It can be due to organic problems such as diabetes and cardiovascular disease, as a result of nerve damage (e.g. after prostate surgery), or as a side effect of various drugs. In some cases, erectile dysfunction is psychological in aetiology.
gynaecomastia	gy-nee-koh-MAS-tee-ah	Gynaecomastia refers to an abnormal enlargement of glandular breast tissues in a male. It is usually due to a hormonal imbalance where the male has an increased amount of oestrogen in relation to levels of androgen and/or testosterone.
hydrocoele	HY-droh-seel	A hydrocoele is a sac of fluid in the testis that can result in a swelling of the scrotum (Fig. 15.3). It can be congenital, occurring in around 10% of male infants, or can develop in adulthood as a result of inflammation or scrotal injury. **Figure 15.3 Hydrocoele** 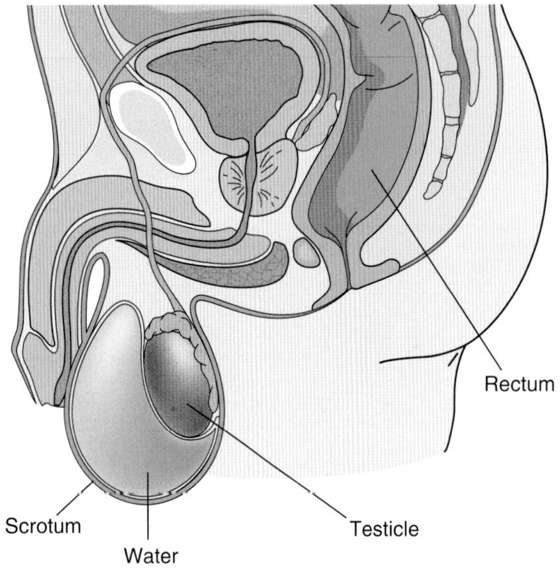 Rectum Scrotum Water Testicle
hypospadias	hy-poh-SPAY-dee-as	Hypospadias is a developmental anomaly where the urethral meatus opens on the underside of the penis. In more severe cases the opening is at the midshaft or base of the penis. Occasionally, the urethral opening is located in or behind the scrotum or on the perineum.
orchitis	or-KY-tis	Orchitis is an acute inflammation and swelling of one or both of the testicles resulting from infection or trauma. Common infections that result in orchitis are mumps, sexually transmitted infections such as gonorrhoea and chlamydia, prostatitis and epididymitis.
paraphimosis	pa-ra-fy-MOH-sis	Paraphimosis is a strangulation of the glans penis due to retraction of a narrowed foreskin. It is not possible to bring the foreskin back to its normal position. Paraphimosis occurs as a result of direct trauma, infection or failure to return the foreskin to its proper position after washing. It is considered an emergency requiring immediate treatment such as circumcision.

Table continued

Term	Pronunciation	Definition
penile cancer	PEE-nyl KAN-sa	Penile cancer almost always occurs in males who are not circumcised. The histology is usually epidermoid or squamous carcinoma that develops from squamous cells. Penile cancer usually presents as a painless wart-like growth or ulcer typically near the end of the penis. It may be related to poor personal hygiene.
phimosis	fy-MOH-sis	Phimosis is the constriction or narrowing of the prepuce (foreskin) over the glans penis. As a result the foreskin cannot be retracted. It can be either congenital or acquired. As with paraphimosis, phimosis occurs only in uncircumcised males.
priapism	PREE-ah-piz-em	Priapism refers to an uncontrolled and prolonged erection, without sexual desire, that can last from several hours to several days causing an enlarged and painful penis. Penile injections that are used to treat erectile dysfunction, some psychiatric medications (e.g. antidepressants) and conditions such as leukaemia or other blood disorders can cause priapism. Priapism can scar the penis and lead to impotence if not treated urgently.
prostate cancer	PROS-tayt KAN-sa	Prostate cancer is one of the most common invasive cancers in men. Usually it is one of the slowest growing malignancies but can be aggressive in a small number of patients. It is frequently asymptomatic for a period of time, with the first symptoms often related to bladder neck obstruction. Prostate cancer tends to metastasise in a predictable pattern – usually to the adjacent lymph nodes and bones in the spine and pelvis.
spermatocele	sper-MAT-oh-seel	A spermatocele is a benign cystic tumour that arises from the epididymis. It contains a milky fluid with spermatozoa. Spermatoceles range from a few millimetres to many centimetres in size. They can be found in the testicles, the ductus deferentes or in the scrotum.
testicular cancer	tes-TIK-yoo-lah KAN-sa	Testicular cancer is a malignant tumour of the testes. The main histological types include seminoma, choriocarcinoma and teratoma. It is the most common malignancy in young men. With early detection by testicular self-examination and treatment with combination chemotherapy, testicular cancer is curable.
testicular torsion	tes-TIK-yoo-lah TOR-shun	Testicular torsion is a rotation or twisting of the testis on the axis of the spermatic cord, cutting off the blood supply. This is an emergency which, if left untreated, can result in gangrene of the testis.
varicocele	VA-rik-oh-seel	A varicocele is a cluster of herniated, dilated veins in the scrotum occurring behind and above the testes. Varicoceles are most often seen on the left side of the scrotum. They usually develop slowly and are more common in young men. Varicoceles are often the cause of male infertility.

TESTS AND PROCEDURES

The following section provides a list of common diagnostic tests and procedures and clinical interventions and surgical procedures that are undertaken for the male reproductive system.

Test/Procedure	Pronunciation	Definition
circumcision	SER-kum-SI-shun	A circumcision is a surgical procedure that involves excising all or some of the foreskin from the penis.
digital rectal examination (DRE)	DIJ-et-al REK-tal ek-zam-in-AY-shun	A DRE is a diagnostic examination involving a doctor gently putting a lubricated, gloved finger of one hand into the rectum to identify abnormalities in the pelvic cavity, such as prostate disorders. **Figure 15.4 Digital rectal examination** (Bonewit-West 2008)
prostate biopsy	PROS-tayt BY-op-see	A prostate biopsy is a procedure that involves inserting a needle into the prostate to remove a small sample of tissue for examination under a microscope. The most common path is via the rectum but can also be via the urethra or the space between the scrotum and anus.
PSA test	pee-es-ay test	A PSA test is a diagnostic test to determine the level of prostate-specific antigen in the blood. A higher level of PSA can be an indicator of prostate disease such as benign prostatic hypertrophy or cancer.
semen analysis	SEE-men a-NAL-e-sis	Semen analysis is a diagnostic test to determine whether a man is infertile. Analysis is undertaken to determine issues with sperm count, motility, autoimmunity and morphology.
transurethral resection of the prostate (TURP)	tranz-yoo-REETH-ral ree-SEK-shun of the PROS-tayt	A TURP is a surgical procedure performed to remove the prostate endoscopically by passing an instrument through the eye of the penis and down the urethra into the area of the prostate. The prostate is removed by electrocautery or sharp dissection.
vasectomy	va-SEK-tom-ee	A vasectomy is a procedure for male sterilisation that involves cutting a segment out of each of the ductus deferens, with the ends being ligated or cauterised.

Exercises

EXERCISE 15.1: LABEL THE DIAGRAM

Using the information provided in this chapter, label the anatomical parts in Figs 15.5a and 15.5b.

1 _____

2 _____

3 _____

4 _____

5 _____

6 _____

7 _____

8 _____

9 _____

10 _____

11 _____

12 _____

13 _____

14 _____

15 _____

16 _____

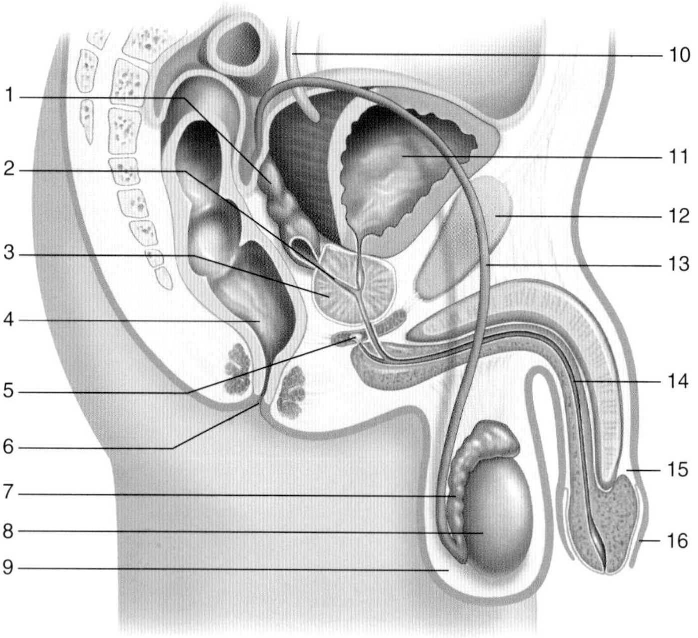

Figure 15.5a Male reproductive organs and associated structures

(Mosby's Dictionary 2014)

1 _____

2 _____

3 _____

4 _____

5 _____

6 _____

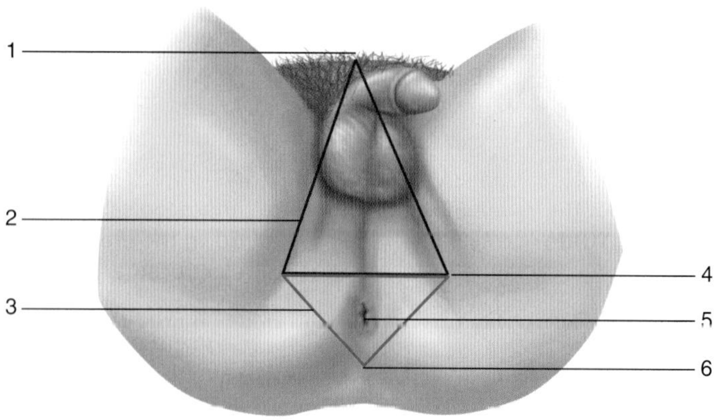

Figure 15.5b External genitals of the male

(Mosby's Dictionary 2014)

EXERCISE 15.2: WORD ELEMENT MEANINGS AND WORD BUILDING

Define the word elements, then use the element correctly in a medical term.

Word Element	Meaning	Medical Term
andr/o		
balan/o		
crypt/o		
epididym/o		
fer/o		
hydr/o		
orch/o		
perine/o		
phall/o		
phim/o		
posth/o		
prostat/o		
semin/i		
sperm/i		
terat/o		
test/i		
urethr/o		
varic/o		
vas/o		
vesicul/o		

EXERCISE 15.3: VOCABULARY BUILDING

Provide the medical term for each of the definitions below.

1. Discharge from the glans penis: _____

2. Enlargement of the prostate: _____

_____

3. Surgical repair of the urethra: _____

_____

4. Formation of sperm: _____

_____

5. Creation of an artificial opening between a ductus deferens and epididymis: _____

_____

6. Inflammation of the epididymis and testes: _____

_____

7. Condition of sperm in urine: _____

_____

8. Pertaining to within the testes: _____

_____

9. An instrument to measure (the size) of the testes: _____

_____

10. Breakdown of sperm: _____

_____

Now provide the meaning for the following terms.

11. seminoma _____

_____

12. vasorrhaphy _____

_____

13. prostatocystotomy _____

_____

14. balanorrhagia _____

_____

15. scrotectomy _____

_____

16. vesiculotomy _____

_____

17. orchialgia _____

_____

18. phallitis _____

_____

19. epididymo-orchitis _____

_____

20. vasovasostomy _____

_____

EXERCISE 15.4: APPLYING MEDICAL TERMINOLOGY

Fill in the blank, select the correct answer or select the correct medical term.

1. The combining form _____ means testicle.
   a) epididym/o
   b) orchid/o
   c) spermat/o
   d) perine/o

2. _____ is a collection of fluid in the testes.
   a) balanitis
   b) hydrocoele
   c) anorchism
   d) seminoma

3. The term that describes scanty production and expulsion of sperm is _____.
   a) azoospermia
   b) hypospadias
   c) oligospermia
   d) dysuria

4. _____ means glans penis.
   a) orchi/o
   b) prostat/o
   c) penile
   d) balan/o

5. A prostatectomy is an incision into the prostate gland
   a) true
   b) false

6. The failure of one or both testes to descend into the scrotum is termed _____.
   a) cryptorchism
   b) orchiectomy
   c) vasectomy
   d) anarchism

7. The urethra helps produce and maintain sperm.
   a) true
   b) false

8. The hormone that is principally responsible for developing male sexual characteristics is _____.
   a) testosterone
   b) follicle-stimulating hormone
   c) luteinising hormone
   d) oestrogen

9. What is the correct anatomical pathway for sperm leaving the body?
   a) epididymis, ductus deferens, urethra, ejaculatory duct
   b) epididymis, ductus deferens, ejaculatory duct, urethra
   c) ductus deferens, ejaculatory duct, ureter, epididymis
   d) ductus deferens, epididymis, ejaculatory duct, ureter

10. Spermatogenesis takes place in the _____.
   a) penis
   b) epididymis
   c) testicles
   d) scrotum

EXERCISE 15.5: EXPAND THE ABBREVIATIONS

Expand the abbreviations to form correct medical terms.

Abbreviation	Expanded Abbreviation
BPH	
DRE	
ED	
HPV	
HSV	
NGU	
NSU	
PSA	
RPR	
STD	
TRUS	
TUNA	
TUR(P)	
VD	

EXERCISE 15.6: VOCABULARY BUILDING

Provide the medical term for each of the definitions below.

1. Absence of a testicle: _____

_____

2. Inflammation of glans penis: _____

_____

3. Strangulation of the glans penis due to a narrowed foreskin: _____

_____

4. Inability to maintain an erection until ejaculation, also called erectile dysfunction: _____

_____

5. Insertion of a device into the prostate via the rectum to remove tissue for microscopic examination: _____

_____

6. Semen without living sperm: _____

_____

7. The gland surrounding the urethra at the base of the urinary bladder: _____

_____

8. Removal of part of the ductus deferens: _____

_____

9. Anastomosis of the ends of a ductus deferens after a vasectomy to attempt to restore function: _____

_____

10. Condition of scanty sperm: _____

_____

EXERCISE 15.7: MATCH MEDICAL TERMS AND MEANINGS

Match the medical term in Column A with its meaning in Column B.

Column A	Answer	Column B
1. ejaculation		A. surgical removal of a testis
2. epididymis		B. release of semen from the urethra
3. hypospadias		C. genital warts
4. orchiectomy		D. duct in the testes
5. papilloma		E. foreskin
6. prepuce		F. herniated veins in the scrotum
7. testicular torsion		G. anomaly where the urethra opens on the underside of the penis
8. varicocele		H. twisting of the spermatic cord

EXERCISE 15.8: PRONUNCIATION AND COMPREHENSION

Read the following paragraph aloud to practise your pronunciation. Using your textbook and a medical dictionary, find the meanings of the underlined medical terms.

A 19 year old male was admitted after having fallen in the straddle position across a brick wall in the garden of his home. He was unable to <u>urinate</u> and passed <u>frank blood per urethra</u> following the injury. He did not have a <u>pelvic fracture</u> but had <u>perineal bruising</u> consistent with <u>urethral</u> trauma in the <u>perineum</u>. He had a <u>suprapubic catheter</u> passed under <u>local anaesthetic</u> and a <u>retrograde urethrogram</u> confirmed leakage from the urethra at the <u>prostatic urethra</u>. <u>Cystoscopy</u> under <u>intravenous</u> sedation (ASA =1NE) showed incomplete disruption of the <u>bulbous urethra</u> 3 cm, below the <u>urogenital diaphragm</u>. It involved a 1 cm segment. A 16 French indwelling catheter was passed <u>cystoscopically</u>, and the <u>scrotal haematoma</u> was drained <u>bilaterally</u>. He was discharged and is to be readmitted in 2 weeks for <u>trial of void</u> after removing his indwelling catheter.

EXERCISE 15.9: CROSSWORD PUZZLE

Complete the puzzle by providing the medical term for each of the clues below.

ACROSS

4. Inflammation of glans penis and foreskin (9)
6. Failure to produce or ejaculate semen (8)
7. A test to determine the level of prostate-specific antigen in blood (3, 4)
8. A cluster of herniated, dilated veins in the scrotum occurring behind and above the testes (10)

DOWN

1. Constriction or narrowing of the prepuce (foreskin) over the glans penis (8)
2. Tube connecting the bladder to the penis for removing fluids (7)
3. Abnormal enlargement of glandular breast tissues in a male (13)
5. A congenital absence of one or both testes (9)

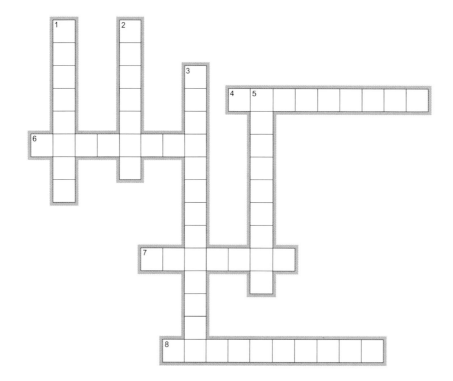

EXERCISE 15.10: ANAGRAMS

Work out each medical term from the jumbled letters below. Then, using the letters in brackets, determine the medical term that matches the description given.

1. spien	__ __ __ __ (__)	the external male reproductive organ
2. ettasrop	__ __ __ __ (__) __ __ __	the gland surrounding the urethra at the base of the bladder
3. comineetp	__ __ __ __ __ (__) __ __ __	erectile dysfunction
4. ctsudu sfreened	__ __ __ __ __ (__) __ __ __ __ __ __ __	the tube that carries sperm from the epididymis
5. hsmsopii	__ __ (__) __ __ __ __ __	a narrowing of the prepuce on the penis
6. atpozroames	__ __ __ __ __ __ (__) __ __ __ __	sperm cells

Rearrange the letters in brackets to form a word that means 'another name for testicle'.

__ __ __ __ __ __

EXERCISE 15.11: APPLYING MEDICAL TERMINOLOGY

Fill in the blank or select the correct medical term.

1. _____ is an inflammation of the prostate gland caused by bacteria.

2. An examination that allows for identification of abnormalities in the pelvis, such as prostate disorders, is known as

   _____ .

3. The _____ transports sperm from the seminiferous tubules to a ductus deferens.

4. A _____ is undertaken to determine fertility levels in a male.

5. _____ is the congenital absence of the upper wall of the urethra.

6. A _____ is a procedure to excise all or some of the foreskin from the penis.

7. The _____ produces a clear sticky fluid known as pre-ejaculate and is also known as the Cowper's gland.

8. A tube that transports sperm from an epididymis to an ejaculatory duct is a _____ .

9. A _____ is a sac of fluid in the testis that can result in a swelling of the scrotum.

10. The condition _____ is strangulation of glans penis due to retraction of narrowed foreskin.

11. _____ is the hormone responsible for male sex characteristics.

12. A male who has abnormally large glandular breast tissues is known to have _____ .

13. _____ is when there is an uncontrolled and prolonged erection, without sexual desire.

14. A _____ test determines the level of prostate-specific antigen in blood.

15. _____ is the procedure to remove the prostate endoscopically.

EXERCISE 15.12: DISCHARGE SUMMARY ANALYSIS

Read the discharge summary below and answer the questions.

UNIVERSITY HOSPITAL DISCHARGE SUMMARY	**UR number:** 323334 **Name:** Alan Hendricks **Address:** 65 Brownley Street, Henley **Date of birth:** 2/2/1946 **Sex:** M **Nominated primary healthcare provider:** Dr Paul Adams
Episode details **Consultant:** Dr Tomkins **Registrar:** Dr Farrow **Unit:** Surgical **Admission source:** Elective **Date of admission:** 1/5/2020	**Discharge details** **Status:** Home **Date of discharge:** 3/5/2020

Reason for admission / Presenting problems:
Long history of poor urinary stream with associated frequency and hesitation. Elevated PSA levels between 8 ng/mL and 10 ng/mL for around 2 years.
Principal diagnosis: Well-differentiated adenocarcinoma of the prostate gland. Gleason score 4/3 in 30% of the prostate.
Comorbidities:
Hypertension, previous MI in 2009
Previous medical history:
Appendicectomy 1967
SCCs right arm and forehead excised 2008
Clinical synopsis:
On DRE, his prostate was found to be significantly enlarged and firm. He proceeded to theatre on 1.5.20 at which time a radical TURP was performed under Da Vinci robotic control. This was performed under a GA. His ASA score was 2NE. Postoperatively, he experienced some scrotal swelling and bruising but otherwise his postoperative period was uncomplicated. His catheter was removed on the day after the procedure and he was voiding and continent at the time of discharge.
Complications:
Clinical interventions:
TURP
Diagnostic interventions:
Histology on the specimen confirmed the presence of well-differentiated adenocarcinoma of the prostate. Gleason score 4/3 in 30% of the prostate. This degree of the disease in a man of his age is well within normal limits.
Medications at discharge:
Ceased medications:
Allergies:
Alerts:

Arranged services:
Recommendations: Will be reassessed at the time of his postoperative outpatient appointment with a view to the need to further investigate him or commence him on further treatment.
Information to patient/relevant parties: Postoperative outpatient appointment in 6 weeks.
Authorising clinician: Dr Farrow
Document recipients: Patient and LMO: Dr Paul Adams

1. **Expand the following abbreviations as found in the discharge summary above.**

   TURP

   ASA

   PSA

   MI

   DRE

2. **Mr Hendricks exhibited some of the most common signs and symptoms of prostate cancer. What were they?**

3. **What is a Gleason score?**

4. **Mr Hendricks had a radical TURP to remove his cancerous prostate gland.**
   List three factors that will determine the type of treatment a patient is given.

5. **List three treatment options other than a TURP that men with prostate cancer may be offered.**

6. **It is stated that Mr Hendricks was voiding and continent at the time of discharge. What does this mean?**

CHAPTER 16

Female Reproductive System

Contents

OBJECTIVES	378
INTRODUCTION	379
NEW WORD ELEMENTS	379
Combining forms	379
Prefixes	380
Suffixes	380
VOCABULARY	380
ABBREVIATIONS	381
FUNCTIONS AND STRUCTURE OF THE FEMALE REPRODUCTIVE SYSTEM	381
Follicular phase	382
Ovulation	382
Luteal phase	383
Menstrual phase	383
Female reproductive organs	383
PATHOLOGY AND DISEASES	385
Benign conditions	385
Malignant tumours	386
Other gynaecological disorders	387
TESTS AND PROCEDURES	388
EXERCISES	392

Objectives

After completing this chapter you should be able to:

1. state the meanings of the word elements related to the female reproductive system

2. build words using the word elements associated with the female reproductive system

3. recognise, pronounce and effectively use medical terms associated with the female reproductive system

4. expand abbreviations related to the female reproductive system

5. describe the structure and functions of the female reproductive system including the uterus, ovaries, fallopian tubes and associated organs and the reproductive process

6. describe common pathological conditions associated with the female reproductive system

7. describe common laboratory tests and diagnostic and surgical procedures associated with the female reproductive system

8. apply what you have learned by interpreting medical terminology in practice.

Demonstrate your knowledge of the female reproductive system by completing the exercises at the end of this chapter.

INTRODUCTION

The female reproductive system consists of the female sexual organs and is involved in sexuality, fertility and propagation of the species. It is a complex system because it also has to support the developing fetus if pregnancy occurs. It is one of the few body systems where a person can function quite well if some organs need to be removed because of disease.

Pregnancy, labour and delivery will be discussed in the obstetrics and neonatology chapter.

NEW WORD ELEMENTS

Here are some word elements related to the female reproductive system. To reinforce your learning, write the meanings of the medical terms in the spaces provided. Use the Glossary of medical terms on page 561 to help you work out the meanings. You may also need to check the meaning in a medical dictionary, but make an attempt yourself first.

Combining forms

Combining Form	Meaning	Medical Term	Meaning of Medical Term
cervic/o	neck, cervix uteri	cervicitis	
colp/o	vagina	colposcope	
culd/o	cul-de-sac	culdoscopy	
endometri/o	endometrium	endometriosis	
episi/o	vulva	episiotomy	
fer/o	carry or bear	lactiferous	
gynaec/o	woman, female	gynaecology	
hyster/o	uterus	hysterectomy	
leiomy/o	smooth muscle	leiomyoma	
mamm/o	breast	mammogram	
mast/o		mastectomy	
men/o	menses, menstruation	oligomenorrhoea	
metr/o	uterus	metroptosis	
metri/o		endometrioma	
my/o	muscle	myomectomy	
o/o	egg, ovum	ooblast	
oophor/o	ovary	oophoropexy	
ov/i	egg, ovum	ovigenesis	
ov/o		ovoid	
ovul/o		ovulatory	
ovari/o	ovary	ovariorrhexis	
perine/o	perineum	perineoplasty	
salping/o	fallopian tube, eustachian (auditory) tube	salpingo-oophorectomy	
uter/o	uterus	uterosalpingography	
vagin/o	vagina	vaginovesical	
vulv/o	vulva	vulvovaginoplasty	

Prefixes

Prefix	Meaning	Medical Term	Meaning of Medical Term
dys-	painful, bad, difficult	dyspareunia	
endo-	within, inside, inner	endocervix	
intra-	within	intrauterine	
pre-	before, in front of	premenstrual	
retro-	backwards, behind	retroversion	

Suffixes

Suffix	Meaning	Medical Term	Meaning of Medical Term
-arche	beginning, first	menarche	
-atresia	closure, occlusion, absence of opening	hysteratresia	
-cele	hernia, swelling	cystocele	
-dynia	condition of pain	vulvodynia	
-rrhoea	discharge, flow	leucorrhoea	
-salpinx	uterine tube	pyosalpinx	

VOCABULARY

The following list provides many of the medical terms used for the first time in this chapter. Pronunciations are provided with each term. As you read the rest of the chapter, make sure you identify each of these terms and understand their meanings.

Term	Pronunciation
aspiration	as-pi-RAY-shun
carcinoma of the breast	kah-sin-O-ma of the brest
carcinoma of the cervix	kah-sin-O-ma of the SER-viks
carcinoma of the ovary	kah-sin-O-ma of the OH-vah-ree
cauterisation	kaw-ter-eye-ZAY-shun
colposcopy	kol-POS-kop-ee
conisation	ko-ny-ZAY-shun
cryosurgery	KRY-oh-ser-ja-ree
culdocentesis	kul-doh-sen-TEE-sis
cystocele	SIS-toh-seel
depot medroxyprogesterone acetate (DPMA) injection	deep-poh med-rok-see-proh-JES-te-rohn ass-e-tate in-JEK-shun
dilation (dilatation) and curettage	dy-LAY-shun (dy-la-TAY-shun) and kyoo-ret-AHJ
endometriosis	en-doh-meet-ree-OH-sis

Table continued

Term	Pronunciation
exenteration	ek-SEN-ter-AY-shun
fibrocystic disease	fy-broh-SIS-tik diz-eez
hysterectomy	his-ter-EK-tom-ee
hysterosalpingography	HIS-ter-oh-sal-ping-GOG-raf-ee
hysteroscopy	his-ter-OS-kop-ee
implanon	IM-plan-on
intrauterine device	in-tra-YOO-ter-yn de-vys
laparoscopy	lap-ah-ROS-kop-ee
large loop excision of transformation zone	larj loop ek-SIZ-shun tranz-for-MAY-shun zone
mammography	ma-MOG-raf-ee
mastectomy	mas-TEK-tom-ee
oophorectomy	oo-for-EK-tom-ee
oral contraceptive	oh-ral kon-trah-SEP-tiv
ovarian cyst	oh-VAIR-ee-an sist
ovarian cystectomy	oh-VAIR-ee-an sis-TEK-tom-ee
Papanicolaou (Pap) smear	pap-a-NIK-ol-ow smear
pelvic inflammatory disease	PEL-vik in-FLAM-a-tor-ee diz-eez
pelvic ultrasonography	PEL-vik ul-tra-son-OG-ra-fee
premenstrual syndrome	pre-MEN-stroo-al SIN-drohm

Table continued

Term	Pronunciation
procidentia	prok-si-DEN-sha
rectocele	REK-toh-seel
salpingo-oophorectomy	sal-ping-goh-oo-for-EK-tom-ee
toxic shock syndrome	TOK-sik shok SIN-drohm
tubal ligation	TYOO-bal ly-GAY-shun
uterine leiomyoma	YOO-ter-yn LY-oh-my-OH-ma
uterine prolapse	YOO-ter-yn PRO-laps

ABBREVIATIONS

The following abbreviations are commonly used in the Australian healthcare environment. Because some abbreviations can have more than one meaning, check the context in which the abbreviation is used before assigning a meaning to it.

Abbreviation	Definition
ACTH	adrenocorticotrophic hormone
BSE	breast self-examination
CIN	cervical intraepithelial neoplasia
CIS	carcinoma in situ
CVS	chorionic villus sampling
cx	cervix
DCIS	ductal carcinoma in situ
D&C	dilation (dilatation) and curettage
DUB	dysfunctional uterine bleeding
FSH	follicle-stimulating hormone
GnRH	gonadotrophin-releasing hormone
gyn, gynae	gynaecology
hCG	human chorionic gonadotrophin
HPV	human papillomavirus
HRT	hormone replacement therapy
HVS	high vaginal swab
IUD	intrauterine device
IVF	in vitro fertilisation
LEEP	loop electrosurgical excision procedure
LLETZ	large loop excision of transformation zone
LH	luteinising hormone
LMP	last menstrual period
MSU	midstream urine
OCP	oral contraceptive pill

Table continued

Abbreviation	Definition
Pap smear	Papanicolaou smear
PID	pelvic inflammatory disease
PMS	premenstrual syndrome
STD	sexually transmitted disease
STI	sexually transmitted infection
TAH	total abdominal hysterectomy
TAHBSO	total abdominal hysterectomy with bilateral salpingo-oophorectomy
TRAM flap	transverse rectus abdominis myocutaneous flap
TSS	toxic shock syndrome
TVH	total vaginal hysterectomy
VAIN	vaginal intraepithelial neoplasia
VDRL	venereal disease research laboratory
VIN	vulval intraepithelial neoplasia

FUNCTIONS AND STRUCTURE OF THE FEMALE REPRODUCTIVE SYSTEM

The female reproductive system is designed for procreation or reproduction. It does this through the production of female gametes or eggs, called ova (singular: ovum) or oocytes, which are released on a monthly basis by the ovaries, where they have been produced and stored. Each ovum is transported through one of the two fallopian tubes to the uterus. If the ovum is fertilised by a spermatozoon from a male, it will implant into the uterus, which has been prepared to support fetal growth until maturity. If the egg is not fertilised, the body will shed the lining of the uterus in a process called menstruation. The female reproductive system produces the female sex hormones, oestrogen and progesterone, that sustain this monthly cycle of creating and discarding the protective environment of the uterus for a growing fetus.

Menarche is the term given to the point during puberty when the female first experiences menstruation. The age at which menarche occurs differs from woman to woman but is generally between the ages of 11 and 14. In later life, around the ages of 45–55, the female reproductive system gradually stops creating the female hormones and the reproductive cycle slows and stops. When there is no longer production of oestrogen and progesterone, ova are no longer produced by the ovaries and a woman is said to be menopausal.

The menstrual cycle, which involves the body's changes associated with the development of an egg and the possibility of pregnancy, is generally around 28 days. However, it can vary from 20 to 40 days. In some women, the length of the menstrual cycle can change or become irregular in reaction to stress, weight changes, excessive physical activity or travelling. The cycle begins on the first day of the menstrual period and ends the day before the next period starts. Each cycle has four phases: follicular phase, ovulation, luteal phase and menstrual phase (Fig. 16.1).

Follicular phase

During the follicular phase, the pituitary gland releases follicle-stimulating hormone (FSH), which instructs the ovary to develop between 10 and 20 follicles or groups of cells, each containing an ovum, or immature egg. The hypothalamus in the brain identifies the rising levels of oestrogen caused by the development of the follicles and releases a chemical called gonadotrophin-releasing hormone (GnRH), which initiates release of luteinising hormone (LH) and more FSH from the pituitary. The oestrogen also triggers a spongy thickening of the endometrium, or lining of the uterus, to around 3 millimetres. In normal circumstances only one of the follicles (the graafian follicle) grows into a mature egg, while the others break down and are reabsorbed by the body.

Ovulation

During the first half of the menstrual cycle, the oestrogen levels rise as the pituitary gland produces

Figure 16.1 **The menstrual cycle**

(Lowdermilk & Perry 2006)

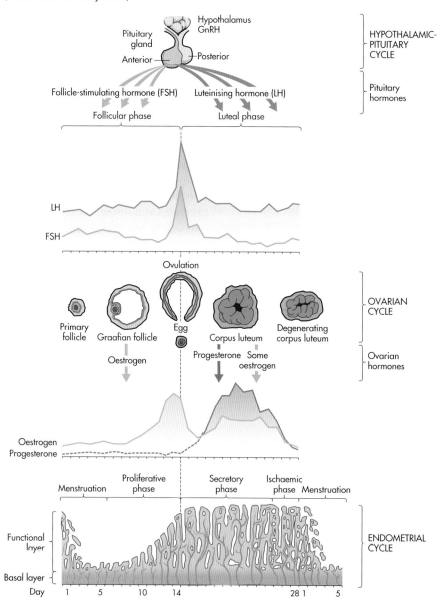

more LH and FSH. The rise in LH causes ovulation, the release of the egg from one of the ovaries. The ovum travels down the fallopian tube, taking about 5 days to reach the uterus if it is fertilised. If it is not fertilised, the ovum will live no longer than 24 hours, and generally between 6 and 12 hours. It will then disintegrate and get reabsorbed.

Luteal phase

The luteal or secretory phase refers to the time when a solid mass called the corpus luteum grows on the surface of the ovary from what is left of the follicle after the egg has been released. The corpus luteum produces hormones, particularly progesterone, which have an important role in preparing the endometrium to accept the fertilised ovum. The increase in progesterone levels also triggers the production of oestrogen by the adrenal glands and suppresses manufacture of FSH and LH. The reduction of these two hormones causes the corpus luteum to then deteriorate and atrophy. In the absence of fertilisation, the progesterone levels continue to fall as the corpus luteum atrophies, initiating breakdown of the endometrial lining leading to menstruation and the start of the next cycle. If the ovum is fertilised, the resulting embryo produces human chorionic gonadotrophin (hCG), which preserves the corpus luteum. hCG is unique to the creation of the embryo and most pregnancy tests look for its presence.

Menstrual phase

Menstruation is the purging of the thickened lining of the endometrium from the body through the vagina. Menstrual fluid contains blood, endometrial cells and mucus. The average length of a menstrual period is 3–7 days, but the length differs from woman to woman.

Female reproductive organs

All the organs of female reproduction are internal except for the vulva (Fig. 16.2).

Vulva – the vulva is the collective name for the external genitalia, consisting of the mons pubis, labia majora, labia minora, clitoris, Bartholin's gland and the perineum. The opening of the urethra is also part of the vulva.

Ovaries – the right and left ovaries are the main female reproductive organs and are located just below the fallopian tubes. Each female infant is born with more than 1,000,000 ovarian follicles, which are small fluid-filled sacs on the outside layer of the ovaries from which the mature ova grow and develop. By the time of menarche, around 40,000 of the follicles remain, with the rest having been absorbed by the body. In addition to producing ova, the ovaries release female hormones (oestrogen and progesterone). The oval-shaped ovaries are situated in the pelvic cavity and are attached to the uterus by ligaments. When a mature ovum bursts out of its follicle around every 28 days, it is picked up by the fimbriae at the end of the fallopian tube and swept down towards the uterus.

Fallopian tubes – after the ovum is released from the ovary and picked up by the fimbriae, it moves to the funnel-shaped end of the fallopian tube called the oviduct. The ovum moves through the fallopian tube through the action of wave-like muscle contractions (peristalsis) and the rhythmic beating of the cilia, microscopic hairs on the walls of the fallopian tubes. The cilia also help spermatozoa swim towards the ovum so that conception (the fertilisation of an ovum with a spermatozoon) occurs most commonly in the part of the fallopian tube closest to the ovary.

Uterus – the uterus is a hollow cavity that plays a vital role in developing a fertilised ovum. The body of the uterus sits low in the pelvic cavity, while above the entrance to the fallopian tubes is the uterine fundus. A narrow passage called the cervix extends from the uterus into the vagina. The uterus has very thick layered walls. The innermost layer is the endometrium, which is where a fertilised egg implants and grows. The muscular middle layer is called the myometrium, and this layer contracts rhythmically during childbirth to help the baby move through the vagina. The outer layer is the perimetrium, a serous membrane that is attached to the peritoneum that lines the organs of the abdominal and pelvic cavities.

Vagina – the vagina is a fibromuscular passage that extends from the cervix to the entrance to the vulva. The vagina accepts semen ejaculated through a male penis during sexual intercourse and provides a path for menstrual blood to leave the body.

Breasts – female breasts are specialised organs located on the anterior chest wall (Fig. 16.3). The main function of the breast is to produce milk for feeding a baby. During puberty, oestrogen and progesterone promote breast growth and maturation. During the final weeks of pregnancy, the breasts start production of milk. Breasts consist of mammary or milk glands (lobules) that produce and supply the milk, lactiferous ducts that transfer the milk from the lobules to the nipple, the nipple and its surrounding pigmented area called the areola (where a baby attaches to suckle), fat and connective tissue.

Figure 16.2 **Female reproductive organs**

(Mosby's Dictionary 2014)

**LATERAL VIEW OF FEMALE REPRODUCTIVE ORGANS
AND ASSOCIATED STRUCTURES**

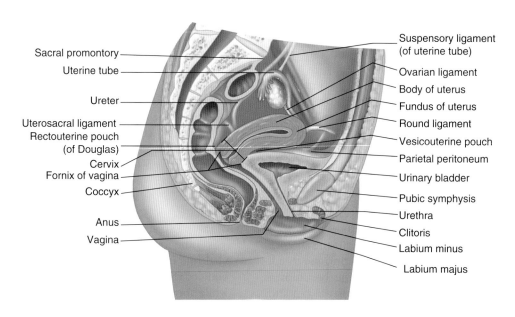

- Sacral promontory
- Uterine tube
- Ureter
- Uterosacral ligament
- Rectouterine pouch (of Douglas)
- Cervix
- Fornix of vagina
- Coccyx
- Anus
- Vagina

- Suspensory ligament (of uterine tube)
- Ovarian ligament
- Body of uterus
- Fundus of uterus
- Round ligament
- Vesicouterine pouch
- Parietal peritoneum
- Urinary bladder
- Pubic symphysis
- Urethra
- Clitoris
- Labium minus
- Labium majus

ANTERIOR VIEW OF FEMALE PELVIC ORGANS

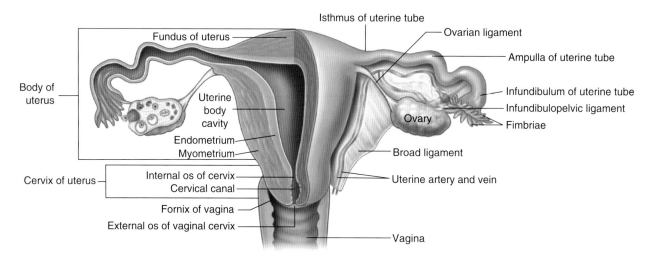

- Isthmus of uterine tube
- Fundus of uterus
- Ovarian ligament
- Ampulla of uterine tube
- Body of uterus
- Uterine body cavity
- Infundibulum of uterine tube
- Infundibulopelvic ligament
- Ovary
- Fimbriae
- Endometrium
- Myometrium
- Broad ligament
- Cervix of uterus
- Internal os of cervix
- Cervical canal
- Uterine artery and vein
- Fornix of vagina
- External os of vaginal cervix
- Vagina

Figure 16.3 Female breast

(Mosby's Dictionary 2014)

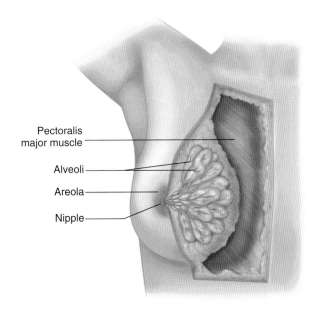

Pectoralis major muscle

Alveoli

Areola

Nipple

PATHOLOGY AND DISEASES

The following section provides a list of common diseases and pathological conditions relevant to the female reproductive system.

Benign conditions

Term	Pronunciation	Definition
fibrocystic disease of the breast	fy-broh-SIS-tik diz-eez	Fibrocystic disease of the breast is a common benign condition characterised by the presence of small sacs of tissue and fluid in the breast. The breasts have a nodular consistency more marked in the upper outer quadrant. Usually there is dull pain and tenderness related to the menstrual cycle, with breast discomfort improving after each menstrual period. Diagnosis is by ultrasound and mammography, but it can be difficult to identify lesions due to the density of breast tissue. In some cases, a surgical biopsy or aspiration may be required to differentiate the condition from breast cancer.
ovarian cyst	oh-VAIR-ee-an sist	An ovarian cyst is a fluid-filled or semi-solid sac located on or in the ovary (Fig. 16.4). The cysts are usually non-neoplastic and can develop any time from puberty to menopause. Often ovarian cysts are asymptomatic, but in some patients, pelvic pain and abdominal swelling may be experienced. There are several different types: follicular, lutein, polycystic and dermoid. If the cysts are not treated, complications may occur. These include amenorrhoea or oligomenorrhoea, secondary dysmenorrhoea or infertility. In some cases, torsion may result in rupture of a cyst. This can lead to peritonitis, intraperitoneal haemorrhage, shock, or even death. Diagnosis is by pelvic examination, ultrasonography and laparoscopy or as an incidental finding during another procedure.

Table continued

Term	Pronunciation	Definition
Figure 16.4 Ovarian cysts Florid cystic endosalpingeosis presenting in an ovarian cyst in a post-menopausal woman (Wong & Lee 2015)		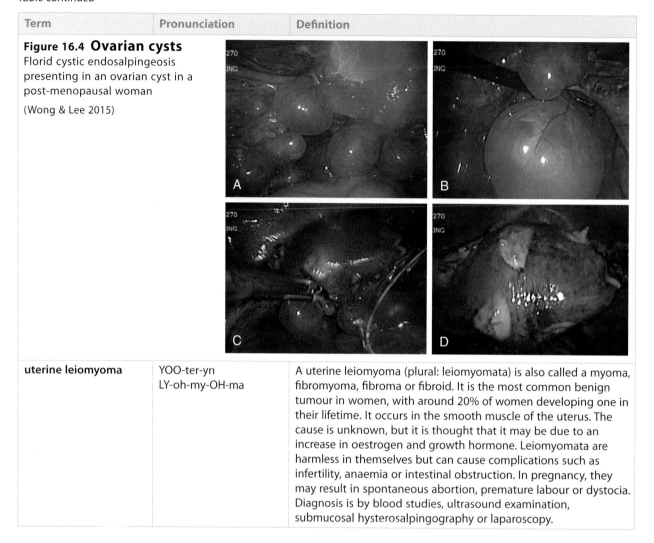
uterine leiomyoma	YOO-ter-yn LY-oh-my-OH-ma	A uterine leiomyoma (plural: leiomyomata) is also called a myoma, fibromyoma, fibroma or fibroid. It is the most common benign tumour in women, with around 20% of women developing one in their lifetime. It occurs in the smooth muscle of the uterus. The cause is unknown, but it is thought that it may be due to an increase in oestrogen and growth hormone. Leiomyomata are harmless in themselves but can cause complications such as infertility, anaemia or intestinal obstruction. In pregnancy, they may result in spontaneous abortion, premature labour or dystocia. Diagnosis is by blood studies, ultrasound examination, submucosal hysterosalpingography or laparoscopy.

Malignant tumours

Term	Pronunciation	Definition
carcinoma of the breast	kah-sin-OH-ma of the brest	Carcinoma of the breast is a malignant tumour of breast tissue. It is one of the leading causes of death in women. The most common type is invasive ductal carcinoma. Other types include inflammatory carcinoma, medullary carcinoma and lobular carcinoma. It is common for carcinoma of the breast to metastasise. Initial spread will be to the axillary lymph nodes, then the chest wall and skin. Secondary spread to brain, bone and other sites can also occur. Breast cancer is often first diagnosed by breast self-examination or mammogram. Diagnosis is confirmed by biopsy – needle core, needle aspiration or surgical specimen.

Table continued

Term	Pronunciation	Definition
carcinoma of the cervix	kah-sin-OH-ma of the SER-viks	Carcinoma of the cervix is a progressive tumour that begins as dysplasia of cervical cells which, without treatment, will become an invasive carcinoma. It is associated with the presence of human papillomavirus (HPV). Cervical cancer is usually asymptomatic in its early stages but is easily detected by a cervical screening test. If diagnosed early, it is curable.
carcinoma of the ovary	kah-sin-OH-ma of the OH-va-ree	Carcinoma of the ovary is a malignant tumour of ovarian tissue. It is sometimes called the 'silent killer' because it is asymptomatic in its early stages and has often metastasised to the liver, pelvis and lungs before any symptoms are experienced. When symptoms do occur, they are non-specific, such as fatigue, lethargy and bloating. Diagnosis is by ultrasound and biopsy of any lesion found.

Other gynaecological disorders

Term	Pronunciation	Definition
cystocele	SIS-toh-seel	A cystocele is a herniation of the urinary bladder into the vagina as a result of trauma or lax pelvic floor muscles and ligaments. Symptoms include urinary frequency, incontinence and pelvic pressure.
endometriosis	en-doh-meet-ree-OH-sis	Endometriosis is a condition where endometrial tissue is found outside the uterus in locations such as the ovaries, fallopian tubes, supporting ligaments, intestine, umbilicus and even, on rare occasions, in the chest cavity. It is caused when portions of menstrual endometrium pass backwards through the lumen of the fallopian tube into the peritoneal cavity during the menstrual cycle. Complications from endometriosis include dysmenorrhoea, pelvic pain, scar tissue, infertility and dyspareunia. Diagnosis is by pelvic examination, ultrasonography and laparoscopy or as an incidental finding during another procedure.
pelvic inflammatory disease	PEL-vik in-FLAM-a-tor-ee diz-eez	Pelvic inflammatory disease is a bacterial infection of the female genital tract that may involve the uterus, ovaries, fallopian tubes and adjacent organs. It usually starts in the vagina often as part of a sexually transmitted infection (e.g. gonorrhoea) and moves up into the uterus, then on to the other organs. Complications include peritonitis, scarring, adhesions, infertility and an increased risk of an ectopic pregnancy.
premenstrual syndrome	pre-MEN-stroo-al SIN-drohm	Premenstrual syndrome is a condition characterised by both physical and emotional manifestations such as irritability, a feeling of depression, headache and breast tenderness. It appears as part of the menstrual cycle, usually a few days before menstruation begins. Severity ranges from mild to debilitating.
toxic shock syndrome (TSS)	TOK-sik shok SIN-drohm	TSS is a severe illness caused by the bacteria *Staphylococcus aureus* or *Streptococcus pyogenes*. It usually only occurs in menstruating women who use tampons. TSS is characterised by high fevers, vomiting, diarrhoea and myalgia, followed by hypotension and potentially shock and death.
rectocele	REK-toh-seel	A rectocele is a herniation of the rectum into the vagina as a result of a weak vaginal wall after pregnancy and childbirth. Symptoms include dyspareunia and difficult defecation.

Table continued

Term	Pronunciation	Definition
uterine prolapse	YOO-ter-yn PRO-laps	A uterine prolapse is a downward displacement of the uterus into the vaginal canal as a result of weakening by vaginal births or a lack of oestrogen after menopause (Fig. 16.5). Chronic constipation and obesity that puts pressure on the pelvic floor can contribute to the prolapse. Symptoms include dyspareunia, frequent urination, protrusion of the uterus/cervix into the vagina and a feeling of heaviness in the pelvis. A complete prolapse is also called a **procidentia** (prok-si-DEN-sha). **Figure 16.5 Uterine prolapse**

TESTS AND PROCEDURES

The following section provides a list of common diagnostic tests and procedures and clinical interventions and surgical procedures that are undertaken for the female reproductive system.

Test/Procedure	Pronunciation	Definition
aspiration	as-pi-RAY-shun	Aspiration is a diagnostic procedure that involves removing fluid from a sac or cavity. For example, aspiration biopsy via a needle can be done of the breast tissue to identify breast disease.
cauterisation	kaw-ter-y-ZAY-shun	Cauterisation is a procedure that involves the destruction of tissue using heat, cold, corrosive chemicals, electricity or laser. It is commonly used to treat cervical dysplasia or erosion.
cervical screening test	ser-VYK-al skree-ning test	The cervical screening test replaced the Papanicolau (Pap) smear in Australia from December 2017. The new screening program is similar to the Pap smear in that a sample of cells is still obtained from the cervix. However, the cervical screening program looks for evidence of HPV infection (which leads to cell changes that cause most forms of cervical cancer) rather than the abnormal cells themselves as in the case of the Pap smear. The new screening process was initiated following the introduction of the HPV vaccination program. If the results of the screening test are normal, subsequent testing is only needed every 5 years.
colposcopy	kol-POS-kop-ee	A colposcopy is a diagnostic procedure that allows for visual examination of the cervix (and vagina) using a colposcope. It is commonly performed as a follow-up procedure when abnormal findings such as dysplasia are found on a Pap smear. It allows for easier identification of the specific areas of the cervical dysplasia.

Table continued

Test/Procedure	Pronunciation	Definition
conisation	ko-ny-ZAY-shun	Also known as a cone biopsy, conisation can be used to diagnose and treat disorders of the cervix. A cone-shaped section of tissue is removed using a laser or scalpel.
contraceptive methods	kon-tra-SEP-tiv meth-odz	Contraceptive or birth control methods can include oral medication, implants or surgical intervention and are all intended to act as a form of fertility control. The methods of contraception include the following:
		• **Depot medroxyprogesterone acetate (DPMA) injections** (dep-poh med-ROK-see-proh-JES-te-rohn ass-e-tate in-JEK-shunz) such as depo-provera and depo-ralovera are fertility control methods that prevent ovulation through the subcutaneous injection of progestogen-like hormones. These are similar to the hormone progesterone produced by the ovaries. The contraceptive effect lasts between 12 and 14 weeks.
		• **Implanon** (IM-plan-on) is a hormone implant containing a progesterone-like hormone. The implant is inserted under the skin and, by gradually releasing the hormone over a period of up to 3 years, prevents ovulation and deters sperm from entering the cervix by thickening the mucus.
		• **Intrauterine device** (in-TRA YOO-ter-yn de-vys) (IUD) is a contraceptive device placed into the uterus. The two types of IUD are copper-containing devices and hormone-containing devices.
		• **Oral contraceptive** (oh-ral kon-trah-SEP-tiv) is a form of fertility control medication that prevents ovulation and thickens the cervical mucus, making it more difficult for sperm to enter the uterus. The lining of the uterus is also changed, making it more difficult for implantation of a fertilised egg.
		• **Tubal ligation** (TYOO-bal ly-GAY-shun) is a procedure for sterilisation performed by clamping, blocking, severing or sealing the fallopian tubes (Fig. 16.6).

Figure 16.6 Tubal ligation
A. A relatively avascular area of the mesosalpinx is identified within the isthmic portion of the tube; **B.** A segment of tube is isolated and removed after double ligation with chromic suture.

(Pfenninger & Fowler 2010)

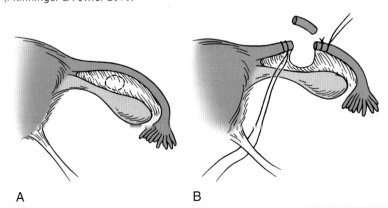

A   B

cryosurgery	KRY-oh-ser-ja-ree	Cryosurgery involves applying extreme cold to destroy tissue. Liquid nitrogen is applied to the tissue using a cryoprobe.
culdocentesis	kul-doh-sen-TEE-sis	A culdocentesis is a procedure to remove fluid from the space just behind the vagina – the cul-de-sac. The fluid is removed by inserting a needle through the vaginal wall.

Table continued

Test/Procedure	Pronunciation	Definition
dilation (dilatation) and curettage (D&C)	dy-LAY-shun (dy-la-TAY-shun) and kyoo-ret-AHJ	A D&C is a surgical procedure that involves widening of the cervix to allow for scraping of the endometrial lining. The cervix is gradually dilated and the lining is gently scraped using a curette. The procedure can be performed to treat conditions such as menorrhagia, incomplete abortion, polyps and uterine infection.
exenteration	ek-SEN-te-RAY-shun	Exenteration is a surgical procedure that involves removing internal organs. Pelvic exenteration involves removing all the organs of the pelvic cavity, including the reproductive organs and the urinary bladder, urethra, rectum and anus (Fig. 16.7).

Figure 16.7 Pelvic exenteration

(Ignatavicius & Workman 2006)

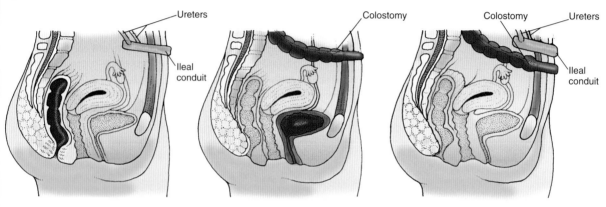

Anterior exenteration is removal of all pelvic organs except the descending colon, rectum, and anal canal.

Posterior exenteration is removal of all pelvic organs except the bladder. A colostomy is created for the passage of faeces.

Total exenteration is removal of all pelvic organs.

Test/Procedure	Pronunciation	Definition
human papilloma virus (HPV) vaccine	hyoo-man pap-il-O-ma vy-rus vak-seen	The HPV vaccine was developed to protect against 9 types of HPV, which account for 90% of all HPV-related cancers of the cervix, anus, vulva, vagina, penis and throat. In Australia the vaccine is offered through schools to both males and females. If the person is under 14 years, they are given two injections 6–12 months apart. If the person is over 15 years or didn't receive the injections 6 months apart, they are given three injections with the doses administered at 0, 2 and 6 months.
hysterectomy	his-ter-EK-tom-ee	A hysterectomy is a surgical procedure to remove the uterus. The different degrees of hysterectomy include: • **total** – removal of uterus and cervix with the fallopian tubes and ovaries preserved • **subtotal** – removal of the body of the uterus, with preservation of the cervix, fallopian tubes and ovaries • **total with a bilateral salpingo-oophorectomy** – removal of the uterus, cervix, fallopian tubes and ovaries. The different surgical approaches for a hysterectomy include: • **vaginal** – the uterus is removed through an incision at the top of the vagina, with no abdominal incisions required • **laparoscopic vaginal** – using a laparoscope, with small incisions into the abdomen, the uterus is detached, then is removed through the vagina • **abdominal** – the uterus is removed through a lower abdominal incision (similar to that performed for a caesarean section).

Table continued

Test/Procedure	Pronunciation	Definition
hysterosalpingography	HIS-ter-oh-sal-ping-GOG-ra-fee	Hysterosalpingography is the process of taking an x-ray examination of a woman's uterus and fallopian tubes using fluoroscopy and contrast medium. The diagnostic procedure allows an evaluation of the shape and structure of the uterus, identification of obstruction of the fallopian tubes and scarring of the uterus or peritoneal cavity.
hysteroscopy	his-ter-OS-kop-ee	A hysteroscopy is a procedure involving a visual examination of the uterine cavity using a hysteroscope. It can be used to identify reasons for infertility, menorrhagia or recurrent miscarriage. It can also be used as a method of approach for removing conditions such as fibroids or polyps.
laparoscopy	lap-ah-ROS-kop-ee	A laparoscopy is a procedure that allows a visual examination of the abdominal and pelvic cavities, via an incision into the abdominal wall and insertion of a scope. Although generally done for diagnostic purposes, it can also be used as a method for treating conditions such as diseased ovaries and for fallopian tube removal.
large loop excision of transformation zone (LLETZ)	larj loop ek-SIZ-shun tranz-for-MAY-shun zone	An LLETZ is performed under the guidance of a colposcope. A fine wire loop charged with electricity is used to shave away abnormal cervical tissue.
mammography	ma-MOG-raf-ee	A mammography is the process of taking a low-dose x-ray image of the breast. It is used as a diagnostic or screening tool to diagnose breast cancer in women with or without symptoms. The Australian Department of Health recommends that women over the age of 50 be screened for breast cancer every 2 years.
mastectomy	mas-TEK-tom-ee	A mastectomy is a surgical procedure that involves the total or partial removal of a breast. The types of mastectomy include: • **simple or total mastectomy** – involves excising the entire breast tissue, overlying skin including the nipple and areola (it does not involve lymph node dissection) • **modified radical mastectomy** – involves excising the breast tissue, the lining of the chest wall muscles and some of the axillary lymph nodes • **radical mastectomy** – involves excising the breast tissue, the chest wall muscle and all of the axillary lymph nodes • **subcutaneous mastectomy** – involves excising breast tissue, preserving the skin and nipple. For those at risk of developing breast cancer due to carrying one of the BRCA gene mutations, a person may decide to undergo prophylactic (or preventative) mastectomies. While most mastectomies performed are for females, they are also performed on men.
ovarian cystectomy	oh-vair-ee-an sis-TEK-tom-ee	An ovarian cystectomy is a surgical procedure that involves removing a cyst on the ovary. The procedure may involve preserving or removing the ovary.
Papanicolaou (Pap) smear (test)	pap-a-NIK-ol-ow smear	A Pap smear is a screening tool used to identify early changes in cervical cells that may lead to cancer. The cells are collected from the cervix and placed (smeared) onto a slide, which is sent for laboratory examination.

Table continued

Test/Procedure	Pronunciation	Definition
pelvic ultrasonography	PEL-vik ul-tra-son-OG-ra-fee	Pelvic ultrasonography is a diagnostic procedure that produces two-dimensional images of the pelvis and its structures. For a pregnant uterus it can be used to determine fetal size, maturity, organ development and fetal and placental position. It can also be used to identify uterine tumours and other pelvic masses.

Exercises

EXERCISE 16.1: LABEL THE DIAGRAM

Using the information provided in this chapter, label the anatomical parts in Fig. 16.8.

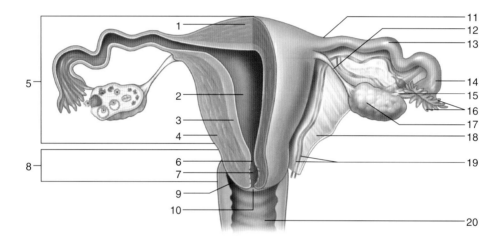

Figure 16.8 Female pelvic organs

(Mosby's Dictionary 2014)

1 _____

2 _____

3 _____

4 _____

5 _____

6 _____

7 _____

8 _____

9 _____

10 _____

11 _____

12 _____

13 _____

14 _____

15 _____

16 _____

17 _____

18 _____

19 _____

20 _____

EXERCISE 16.2: WORD ELEMENT MEANINGS AND WORD BUILDING

Define each combining form, then use the element correctly in a medical term.

Word Element	Meaning	Medical Term
colp/o		
culd/o		
endometri/o		
episi/o		
fer/o		
gynaec/o		
hyster/o		
leiomy/o		
mamm/o		
mast/o		
men/o		
metr/o		
my/o		
oophor/o		
ov/i		
ovari/o		
salping/o		
uter/o		
vagin/o		
vulv/o		

EXERCISE 16.3: CIRCLE THE CORRECT SPELLING

Circle the correctly spelled medical term from the options provided.

meenorrhagia	menorhagia	menorrhagia	mennorhagia
culdoscopy	culdoscoopy	culdoscopee	culldoscopy
mymectomy	myoomectomy	myomectomy	myemectomy
salpingorrhafy	salpingorrhaphy	salpingorhaphy	salpingoorrhaphy
oofoorectomy	ophorectomy	oophorectomy	oopherectomy
histeroscopy	histuroscopy	hystaoscopy	hysteroscopy
rectocele	rectoceel	rectosele	reectocele
hypomenorhoea	hypomenorhea	hypomenorrhea	hypomenorrhoea
endomeetriosis	endomeatriosis	endometriosis	endometreosis
fybromyoma	fibromyoma	fibromioma	fibromyeoma

EXERCISE 16.4: WORD ANALYSIS AND MEANING

Break up the medical terms below into their component parts (prefixes, suffixes, combining forms). Provide the meaning for each word element and each term as a whole.

Example:
amenorrhoea

a = no, not, without, absence of

men/o = menses, menstruation

-rrhoea = discharge, flow

Meaning = discharge or flow of no menses (no menstrual flow or discharge)

1. mastectomy _____

_____

_____

2. menarche _____

_____

_____

3. oligomenorrhoea _____

_____

_____

4. ooblast _____

_____

_____

5. cervicitis _____

_____

_____

6. hymenotomy _____

_____

_____

7. hysterotomy _____

_____

_____

8. mammogram _____

_____

_____

9. metroptosis _____

_____

_____

10. uterosalpingography _____

_____

_____

EXERCISE 16.5: EXPAND THE ABBREVIATIONS

Expand the abbreviations to form correct medical terms.

Abbreviation	Expanded Abbreviation
BSE	
CIN	
CIS	
Cx	
D&C	
DUB	
FSH	
HPV	

Abbreviation	Expanded Abbreviation
HRT	
IUD	
IVF	
LEEP	
LH	
LMP	
PID	
STI	
TAH	
TAHBSO	
TRAM flap	
VAIN	

EXERCISE 16.6: MATCH THE FEMALE REPRODUCTIVE ORGAN WITH ITS DESCRIPTION

Match the female reproductive organ in Column A with its description in Column B.

Column A	Answer	Column B
1. labia		A. fringe-like ends of the fallopian tubes
2. fallopian tube		B. fold of skin in front of the clitoris
3. hymen		C. neck of uterus
4. fundus		D. uterine muscle layer
5. myometrium		E. produce mucus for lubrication of vagina
6. fornix		F. membrane across the opening of the vagina
7. prepuce		G. rounded section of the uterus
8. fimbriae		H. tube to transport ovum from ovary to uterus
9. cervix		I. lip-like folds of skin of the vulva
10. Bartholin's glands		J. deepest part of the vagina

EXERCISE 16.7: APPLYING MEDICAL TERMINOLOGY

Fill in the blank or select the correct medical term.

1. The inner lining of the uterus is called the
   _____.
   a) myometrium
   b) endometrium
   c) fundus
   d) cervix

2. The term meaning painful intercourse is _____.
   a) amenorrhoea
   b) anovulation
   c) dysmenorrhoea
   d) dyspareunia

3. A follicular cyst is found in the _____.
   a) ovary
   b) uterus
   c) vagina
   d) vulva

4. The endoscope used to examine within the vagina is
   called a(n) _____.
   a) hysteroscope
   b) colposcope
   c) laparoscope
   d) proctoscope

5. Which of the following is the term for the pouching of
   the rectum into the vagina?
   a) enterocele
   b) cystocele
   c) urethrocele
   d) rectocele

6. Which of the following is a malignant tumour of
   glandular breast tissue?
   a) amastia
   b) fibrocystic breasts
   c) adenocarcinoma of the breast
   d) hypermastia

7. Which of the following includes removal of all the
   axillary lymph nodes?
   a) radical mastectomy
   b) simple mastectomy
   c) mammoplasty
   d) lumpectomy

8. The ring of colour around the nipple is known as
   _____.
   a) alveoli
   b) areola
   c) vulva
   d) areolia

9. Bleeding after the menstrual cycle has ceased is called
   _____.
   a) premenopausal bleeding
   b) menomenorrhagia
   c) hypomenorrhagia
   d) postmenopausal bleeding

10. _____ is when the uterus 'slips' outwards into
    the vagina and outside the body.
    a) uterine lapse
    b) uterine prolapse
    c) uterine fall
    d) uterine collapse

EXERCISE 16.8: PRONUNCIATION AND COMPREHENSION

Read the following paragraph aloud to practise your pronunciation. Using your textbook and a medical dictionary, find the meanings of the underlined medical terms.

A 48-year-old woman was admitted for a <u>hysteroscopy</u> and <u>dilation and curettage</u> (D&C) because of irregular periods and <u>intermenstrual</u> bleeding – that is, <u>dysfunctional uterine bleeding</u>. She had a Pap smear in July of this year, which had apparently shown <u>atypical squamous cells</u>. She underwent a hysteroscopy with an <u>endometrial biopsy</u>, a D&C, as well as a biopsy of her <u>cervix</u> because of an unusual-looking area on her <u>anterior lip</u>. This identified moderate <u>cervical dysplasia</u> and <u>human papillomavirus</u>. A general <u>anaesthetic</u> was administered (ASA = 1NE). There were no postoperative complications and she was discharged home to be reviewed soon in <u>gynaecology</u> outpatients.

EXERCISE 16.9: CROSSWORD PUZZLE

Complete the puzzle by providing the medical term for each of the clues below.

ACROSS

1. Visual examination of the uterine cavity (12)
4. Downward displacement of the uterus into the vaginal canal (7, 8)
7. Visual examination of the cervix (and vagina) (10)
8. Surgical removal of the uterus (12)
9. A condition where endometrial tissue is found outside the uterus (13)
10. Also known as PMS (12, 8)

DOWN

2. A fluid-filled or semi-solid sac located on or in the ovary (7, 4)
3. A benign condition characterised by the presence of small sacs of tissue and fluid in the breast (11, 7)
5. Removal of fluid from a sac or cavity (10)
6. Removal of fluid from the space just behind the vagina, the cul-de-sac (13)

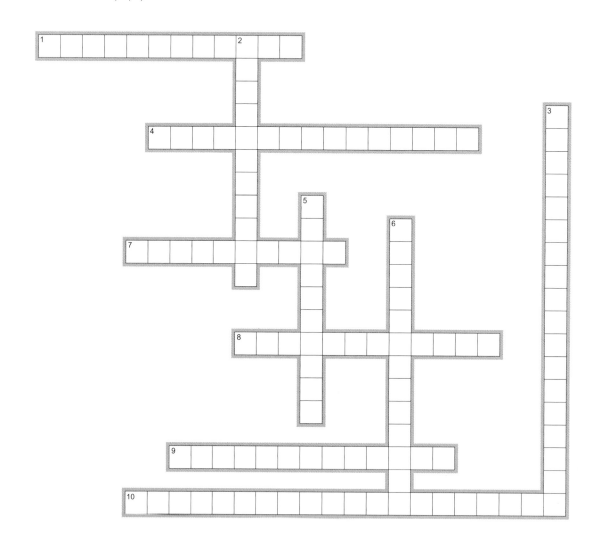

EXERCISE 16.10: ANAGRAMS

Work out each medical term from the jumbled letters below. Then, using the letters in brackets, determine the medical term that matches the description given.

1. nhecemra	__ __ __ __ (__) __ __ __	first menstrual period
2. bliaa	__ __ (__) __ __	lips of the vagina
3. royav	(__) __ __ __ __	almond-shaped organ that produces ova
4. vccteisiir	__ __ __ __ __ __ (__) __ __ __	inflammation of the cervix
5. ltuonoiva	__ __ __ __ __ __ (__) __ __	the release of an ovum
6. raiimfbe	(__) __ __ __ __ __ __ __	finger-like projections on the end of the fallopian tubes
7. praeynuiasd	(__) __ __ __ __ __ __ __ __ __	painful intercourse

Rearrange the letters in brackets to form a word that means 'a benign tumour in the uterus, also called a leiomyoma'.

— — — — — — —

EXERCISE 16.11: DISCHARGE SUMMARY ANALYSIS

Read the discharge summary below and answer the questions.

UNIVERSITY HOSPITAL DISCHARGE SUMMARY	**UR number:** 353637 **Name:** Andrea Preston **Address:** 36 High Street, Mossley **Date of birth:** 31/3/1969 **Sex:** F **Nominated primary healthcare provider:** Dr Patricia Norris
Episode details **Consultant:** Dr Johnstone **Registrar:** Dr Michaelson **Unit:** Gynaecology **Admission source:** Elective **Date of admission:** 5/4/2020	**Discharge details** **Status:** Home **Date of discharge:** 10/4/2020

Reason for admission / Presenting problems: Routine admission for TAH/BSO
Principal diagnosis: Fibroids
Comorbidities: Endometriosis
Previous medical history: Mrs Preston has had bilateral breast malignancies treated with lumpectomies and axillary clearance in the past, and also TCC of the bladder treated by resection. Because her breast malignancies were oestrogen-receptor positive, it was decided to perform a bilateral oophorectomy at the same time as the hysterectomy.
Clinical synopsis: A routine admission for a total abdominal hysterectomy and bilateral salpingo-oophorectomy in a woman with menorrhagia, dyspareunia, endometriosis and uterine fibroids evident on recent laparoscopy. **Complications:** During the postoperative period, she had a low-grade temperature, which appeared to be due to a wound infection. This was treated with oral flucloxacillin.

Clinical interventions:
TAH and BSO performed on 7 April under GA (ASA = 1NE) and an anteverted uterus with a pedunculated fibroid was noted. The ovaries were minimally enlarged with multiple small cysts.

Diagnostic interventions:
Histology showed chronic cervicitis, a proliferative pattern to the endometrium with a fundal glandular cystic endometrial polyp and leiomyomata in the myometrium. Histology of the ovaries showed cortical stromal hyperplasia. MSU and HVS were both clear.

Medications at discharge:
Dixarit for symptomatic relief of any menopausal symptoms.

Ceased medications:

Allergies:

Alerts:

Arranged services:

Recommendations: Review in outpatients in 6 weeks.

Information to patient/relevant parties:

Authorising clinician: Dr Michaelson

Document recipients:
Patient and LMO: Dr Patricia Norris

1. **Expand the following abbreviations as found in the discharge summary above.**

   BSO

   HVS

   MSU

   TAH

   TCC

2. **Explain why Mrs Preston had her ovaries removed at the same time as her hysterectomy.**

3. **Mrs Preston's discharge summary has endometriosis listed as a comorbidity.**

   What is meant by comorbidity?

   What is endometriosis?

   Why is it important to treat endometriosis?

4. **Mrs Preston's principal diagnosis was fibroids.**

   What is the medical term for fibroid?

   What are the common symptoms of fibroids?

   Which of those fibroid-related symptoms did Mrs Preston experience as documented in her discharge summary? Explain what her symptoms mean.

CHAPTER 17
Obstetrics and Neonatology

Contents

OBJECTIVES 401

INTRODUCTION 402

NEW WORD ELEMENTS 402
  Combining forms 402
  Prefixes 403
  Suffixes 403

VOCABULARY 403

ABBREVIATIONS 404

FUNCTIONS AND STRUCTURE RELATED TO OBSTETRICS AND NEONATOLOGY 405
  First trimester 405
  Second trimester 406
  Third trimester 407
  Labour and delivery 407
  Presentation for delivery 408
  Definitions related to obstetrics and neonatology 409

PATHOLOGY AND DISEASES 409
  Pathological conditions and diseases related to obstetrics 410
  Pathological conditions and diseases related to neonatology 411

TESTS AND PROCEDURES 415

EXERCISES 420

Objectives

After completing this chapter you should be able to:

1. state the meanings of the word elements related to obstetrics and neonatology

2. build words using the word elements associated with obstetrics and neonatology

3. recognise, pronounce and effectively use medical terms associated with obstetrics and neonatology

4. expand abbreviations related to obstetrics and neonatology

5. describe the obstetric sequence from conception, through pregnancy, labour, delivery and the puerperium and describe specific issues related to neonatology

6. describe common pathological conditions associated with obstetrics and neonatology

7. describe common laboratory tests and diagnostic and surgical procedures associated with obstetrics and neonatology

8. apply what you have learned by interpreting medical terminology in practice.

Demonstrate your knowledge of obstetrics and neonatology by completing the exercises at the end of this chapter.

INTRODUCTION

Previous chapters in this textbook have discussed specific body systems. This chapter is different in that it does not relate to a specific system. Obstetrics is concerned with the management of childbirth from the mother's perspective. It covers the sequence of pregnancy, labour, delivery and the puerperium. Neonatology is about birth and the first 4 weeks of life from the baby's perspective. Terminology from both aspects is discussed in this chapter. A number of the conditions that may affect the mother or the newborn baby are also discussed in the body system chapters.

NEW WORD ELEMENTS

Here are some word elements related to obstetrics and neonatology. To reinforce your learning, write the meanings of the medical terms in the spaces provided. Use the Glossary of medical terms on page 561 to help you work out the meanings. You may also need to check the meaning in a medical dictionary, but make an attempt yourself first.

Combining forms

Combining Form	Meaning	Medical Term	Meaning of Medical Term
amni/o	amnion, amniotic fluid	amniocentesis	
blast/o	embryonic or developing cell	blastolysis	
cephal/o	head	cephalometry	
chori/o	chorion	chorioamnionitis	
chorion/o		chorionic	
cyes/i	pregnancy	cyesiology	
cyes/o		cyesis	
embry/o	embryo, fetus	embryogenic	
encephal/o	brain	anencephalic	
episi/o	vulva	episiotomy	
fet/o	fetus	fetology	
galact/o	milk	galactopoiesis	
lact/i	milk	lactiferous	
lact/o		lactorrhoea	
mening/o	meninges	meningocele	
nat/i	birth	natimortality	
nat/o		prenatal	
obstetr/o	midwife	obstetrician	
omphal/o	umbilicus	omphalitis	
paed/o	child	paediatric	
part/o	bear, give birth to	parturition	
pelv/i	pelvis	pelvimetry	
pelv/o		pelvocaliectasis	
perine/o	perineum	perineorrhaphy	
placent/o	placenta	placentogram	
puerper/o	childbirth	puerperium	
terat/o	monster, malformed	teratoma	
tox/o	poison, toxin	toxaemia	
troph/o	nourishment, development	trophoblast	
zyg/o	union, joined, fusion	zygogenesis	

Prefixes

Prefix	Meaning	Medical Term	Meaning of Medical Term
ante-	before, forward	antenatal	
con-	together, with	congenital	
dys-	bad, painful, difficult	dystocia	
hyper-	above, excessive	hyperemesis	
macro-	large	macrosomia	
micro-	small	microcephalus	
multi-	many, much	multipara	
neo-	new	neonatal	
nulli-	none	nulligravida	
oligo-	scanty, deficiency, few	oligohydramnios	
oxy-	quick, sharp	oxytocia	
post-	after, behind	postpartum	
primi-	first	primiparous	
pseudo-	false	pseudocyesis	
tetra-	four	tetralogy of Fallot	

Suffixes

Suffix	Meaning	Medical Term	Meaning of Medical Term
-amnios	amnion, amniotic fluid	polyhydramnios	
-blast	embryonic or developing cell	osteoblast	
-cyesis	pregnancy	salpingocyesis	
-gravida	pregnancy	secundigravida	
-icterus	jaundice	kernicterus	
-para	to bear, bring forth	nullipara	
-parous		primiparous	
-partum	childbirth, labour	antepartum	
-rrhexis	rupture	hysterorrhexis	
-schisis	split	gastroschisis	
-tocia	condition of labour, condition of childbirth	eutocia	
-version	to turn	retroversion	

VOCABULARY

The following list provides many of the medical terms used for the first time in this chapter. Pronunciations are provided with each term. As you read the rest of the chapter, make sure you identify each of these terms and understand their meanings.

Term	Pronunciation
abnormal fetal presentation	ab-NOR-mal FEE-tal prez-en-TAY-shun
abortion	a-BOR-shun

Table continued

Term	Pronunciation
amniocentesis	am-nee-oh-sen-TEE-sis
APGAR score	ap-gar score
artificial insemination (AI)	art-e-FISH-al in-sem-in-AY-shun
augmentation of labour	org-men-TAY-shun of LAY-ba
bronchiolitis	BRON-ky-ol-EYE-tis
caesarean section	se-ZAIR-ee-an SEK-shun

Table continued

Term	Pronunciation
chorionic villus sampling	KO-ree-ON-ik VIL-us sam-pling
colic	KOL-ik
Down syndrome	down SIN-drohm
ectopic pregnancy	ek-TOP-ik PREG-nan-see
embryo transfer to uterus	EM-bree-oh tranz-fur to YOO-ter-us
episiotomy	e-PEEZ-ee-o-tom-ee
erythroblastosis fetalis	e-REETH-roh-blah-STOH-sis fee-TAH-lis
fetal monitoring	FEE-tal MON-i-tor-ing
gamete intrafallopian transfer (GIFT)	gam-eet in-tra-fal-O-pee-an tranz-fur
gastroschisis	GAS-troh-shee-sis
haemorrhagic disease of newborn	heem-or-AY-jik dis-eez of nyoo-bawn
hydrocephalus	HY-droh-KEF-a-lus
hyperemesis gravidarum	HY-per-EM-ee-sis grav-i-DAR-um
induction of labour	in-DUK-shun of lay-BA
intracytoplasmic sperm injection (ICSI)	in-tra-syt-o-PLAS-mik sperm in-JEK-shun
intrauterine insemination (IUI)	in-tra-YOO-te-ryn in-sem-in-AY-shun
intrauterine growth retardation	in-tra-YOO-te-ryn growth re-tar-DAY-shun
in vitro fertilisation (IVF)	in VIT-roh fur-til-eye-ZAY-shun
jaundice	JORN-dis
meconium aspiration syndrome	mek-OWN-ee-um as-per-AY-shun SIN-drohm
necrotising enterocolitis	NEK-rot-eye-zing en-ter-o-kol-EYE-tis
neuraxial block	nyoo-RAK-see-al block
oral cleft	o-ral kleft
ovarian hyperstimulation	oh-VAIR-ee-an hy-per-stim-yoo-LAY-shun
ovulation induction	ov-yoo-LAY-shun in-DUK-shun
pelvimetry	pel-VIM-et-ree
phenylketonuria	fen-el-kee-ton-YOO-ree-a
placenta abruptio	pla-SEN-ta ab-RUP-tee-oh
placenta praevia	pla-SEN-ta PREE-vee-a
pre-eclampsia	pre-ek-LAMP-see-a
pyloric stenosis	py-LOR-ik sten-O-sis
respiratory distress syndrome	res-PIR-at-or-ee dis-TRESS SIN-drohm

Table continued

Term	Pronunciation
spina bifida	SPY-na BIF-id-a
transient tachypnoea of newborn	TRANZ-ee-ent tak-ee-NEE-a of NYOO-bawn
transvaginal oocyte retrieval	tranz-vaj-EYE-nal o-o-syt ree-TREE-val
vacuum extraction	VAC-yoom ek-STRAK-shun

ABBREVIATIONS

The following abbreviations are commonly used in the Australian healthcare environment. Because some abbreviations can have more than one meaning, check the context in which the abbreviation is used before assigning a meaning to it.

Abbreviation	Definition
AFP	alpha fetoprotein
AI	artificial insemination
APH	antepartum haemorrhage
ARM	artificial rupture of membranes
ART	assisted reproductive technology/ treatment
ASD	atrial septal defect
BF	breastfeeding
BPD	bronchopulmonary dysplasia
CCS	classical caesarean section
CHD	congenital heart disease
CPD	cephalopelvic disproportion
CTG	cardiotocograph
CVS	chorionic villus sampling
DIC	disseminated intravascular coagulation
EBM	expressed breast milk
ECV	external cephalic version
EDC/EDD	estimated date of confinement/ delivery
FH	fundal height
FHR	fetal heart rate
FTP	failure to progress
G	gravida (the number of times a woman has been pregnant)
hCG	human chorionic gonadotrophin
HELLP	haemolysis, elevated liver enzymes, low platelets
HIE	hypoxic ischaemic encephalopathy
HMD	hyaline membrane disease

Table continued

Abbreviation	Definition
ICSI	intracytoplasmic sperm injection
IUCD	intrauterine contraceptive device
IUI	intrauterine insemination
IUD	intrauterine death
IOL	induction of labour
IUGR	intrauterine growth retardation
IVF	in vitro fertilisation
L&D	labour and delivery
LBW	low birth weight
LGA	large for gestational age
LMP	last menstrual period
L(U)SCS	lower (uterine) segment caesarean section
MROP	manual removal of placenta
NEC	necrotising enterocolitis
NND	neonatal death
NNJ	neonatal jaundice
NVD	normal vaginal (or vertex) delivery
OA	occipitoanterior
O&G	obstetrics and gynaecology
OCP	oral contraceptive pill
OT	occipitotransverse
P	para (the outcome of previous pregnancies)
PDA	patent ductus arteriosus
PET	pre-eclamptic toxaemia
PIH	pregnancy-induced hypertension
POC	products of conception
(P)OP	(persistent) occipitoposterior
PPH	postpartum haemorrhage
PPROM	persistent (or preterm) premature rupture of membranes
PROM	premature rupture of membranes
RPOC	retained products of conception
RDS	respiratory distress syndrome
SGA	small for gestational age
SIDS	sudden infant death syndrome
SROM	spontaneous rupture of membranes
SUDI	sudden unexpected death in infancy
SVD	spontaneous vaginal delivery
TOL	trial of labour
TOP	termination of pregnancy
TTN	transient tachypnoea of newborn
VBAC	vaginal birth after caesarean

Table continued

Abbreviation	Definition
VE	vaginal examination
	vacuum (or ventouse) extraction
VSD	ventricular septal defect

FUNCTIONS AND STRUCTURE RELATED TO OBSTETRICS AND NEONATOLOGY

Conception, or the beginning of pregnancy, occurs when there is a joining of the gametes – 23 chromosomes from the male parent and 23 from the female parent – in a process called fertilisation. When a female ovulates at about the midway point in her menstrual cycle, the ovum moves into the fallopian tube where it may meet spermatozoa ejaculated from a male. When the ovum is released and there are spermatozoa in the fallopian tube, a pregnancy results in about 25% of cases. The spermatozoon produces enzymes that allow it to channel into the ovum. A number of strong spermatozoa may enter the outer lining of the ovum, but once one spermatozoon reaches the inner layers, a chemical reaction causes the ovum to become impenetrable to other spermatozoa. The plasma from both the ovum and spermatozoon join and the fertilisation occurs. The zygote, as the fertilised ovum is called, then travels down the fallopian tube to the uterus where it implants into the uterine wall and begins to grow through a process of cell division, replication and specialisation.

Normally only one ovum is released at a time. However, non-identical twins, triplets or other multiples may be conceived if two or more ova are released and fertilised at the same time. Release of multiple ova is an inherited trait, so that non-identical twins are said to 'run in the family'. Identical twins can only occur when a single fertilised ovum splits into two developing fetuses. It is not known why this occurs, but the occurrence is less common than conceiving non-identical twins.

A normal pregnancy lasts between 37 and 42 weeks. The number of weeks is calculated from the first day of a woman's last menstrual period. Typically, the pregnancy is divided into three trimesters, each of which has a different role in the growth and development of the fetus.

First trimester
The first trimester starts at the time of conception and lasts for 12 weeks. Within a few hours of conception, the fertilised ovum, or **zygote,** divides into two identical

cells, then into four, then eight and so on. By the fifth day of life, these identical cells start to differentiate and prepare to carry out their own specialised functions as different organs and parts of the body. During this period, the developing fetus is called a **blastocyst** and is nourished by a yolk sac. The outside of the developing blastocyst divides into two layers, an outer layer (the chorion) grows villi that infiltrate the uterine endometrium and form the beginning of the placenta. The inner layer or amnion becomes the amniotic sac, which fills with amniotic fluid to create a protective temperature-controlled environment. At this stage, usually by day 10–12, the developing blastocyst is called an **embryo** (Fig. 17.1).

By around day 20 the embryo is about 1.5 millimetres in length and has a regular heartbeat, although the heart will not be fully developed until about the 10th week after conception. Its spinal cord and brain begin to form and buds of arms and legs appear. From the end of the eighth week the developing embryo is called a **fetus**. All of its organs are present and growing, although they remain immature.

The yolk sac begins to be absorbed by the maternal body as the placenta is formed. The placenta connects the mother and developing fetus via the umbilical cord, which has two arteries and one vein that perfuse nutrients and oxygen between mother and fetus and remove waste products from the fetus. The placenta also secretes the hormone human chorionic gonadotrophin (hCG), which instructs the corpus luteum to continue to release oestrogen and progesterone to maintain the endometrial lining, allowing the uterus

to grow and expand. It also begins the process of maternal breast development, the change in colour of the areola and nipples and lactation. The presence of hCG in the blood or urine is indicative of pregnancy.

During this period of rapid fetal development, the mother may feel tired as her body works to produce sufficient blood to nurture the growing fetus. Another symptom of pregnancy for some women is hyperemesis gravidarum, or 'morning sickness', which is a reaction to the hormones being released to manage the pregnancy. The threat of miscarriage is most common in these early weeks of pregnancy.

Second trimester

The 13th to 28th weeks of pregnancy are known as the second trimester. The growing fetus has all of its organs and this is the time of maturation and growth. In Australia, if a baby is born alive or still born at any time after the 20th week, the birth must be registered with a Registry of Births, Deaths and Marriages, although babies born earlier than 24 weeks are less likely to survive. Prior to the 20th week, a fetus that is not alive at birth is regarded as a miscarriage.

During the second trimester, the fetus gains about three-quarters of its total body weight. The fetus may be felt to move as it floats around in its amniotic fluid. The fetal heartbeat can be auscultated. The mother's breasts may leak colostrum, a creamy yellow fluid that is created in the lead-up to breast milk.

The fetus has translucent skin that appears wrinkly and fine. The blood vessels under the skin give the fetus a reddish-purple appearance. It does not yet have a

Figure 17.1 The uterus of a pregnant woman

(Based on LaFleur Brooks 2005)

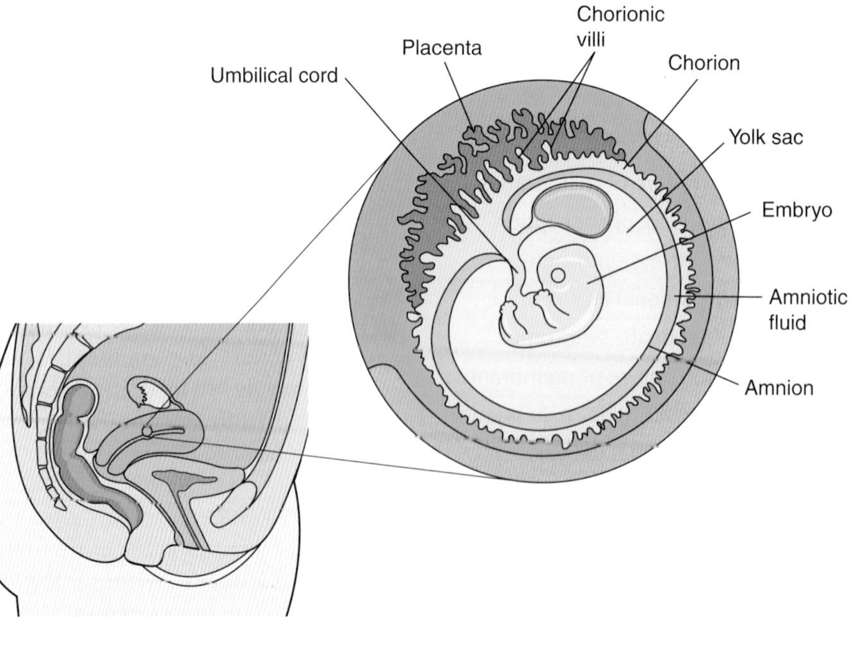

layer of subdermal fat but is covered with a fine layer of hair called lanugo. This is generally shed in the weeks before birth. During the latter part of the trimester, the body is covered in a thick wax-like material called the vernix, which protects it from the effects of its watery environment. At about 24 weeks the lungs start to produce surfactant, a substance that coats the inside of the lungs and assists breathing when the baby is born.

Third trimester

The third trimester begins at the end of the 28th week of pregnancy and lasts until delivery. These final weeks are the period in which the fetus grows and its organs mature in preparation for life apart from its mother (Fig. 17.2). The bone marrow begins production of its own blood supply and the liver stores iron delivered from the mother. The lungs are fully mature at about 36 weeks. The fetus does not grow very much in length

Figure 17.2 **Lateral view of developing pregnancy**

(Based on Stoy et al 2007)

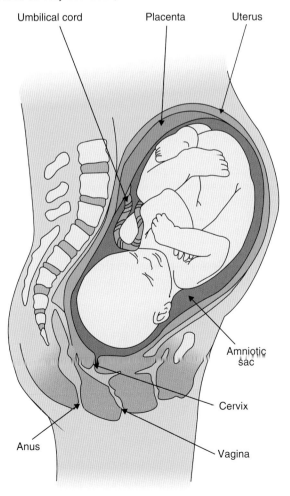

Umbilical cord   Placenta   Uterus

Amniotic sac

Cervix

Anus

Vagina

in the latter part of this trimester but puts on weight at a rate of about 230 grams per week.

The placenta now covers about one-third of the uterus and processes approximately 12 litres of blood every hour. The mother may experience Braxton Hicks contractions, although these are not a sign of true labour. About midway through this trimester, the fetus moves into position for birth, typically head down. When the head descends into the pelvic area, this is known as engagement. An Australian or New Zealand baby born at term weighs about 3300 grams on average and is approximately 50 centimetres in length from head to toe.

Only about 5% of all babies arrive on their 'due date' and the length of pregnancy differs from woman to woman.

Labour and delivery

There are three possible signs that a woman has gone into labour. The first of these is rupture of the membranes and leakage of amniotic fluid. About 25% of all deliveries begin this way.

The second is a slow beginning of contractions, which gradually become stronger and more frequent. The interval between contractions shortens from 20 to 5 minutes. The hormone oxytocin is responsible for the uterine contractions.

A 'show' is the third sign that labour has begun. It refers to the discharge of a small amount of blood and expulsion of the mucus plug from the uterine cervix.

As labour progresses it moves through three stages. Stage one of labour is when the cervix thins and softens and dilates to about 10 centimetres to accommodate delivery of the baby. The beginning of this stage is known as the latent phase and can occur over hours or days or even weeks. The active part of the stage occurs as the contractions become stronger and more painful and are closer together, as the cervix dilates to about 7 centimetres. The last hour or so of stage one occurs as the contractions become stronger and closer together. This is caused by the tightening and relaxation of the uterine muscles, which begin in the upper segment of the uterus and move in a spiral direction towards the lower segment. This is known as the transition phase as the cervix dilates to its greatest width of around 10 centimetres. The duration of this phase differs but is typically about 8 hours in nulliparous women and about 4 hours in women who have previously given birth.

The second stage of labour occurs when the cervix is fully dilated and ends when the baby is born. The contractions are frequent and regular and the urge to push appears with the advent of each contraction. The baby's head moves through the vaginal canal. The point when it becomes visible is called crowning. As the head emerges, the rest of the body turns and slips out. The second stage typically lasts between 15 minutes and an hour (Fig. 17.3).

The third stage of labour is the time from delivery of the baby to expulsion of the placenta. The uterus contracts and pushes the placenta out of the vagina. The umbilical cord may be clamped or left to close naturally.

Presentation for delivery

During pregnancy, the developing fetus may move around in the amniotic sac and may change its position frequently. However, during the final few weeks it determines the most appropriate presentation to facilitate delivery. The term presentation refers to the position of the fetus as it moves into the birth canal ready for delivery. The fetus' position is also described in terms of its 'lie'. This describes the relationship between the long axis of the fetus and the long axis of the mother.

The majority of babies are born in the vertex position – in other words, they are positioned head down with the head flexed so that the occiput or

back of the head presents anteriorly facing the spine and the chin is tucked in towards the chest. The position may be described as left occipitoanterior or right occipitoanterior, depending on the position of the occiput in relation to the mother's pelvis. This is the easiest path around the maternal pelvic curve for delivery. In cases where the occiput remains posterior, instruments may be required to assist the birth. This is known as a persistent occipitoposterior presentation (POP).

If the head is extended rather than flexed, the face, chin or forehead presents first. Because this means that the smallest part of the head is not leading the way, it may be necessary for obstetric intervention such as forceps or vacuum extraction.

In about 5% of all births, the presentation of the baby is not vertex. A breech presentation occurs when the feet or buttocks are the presenting part, not the occiput (Fig. 17.4). Of all breech presentations, frank breech occurs in 50–70% of occurrences. This is where the hips are flexed and the knees extended. A complete breech presentation, where both hips and knees are flexed, occurs in a further 5–10% of breech births. Footling or incomplete breech presentations occur in 10–30% of breech deliveries, with one or both hips extended or one or both feet presenting.

In a breech position, it may be possible for a vaginal birth to occur, with or without the use of instrumentation, but many women opt for a caesarean section.

A fetus that is lying horizontally across the maternal uterus may present shoulder, trunk or arm first. This is relatively uncommon and generally results in an instrumental or caesarean birth.

A fetus positioned for delivery is also described in terms of its 'station' or position within the birth canal. The station is the relationship between the presenting part of the fetus and the area of the mother's pelvis called the ischial spines. The ischial spines are the

Figure 17.3 **Process of labour and delivery**

(Moore & Persaud 2008)

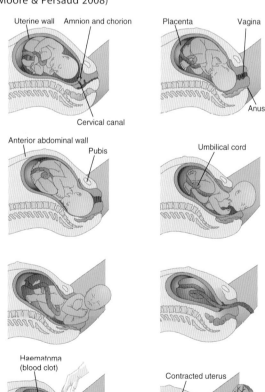

Figure 17.4 **Breech presentation**

(Slone McKinney et al 2000)

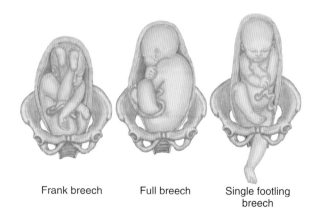

Frank breech   Full breech   Single footling breech

narrowest part of the pelvis and are used as the point for measuring progress of the delivery. If the presenting part of the fetus lies above the ischial spines, it is reported at a station using a negative number from −1 to −5 centimetres. If the presenting part lies below the ischial spines, the station is a positive number from +1 to +5. The fetus is said to be 'engaged' in the pelvis when it is parallel with the ischial spines at 0 centimetres.

Definitions related to obstetrics and neonatology

The World Health Organization publishes definitions relevant to obstetrics and neonatology in the *International Statistical Classification of Diseases and Related Health Problems* (ICD-11). The purpose of these definitions is to standardise the way that obstetric events are counted (see: https://icd.who.int/icd11refguide/en/index.html #2.28.4StandardsAndReporting|standards-and-reporting-requirements-for-mortality-in-perinatal-and-related-periods|c2-28-4).

Live birth

Live birth is the complete expulsion or extraction from its mother of a product of conception, irrespective of the duration of the pregnancy, which, after such separation, breathes or shows any other evidence of life such as beating of the heart, pulsation of the umbilical cord or definite movement of voluntary muscles, whether or not the umbilical cord has been cut or the placenta is attached; each product of such a birth is considered liveborn.

Fetal death (deadborn fetus)

Fetal death is death prior to the complete expulsion or extraction from its mother of a product of conception, irrespective of the duration of pregnancy; the death is indicated by the fact that after such separation the fetus does not breathe or show any other evidence of life such as beating of the heart, pulsation of the umbilical cord or definite movement of voluntary muscles.

Birth weight

The first weight of the fetus or newborn obtained after birth.

LOW BIRTH WEIGHT

Less than 2500 g (up to and including 2499 g).

VERY LOW BIRTH WEIGHT

Less than 1500 g (up to and including 1499 g).

EXTREMELY LOW BIRTH WEIGHT

Less than 1000 g (up to and including 999 g).

Gestational age

The duration of gestation is measured from the first day of the last normal menstrual period. Gestational age is expressed in completed days or completed weeks (e.g. events occurring 280–286 completed days after the onset of the last normal menstrual period are considered to have occurred at 40 weeks of gestation).

PRE-TERM

Less than 37 completed weeks (less than 259 days) of gestation.

TERM

From 37 completed weeks to less than 42 completed weeks (259–293 days) of gestation.

POST-TERM

42 completed weeks or more (294 days or more) of gestation.

Perinatal period

The perinatal period commences at 22 completed weeks (154 days) of gestation (the time when birth weight is normally 500 g) and ends 7 completed days after birth.

Neonatal period

The neonatal period commences at birth and ends 28 completed days after birth. Neonatal deaths (deaths among live births during the first 28 completed days of life) may be subdivided into *early neonatal deaths*, occurring during the first 7 days of life and *late neonatal deaths*, occurring after the seventh day but before 28 completed days of life.

PATHOLOGY AND DISEASES

The following section provides a list of common diseases and pathological conditions relevant to obstetrics and neonatology.

Pathological conditions and diseases related to obstetrics

Term	Pronunciation	Definition
abnormal fetal presentation	ab-NOR-mal FEE-tal prez-en-TAY-shun	The normal fetal presentation is cephalic, with the occiput as the leading part. Sometimes other body parts such as the feet, buttocks, a shoulder, an arm or a combination of more than one of these will present first, meaning that the delivery is more difficult. A caesarean section may be required for certain presentations.
abortion	a-BOR-shun	An abortion is the expulsion of the fetus from the uterus before viability, usually before 20 weeks' gestation or when the fetus weighs less than 400 grams. A **spontaneous abortion** is the termination of a pregnancy that occurs naturally. It is commonly called a **miscarriage.** It may be either complete (all products of conception are expelled) or incomplete (some products of conception remain in the uterus and must be removed by dilation and curettage). A **threatened abortion** occurs when there is uterine bleeding with the threat of miscarriage. A **missed abortion** occurs when the fetus has died in utero but has not been expelled after death. A woman who has three or more consecutive pregnancies that end in spontaneous abortion is termed a **habitual aborter.**
ectopic pregnancy	ek-TOP-ik PREG-nan-see	An ectopic pregnancy occurs when a fertilised egg implants outside the uterus. The most common site is the fallopian tubes. However, ectopic pregnancies can also occur in the ovary, abdominal cavity, wall of the colon or cervix. An ectopic pregnancy is often caused by hormonal factors or an abnormality in the fallopian tubes that blocks or slows the movement of the fertilised egg to the uterus. This type of pregnancy is generally not viable or constitutes a danger to the mother and needs to be surgically removed.
hyperemesis gravidarum	hy-per-EM-e-sis grav-ee-DAH-rum	Hyperemesis gravidarum is a pregnancy-related condition characterised by excessive vomiting and nausea that can lead to severe dehydration in both the mother and fetus.
placenta abruptio	pla-SEN-ta ab-RUP-tee-oh	Placenta abruptio is the premature detachment of a normally located placenta from the uterine wall prior to delivery of the fetus (Fig. 17.5). It can occur as a result of a direct injury. Other risk factors include hypertension, maternal diabetes, multiple pregnancies and an older mother, but usually no cause is found. Symptoms include severe haemorrhage, abdominal pain and contractions. It is considered an obstetric emergency and requires close monitoring of the mother and fetus. Total bed rest is indicated and a caesarean section will be performed when safe to do so.
placenta praevia	pla-SEN-ta PREE-vee-a	Placenta praevia occurs when the placenta is attached to the lower section of the uterus and covers all or part of the opening to the cervix (Fig. 17.5). As the fetus grows, stress is put on the placenta. This can lead to sudden vaginal bleeding that often occurs near the end of the second trimester or beginning of the third trimester. This bleeding can be severe and can be life threatening to the mother. Total bed rest is indicated and a caesarean section will generally be performed when the fetus is viable.

Table continued

Term	Pronunciation	Definition
Figure 17.5 Types of placenta abruptio and placenta praevia		

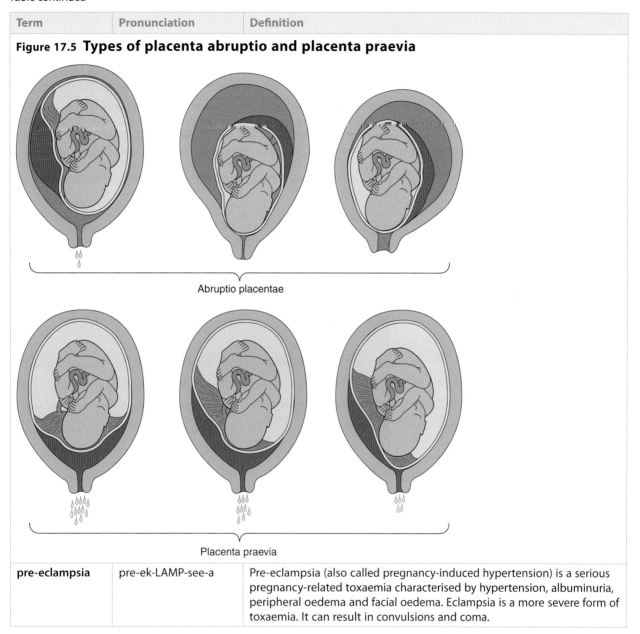

Abruptio placentae

Placenta praevia

Term	Pronunciation	Definition
pre-eclampsia	pre-ek-LAMP-see-a	Pre-eclampsia (also called pregnancy-induced hypertension) is a serious pregnancy-related toxaemia characterised by hypertension, albuminuria, peripheral oedema and facial oedema. Eclampsia is a more severe form of toxaemia. It can result in convulsions and coma.

Pathological conditions and diseases related to neonatology

Term	Pronunciation	Definition
bronchiolitis	BRON-ky-ol-EYE-tis	Bronchiolitis is a viral condition that occurs when the bronchioles, the smallest airways in the lungs, are infected. This causes them to fill with mucus and to swell, making breathing difficult. About one-third of all babies suffer from bronchiolitis during their first year of life.
colic	KOL-ik	Colic is the term given to babies who cry for several hours each day for no apparent reason. Generally manifesting in the first 4 months of age, colic affects about one-third of all babies and often occurs in the late afternoon or early evening period. The baby appears to be suffering from abdominal pain, frowning and grimacing with a red face and inconsolable crying and screaming. The baby seems to recover spontaneously and suffers no long-term effects.

Table continued

Term	Pronunciation	Definition
Down syndrome	down sin-drohm	Also known as trisomy 21, Down syndrome is a chromosomal abnormality that results in distinctive physical abnormalities such as sloping forehead, flat nose, low-set ears and stunted growth as well as mild to severe mental retardation. It occurs more often in babies of older mothers.
erythroblastosis fetalis	e-REETH-roh-blah-STOH-sis fee-TAH-lis	Erythroblastosis fetalis is a condition resulting in the destruction (haemolysis) of erythrocytes in a newborn. It is due to an incompatibility between the baby's blood and mother's blood occurring when the baby has Rh-positive blood and the mother has Rh-negative blood. It is also caused by an ABO incompatibility. It may be treated by an in-utero blood transfusion. Erythroblastosis fetalis is also known as haemolytic disease of the newborn.
gastroschisis	GAS-troh-shee-sis	Gastroschisis is a congenital abnormality that involves a defect on one side of the umbilical cord (Fig. 17.6). This results in failure of the abdominal wall to close as the fetus develops, causing protrusion of the abdominal organs. **Figure 17.6 Gastroschisis in a newborn** (Moore et al 2000) 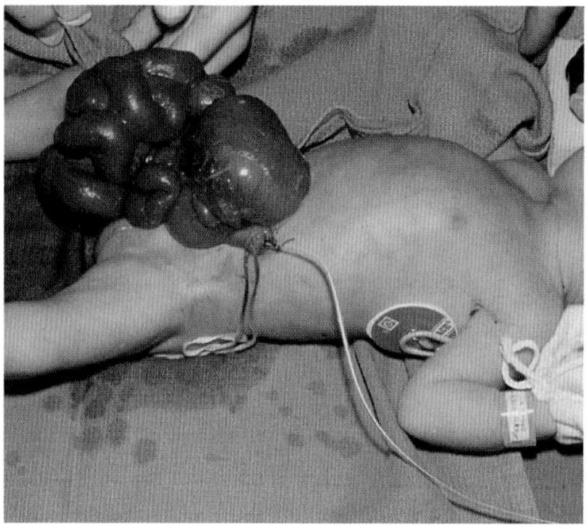
haemorrhagic disease of newborn (vitamin K deficiency syndrome)	hem-or-RAY-jik dis-eez of nyoo-bawn	Haemorrhagic disease of the newborn (vitamin K deficiency syndrome) is a condition causing blood coagulation problems caused by a lack of vitamin K. As a result, there is an increased risk of haemorrhage, most commonly in the gastrointestinal tract, mucosal and cutaneous tissue and the umbilical stump. Most newborns are given a prophylactic dose of vitamin K shortly after delivery.
hydrocephalus	HY-droh-KEF-a-lus	Hydrocephalus is an abnormal build-up of cerebrospinal fluid in the ventricles in the brain (Fig. 17.7). This causes the sutures in the cranial bones to separate, resulting in an enlarged head. Insertion of a shunt to drain the excess fluid is required to prevent the development of neurological complications. The shunt redirects the flow of cerebrospinal fluid from the central nervous system to another area of the body (commonly the abdomen), where it can be absorbed as part of the normal circulatory process.

Table continued

Term	Pronunciation	Definition
		Figure 17.7 Fetus with severe hydrocephalus (Carlson 2004)
intrauterine growth retardation (IUGR)	in-tra-YOO-te-ryn growth re-tar-DAY-shun	IUGR is the term given to a lack of growth of the fetus compared with that expected in the population. This may be due to maternal causes such as a lack of adequate nutrition, alcohol or drug use, smoking, conditions such as hypertension, diabetes and anaemia or lack of sufficient oxygen supply to the baby. It may also be caused by pre-eclampsia, multiple pregnancy, intrauterine infection or due to a congenital abnormality in the baby.
jaundice	JORN-dis	Jaundice is a yellow colouring of the skin and sclera caused by raised levels of bilirubin in the blood of the neonate. It may be due to prematurity, rhesus incompatibility or biliary obstruction.
meconium aspiration syndrome	mek-OWN-ee-um as-per-AY-shun SIN-drohm	Meconium is a form of fetal faeces made up of materials such as intestinal epithelial cells, lanugo, mucus, amniotic fluid, bile and water that the infant ingests while in utero. Although meconium is generally excreted in the first few days of life, it may be eliminated into the amniotic fluid during delivery, causing fetal distress when the baby inhales it. When the baby is born, it shows signs of respiratory distress such as a low APGAR score, rapid or difficult breathing, cyanosis, slow heartbeat and a barrel-shaped chest.
necrotising enterocolitis	NEK-rot-eye-zing en-ter-oh-kol-EYE-tis	Necrotising enterocolitis is a condition seen in premature babies that causes intestinal ischaemia. It occurs most commonly in the right colon, caecum, terminal ileum and appendix, but the entire gastrointestinal tract may be affected. No definitive cause has yet been identified and the condition results in a significant rate of mortality.
oral cleft	o-ral kleft	Oral cleft is a collective term for a group of developmental disorders that include cleft lip, cleft palate and combination cleft lip and palate (Fig. 17.8). The actual cause of oral clefts is not known, but environmental factors and genetic influences are believed to play a part. In a cleft lip, the lip does not join completely during fetal development. In a cleft palate, the roof of the mouth does not fuse completely leaving an open space or cleft. Cleft lip and cleft palate often occur together and can be either on one side of the mouth (unilateral) or both sides (bilateral). Usually there is only involvement of soft tissues, but in more severe cases bone can also be involved. Oral clefts occur in approximately one in 600 live births. Initially treatment will involve special feeding techniques until the baby is old enough for surgery. A cleft lip is usually surgically repaired at 3–6 months of age and a cleft palate at around 9–12 months of age, before the child starts to speak. Subsequent speech therapy is often necessary.

Table continued

Term	Pronunciation	Definition

Figure 17.8 **Oral clefts**

(Wang et al 2014)

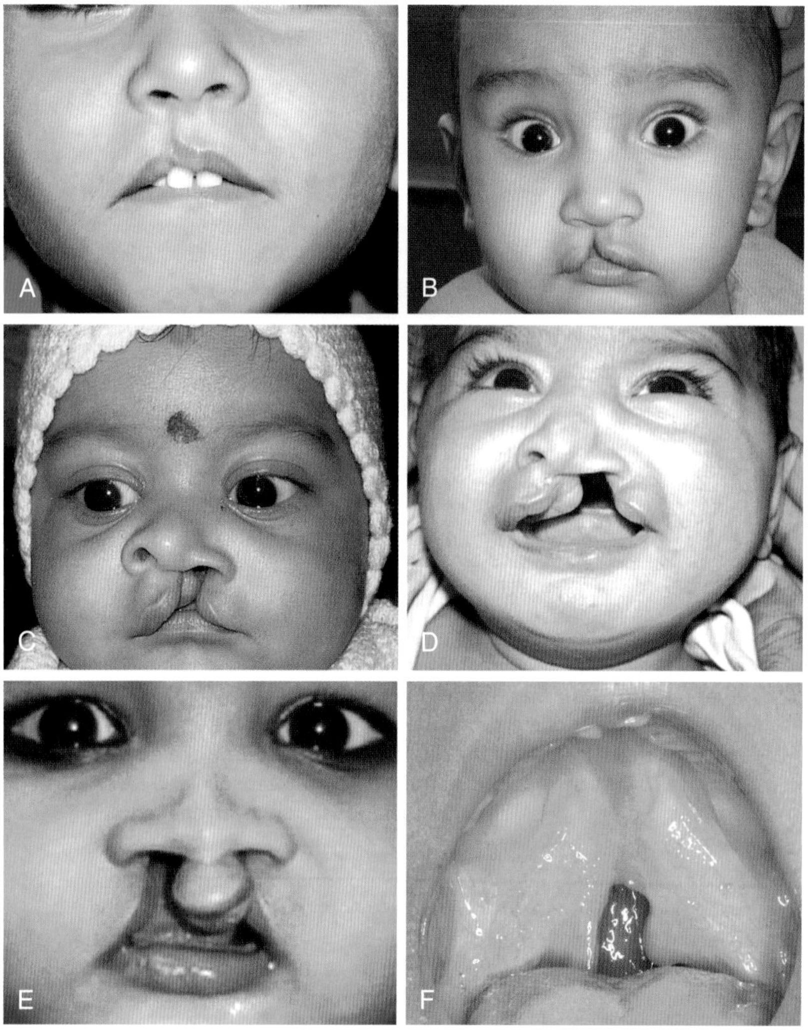

pyloric stenosis	py-LOR-ik sten-O-sis	Pyloric stenosis is a congenital narrowing of the pyloric sphincter that results in obstruction so that food cannot flow into the duodenum. Babies with this condition will have projectile vomiting.
respiratory distress syndrome (RDS)	res-PIR-a-tor-ee dis-TRESS SIN-drohm	Also called hyaline membrane disease, RDS occurs most frequently in premature babies. It is due to a lack of surfactant (a protein lubricant) in the lungs, causing them to collapse. When a fetus must be delivered prematurely, the likelihood of RDS occurring can be reduced by giving betamethasone to the mother for at least 24 hours before delivery to stimulate the fetus' production of surfactant.
spina bifida	SPY-na BIF-id-a	Spina bifida is a congenital malformation of the vertebral column that occurs when there is an incomplete closure of the neural tube during fetal development (Fig. 17.9). This results in a herniation of the meninges and/or spinal cord through the gap in the bones. The term for this is meningocele if the meninges herniate or myelomeningocele if both the meninges and spinal cord are affected.

Table continued

Term	Pronunciation	Definition

Figure 17.9 Spina bifida

(Thompson 2014)

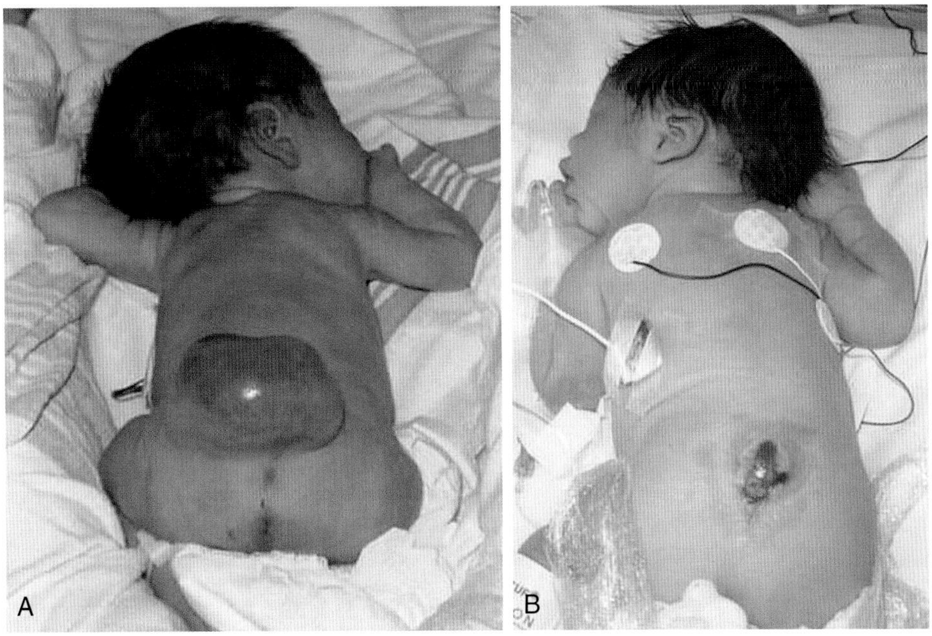

A   B

transient tachypnoea of newborn (TTN)	TRANZ-ee-ent tak-ee-NEE-a of NYOO-bawn	TTN is a common cause of respiratory distress seen soon after delivery. It is generally caused by retained fluid in the baby's lung, causing rapid breathing. It is generally treated with oxygen therapy and resolves within 48 hours.

TESTS AND PROCEDURES

The following section provides a list of common diagnostic tests and procedures and clinical interventions and surgical procedures that are undertaken for obstetrics and neonatology.

Test/Procedure	Pronunciation	Definition
abortion	a-BAW-shun	An abortion is the medical term for the intentional termination of a pregnancy before fetal viability. An abortion can be performed for non-medical or social reasons. It may also be a therapeutic procedure, generally performed for fetal abnormalities or when there are concerns for the mother's health if the pregnancy continues. Methods of abortion include surgical (D&C, vacuum aspiration) or medical (administration of drugs or stimulation of uterine contractions by injection of saline into the amniotic cavity). The legal status and prevalence of abortions differs among different cultural and religious groups.

Table continued

Test/Procedure	Pronunciation	Definition
amniocentesis	am-nee-oh-sen-TEE-sis	Amniocentesis is a diagnostic procedure that involves aspiration of fluid from the amniotic sac for laboratory examination (Fig. 17.10). The procedure can assist in identifying conditions such as chromosomal abnormalities in the fetus. **Figure 17.10 Amniocentesis** 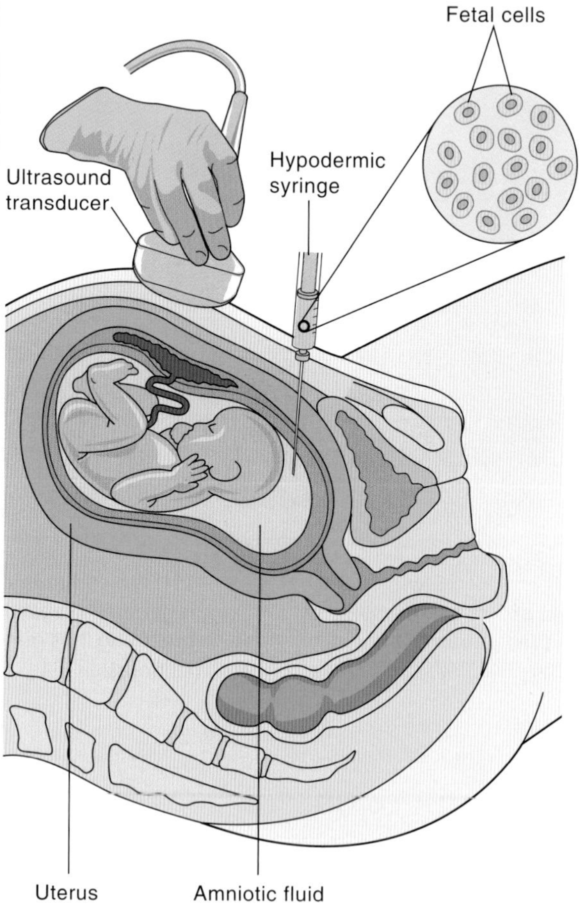
APGAR score	AP-gar scaw	The APGAR test is the first test given to a newborn and stands for Activity, Pulse, Grimace, Appearance and Respiration. A score between 0 and 2 (2 being the highest) is given to each of these five factors. The score is then added together to give a total out of 10. The test will be done at 1 and 5 minutes post-delivery and gives a summary measure of the health of the newborn.
assisted reproductive technology/treatment (ART)		ART is a collective term that refers to treatments for infertility. As well as potentially using ova or spermatozoa from the infertile couple, ART can also involve the use of donor eggs, donor spermatozoa or previously frozen embryos. ART includes a wide range of treatments, some of which are discussed below.
– embryo transfer to uterus	EM-bree-o tranz-fur to YOO-ter-us	An embryo transfer to uterus is part of an IVF procedure. In IVF, ova are retrieved from the woman then fertilised with spermatozoa from her partner or a donor. The resulting embryos are kept in culture media in the laboratory until required for transfer. The embryo transfer to uterus stage involves placing one or more embryos into the female with the intent of establishing a pregnancy. A soft catheter is loaded with the embryos, and inserted through the cervical canal into the uterine cavity. The contents of the catheter are deposited into the uterus.

Table continued

Test/Procedure	Pronunciation	Definition
– gamete intrafallopian transfer (GIFT)	gam-eet in-tra fall-O-pee-an tranz-fur	GIFT is a form of reproductive technology that involves retrieving an oocyte and placing it in the fallopian tube. Spermatozoa are also placed in the fallopian tube at the time of the transfer to allow for fertilisation. GIFT is not commonly used anymore. However, for women with healthy fallopian tubes it is an alternative treatment option if they prefer not to use IVF.
– intracytoplasmic sperm injection (ICSI)	in-tra-syt-o-PLAS-mik sperm in-JEK-shun	ICSI is used to improve the chances of fertilisation occurring where there are issues with spermatozoa such as motility and ability to penetrate an ovum. A number of mature ova are collected from the woman and a single spermatozoon is injected directly into each ovum in a petri dish. The ova and spermatozoa are then left in the laboratory for several days to allow fertilisation to take place, before one (or two) are placed into the uterus. Normal cellular events of fertilisation still need to occur so therefore fertilisation is not assured.
– intrauterine insemination (IUI)	in-tra-YOO-te-ryn in-sem-in-AY-shun	IUI, previously called artificial insemination, is a type of ART in which spermatozoa are directly introduced into a woman's uterus via the cervix around the time of ovulation to improve the chances of conception occurring. The spermatozoa are either fresh from the partner or frozen from the partner or a donor. IUI may be used in combination with ovulation induction if the woman has irregular menstrual cycles.
– in vitro fertilisation (IVF)	in VIT-roh fur-til-eye-ZAY-shun	IVF is the most commonly used form of ART. It involves collecting ova from a woman's ovary after the ovaries have been artificially stimulated to increase production of ova. Fertilisation then takes place by combining the ova with spermatozoa in a sterile environment, generally in a petri dish. If successful, the resulting embryos are allowed to develop for 2–5 days in the laboratory and are then transferred to the woman's uterus. The difference between this technique and ICSI is that the spermatozoa are not injected into the middle of the ova.
– ovarian hyperstimulation	oh-VAIR-ee-an hy-per-stim-yoo-LAY-shun	Ovarian hyperstimulation or controlled ovarian hyperstimulation involves stimulating the ovaries to produce multiple follicles during a single cycle for IVF. Medications such as follicle-stimulating hormones are used to encourage the ovaries to produce more follicles.
– ovulation induction	ov-yoo-LAY-shun in-DUK-shun	Ovulation induction is a simple form of ART that may assist women who have problems with ovulation. It involves the woman taking medication to stimulate the development of one or more ovarian follicles. When the follicles are large enough, another medication is administered to stimulate the release of the ova from the follicles. This process is tracked with blood tests and ultrasound to identify the best time to conceive either by intercourse or IUI.
– transvaginal oocyte retrieval	tranz-vaj-EYE-nal oo-syt ree-TREE-val	A transvaginal oocyte retrieval is a procedure performed under ultrasound guidance to remove oocytes (ova) for fertilisation outside of the uterus using ART. A needle is inserted through the vagina into the follicle so the ova and follicular fluid can be aspirated. This process is commonly known as egg collection.
augmentation of labour	org-men-TAY-shun of LAY-ba	Augmentation of labour involves using medication (oxytocins) or other interventions (artificial rupture of membranes) to 'speed up' labour that has commenced spontaneously. It may be undertaken when the health of the fetus or mother is at risk or in abnormal or difficult labour.

Table continued

Test/Procedure	Pronunciation	Definition
caesarean section	se-ZAIR-ee-an SEK-shun	A caesarean section is a surgical procedure that involves an incision into the abdominal wall and uterus to allow delivery of a fetus (Fig. 17.11). A caesarean section may be performed when there is fetal distress, cord prolapse, failure of labour to progress, abnormal fetal presentation, cephalopelvic disproportion, placental abruption or placenta praevia. There are two types of incisions performed on the uterus for a caesarean section: 1. **Lower uterine segment caesarean section** – the most common type of incision involving a horizontal cut through both the abdominal wall and the lower segment of the uterus. This method results in less bleeding, better healing and is less likely to cause problems in future pregnancies. The incision is commonly known as a bikini line incision. 2. **Classical caesarean section** – this involves a vertical incision into the uterus and either a horizontal or vertical incision into the abdominal wall. Indications for this method include if the placenta is lying low or the fetus is lying sideways, or if there is an abnormal or poorly developed lower segment.

Figure 17.11 Caesarean delivery

(Lowdermilk & Perry 2004)

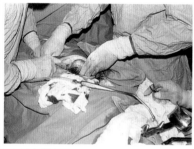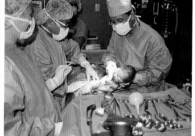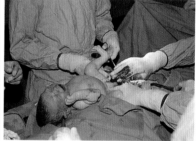

Test/Procedure	Pronunciation	Definition
chorionic villus sampling (CVS)	KO-ree-ON-ik VIL-us sam-pling	CVS is a diagnostic procedure that involves removing placental tissue, generally by way of a needle biopsy via a transabdominal approach, for laboratory examination. The test is used to detect specific conditions such as Down syndrome and cystic fibrosis.
episiotomy	e-PEEZ-ee-OT-oh-mee	An episiotomy is performed by making an incision into the perineum (the space between the vagina and the anus) to enlarge the vaginal opening to help deliver the fetus.
fetal monitoring	FEE-tal MON-i-tor-ing	Fetal monitoring involves measuring the fetal heart rate during labour. It can be external (where the monitor is attached to the mother's abdomen so that the fetal heart rate can be detected) or internal (where the monitor is directly attached to the baby's scalp).
forceps delivery	FOR-seps de-LIV-e-ree	Forceps are large tong-like instruments that are placed around a baby's head to support or pull it from the birth canal. Forceps have various shapes depending on the delivery and are named according to the station at which the baby is located when the forceps are applied. Outlet forceps are applied when the fetal head has reached the perineal floor and is visible between contractions. A low-forceps delivery occurs when the baby's head is at +2 station or lower. Mid-forceps refers to forceps used when the baby's head is above +2 station. High-forceps deliveries are no longer performed in modern medical practice but were historically used when the baby's head was not engaged (Fig. 17.12).

Table continued

Test/Procedure	Pronunciation	Definition
		Figure 17.12 Forceps delivery (Greer et al 2001) 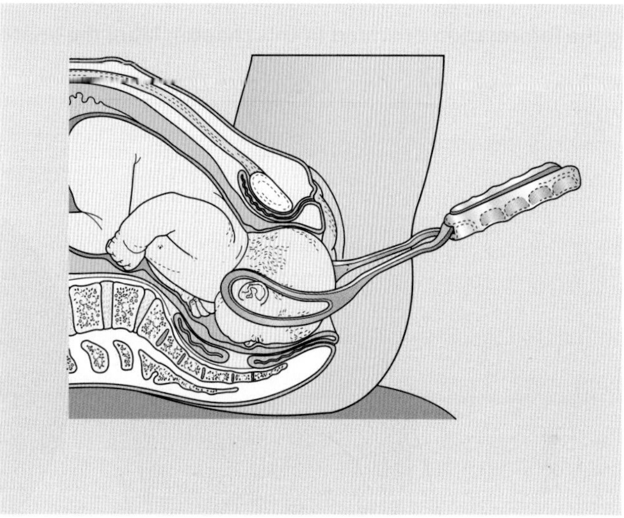
induction of labour	in-DUK-shun of LAY-ba	Induction of labour is a process to artificially start the labour process. Labour is induced most commonly for distress in the fetus, health concerns with the mother, when the pregnancy has gone beyond 41 weeks or if the amniotic waters have broken but labour has not begun. The labour is induced by one or a combination of the following methods: prostaglandin (a hormone-like substance that helps with contraction and relaxation of uterine muscle); cervical ripening balloon catheter to dilate the cervix; or use of the hormone oxytocin or by artificially breaking the amniotic sac.
neuraxial block	nyoo-RAK-see-al block	A neuraxial block (spinal or epidural injection) is a common method used for pain relief during labour. It involves inserting a small needle into the lower back and a catheter through the needle into the epidural space. The needle is then removed, leaving the catheter in place to allow anaesthesia to be administered.
pelvimetry	pel-VIM-e-tree	Pelvimetry involves assessing the measurements of the female pelvis to determine the possibility of a vaginal delivery. Pelvimetry assists in determining if a baby's skull is too big for the mother's pelvic outlet, a condition known as cephalopelvic disproportion.
phenylketonuria (PKU) test	fen-el-kee-ton-YOO-ree-a test	A PKU test is undertaken on newborns to detect the presence of phenylketones in the urine (phenylketonuria). If phenylketonuria is present in the newborn, the body cannot break down an amino acid in food called phenylalanine. Build up of this substance in the blood causes brain damage. Early detection and providing a special diet that excludes phenylalanine can prevent intellectual disability.
vacuum extraction	VAK-yoom ek-STRAK-shun	A vacuum extraction is a method of assisting the delivery of a fetus using a vacuum-suction device attached to the baby's head to assist with pulling it out of the birth canal when labour has not progressed.

Exercises

EXERCISE 17.1: LABEL THE DIAGRAM

Using the information provided in this chapter, label the anatomical parts in Fig. 17.13.

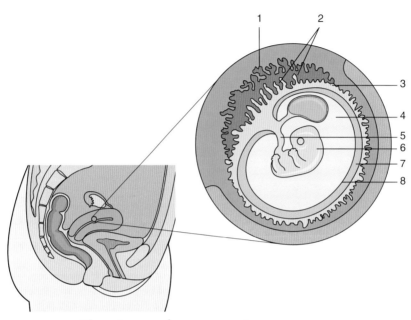

Figure 17.13 The uterus of a pregnant woman

(Based on LaFleur Brooks 2005)

1 _____

2 _____

3 _____

4 _____

5 _____

6 _____

7 _____

8 _____

EXERCISE 17.2: MATCH WORD ELEMENTS AND MEANINGS

Match the prefix, suffix or combining form in Column A with its meaning from Column B.

Column A	Answer	Column B
1. omphal/o		A. birth
2. galact/o		B. head
3. embry/o		C. meninges
4. macro-		D. pregnancy
5. cephal/o		E. split
6. paed/o		F. umbilicus
7. amni/o		G. before
8. primi-		H. monster, malformed
9. epis/o		I. fetus
10. -cyesis		J. embryo, fetus
11. mening/o		K. bear, give birth to
12. -icterus		L. vulva
13. -rrhexis		M. large
14. nat/i		N. milk
15. neo-		O. first
16. ante-		P. amnion, amniotic fluid
17. terat/o		Q. new
18. -schisis		R. child
19. fet/o		S. jaundice
20. part/o		T. rupture

EXERCISE 17.3: VOCABULARY BUILDING

Provide the medical term for each of the definitions below.

1. A woman who has never been pregnant: _____

2. Pertaining to the production of milk: _____

3. Pertaining to before birth: _____

4. Pertaining to after birth: _____

5. (A woman who gives birth to her) first child: _____

6. A false pregnancy: _____

7. A quick labour: _____

8. Inflammation of the umbilicus: _____

9. (A woman who has had) many deliveries: _____

10. Aspiration of amniotic fluid: _____

11. The premature detachment of a normally located placenta prior to delivery of the fetus is known as _____

_____.

12. An _____ occurs when a fertilised egg implants outside the uterus.

13. _____ occurs when the back part of the head remains in a posterior presentation during delivery.

14. _____ is a yellow colouring of the skin and sclera caused by raised levels of bilirubin in the blood of the neonate.

15. _____ is a congenital malformation of the vertebral column occurring when there is an incomplete closure of the neural tube during fetal development.

16. _____ occurs when the placenta is attached to the lower section of the uterus and covers all or part of the opening to the cervix.

17. _____ is a condition resulting in the destruction of erythrocytes in a newborn.

18. An abnormal build-up of cerebrospinal fluid in the ventricles in the brain of the fetus or newborn is known as _____

_____.

19. Congenital narrowing of the pyloric sphincter is called _____.

20. _____ is a chromosomal abnormality that results in distinctive physical abnormalities such as sloping forehead, flat nose, low-set ears and retarded growth as well as mild to severe mental retardation.

EXERCISE 17.4: WORD ANALYSIS AND MEANING

Break up the medical terms below into their component parts (prefixes, suffixes, combining forms). Provide the meaning for each word element and each term as a whole.

Example:

lactorrhoea

lact/o = milk

-rrhoea = discharge, flow

Meaning = discharge of milk

1. oligohydramnios _____

_____

2. pelvimetry _____

_____

3. primigravida _____

_____

4. macrosomia _____

_____

5. neonatal _____

_____

6. hyperemesis _____

_____

7. microcephalic _____

_____

8. perineorrhaphy _____

_____

9. chorioamnionitis _____

_____

10. gastroschisis _____

_____

EXERCISE 17.5: EXPAND THE ABBREVIATIONS

Confirm whether each of the following abbreviations is related to obstetric or neonatal matters and expand it to form the correct medical term.

Abbreviation	Is This Obstetric or Neonatal?	Expanded Abbreviation
APH		
BF		
DIC		
EDC/EDD		
HIE		
IUD		
IOL		
LGA		
NND		
OT		

Abbreviation	Is This Obstetric or Neonatal?	Expanded Abbreviation
PIH		
POC		
SGA		
SIDS		
TOP		

EXERCISE 17.6: CORRECT THE SPELLING AND IDENTIFY THE INCORRECT TERMS

Identify the medical terms spelled incorrectly or words used inappropriately below. Provide the correct terms.

1. He had been a cephallic OA presentation delivered by urgent LSSCS because of fetel distress identified during labur.

2. The baby underwent elective endotracheel intubetion in neonatal intinsive care.

3. Her birth wieght was 3060 kg and birth head circumference was 34.4 m. Her blood group was O positive.

4. The baby made good progress, being rapidly weened down on ventilater settings so that it was possible to extubayte the baby on day 5.

5. This was a twin pregnancy and following spontanous onset of labuor at 34 weeks' gesstation, a ceesarean section was performed, as a previous delivery had been by cesarean section for feetal distress.

6. Chest x-ray indicated hialine membrane disease consistent with gesstational age. He also had a small shignon as a result of the delivery.

7. Initial blood gas showed combined meetabolic and respratory acidiosis.

8. She was born by caesaren section with a congenital disloccation of both hips, having been in breach position from 31 weeks until birth.

9. Her baby boy was delivered by vaccum extraction because of a delay in the second stage of laybor. The delivery was complicated by a post-partuum hemorhage of 900 mL, but she was not transfused. An epidural anestetic was administered during labour to relieve pain.

10. Labor was induced by artifccial rupture of membranes and syntoccinon due to hypertension/pre-eclampsea at 34 weeks' gestaytion.

EXERCISE 17.7: PRONUNCIATION AND COMPREHENSION

Read the following paragraph aloud to practise your pronunciation. Using your textbook and a medical dictionary, find the meanings of the underlined medical terms.

This baby was born at 31.5 weeks' <u>gestation</u> and had a nursery stay of 11 days. Her birth weight was 1630 grams and birth head circumference was 28.4 cm. Her blood group was O positive. She was a <u>cephalic occipitoanterior presentation</u> but was delivered by an urgent <u>caesarean</u> section because of severe maternal <u>pre-eclamptic toxaemia</u>. The mother had been transferred to this hospital from a rural hospital prior to delivery. The baby required mask oxygen-only <u>resuscitation</u>. Her final diagnoses included: prematurity, retained lung fluid, <u>non-haemolytic jaundice</u>, with the highest total <u>bilirubin</u> concentration being 173 micromoles/L. Her management during the admission included supplemental oxygen, highest oxygen concentration 35%; total duration of oxygen therapy 14 hours; <u>peripheral intravenous therapy</u>; <u>phototherapy</u> and <u>cranial ultrasound</u> – 30/6 L colloid cyst. She was transferred back to her local rural hospital at 11 days of age.

EXERCISE 17.8: CROSSWORD PUZZLE

Complete the puzzle by providing the medical term for each of the clues below.

ACROSS

3. A chromosomal abnormality that results in distinctive physical abnormalities such as sloping forehead, flat nose and low-set ears (4, 8)

7. The premature detachment of a normally located placenta prior to delivery of the fetus (8, 8)

8. Pregnancy-related toxaemia (12)

9. An incision in the perineum to assist the delivery of the fetus (10)

10. A test for newborns that measures for activity, pulse, grimace, appearance and respiration (5, 5)

11. *See 4 down*

DOWN

1. A lack of surfactant in the lungs of premature babies, causing them to collapse (11, 8, 8)

2. Excessive vomiting and nausea during pregnancy (11, 10)

4. Down & 11 across. A condition resulting in the destruction (haemolysis) of erythrocytes in a newborn (16, 7)

5. A common method for pain relief during labour (9, 5)

6. Yellow colouring of the skin and sclera caused by raised levels of bilirubin (8)

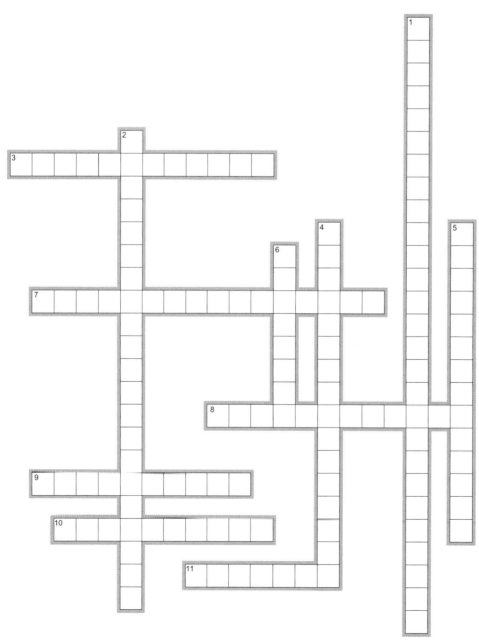

EXERCISE 17.9: DISCHARGE SUMMARY ANALYSIS

Read the discharge summary below and answer the questions.

UNIVERSITY HOSPITAL DISCHARGE SUMMARY	**UR number:** 373839
	Name: Chloe Fingle
	Address: 17 The Esplanade, Anglers Haven
	Date of birth: 15/09/1983
	Sex: F
	Nominated primary healthcare provider: Dr Sally Porter

Episode details	**Discharge details**
Consultant: Dr Reading	**Status:** Home
Registrar: Dr Planter	**Date of discharge:** 30/10/2020
Unit: Maternity	
Admission source: Antenatal clinic	
Date of admission: 16/10/2020	

Reason for admission / Presenting problems:

Pregnancy-induced hypertension with associated proteinuria

Principal diagnosis: Pregnancy-induced hypertension with associated proteinuria

Comorbidities:

Twin pregnancy identified at 18 weeks

Renal impairment

Previous medical history:

Migraines

Clinical synopsis:

Patient was admitted on 16 October 2020 under the care of Dr Reading. It had been identified at 18 weeks that she was expecting twins. PIH with associated proteinuria was present. The hypertension was complicated by renal impairment. The maternal blood group was O Pos. Labour was induced by ARM and IV syntocinon due to hypertension/pre-eclampsia, at 34 weeks' gestation.

Her twins – identical girls – were delivered on 24 October 2020 at 01.38 and 01.40 by emergency LSCS. The indication for caesarean section was fetal distress in twin number one. A general anaesthetic was administered (ASA = 1E). The babies' birth weights were 1327 grams and 1642 grams.

Complications:

Clinical interventions:

LSCS

ARM

Diagnostic interventions:

Medications at discharge:

Ceased medications:

Allergies: Bandaids

Alerts:

Arranged services:

Recommendations:

Information to patient/relevant parties:

The mother has been discharged from hospital, but the babies remain in SCN.

Follow-up by her LMO 1 week post discharge.

Authorising clinician: Dr Planter

Document recipients:

Patient and LMO: Dr Sally Porter

1. Expand the following abbreviations as found in the discharge summary above.

   PIH

   LSCS

   ARM

   IV

   LMO

   SCN

2. What is pregnancy-induced hypertension with proteinuria?
   Why is it an indication for induction of labour?

3. Chloe's labour was induced at 34 weeks by ARM and IV syntocinon. What does this mean?

4. What is the difference between an emergency caesarean section and an elective caesarean section?

5. Why did the babies have to stay in the SCN?

Contents

OBJECTIVES   429

INTRODUCTION   430

NEW WORD ELEMENTS   430

   Combining forms   430

   Prefixes   431

   Suffixes   431

VOCABULARY   431

ABBREVIATIONS   432

MENTAL HEALTH DISORDERS   432

GLOSSARY OF MENTAL
HEALTH TERMS   433

SPECIFIC MENTAL HEALTH
DISORDERS   434

   Disorders usually first diagnosed
in infancy, childhood or
adolescence   434

   Delirium, dementia and amnesic
and other cognitive disorders   434

   Substance-related disorders   435

   Schizophrenia and other
psychotic disorders   435

   Mood disorders   436

   Anxiety disorders   437

   Some common (and not so
common) phobias   438

   Factitious disorders   438

   Dissociative disorders   439

   Sexual and gender identity
disorders   439

   Eating disorders   440

   Personality disorders   440

THERAPEUTIC INTERVENTIONS   441

   Psychological and psychosocial
therapies   441

   Psychopharmacology   442

   Other therapeutic methods   443

EXERCISES   443

Objectives

After completing this chapter you should be able to:

1. state the meanings of the word elements related to mental health

2. build words using the word elements associated with mental health

3. recognise, pronounce and effectively use medical terms associated with mental health

4. expand abbreviations related to mental health

5. describe common mental health disorders

6. describe common laboratory tests, diagnostic and surgical procedures associated with mental health

7. apply what you have learned by interpreting medical terminology in practice.

Demonstrate your knowledge of mental health by completing the exercises at the end of this chapter.

INTRODUCTION

A person's mental health status can be affected by a variety of social, environmental, biological and psychological factors. Our mental health determines how we handle stress, relate to others, make choices and function on a daily level.

As a medical specialty, mental health is concerned with diagnosing, treating and preventing disorders of the mind. It treats a wide range of disorders that can result in a significant impairment of a person's thinking, functioning, cognitive abilities and emotional wellbeing.

The discipline of mental health was previously called psychiatry. The name was changed to promote a more positive focus and to be more inclusive. Knowledge of mental health is frequently changing as more is learned about how the mind works and about disorders that can affect it. The meaning of some medical terms in this discipline has had to change to keep pace. For example, a person with schizophrenia was once believed to have a split personality (schiz/o = split). Although it is now known that this is not true, the term is still used with a modified meaning.

This chapter will look at the terminology associated with mental health and discuss some of the more common mental health disorders and treatments.

NEW WORD ELEMENTS

Here are some word elements related to mental health. To reinforce your learning, write the meanings of the medical terms in the spaces provided. Use the Glossary of medical terms on page 561 to help you work out the meanings. You may also need to check the meaning in a medical dictionary, but make an attempt yourself first.

Combining forms

Combining Form	Meaning	Medical Term	Meaning of Medical Term
anxi/o	uneasy, distressed	anxious	
cycl/o	circle, recurring, ciliary body of eye	cyclothymia	
geront/o	old age, the aged	gerontology	
hallucin/o	hallucination, to wander in the mind	hallucinosis	
hypn/o	sleep	hypnotherapy	
iatr/o	physician, medicine, treatment	psychiatrist	
klept/o	steal	kleptomania	
ment/o	mind	mental	
morph/o	form, shape	dysmorphophobia	
neur/o	nerve	neurosis	
phil/o	attraction to, love	necrophilia	
phob/o	fear, sensitivity	gerontophobia	
phor/o	carry, bear	dysphoric	
phren/o	mind, diaphragm	phrenology	
pol/o	extreme	bipolar	
psych/o	mind	psychologist	
pyr/o	fire, heat	pyromania	
schiz/o	split	schizophrenia	
somat/o	body	psychosomatic	
xen/o	foreign, strange	xenophobia	

Prefixes

Prefix	Meaning	Medical Term	Meaning of Medical Term
a-, an-	no, not, without, absence of	apathy	
agora-	marketplace, open space	agoraphobia	
cata-	down, lower	catatonic	
electro-	electricity, electrical activity	electroencephalogram	
eu-	normal, good	euphoria	
hypo-	below, under, deficient, less than normal	hypochondriac	

Suffixes

Suffix	Meaning	Medical Term	Meaning of Medical Term
-genic	pertaining to formation, producing	psychogenic	
-lalia	disorder of speech	coprolalia	
-leptic	type of seizure	narcoleptic	
-mania	state of mental disorder, frenzy	trichotillomania	
-philia	attraction for	paedophilia	
-phobia	condition of fear	nyctophobia	
-phoria	feeling, emotional state	dysphoria	
-thymia	condition of mind, emotion	dysthymia	

VOCABULARY

The following list provides many of the medical terms used for the first time in this chapter. Pronunciations are provided with each term. As you read the rest of the chapter, make sure you identify each of these terms and understand their meanings.

Term	Pronunciation
anorexia nervosa	an-o-REK-see-ah ner-VOH-sa
anti-anxiety and anti-panic agent	an-tee-ang-ZY-et-ee and an-tee-PAN-ik ay-jent
antidepressant	an-tee-de-PRESS-ant
antipsychotic (neuroleptic)	an-tee-sy-KOT-ik (nyoo-roh-LEP-tik)
attention-deficit (hyperactivity) disorder	a-ten-shun-DEF-is-it (hy-per-ak-TIV-it-ee) dis-OR-da
autism spectrum disorder	OR-tiz-em SPEK-trum dis-OR-da
bipolar disorder	by-POH-lah dis-OR-da
bulimia nervosa	byoo-LEEM-ee-a ner-VOH-sa

Table continued

Term	Pronunciation
cognitive behaviour therapy	KOG-ni-tiv bee-HAYV-ya THER-a-pee
delirium	de-LEE-ree-um
dementia	de-MEN-cha
depressive disorder	de-PRESS-iv dis-OR-da
dissociative disorder	di-SOH-see-at-iv dis-OR-da
electroconvulsive therapy	ee-LEK-tro-kon-VUL-siv THER-a-pee
family therapy	FAM-il-ee THER-a-pee
gender identity disorder	JEN-da eye-DEN-tit-ee dis-OR-da
generalised anxiety disorder	JEN-er-al-yzed ang-ZY-it-ee dis-OR-da
group therapy	groop THER-a-pee
hypnosis	hip-NOH-sis
hypnotics	hip-NOT-iks
insight-oriented psychotherapy	IN-syt-OR-ee-en-ted sy-ko-THER-a-pee
mood stabilisers	mood STAY-bil-eyez-erz
Munchausen's syndrome	MUN-chow-zunz SIN-drohm

Table continued

Term	Pronunciation
Munchausen's syndrome by proxy	MUN-chow-zunz SIN-drohm by PROK-see
obsessive-compulsive disorder	ob-SES-iv kom-PUL-siv dis-OR-da
panic disorder	pan-ik dis-OR-da
paraphilia	pa-ra-FIL-ee-a
phobia	FO-bee-a
play therapy	play THER-a-pee
post-traumatic stress disorder	post traw-MAT-ik stress dis-OR-da
psychoanalysis	sy-koh-a-NAL-a-sis
psychosis	sy-KOH-sis
schizophrenia	skit-soh-FREN-ee-a
seasonal affective disorder	SEEZ-on-al a-FEK-tiv dis-OR-da
sex therapy	seks THER-a-pee
sexual disorder	seks-yoo-al dis-OR-da
stimulant	STIM-yoo-lant
substance-related disorder	SUB-stans ree-LAY-ted dis-OR-da
supportive psychotherapy	sup-PAW-tiv sy-koh-THER-a-pee

Table continued

Abbreviation	Definition
GCS	Glasgow Coma Scale
IQ	intelligence quotient
LOC	loss of consciousness
MA	mental age
MAOI	monoamine oxidase inhibitor
MDD	major depressive disorder
MMPI	Minnesota Multiphasic Personality Inventory
MMSE	Mini-Mental State Examination
MSE	Mental State Examination
MSQ	Mental Status Questionnaire
OCD	obsessive-compulsive disorder
OD	overdose
PTSD	post-traumatic stress disorder
SAD	seasonal affective disorder
SUD	substance use disorder
SSRI	selective serotonin reuptake inhibitor
WAIS	Wechsler adult intelligence scale
WISC(-R)	Wechsler intelligence scale for children (revised)
Ψ	symbol for psychiatry/psychology
ΨRx	symbol for psychotherapy

ABBREVIATIONS

The following abbreviations are commonly used in the Australian healthcare environment. Because some abbreviations can have more than one meaning, check the context in which the abbreviation is used before assigning a meaning to it.

Abbreviation	Definition
AD	Alzheimer's disease
AD(H)D	attention-deficit (hyperactivity) disorder
ADL	activities of daily living
ASD	autism spectrum disorder
CA	chronological age
CBT	cognitive behaviour therapy
DSM-5	*Diagnostic and Statistical Manual of Mental Disorders* (American Psychiatric Association, 5th edition, 2013)
DT	delirium tremens
ECT	electroconvulsive therapy
ETOH	ethanol (or alcohol)
GAD	generalised anxiety disorder

MENTAL HEALTH DISORDERS

The World Health Organization defines mental health as 'a state of well-being in which every individual realizes his or her own potential, can cope with the normal stresses of life, can work productively and fruitfully, and is able to make a contribution to her or his community' (www.who.int/features/factfiles/mental_health/en/).

Mental health is concerned with the emotional, social and behavioural wellbeing of an individual. The mental health of a person is determined by an assortment of social, psychological and biological factors that may affect the individual in various ways at different points in time. Some of the pressures that may predispose an individual to mental health disorders include exposure to violence, persistent socioeconomic pressures, human rights infringements, experiencing rapid changes in social circumstances, stressful work environments, discrimination in various forms, social exclusion and persistent poor physical health. As factors in the external environment can affect a person's wellbeing, good mental health requires a balance between the external environment and the individual's internal wellbeing.

Under certain circumstances (substance abuse, social factors, genetics, environmental changes), this balance can be disturbed. If it is disturbed to such a degree that the individual can no longer cope with life's stressors, the person is considered to have a mental illness. Mental illness is a general term used to describe all diagnosable mental health disorders. The term 'mental health disorders' describes the myriad conditions that can adversely affect a person's mental wellbeing. Alterations in thinking, mood, function, judgement or behaviour are common manifestations of mental health disorders.

As a specialty, mental health is the branch of medicine that deals with the achievement and maintenance of emotional, cognitive and psychological health and the treatment of mental illness.

It is common practice to refer to mental health disorders according to the diagnostic category into which they are grouped. The *Diagnostic and Statistical Manual of Mental Disorders*, 5th edition (DSM-5) is the current classification of mental health disorders and contains more than 300 diagnostic categories with specific criteria for inclusion. The structure of the following section is based on these DSM-5 categories. It is beyond the scope of this book to discuss all mental health disorders, so only those that occur frequently or are of specific interest have been included.

The following section provides a list of common diseases and pathological conditions relevant to mental health.

GLOSSARY OF MENTAL HEALTH TERMS

The following terms are often encountered in mental health. You may see some of these terms in the following discussion on mental health disorders.

Term	Pronunciation	Meaning
affect	A-fekt	Affect is the external expression of an emotional feeling or mood.
amnesia	am-NEE-see-a	Amnesia is a loss of memory caused by brain trauma or a severe emotional trauma.
apathy	AP-a-thee	Apathy is a demonstrated lack of interest or emotions.
compulsion	kom-PUL-shun	A compulsion is an uncontrollable need to perform an action persistently.
counsellor	KOWN-sel-a	A healthcare counsellor is a therapist who gives advice on lifestyle, personal, health or psychological problems.
defence mechanism	de-FENS mek-an-iz-em	A defence mechanism is a strategy (often unconscious) that a person uses to cope with a difficult situation or to conceal anxiety.
delusion	de-LOO-shun	A delusion is a false belief that has no basis in reality.
dissociation	dis-OS-ee-AY-shun	Dissociation is a state of mind where perception of the environment, thoughts, emotions or memories are separated from the conscious mind because they have become too difficult to assimilate.
DSM-5	dee-ess-em-5	The *Diagnostic and Statistical Manual of Mental Disorders*, 5th edition (DSM-5) is a classification used by clinicians and psychiatrists to classify mental health disorders. It describes symptoms, statistics and treatments. It is regularly updated by the American Psychiatric Association.
fugue	fyoog	A fugue is an episode of amnesia in which the person is unable to recall some or all of his or her past. It is usually associated with the person leaving their home environment to create a new identity and life. During the fugue state the person has no memory of their previous life. Conversely, after recovery the person has no memory of what happened during the fugue state.
hallucination	hal-OO-sin-AY-shun	An hallucination is a false sensory perception (visual, auditory, tactile, olfactory or gustatory) that occurs without external stimulation and has no basis in reality but feels very real to the person experiencing it.
ideation	EYE-dee-AY-shun	Ideation is the ability to form thoughts or ideas that may become an action or plan.

Table continued

Term	Pronunciation	Meaning
neurosis	nyoo-RO-sis	A neurosis is a mental health disorder in which anxiety is the main component and is distressing to the patient. Reality testing is intact and there is no apparent organic explanation.
obsession	ob-SES-shun	An obsession is a fixation on a particular thing or activity, a persistent thought or idea that does not go away.
psychiatrist	sy-KY-a-trist	A psychiatrist is a medical doctor who specialises in the diagnosis, treatment and prevention of mental disorders.
psychiatry	sy-KY-a-tree	Psychiatry is the medical specialty that deals with the diagnosis, treatment and prevention of mental disorders.
psychologist	sy-KOL-o-jist	A psychologist is a health professional who specialises in the study of human behaviour and the mind and its disorders. A psychologist does not require medical training.
psychology	sy-KOL-o-jee	Psychology is the study of human behaviour and the mind and its disorders.
psychosis	sy-KOH-sis	A psychosis is a mental health disorder in which reality becomes distorted, leading to an inability to function and relate to people.

SPECIFIC MENTAL HEALTH DISORDERS

Disorders usually first diagnosed in infancy, childhood or adolescence

Term	Pronunciation	Definition
autism spectrum disorder	OR-tiz-em SPEK-trum dis-OR-da	Autism spectrum disorder, also called pervasive developmental disorder, refers to a group of disorders including autism, Asperger's syndrome, childhood disintegrative disorder and Rett disorder. People with any of these disorders have varying degrees of impaired verbal and non-verbal communication, impaired social interaction, hypersensitivity to sensory stimuli, may exhibit repetitive behaviours such as rocking or hand wringing and have restricted interests. The exact cause of autism spectrum disorder is not known, but there is a strong genetic link. Environmental, immunological and metabolic factors also influence the development of the disorder. Symptoms usually appear before 3 years of age.
attention-deficit (hyperactivity) disorder (ADHD)	at-ten-shun DEF-is-it (hy-per-ak-TIV-it-ee) dis-OR-da	ADHD is a condition that is characterised by poor attention span, distractibility and/or hyperactive and impulsive behaviours. Difficulties with concentration, mental focus and inhibition of impulses and behaviours are chronic and persistent. It is one of the most common mental disorders that develops in children. Symptoms may continue into adolescence and adulthood. If left untreated, ADHD can lead to poor performance at school, difficulty forming social relationships and low self-esteem. The exact cause of ADHD has not been determined; however, the condition is thought to have genetic and biological elements.

Delirium, dementia and amnesic and other cognitive disorders

Term	Pronunciation	Definition
delirium	de-LEER-ee-um	Delirium is a sudden, acute impairment of cognitive functioning caused by a physical or mental illness or by the ingestion of drugs or alcohol. The patient exhibits signs of mental confusion and disorientation, an inability to focus, and fluctuations in their state of awareness. Depending on the actual cause, delirium can usually be completely reversed or controlled.

Table continued

Term	Pronunciation	Definition
dementia	de-MEN-cha	Dementia is an irreversible, progressive, cognitive brain disorder that results from damage to the brain's structure. Patients with dementia will demonstrate a gradual loss of intellectual abilities, impaired judgement and memory and personality changes. They lose their ability to process information and make decisions. Social situations can be very stressful because their behaviour can be inappropriate. Dementia can be caused by Alzheimer's disease, Parkinson's disease, cerebrovascular accidents and brain tumours. These conditions are discussed separately in Chapter 12 Nervous System.

Substance-related disorders

Term	Pronunciation	Definition
dependence (substance use disorder)	de-PEN-dens	Dependence (or substance use disorder) refers to a cluster of behavioural, cognitive and physiological phenomena that develop after repeated substance use and that typically include a strong desire to take the substance, difficulties in controlling its use, a subjective feeling of craving or urge to use the substance despite harmful consequences. A higher priority is given to substance use than to other activities and obligations, with increased tolerance and sometimes a physical withdrawal state (*International Statistical Classification of Diseases and Related Health Problems* (ICD-11)).
substance-related disorders	sub-stans ree-LAY-ted dis-OR-da	Substance-related disorders include side effects of medications, exposure to toxins and use of drugs of addiction. Drugs of addiction include alcohol, amphetamines, cannabis, cocaine, hallucinogens, opioids, sedatives and tobacco. A person may be a casual user or have a psychological or physical dependence on the substance. Substance-related disorders fall into two categories: **substance use disorders**, which includes dependence on and abuse of the substance; and **substance-induced disorders**, which include intoxication, withdrawal and other physical and psychological conditions and are caused by the exposure to the substance. These conditions are usually reversible when the substance use has ceased. Alcoholism is an example of a substance use disorder. Drug-induced paranoia is an example of a substance-induced disorder.

Schizophrenia and other psychotic disorders

Term	Pronunciation	Definition
psychosis	sy-KOH-sis	Psychosis is a group of symptoms that represent a major mental health disorder such as schizophrenia, schizoaffective disorder, delusional disorder, brief reactive psychosis, bipolar disorder and psychotic depression. Common to all of these is a disturbance of perception and thought processes. The person's ability to interpret reality and behave appropriately is impaired. The most common manifestations of psychosis are hallucinations, delusions, disordered thinking and disordered behaviour. Hallucinations are seeing, hearing, smelling, feeling or tasting things that are not really there. Delusions are false beliefs despite evidence to the contrary. For example, a person may believe that someone is trying to hurt them (paranoia) or that they possess special powers. There are many different types of psychoses including drug-induced psychosis and brief reactive psychosis, which can occur after a stressful situation. Bipolar disorder can have periods of psychosis as part of the condition, as can severe depression and schizophrenia.

Table continued

Term	Pronunciation	Definition
schizophrenia	skit-soh-FREN-ee-ah	Schizophrenia is a type of psychotic disorder in which there is dissociation from reality. The most common symptom is psychosis, which is often experienced in short, intense bursts. Patients may withdraw from reality into an inner world. The condition manifests with symptoms such as delusions of harm, hallucinations (especially hearing voices and seeing things that are not present), disordered thought processes, decreased emotional expressiveness and impaired social skills. Anxiety and depression may also be present. There are four main types of schizophrenia: 1. **Disorganised schizophrenia** – patients become easily confused and have irrational thoughts. Their behaviour is disordered; they are emotionally flat and have difficulty functioning in society. 2. **Paranoid schizophrenia** – patients have delusions of grandeur and/or persecution. Hallucinations are common. 3. **Residual schizophrenia** – patients experience at least one schizophrenic episode but are left with relatively mild symptoms and can function quite well. 4. **Catatonic schizophrenia** – patients become completely unresponsive (catatonic) with rigidity and stupor but can also become frenzied. Schizophrenia is treated with psychotherapy, cognitive behaviour therapy and antipsychotic drugs. However, compliance with taking the medication can be a problem for many patients.

Mood disorders

Term	Pronunciation	Definition
bipolar disorder	by-PO-lah dis-OR-da	Bipolar disorder (previously called manic depression) is a disorder characterised by severe mood swings with manic episodes (highs) followed by depressive episodes (lows). During the manic phase, the person will speak rapidly, have excessive energy, insomnia, delusions, hallucinations and often bizarre and inappropriate thought processes. During the depressive phase, the person will appear withdrawn, have a poor appetite, a flat demeanour and a disturbed sleep pattern. The cause of bipolar disorder is believed to be a combination of heredity and changes to chemical exchanges in the brain. Patients with bipolar disorder may experience an episode of mania or depression if they are exposed to an event that they find stressful. Medication to treat both phases is given in conjunction with psychotherapy.
depressive disorder	de-PRESS-iv dis-OR-da	The terms *major depression*, *major depressive illness* and *clinical depression* are all synonyms for the term **depressive disorder**. A depressive disorder refers to a major depressive episode without mania. It involves feelings of severe dysphoria (deep sadness, worry and hopelessness), appetite disturbance, altered sleep patterns, feelings of worthlessness and a lack of interest in one's surroundings. Depression may be a genetic condition caused by an electrochemical imbalance in the brain or may be caused by a reaction to a stressful event. Antidepressant medication and cognitive behaviour therapy are common treatments.

Table continued

Term	Pronunciation	Definition
seasonal affective disorder (SAD)	SEEZ-on-al a-FEK-tiv dis-OR-da	SAD is an affective disorder characterised by periods of depression, especially during the winter months. The symptoms disappear during the spring and summer. It is thought to be caused by an increase in the secretion of melatonin as a result of a lack of natural sunlight. Exposure to artificial sunlight helps to alleviate some of the symptoms.

Anxiety disorders

Term	Pronunciation	Definition
generalised anxiety disorder (GAD)	JEN-er-a-lyzed ang-ZEYE-it-ee dis-OR-da	GAD refers to a condition characterised by chronic repeated episodes of severe worry about problems that may or may not exist. Patients worry about unlikely major disasters and everyday issues like health, money and family. GAD can result in physical symptoms such as headaches, fatigue, muscle tension, insomnia and hypertension. Medication, psychotherapy and relaxation are common treatments. Physical symptoms may also be treated.
panic disorder	PAN-ik dis-OR-da	Panic disorder is also known as a panic attack. It refers to a sudden episode of intense feeling that something bad will occur or anxiety about being in a situation where an escape may be difficult, such as being in a plane or in a crowd. A panic attack begins suddenly, peaks within 10–20 minutes and can last for an hour or more. Because it can also cause discomforting physical symptoms, such as chest pain, breathlessness and palpitations, a panic attack may be mistaken for a heart attack. Treatment includes antidepressant medication and cognitive behaviour therapy.
phobia	FOH-bee-a	A phobia is an exaggerated, irrational fear associated with a specific object or situation. When the object or situation is encountered, a high level of anxiety is generated. Specific phobias are named after the object that is feared. See the following table for some common (and not so common) phobias.
obsessive-compulsive disorder (OCD)	ob-SES-iv kom-PULS-iv dis-OR-da	OCD is an anxiety disorder characterised by recurrent unwanted thoughts (obsessions) and repetitive actions, rituals or behaviours that the person feels they must carry out in the belief they will prevent a feared event or situation and/or will reduce anxiety (compulsions). Repetitive behaviour includes actions such as repeated handwashing, checking locks, excessive neatness, counting and switching lights on and off. OCD can have serious lifestyle implications because of the time taken to repeatedly perform the rituals. OCD often prevents patients from leading normal lives. A combination of psychotherapy, stress reduction, hypnotherapy and medication are needed for treatment.
post-traumatic stress disorder (PTSD)	pohst traw-MAT-ik stress dis-OR-da	PTSD is an anxiety disorder that is a response to exposure to a traumatic event, in particular where the person's safety or life has been threatened. It is common in military personnel who have been to war, in victims of violent attacks such as sexual assault and in survivors of a natural disaster. People suffering from PTSD experience dysphoria, flashbacks of the incident, have problems sleeping and feel emotionally numb. Treatment includes medication for the anxiety/depression and cognitive behaviour therapy.

Some common (and not so common) phobias

Table continued

Phobia	Meaning
acrophobia	fear of heights
agoraphobia	fear of open places
androphobia	fear of men
arachibutyrophobia	fear of peanut butter sticking to the roof of the mouth
arachnophobia	fear of spiders
belonephobia	fear of needles
brontophobia	fear of thunder and lightning
claustrophobia	fear of confined spaces
coulrophobia	fear of clowns
cynophobia	fear of dogs
gamophobia	fear of marriage
gynaephobia	fear of women
haemophobia	fear of blood

Phobia	Meaning
hypnophobia	fear of sleep
iatrophobia	fear of going to the doctor
laliophobia	fear of stuttering
mysophobia	fear of infection or contamination
ornithophobia	fear of birds
pathophobia	fear of disease
pyrophobia	fear of fire
sesquipedalophobia	fear of long words
thalassophobia	fear of the sea
trichophobia	fear of hair
triskaidekaphobia	fear of the number 13
xenophobia	fear of strangers
zoophobia	fear of animals

Factitious disorders

Term	Pronunciation	Definition
Munchausen's syndrome	MUN-chow-zunz SIN-drohm	Munchausen's syndrome (named after Baron von Munchausen, an 18th century German officer who liked to exaggerate his stories) is the most common factitious disorder. It is a condition where a person deliberately embellishes medical symptoms just to seek a sick role. The patient may injure themselves, alter diagnostic tests (e.g. by contaminating a urine sample) and seek to undergo unnecessary procedures and operations. This is done to gain the special attention given to people who are actually ill. Despite actively seeking medical treatment and attention, a person with Munchausen's syndrome is often unwilling to admit to, and seek treatment for, the syndrome itself.
Munchausen's syndrome by proxy	MUN-chow-zunz SIN-drohm by PROK-see	Munchausen's syndrome by proxy is a condition in which the primary caregiver for a dependent person (commonly a child) fakes illnesses or symptoms in that person. The dependant may be deliberately made to seem sick by induction of symptoms or by the caregiver convincing others that he or she is sick by reporting fictitious episodes of illness. As a result, the dependant will have unnecessary treatments and even surgery to try to determine the cause of the symptoms. The caregiver appears concerned and caring about the dependent person while in reality feeling satisfied by gaining the attention and sympathy of the doctors and nurses who are looking after them. Munchausen's syndrome by proxy is also known as fabricated or induced illness by carers (FIIC).

Dissociative disorders

Term	Pronunciation	Definition
dissociative disorder	dis-SOH-see-at-iv dis-OR-da	Traumatic events in a person's life can lead to a dissociative disorder. People cope with difficult situations in different ways. Sometimes dissociating from a difficult situation – choosing to forget that it happened – is a way of coping with trauma.
		Dissociative disorders can be classified into the following types.
		Dissociative amnesia – an inability to remember significant personal information as a result of an emotional trauma. The individual blocks information that might be traumatic and stressful in nature.
		Dissociative fugue – an individual forgets all about their past, including their identity, and simply walks away from their life, often travelling a long distance in a state of confusion. Afterwards, there is little recollection of what occurred during the fugue phase.
		Dissociative identity disorder (DID) – DID was formerly called multiple personality disorder. It is the best known of the dissociative disorders thanks to the popular media. In DID, patients assume alternate personalities (called alters). Two or more distinct personalities co-exist within the person. Each personality is unique and can be of any age, gender or status. They may not know of each other's existence. The patient experiences amnesia and appears to forget events, personal information or traumatic episodes.
		Depersonalisation disorder – in this disorder, the patient feels detached from their mind, body and the environment. It is like being in a dream. The person watches life events as if from the sidelines. This condition commonly occurs in psychosis and severe depression.

Sexual and gender identity disorders

Term	Pronunciation	Definition
gender dysphoria	JEN-da dis-FOR-ee-ah	Gender dysphoria is the existence of persistent feelings in a person that their biological sex is wrong and does not represent their actual gender identity. People with gender dysphoria feel they have been born in the wrong sex and therefore seek to alter their physical and sexual identities. They often dress as the other gender and prefer to be seen in public as a member of the other sex. They may exhibit feelings and reactions typical of the other gender. Some people feel they are not male or female but might identify as being somewhere in between. Gender dysphoria is itself not a mental illness but may cause severe anxiety and depression in the affected individual.
paraphilia	pa-ra-FIL-ee-a	Paraphilia is a form of sexual dysfunction that includes attraction to unusual objects, sexual deviation or perversion or a disorder of sexual preference. It involves repeated, intense sexual arousal to socially unacceptable stimuli such as non-human objects, children and non-consenting adults. Some of the more common paraphilias include paedophilia (children), exhibitionism (exposing one's genitals) fetishism (attraction to specific objects such as latex or underwear), frotteurism (rubbing against strangers), sexual masochism (hurting one's self, autoerotic asphyxia), sexual sadism (hurting someone else), voyeurism (peeping at unsuspecting victims) or zoophilia (sexual acts with animals).

Table continued

Term	Pronunciation	Definition
sexual disorder	seks-yoo-al dis-OR-da	Sexual disorders often relate to physical sexual dysfunction and include conditions such as hypoactive sexual desire disorder where there is a lack of interest in sexual activity, sexual arousal disorders such as psychological impotence, orgasmic disorders such as premature ejaculation in a man or the inability to reach an orgasm in a female and vaginismus in which there are painful spasms in the vagina.

Eating disorders

Term	Pronunciation	Definition
anorexia nervosa	an-o-REK-see-a ner-VOH-sa	Anorexia nervosa is a persistent quest for slimness, despite the person already being extremely thin or emaciated. A person with anorexia often begins dieting to lose weight. Over time, the weight loss becomes a sign of control over their body. The characteristics of someone with anorexia nervosa include an obsessive attitude towards eating, restrictive eating of particular foods, frequent weighing and excessive exercising. Often people with anorexia will take large numbers of diet pills, diuretics and laxatives. Even with treatment, relapses are common. As well as being a psychological disorder, anorexia nervosa can have a serious physical impact on the body, with cardiac problems such as palpitations, arrhythmias, bradycardia and hypotension being common. Amenorrhoea is also associated with anorexia nervosa.
bulimia nervosa	byoo-LEEM-ee-a ner-VOH-sa	Bulimia nervosa is characterised by binge eating followed by vomiting. People with bulimia nervosa have a disturbance in perception of their body size and shape. Despite eating excessively, a bulimic person's body weight is usually in the normal range due to their frequent purging, use of laxatives and/or excessive exercising. As well as being a psychological disorder, bulimia nervosa can have a serious physical impact on the body, with heart palpitations, cardiac arrest, tooth decay, inflamed sore throat, dehydration and kidney disease being common consequences.

Personality disorders

Term	Pronunciation	Definition
personality disorder	per-son-AL-it-ee dis-OR-da	Personality disorders are a group of disorders characterised by chronic, maladaptive patterns of thoughts and behaviours that cause difficulties with interpersonal relationships, fitting into society and the ability to work. People with personality disorders have trouble dealing with everyday stresses and problems. The most noticeable and significant feature of these disorders is their negative effect on interpersonal relationships. The exact cause of personality disorders is unknown. However, genetics and childhood experiences may play a role. Symptoms vary widely depending on the specific type of personality disorder. Treatment usually includes psychotherapy and sometimes medication. There are several different personality disorders: **Antisocial personality disorder** – a disorder characterised by a chronic tendency to violate the rights and safety of others. Sufferers tend to be chronic liars, aggressive and rarely show remorse for their actions. Many criminals have this disorder.

Table continued

Term	Pronunciation	Definition
		Borderline personality disorder – a disorder characterised by emotional instability, leading to stress and other problems. People with this disorder desire loving relationships but tend to alienate others with their anger, impulsivity and frequent mood swings.
		Histrionic personality disorder – a disorder characterised by very emotional and dramatic behaviour by an individual in a way that draws attention to themselves. There is a need to be the centre of attention. These patients constantly seek reassurance or approval. People with this disorder are usually able to function at a high level and can be successful socially and at work.
		Narcissistic personality disorder – a disorder characterised by an inflated sense of self-importance and an extreme preoccupation with self. People with this condition are likely to disregard the feelings of others, have little ability to feel empathy and have a strong need for constant attention and admiration. Paradoxically, they are generally lacking in self-esteem and are emotionally delicate.
		Paranoid personality disorder – a disorder characterised by longstanding paranoia, distrust and suspicion against people, social isolation and hostility. Symptoms of this disorder include great difficulty in maintaining interpersonal relationships because of the suspicion and distrust. Despite these symptoms, the person does not have a full-blown psychotic disorder such as schizophrenia.
		Schizoid personality disorder – a disorder characterised by extreme shyness, detachment and introversion. People with this disorder will avoid social activities and interaction with others. They are seen as loners and have difficulty forming personal relationships.

THERAPEUTIC INTERVENTIONS

Treatment of mental health disorders falls into the following types of therapies: psychological and psychosocial therapies, psychopharmacology and other therapeutic methods.

Psychological and psychosocial therapies

These methods of treatment, collectively called psychotherapy, involve the use of one or more of a range of psychological techniques by psychiatrists, psychologists and other mental health professionals. In psychotherapy, the mental health professional uses encouragement and techniques to positively reinforce the patient's adaptive patterns of thought and behaviours to assist them through conflict.

Type of Therapy	Pronunciation	Definition
cognitive behaviour therapy (CBT)	KOG-ni-tiv bee-HAYV-ya THER-a-pee	CBT is based on the premise of changing the patient's patterns of behaviour by assisting them to identify and modify unhealthy or unhelpful thoughts or actions. CBT may be useful in treating depression, anxiety disorders and psychotic disorders.

Table continued

Type of Therapy	Pronunciation	Definition
interpersonal psychotherapy – family therapy – group therapy	in-ter-PER-son-al THER-a-pee FAM-i-lee THER-a-pee groop THER-a-pee	This form of treatment seeks to examine how a person interacts with others and how these interactions relate to their own thoughts and actions. Family therapy looks at the network of relationships and the individuals themselves to understand the basis of the conflicts and identify resolutions. Group therapy, with the aid of a mental health professional, provides the avenue for group discussions and the opportunity for patients to examine and explore issues.
play therapy	play THER-a-pee	Play therapy is a method in which a child uses toys to communicate and resolve psychological problems.
psychoanalysis	sy-koh-a-NAL-a-sis	Psychoanalysis has been a dominant form of therapy since its development by Sigmund Freud. Through the use of techniques such as free discussion, dream interpretation and free association, the patient's awareness of underlying psychic conflicts and defences is raised.

Psychopharmacology

The following table provides a summary of the medications used to treat mental disorders, grouped according to the types of conditions that are being treated.

Type of Drug	Definition
anti-alcoholics	Drugs used to suppress the desire to consume alcohol or to treat alcohol-related withdrawal symptoms.
anti-anxiety and anti-panic agents	Anti-anxiety and anti-panic agents are used to treat patients with anxiety, tension and agitation, particularly when associated with panic attacks.
antidepressants	Drugs for alleviating the symptoms of depression and to improve functional capacity, particularly for patients with major depression, panic disorders and obsessive compulsive disorders.
antipsychotics	Drugs used to manage psychotic symptoms such as hallucinations and delusions in disorders such as schizophrenia and bipolar disorder.
hypnotics	Drugs used in insomnia to promote sleep but may also be used in surgical anaesthesia.
mood stabilisers	Drugs to prevent acute mood shifts and to balance the activities of neurotransmitters in the brain.
sedatives, sedative-hypnotics	Drugs that apply a calming effect on the patient, with or without inducing sleep.
stimulants	Drugs to increase alertness, attention and energy.

Other therapeutic methods

Type of Therapy	Pronunciation	Definition
electroconvulsive therapy (ECT)	ee-LEK-troh-kon-VUL-siv THER-a-pee	ECT is a medical procedure that is used to treat mental illnesses such as severe depression and some forms of mania and schizophrenia. This form of treatment is usually used when other forms of therapy have not been effective. However, in emergency or life-threatening situations (e.g. threatened suicide), it can be the first line of treatment. The procedure involves placing electrodes at strategic points on the patient's skull, either unilaterally or bilaterally. The brain is then stimulated through a series of low-frequency electrical pulses that stimulate a convulsion. As the patient is under general anaesthetic and has had muscle relaxants administered, the intensity of the resultant muscle spasms is minimised. Some patients experience temporary confusion, headaches and memory loss after an ECG. Administering an ultrabrief pulse on the right side is now a more commonly used treatment method that can potentially combine effectiveness with fewer cognitive side effects.
hypnosis	hip-NOH-sis	Hypnosis involves the patient being put into a trance-like state, making them more susceptible to suggestion, and providing the opportunity to alter existing behaviours.

Exercises

EXERCISE 18.1: WORD ELEMENT MEANINGS AND WORD BUILDING

Define each word element below, then use the element correctly in a medical term.

Combining Forms	Meaning	Medical Term
cycl/o		
hallucin/o		
iatr/o		
klept/o		
morph/o		
neur/o		
phil/o		
phor/o		
pol/o		
psych/o		
schiz/o		

Combining Forms	Meaning	Medical Term
somat/o		
xen/o		
agora-		
cata-		
electro-		
eu-		
-lalia		
-leptic		
-mania		
-philia		

EXERCISE 18.2: WORD ANALYSIS AND MEANING

Break up the medical terms below into their component parts (prefixes, suffixes, combining forms). Provide the meaning for each word element and each term as a whole.

Example:

necrophilia

necro = death

phil/o = attraction to, love

-ia = condition

Meaning = condition of attraction to death

1. kleptomania _____

    _____

2. gerontophobia _____

    _____

3. hypochondriac _____

    _____

4. dysmorphophobia _____

    _____

5. schizophrenia _____

_____

6. neurosis _____

_____

7. dysthymia _____

_____

8. coprolalia _____

_____

9. narcoleptic _____

_____

10. trichotillomania _____

_____

EXERCISE 18.3: VOCABULARY BUILDING

Provide the medical term for each of the definitions below.

1. A condition of wandering in the mind: _____

2. A doctor who specialises in the treatment of the mind: _____

3. Pertaining to two extremes: _____

4. A bad emotional state: _____

5. A fear of the night: _____

6. Fire frenzy: _____

7. Pertaining to the mind: _____

8. A fear of the open space: _____

9. No emotion: _____

10. Abnormal condition of sleep: _____

EXERCISE 18.4: MATCH THE ABBREVIATIONS WITH THE EXPANDED FORM

Match the abbreviation in Column A with its expanded form in Column B.

Column A	Answer	Column B
1. AD		A. selective serotonin reuptake inhibitor
2. OCD		B. Mental State Examination
3. MDD		C. seasonal affective disorder
4. SSRI		D. autistic spectrum disorder
5. CBT		E. mental age
6. MSE		F. obsessive compulsive disorder
7. ETOH		G. Alzheimer's disease
8. SAD		H. cognitive behaviour therapy
9. ASD		I. ethanol
10. MA		J. major depressive disorder

EXERCISE 18.5: MATCH THE THERAPY WITH ITS MEANING

Match the type of mental health therapy in Column A with its meaning in Column B.

Column A	Answer	Column B
1. psychoanalysis		A. Uses group discussion to explore issues
2. family therapy		B. Puts a patient in a trance-like state to make them susceptible to change
3. psychotherapy		C. Modifies the patterns of thought and behaviour
4. group therapy		D. Uses toys to communicate and resolve psychological problems
5. hypnosis		E. Uses free association and dream interpretation to raise awareness of conflicts
6. play therapy		F. Looks at the network of relationships and the individual
7. cognitive behaviour therapy		G. Looks at how a person interacts with others and how this relates to their own thoughts and actions

EXERCISE 18.6: PRONUNCIATION AND COMPREHENSION

Read the following paragraphs aloud to practise your pronunciation. Using your textbook and a medical dictionary, find the meanings of the underlined medical terms.

This 28-year-old woman was admitted following an overdose of 30 × 25 mg of Prothiaden (dothiepin hydrochloride) and alcohol. She suffers from chronic depression, but she claims that this overdose was an accident.

In the emergency department she was found to be drowsy but extremely agitated with a rapidly deteriorating mental state and, as we had seen her approximately 2 hours after her ingestion, it was thought best to administer intravenous sedation (ASA = 1NE), then intubate her and perform a gastric lavage. She was given intravenous haloperidol and was subsequently intubated by the anaesthetist. Lavage showed large numbers of orange-coloured tablets. She was also given charcoal through the nasogastric tube.

She was admitted to intensive care and observed overnight. The following day she was reviewed by the hospital psychiatrist and was felt to be safe for discharge. She will be followed up by her LMO and her own psychiatrist.

EXERCISE 18.7: CROSSWORD PUZZLE

Complete the puzzle by providing the medical term for each of the clues below.

ACROSS

1. Fear of the number 13 (17)
3. Fear of going to the doctor (11)
5. Fear of needles (12)
6. Fear of long words (18)
7. Fear of thunder and lightning (12)
9. Fear of marriage (10)
10. Fear of dogs (10)

DOWN

2. Fear of heights (10)
4. Fear of infection or contamination (10)
8. Fear of men (11)

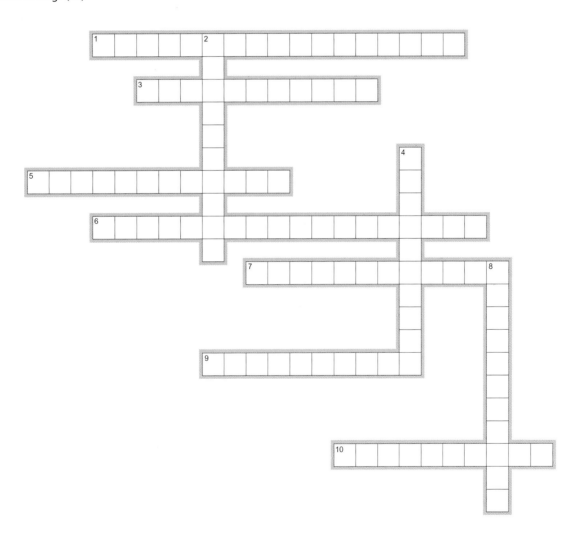

EXERCISE 18.8: DISCHARGE SUMMARY ANALYSIS

Read the discharge summary below and answer the questions.

UNIVERSITY HOSPITAL DISCHARGE SUMMARY	**UR number:** 010203 **Name:** Christine Harris **Address:** 55 Longley Crescent, Frankstown **Date of birth:** 25/5/1970 **Sex:** F **Nominated primary healthcare provider:** Dr John Smart
Episode details **Consultant:** Dr Godfrey **Registrar:** Dr Bresslin **Unit:** Psychiatric ward **Admission source:** Psychiatric OPD **Date of admission:** 18/11/2020	**Discharge details** **Status:** Home **Date of discharge:** 3/12/2020

Reason for admission / Presenting problems:

Four-year history of depression

Principal diagnosis: Depression

Comorbidities: Atypical seizures

Previous medical history: Abnormal TFTs October 2019

Clinical synopsis:

This 50-year-old woman was admitted for management of her depression. History from her husband was that she had become increasingly depressed over the past 4 years and was having difficulty coping at home. She was currently totally cared for by her husband and his mother. She did not cook or do any of the household tasks. She had been requiring supervision to go to the toilet and had been incontinent of faeces in the bed. She was even becoming unable to hold a conversation. She had had a previous admission in October of last year. At that time she had had abnormal TFTs but these were thought to be consistent with a low thyroid binding globulin and that no further investigations at that time were required.

She was admitted for further assessment and urgent family respite.

On examination she was unable to hold a lucid conversation. Her MSQ, however, was 9/10. She obeyed commands and appeared appropriate in her actions. Her affect was flat. There were no psychotic features. There was no formal thought disorder and she was not suicidal. There were no neurological deficits on examination.

Psychiatric review: history from the patient suggests an episode of unconsciousness 2 days prior to admission. There was no preceding aura. She was drowsy following this, but otherwise normal. She was given Prozac and continued on Prothiaden. A 24-hour Holter EEG was performed. This was normal.

She was slowly improving on the above medications and then discharged home to be followed up in outpatients. She was reviewed by the neurologist, who felt that on the history and information available, the seizures were not organic in nature and that they required no further investigations at present.

Complications:

Clinical interventions: Holter EEG

Diagnostic interventions:

Screening tests involving a full blood count, B_{12}, folate, coag profile, syphilis serology, SMA and liver function tests were all normal. Repeat thyroid function tests were normal.

Medications at discharge: Sinequan 150 mg nocte

Ceased medications: Nil

Allergies: Nil

Alerts: Nil

Arranged services: Nil
Recommendations: Psychiatric OPD review
Information to patient/relevant parties:
Authorising clinician: Dr Bresslin
Document recipients:
Patient and LMO: Dr John Smart

1. **Expand the following abbreviations as found in the discharge summary above.**

   B_{12}

   EEG

   MSQ

   SMA

   TFTs

2. **On discharge Mrs Harris was prescribed Sinequan. When should she be taking the drug?**

3. **Under diagnostic interventions the patient had syphilis serology performed. What is the purpose of this test?**

4. **What is the purpose of performing the Holter EEG in this case study?**

5. **Explain the term atypical seizures.**

MODULE 4

Systemic Conditions

CHAPTER 19

Oncology

Contents

OBJECTIVES   452

INTRODUCTION   453

NEW WORD ELEMENTS   453

    Combining forms   453

    Prefixes   454

    Suffixes   454

VOCABULARY   454

ABBREVIATIONS   455

CANCERS AND TUMOURS   456

    Differences between malignant
    and benign tumours   456

    Primary tumours versus
    metastatic (secondary)
    tumours   458

    Common sites for metastatic
    spread   458

    Causes of cancer   458

    Types of cancers   458

    Grading and staging systems   460

    Cancer in Australia and New
    Zealand   461

TESTS AND PROCEDURES   462

    Diagnostic tests and
    procedures   462

    Surgical interventions   464

    Radiotherapy   464

    Chemotherapy   465

EXERCISES   467

Objectives

After completing this chapter you should be able to:

1. state the meanings of the word elements related to oncology

2. build words using the word elements associated with oncology

3. recognise, pronounce and effectively use medical terms associated with oncology

4. expand abbreviations related to oncology

5. describe the different types of tumours, the differences between malignant and benign tumours, the various grading and staging systems and the causes of cancer

6. describe common laboratory tests and diagnostic and surgical procedures associated with oncology

7. apply what you have learned by interpreting medical terminology in practice.

Demonstrate your knowledge of oncology by completing the exercises at the end of this chapter.

INTRODUCTION

As a specialty, oncology is concerned with the study and treatment of neoplasms. Neoplasm means 'new growth'. Neoplasms can be either benign (non-cancerous), in situ (pre-cancerous) or malignant (cancerous). Cancer is the general term given to a range of malignant neoplasms, occurring when a group of cells grows and multiplies uncontrollably. Neoplasms can occur in any body tissue, at any age and in anyone.

This chapter discusses the causes of cancer, the different types of neoplasms, grading and staging systems and the many types of treatment.

General discussion about different cancers is included in this chapter, but tumours specific to particular body systems are discussed in the relevant body system chapters.

NEW WORD ELEMENTS

Here are some word elements related to oncology. To reinforce your learning, write the meanings of the medical terms in the spaces provided. Use the Glossary of medical terms on page 561 to help you work out the meanings. You may also need to check the meaning in a medical dictionary, but make an attempt yourself first.

Combining forms

Combining Form	Meaning	Medical Term	Meaning of Medical Term
aden/o	gland	adenocarcinoma	
astr/o	star	astrocytoma	
blast/o	embryonic or developing cell	retinoblastoma	
cac/o	ill, unpleasant, bad, abnormal	cachexia	
cancer/o	cancer	cancerous	
carcin/o	cancerous, malignant	carcinogenesis	
cauter/o	heat, burn	cautery	
chem/o	chemical, drug	chemoprophylaxis	
chondr/o	cartilage	osteochondroma	
cry/o	cold	cryosurgery	
cyt/o	cell	cytogenic	
fibr/o	fibres	neurofibroma	
gli/o	glue	glioblastoma	
gnos/o	knowledge	prognosis	
hist/o	tissue	histopathology	
histi/o		histiocytosis	
immun/o	protection	immunotherapy	
leuc/o	white	leucocyte	
leuk/o		leukaemia	
(Note that the CF leuk/o is used in Australia for the word leukaemia and derivative terms only)			
melan/o	black	melanoma	
mut/a	genetic change	mutation	
onc/o	tumour	oncologist	
papill/o	nipple-shaped projection	papillary	
plas/o	formation	neoplasia	

Table continued

Combining Form	Meaning	Medical Term	Meaning of Medical Term
polyp/o	polyp	polyposis	
radi/o	x-rays, radius	radiation	
rhabd/o	rod-shaped, striated (skeletal) muscle	rhabdomyosarcoma	
sarc/o	flesh	sarcoma	
scirrh/o	hard	scirrhoid	

Prefixes

Prefix	Meaning	Medical Term	Meaning of Medical Term
ana-	up, towards, apart	anaplastic	
brachy-	short	brachytherapy	
epi-	above, upon, on	epidermoid	
meta-	change, beyond	metastasis	
neo-	new	neoplasm	
pleio-	more	pleiotrophy	
pleo-		pleomorphic	
tele-	distant, end, far, complete	telediagnosis	

Suffixes

Suffix	Meaning	Medical Term	Meaning of Medical Term
-blastoma	immature tumour	neuroblastoma	
-genesis	pertaining to formation, producing	oncogenesis	
-oma	tumour, collection, mass, swelling	adenoma	
-plasia	formation, development, growth	dysplasia	
-plasm	growth, formation, substance	cytoplasm	
-suppression	to stop	immunosuppression	
-therapy	treatment	chemotherapy	

VOCABULARY

The following list provides many of the medical terms used for the first time in this chapter. Pronunciations are provided with each term. As you read the rest of the chapter, make sure you identify each of these terms and understand their meanings.

Term	Pronunciation
alkylating agent	AL-kil-ay-ting AY-jent
anaplastic	an-a-PLAS-tik
antimetabolite	an-tee-me-TAB-oh-lite

Table continued

Term	Pronunciation
antimicrotubules	an-tee-MY-kroh-tyoob-yoolz
apoptosis	a-po-TOH-sis
benign	be-NYN
bone marrow biopsy	bohn MA-roh BY-op-see
brachytherapy	bray-kee-THER-a-pee
carcinogenesis	kah-SIN-o-JEN-e-sis
carcinoma	kah-sin-O-ma
cell differentiation	sell dif-er-ENT-shee-AY-shun

Table continued

Term	Pronunciation
cytotoxic antibiotics	sy-toh-TOK-sik an-tee-by-OT-iks
exfoliative cytology	eks-FOH-lee-ay-tiv sy-TOL-o-jee
fibreoptic colonoscopy	fy-ber-OP-tik kol-on-OS-kop-ee
Gleason system	glee-son SIS-tem
grading	GRAY-ding
hormonal agent	haw-MOHN-al AY-jent
immunotherapy	im-YOON-oh-THER-a-pee
in situ	in SYT-yoo
laparoscopy	lap-ah-ROS-kop-ee
malignant	ma-LIG-nant
mammography	mam-MOG-raf-ee
metastasis (metastases)	me-TAS-tah-sis (me-TAS-tah-seez)
metastasise	me-TAS-tah-syz
metastatic	me-tas-TAT-ik
morphology	mor-FOL-oh-jee
myeloma	my-el-O-ma
needle biopsy	NEE-del BY-op-see
neoplasm	NEE-o-plaz-em
oncogene	ON-koh-jeen
platinum analogue	PLAT-in-um an-a-log
protein marker test	pro-teen mah-ka test
radionuclide scan	ray-dee-o-NYOO-klyd skan
sarcoma	sah-KOH-ma
staging	STAY-jing
topoisomerase inhibitors	to-poy-SOM-er-ayz in-HIB-it-orz
tumour	TYOO-mah
undifferentiated	un-dif-er-ENT-shee-AY-ted
well differentiated	well dif-er-ENT-shee-AY-ted

ABBREVIATIONS

The following abbreviations are commonly used in the Australian healthcare environment. Because some abbreviations can have more than one meaning, check the context in which the abbreviation is used before assigning a meaning to it.

Abbreviation	Definition
ABC	advanced breast cancer
ABMT	autologous bone marrow transplant

Table continued

Abbreviation	Definition
adj	adjuvant therapy
AFP	alphafetoprotein
AI	aromatase inhibitor
ALL	acute lymphoblastic leukaemia
	acute lymphocytic leukaemia
AML	acute myeloid leukaemia
BCC	basal cell carcinoma
BM	bone marrow
BRCA1, BRCA2	breast cancer 1, breast cancer 2 are genes, prone to multiple mutations, involved in about 5% of breast cancers
BSE	breast self-examination
bx	biopsy
Ca	cancer, carcinoma
CT, CAT	computed tomography, computerised axial tomography
chemo	chemotherapy
CLL	chronic lymphocytic leukaemia
CML	chronic myeloid leukaemia
CMML	chronic myelomonocytic leukaemia
CST	cervical screening test
DCIS	ductal carcinoma in situ
DRE	digital rectal examination
FAP	familial adenomatous polyposis
FIGO	International Federation of Gynecology and Obstetrics – gynaecological staging system
FNA(B)	fine-needle aspiration (biopsy)
FOBT	faecal occult blood test
GIST	gastrointestinal stromal tumour
Gy	gray (unit of radiation equal to 100 RAD)
HER2	human epidermal growth factor receptor
HPV	human papillomavirus
LMP	low malignant potential
mets	metastases
MOAB	monoclonal antibody
MRI	magnetic resonance imaging
NED	no evidence of disease
NHL	non-Hodgkin lymphoma
NK	natural killer (cells)
NMSC	non-melanoma skin cancer
Pap smear	Papanicolaou smear

Table continued

Abbreviation	Definition
PET	positron emission tomography
PSA	prostate-specific antigen
RAD	radiation absorbed dose
SCC	squamous cell carcinoma
SNB	sentinel node biopsy
SSM	superficial spreading melanoma
SPECT	single-photon emission computed tomography
TCC	transitional cell carcinoma
TNM	tumour, node, metastasis – staging system for tumours

CANCERS AND TUMOURS

Cancer is the common term used for all types of malignant tumours. There are approximately 200 different types of cancer that can differentially affect nearly all the organs and tissues in the body. A tumour is an abnormal growth of cells and tissues in the body. Every cell in the body has the potential to be affected by a tumour. Also known as a neoplasm (meaning 'new growth'), a tumour can be benign, in situ or malignant, with the difference due to degrees of cell differentiation, rate of growth, invasion to adjacent tissue and ability to metastasise. Normally, the body creates cells at the rate required to replace those that die in a process known as apoptosis, or as necessary to assist in growth and development. However, sometimes cells begin to grow and divide in a way that is unregulated by normal body control mechanisms. It is not known what triggers this abnormal growth. Malignant tumours may be in situ ('in place'), meaning they are localised in their tissue of origin, or may invade surrounding tissues and can then spread to other body sites, making them more dangerous than benign tumours, which do not invade and spread. Oncology (Greek 'oncos' = tumour) is the study of tumours or cancers.

A benign tumour is generally well defined, with regular cell boundaries or a surrounding capsule that expands in size, although generally this growth is slow and the tumour may even stop growing when it reaches a certain diameter. The growth can cause problems if the tumour causes the surrounding tissue to push up against a solid surface in the body. For example, a benign brain tumour may grow so that it compresses surrounding brain tissue against the skull, resulting in differing effects depending on the affected tissue. The tumour may therefore cause symptoms such as paralysis, dizziness or loss of hearing or sight. Benign tumours may also cause problems if they are physiologically active – for example, if they produce hormones.

Benign tumours consist of cells that are 'well differentiated'. In other words, the tumour cells closely resemble the normal cells from which they have originated both in terms of morphology (structure) and function. The tumour tissues remain ordered and organised. The more similar the structure of the tumour cell is to that of a normal cell structure, the better it is differentiated. Most benign tumours grow slowly and remain localised to their point of origin.

In contrast, a malignant tumour or cancer consists of cells that range from well differentiated to poorly differentiated to undifferentiated or anaplastic. The increasing lack of differentiation is characteristic of malignant transformation and is accompanied by structural and functional changes. The neoplastic cells and their nuclei are typically pleomorphic, meaning they vary in size and shape and are less similar to normal body cells. The neoplastic cells grow rapidly in a disorganised fashion, although their rate of growth may change over time, being affected by such things as hormone dependence and blood supply. The growth of malignant tumours generally begins by changes in one cell in which the genes in the cell's DNA that control growth and differentiation are altered (Fig. 19.1). Cancers that are in situ are still classified as malignant although they are pre-invasive and have not yet spread beyond their cells of origin. However, in time the mutant genetic changes are passed on to subsequent cells arising from the original transformed cell. Through reproduction, these mutant cells progress from the primary site to infiltrate, invade and ultimately obliterate surrounding tissue and regional lymph nodes. Increasing changes in the abnormal cells' DNA may cause the cells to leave their site of origin and travel via blood or lymph to distant sites. This process is known as metastatic spread (Fig. 19.2), causing the growth of secondary tumours (or metastases) with similar characteristics in other organs and tissues.

Differences between malignant and benign tumours

Malignant Tumours	Benign Tumours
Grow rapidly	Grow slowly
Invasive and infiltrative into adjacent organs	Encapsulated so they don't invade surrounding tissue
Cells are undifferentiated (anaplastic)	Cells are well differentiated and resemble normal tissue
Tumour can metastasise to distant sites via blood or lymph	Tumour does not metastasise to distant sites

Figure 19.1 **Progression of tumour growth**

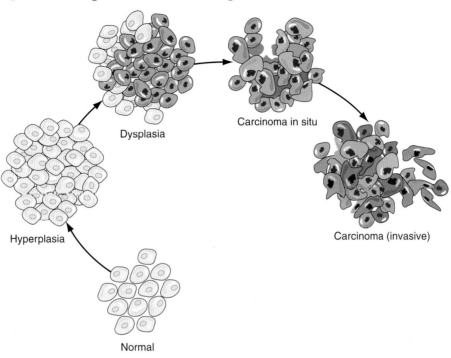

Dysplasia

Carcinoma in situ

Carcinoma (invasive)

Hyperplasia

Normal

Figure 19.2 **Process of metastatic spread**

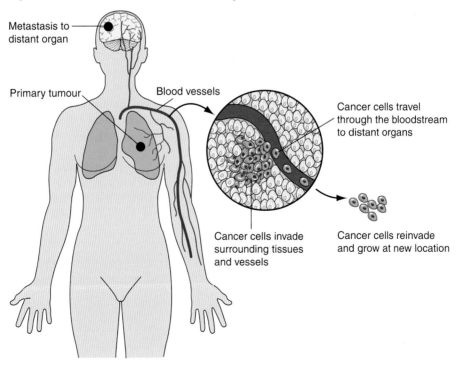

Metastasis to distant organ

Primary tumour

Blood vessels

Cancer cells travel through the bloodstream to distant organs

Cancer cells invade surrounding tissues and vessels

Cancer cells reinvade and grow at new location

Primary tumours versus metastatic (secondary) tumours

The term 'primary tumour' refers to the original tumour in the body – the site where the cancer first started. It is important for this site to be identified so that treatment and prevention strategies can be developed. Some tumours will remain at the site of origin, others may spread into the surrounding tissue, while other tumours will spread to distant sites via the bloodstream, lymphatic system or through a body cavity. The tumour in a site other than its site of origin is called a metastatic tumour or metastasis. It can also be called a secondary tumour. Metastatic cancer has the same morphological name and the same histological composition as the primary tumour. For example, prostate cancer that spreads to the bones and forms a metastatic tumour is metastatic prostate cancer, not bone cancer.

Primary tumours can spread to many different metastatic sites in the body but most commonly spread to the lymph nodes, lungs, bones, brain and liver. There is a tendency for specific solid tumours to metastasise to particular organs. The following table shows the most frequent sites of metastasis for some common primary sites of cancer.

Common sites for metastatic spread

Body Site of Primary Tumour	Common Metastatic Sites
breast	lungs, liver, bones, brain, lymph nodes
colon	liver, peritoneum, lungs, lymph nodes
kidney	lungs, liver, bones, brain, adrenal gland, lymph nodes
lungs	adrenal gland, liver, other lung, brain, bones, lymph nodes
melanoma	lungs, brain, liver, bone, lymph nodes
ovary	peritoneum, liver, lungs, lymph nodes
pancreas	liver, lungs, peritoneum, lymph nodes
prostate	bones, lungs, liver, adrenal glands, lymph nodes
rectum	liver, lungs, peritoneum, lymph nodes
stomach	liver, peritoneum, lungs, lymph nodes

Table continued

Body Site of Primary Tumour	Common Metastatic Sites
thyroid	lungs, liver, bones, lymph nodes
uterus	liver, lungs, peritoneum, bone, vagina, lymph nodes

Causes of cancer

Carcinogenesis is the term used to describe the transformation of normal cells into cancerous cells. When the normal equilibrium between cell creation and cell death is disturbed by mutation in the cell DNA, a tumour results. Some of these tumours will remain benign, but others will undergo malignant transformation. The affected genes are divided into two broad categories: oncogenes, which promote cell growth and reproduction, and tumour suppressor genes, which hamper cell division and survival. Malignant transformation begins through developing abnormal oncogenes, or an unusual proliferation of normal oncogenes, or by the tumour suppressor genes being disabled.

There are several risk factors relating to carcinogenesis. In general, anything that can cause a DNA mutation can cause cancer. Differential exposures to the various risk factors can cause distinctive types of cancers in various body sites. Some cancers have a familial or genetic component, but others do not.

Around 30% of all cancers can be prevented by avoiding certain risk factors. Some of the common risk factors for different cancers include:

- smoking, particularly of tobacco products
- exposure to radiation, including ultraviolet (UV) radiation, x-rays and radioactive substances
- chemicals and certain drugs
- alcohol
- exposure to environmental carcinogens such as chemicals, dyes and insecticides
- poor diet, high in fats and highly processed foods and low in fruit and vegetables
- lack of exercise and weight control
- viruses
- heredity and genetics (Fig. 19.3).

Types of cancers

There are six main categories into which all types of malignancies fall. The categories relate to the form and structure of the tissues in which the cancer arises. This is called the morphology of the tumour. The table on the following page shows the different morphologies of tumours and the specific characteristics of each.

Figure 19.3 Environmental and hereditary agents as causes of cancer

Environmental agents	Diet Tobacco Chemicals Radiation Viruses Alcohol Other lifestyle factors	DNA mutation causing premalignant changes	Malignancy (in situ, malignant primary, metastic)
Inherited agents	Ova Sperm		

Type of Cancer	General Description	Common Subtypes of the Cancer
carcinoma	Carcinomas are solid tumours that arise from epithelial tissue. They are commonly found in the skin, lungs, breast, colon, liver, prostate and stomach. Most cancers are carcinomas.	Based on the type of cell or structure the carcinoma arises in, common subtypes are: • adenocarcinoma • basal cell carcinoma • large cell carcinoma • renal cell carcinoma • small cell carcinoma • squamous cell carcinoma • transitional cell carcinoma.
leukaemia	Leukaemia is a malignancy of the blood-forming cells in the bone marrow. There is an overproduction of abnormal leucocytes that congest the bone marrow, preventing the production of erythrocytes and platelets. The abnormal cells are carried in the blood to organs such as the liver, spleen, lungs and kidneys.	Based on the type of cell the leukaemia arises in and whether it is acute or chronic: • acute lymphocytic leukaemia (ALL) • chronic lymphocytic leukaemia (CLL) • acute myeloid leukaemia (AML) • chronic myeloid leukaemia (CML).
lymphoma	Lymphomas are tumours arising in immune cells or lymphocytes in the lymphatic system. They frequently originate in lymph nodes, where the node appears enlarged due to the presence of tumour. Lymphomas can also occur in other organs such as the brain or colon. Lymphomas are the most common type of haematopoietic cancer.	There are many types of lymphomas. These types are based on the type of cell or the site the lymphoma arises in. Some of the more commonly occurring ones are: • Burkitt's lymphoma • extranodal lymphoma • Hodgkin lymphoma • non-Hodgkin lymphoma.
mixed types	This is cancer composed of more than one type of neoplastic tissue such as combinations of different epithelial and connective tissue types.	Common mixed cell tumours include: • germ cell tumours occurring in the cells that make up the reproductive system in males and females, particularly ovaries and testicles • mixed small-cell and large-cell tumours arising in the lungs.

Table continued

Type of Cancer	General Description	Common Subtypes of the Cancer
myeloma	Myeloma is a tumour consisting of antibody-producing plasma cells (a form of lymphocyte), generally arising in bone marrow. Myeloma usually arises in multiple sites and causes destruction of the bone.	Based on the type of cell or site the myeloma arises in, common subtypes are: · endothelial myeloma · extramedullary myeloma · giant cell myeloma · multiple myeloma · osteogenic myeloma.
sarcoma	Sarcomas arise from connective tissue such as bone, cartilage, skeletal muscle, fibrous tissue, fat, blood vessels, lymphatic tissue and haematopoietic tissue.	Based on the type of cell, connective tissue, or structure the sarcoma arises in, common subtypes are: · angiosarcoma · chondrosarcoma · Ewing's sarcoma · fibrosarcoma · Kaposi's sarcoma · leiomyosarcoma · liposarcoma · malignant schwannoma · neurofibrosarcoma · osteosarcoma.

Grading and staging systems

The grade and stage of a tumour are the most important predictors for long-term prognosis and for determining the most effective treatment following a cancer diagnosis.

The grade of a tumour refers to how quickly, or how aggressively, it is growing. It describes the degree of cell differentiation when viewed microscopically. The specific factors used to determine the grade of a tumour differ depending on the type of cancer and the grading classifications used for different cancer types. However, most commonly four levels of grading are used, with grade 1 being cancers that are well differentiated, grade 2 being moderately differentiated, grade 3 being poorly differentiated and grade 4 being undifferentiated or anaplastic.

Specific grading systems include the Gleason system to describe the degree of differentiation of prostate cancer cells. The Gleason system has scores ranging from 2 to 10, with lower Gleason scores indicating well-differentiated and less aggressive tumours with a higher survival rate and, conversely, higher scores describing poorly differentiated, more aggressive tumours.

The stage of a cancer relates to the size of the tumour and whether it has spread throughout the body. Some staging systems relate to several types of cancer, while others are specific to a cancer type.

The elements most commonly considered in staging cancers are:

- site of the primary tumour
- tumour size and number of tumours
- lymph node involvement
- cell type and tumour grade
- the presence or absence of metastases.

Staging can be done on clinical examination, or by using imaging, pathology tests or surgical examination. The most common method to describe solid tumours is the TNM staging system, which has four main categories (I, II, III, IV); these are subdivided into more specific staging groups (IIa, IIb, IIIa, IIIb). The TNM system describes the size of the primary tumour (T, tumour), whether any cancer cells have spread from the primary site to reach nearby lymph nodes (N, node), and whether the cancer cells have spread further around the body (M, metastasis). The TNM system classifies tumours as follows:

Primary tumour (T)

TX   Primary tumour cannot be evaluated
T0   No evidence of primary tumour
TIS   Carcinoma in situ
T1, T2, T3, T4   Size and/or extent of the primary tumour

Regional lymph nodes (N)

NX   Regional lymph nodes cannot be evaluated

N0   No regional lymph node involvement

N1, N2, N3   Involvement of regional lymph nodes (number of lymph nodes and/or extent of spread)

Distant metastasis (M)

MX   Distant metastasis cannot be evaluated

M0   No distant metastasis

M1   Distant metastasis is present

The various stages of lymphomas are classified differently. They are classified according to how many groups of lymph nodes are affected:

- **Stage I** – tumour is found in a single group of lymph nodes or a single extralymphatic organ.
- **Stage II** – tumour is found in two or more groups of lymph nodes on the same side of the diaphragm, or tumour is found in one group of lymph nodes plus a single extralymphatic organ on the same side of the diaphragm.
- **Stage III** – tumour is found in groups of lymph nodes on both sides of the diaphragm. It may have also spread to an extralymphatic organ or to the spleen, or both.
- **Stage IV** – tumour has disseminated within or outside the lymphatic system and can be found in organs such as the liver, lungs and bone marrow.

In Australia, the staging system for colorectal (bowel) cancer (Fig. 19.4) is the Australian Clinico-Pathological Staging (ACPS) System:

- **Stage A0 (carcinoma in situ)** – the cancer is found only in the innermost lining of the colon. Stage A0 cancer is also called carcinoma in situ.

- **Stage A** – the cancer has spread beyond the innermost tissue layer of the colon but is confined to the inside of the bowel wall.
- **Stage B** – the cancer has spread to the outer surface of the colon wall.
- **Stage C** – the cancer is found in the lymph nodes in the area of the colon.
- **Stage D** (also known as metastatic bowel cancer) – the cancer has spread from where it started in the colon or rectum to other organs, especially the liver or lungs.

Reference: https://www.bowelcanceraustralia.org/bowel-cancer-staging

Cancer in Australia and New Zealand

In Australia, an estimated 144,000 new cancers (excluding non-melanoma skin cancers) were diagnosed in 2019, with an overall risk of being diagnosed with cancer before the age of 85 years of 1 in 2 for males and females. In New Zealand, about 22,000 new cancers are diagnosed annually.

The most recently available data estimates that the most commonly diagnosed cancers in Australia in 2019 were:

- breast cancer
- prostate cancer
- colorectal cancer
- melanoma of the skin
- lung cancer.

Reference: https://www.aihw.gov.au/reports-data/health-conditions-disability-deaths/cancer/overview

When looking at deaths from cancer in Australia, the order is different. There are about 46,000 deaths

Figure 19.4 Staging of colon cancer
A: Stage A0; B: Stage B; C: Stage D

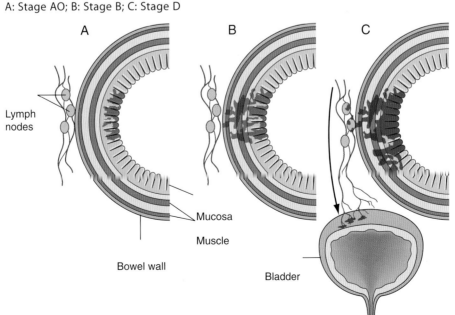

from cancer in Australia annually. The most recently available data for 2017 identifies the most common sites for mortality from cancer as:

- lung cancer
- colorectal cancer
- prostate cancer
- breast cancer
- pancreatic cancer.

Reference: http://www.abs.gov.au/ausstats/abs@.nsf/mf/3303.0

The difference between the figures demonstrates the success of many of the screening programs and treatments now available.

In 2016 in New Zealand, the most common cancers were prostate, followed by breast cancer, colorectal cancer, melanoma and lung cancer. Lung cancer was the most common cause of cancer deaths. Colorectal cancer was the next most common cause of death from cancer, followed by breast, prostate and pancreatic cancers.

Reference: https://www.health.govt.nz/nz-health-statistics/health-statistics-and-data-sets/cancer-data-and-stats

TESTS AND PROCEDURES

The following section provides a list of common diagnostic tests and procedures and clinical interventions and surgical procedures that are undertaken for oncology.

Diagnostic tests and procedures

The following table provides a list of tests and procedures that are used to diagnose tumours.

Test/Procedure	Pronunciation	Definition
bone marrow biopsy	bohn MA-roh BY-op-see	A bone marrow biopsy is a diagnostic procedure that is useful in diagnosing leukaemia and myeloma. The procedure is performed by introducing a needle into the bone marrow cavity and aspirating a small amount of marrow for examination under a microscope.
exfoliative cytology	eks-FOH-lee-ay-tiv sy-TOL-o-jee	Exfoliative cytology involves the microscopic examination of cells that have been removed from a body surface or lesion through aspiration, scraping, smearing or washing to identify malignant cells.
fibreoptic colonoscopy	fy-ber-OP-tik kol-on-OS-kop-ee	A procedure that involves a visual examination of the colon via fibreoptic colonoscope. It is a key screening process for cancer and pre-malignant polyps.
laparoscopy	lap-ah-ROS-kop-ee	Laparoscopy is a visual examination of the abdominal and pelvic cavities via an incision and insertion of a scope through the abdominal wall. It is used for diagnostic purposes and can also be used as a method for accessing abdominopelvic organs for treatment.
mammography	ma-MOG-raf-ee	Mammography is the process of taking a mammogram – a diagnostic procedure that uses low-dose x-ray for imaging of the breast (Fig. 19.5). It is used as a screening tool to diagnose breast cancer in women with or without symptoms (Fig. 19.6). In Australia, it is recommended that women over the age of 50 be screened for breast cancer every 2 years. Reference: http://www.cancer.org.au/preventing-cancer/early-detection/screening-programs/breast-cancer-screening.html

Table continued

Test/Procedure	Pronunciation	Definition
		Figure 19.5 Mammography (Frank et al 2007) 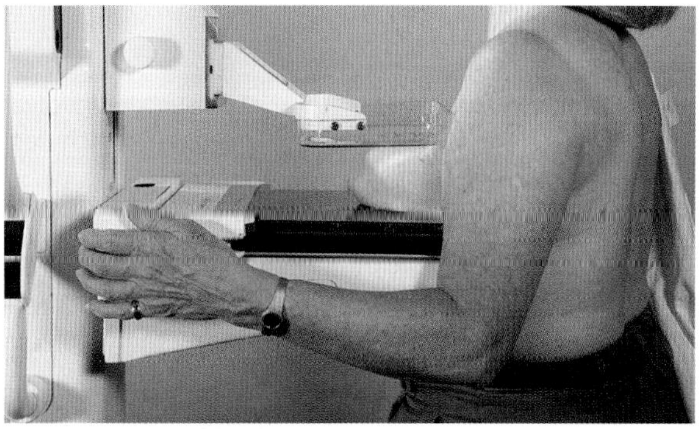 **Figure 19.6 Mammogram showing small invasive breast carcinoma** (Courtesy of Peter Farkas, Royal Darwin Hospital) 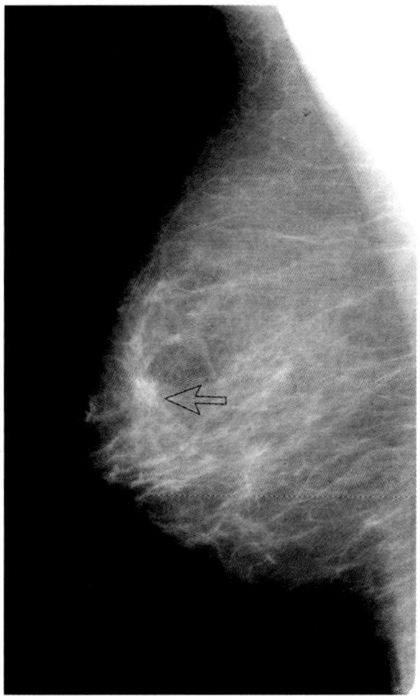
needle biopsy	NEE-del BY-op-see	A needle biopsy is a diagnostic procedure that involves removing fluid or tissue from a cavity or tumour mass for laboratory examination.
radionuclide scan	ray-dee-oh-NYOO-klyd skan	A radionuclide scan is a diagnostic procedure that involves intravenous injection of radionuclides (radioactive substances) so that images can be taken of organs to identify tumours or metastases. Different types of radionuclide are used for different parts of the body. For example, radioactive iodine injected into a vein will be taken up by the thyroid gland.
protein marker tests	pro-teen mah-ka tests	The purpose of the protein marker test is to diagnose cancer (either initial diagnosis or a recurrence). The level of the protein on the surface of a tumour cell or in the blood is measured. Some examples are: CA125 (ovarian cancer), oestrogen receptor (breast cancer) and prostate-specific antigen (PSA) (prostate cancer).

Surgical interventions

The type of surgical intervention that is undertaken to remove a tumour will depend on the nature of the tumour and the extent of organ or tissue involvement. Listed below are common methods of removing tumours or medical or surgical interventions in the treatment of tumours.

Surgical Intervention	Pronunciation	Definition
cryosurgery	kry-o-SER-ja-ree	Cryosurgery involves freezing a lesion using a cryogen such as liquid nitrogen, which destroys the tissue.
electrocauterisation	ee-LEK-troh kaw-ter-y-ZAY-shun	Electrocauterisation involves the destruction of tissue using electric currents.
en bloc resection	on blok re-SEK-shun	En bloc resection involves completely removing an organ and the surrounding tissue, including the lymph nodes (e.g. radical mastectomy, colectomy, gastrectomy).
excisional biopsy	ek-SI-shun-al BY-op-see	An excisional biopsy involves removing an entire lesion from a structure or organ, along with a margin of surrounding tissue. The lesion is sent for histological analysis.
exenteration	ek-SEN-ter-AY-shun	Exenteration is a surgical procedure for removing internal organs. Pelvic exenteration involves removing the organs of the pelvic cavity including the reproductive organs and the urinary bladder, urethra, rectum and anus.
fulguration	ful-ger-AY-shun	Fulguration is the destruction of tissue, usually malignant, using high-frequency electric current via a needle-like electrode.
incisional biopsy	in-SI-shun-al BY-op-see	Incisional biopsy involves removing a sample of tissue or tumour from an organ or structure for histological analysis and diagnosis.
bone marrow or stem cell transplant	bohn MA-roh or stem sel TRANS-plant	Bone marrow transplant is a two-step process that involves aspirating the bone marrow from a compatible donor (a donor whose tissues and blood cells closely match the recipient) and transfusing it into the recipient. Prior to intravenous transfusion of the marrow into the recipient, the patient generally undergoes chemotherapy or total body radiation. Once the transfusion has occurred, the donor marrow repopulates the patient's marrow space with normal cells. Complications that can occur include infection, graft-versus-host disease and relapse of the original disease. Stem cell transplant is the harvesting of the undifferentiated cells from the peripheral blood of the patient. Infusion of the stem cells is undertaken following chemotherapy. Stem cells are primitive blood-forming cells that can divide and mature into all the different types of blood cells.

Radiotherapy

Radiotherapy can be used as the sole method of treating a cancer or as an adjunct to surgery or chemotherapy. Through the administration of radiation, the aim of radiotherapy is to destroy or injure cancer cells so they do not multiply. The table below provides a list of common terms used in treating cancers involving radiotherapy.

Procedure	Pronunciation	Definition
brachytherapy	bray-kee-THER-a-pee	Brachytherapy involves placing radioactive material next to or inside a tumour to allow for a high dose of radiation to treat a small area (Fig. 19.7). The radioactive substance (seeds or pellets) can be placed permanently in the tumour. Over time the level of radioactivity of the implant reduces to nothing. Alternatively, the radioactive substance may be placed for a specified period and then removed.

Table continued

Procedure	Pronunciation	Definition

Figure 19.7 Brachytherapy for prostate cancer

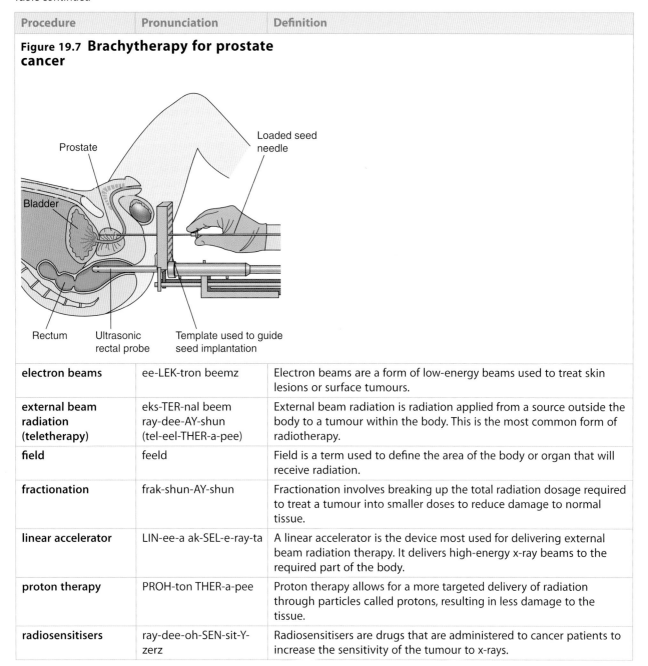

electron beams	ee-LEK-tron beemz	Electron beams are a form of low-energy beams used to treat skin lesions or surface tumours.
external beam radiation (teletherapy)	eks-TER-nal beem ray-dee-AY-shun (tel-eel-THER-a-pee)	External beam radiation is radiation applied from a source outside the body to a tumour within the body. This is the most common form of radiotherapy.
field	feeld	Field is a term used to define the area of the body or organ that will receive radiation.
fractionation	frak-shun-AY-shun	Fractionation involves breaking up the total radiation dosage required to treat a tumour into smaller doses to reduce damage to normal tissue.
linear accelerator	LIN-ee-a ak-SEL-e-ray-ta	A linear accelerator is the device most used for delivering external beam radiation therapy. It delivers high-energy x-ray beams to the required part of the body.
proton therapy	PROH-ton THER-a-pee	Proton therapy allows for a more targeted delivery of radiation through particles called protons, resulting in less damage to the tissue.
radiosensitisers	ray-dee-oh-SEN-sit-Y-zerz	Radiosensitisers are drugs that are administered to cancer patients to increase the sensitivity of the tumour to x-rays.

Chemotherapy

Chemotherapy involves administering cytotoxic agents to impair cancer cells' ability to replicate. The table following provides common groupings of cytotoxic agents, selected types of drugs and which cancers they are used to treat.

Type of Chemotherapeutic Agent	Pronunciation	Definition	Type of Cancer
alkylating agent	AL-kil-ay-ting AY-jent	An alkylating agent forms cross-bridges between DNA strands, interfering with cellular replication.	Brain
			Chronic lymphocytic leukaemia
			Lymphoma
			Hodgkin lymphoma
			Multiple myeloma
platinum analogues	plat-in-um an-a-logz	Platinum analogues form cross-linkages with DNA, acting in a similar manner to alkylating agents.	Small cell and non-small cell lung cancer
			Stomach
			Oesophageal
			Ovarian
cytotoxic antibiotics	sy-toh-tok-sik an-tee-by-OT-iks	Cytotoxic antibiotics are derived from bacteria or fungi and cause DNA strand breakage by binding to the DNA in a cell.	Testicular
			AML
			Lung
antimetabolites	an-tee-me-TAB-o-lites	Antimetabolites work to either inhibit folic acid conversion or to interfere with purine synthesis or pyrimidine synthesis.	Pancreatic
			Stomach
			Oesophageal
			Hairy cell leukaemia
			AML
			CLL
			Colorectal
			ALL
antimicrotubules	an-tee-my-kroh-TYOOB-yoolz	Antimicrotubule drugs are derived from plants and freeze or prevent the formation of the spindle in a cell, halting the process of mitosis.	Breast
			Hodgkin lymphoma
			Lung
topoisomerase inhibitors	to-poy-som-er-ayz in-HIB-it-orz	Topoisomerase inhibitors work to inhibit the enzyme that helps to regulate DNA structure.	Breast
			Stomach
			Oesophageal
hormonal agents	haw-mohn-al AY-jents	Hormonal agents act by removing the presence of a hormone that is required by some tumours to grow.	Breast
			Lymphoma
			Prostate
			ALL

IMMUNOTHERAPY

Normally, the body's immune system works to detect and destroy abnormal cells, which prevents some cancers from developing. However, certain cancer cells can hide from the immune system or are not destroyed by the immune system or the immune system may not be strong enough to stop them growing and multiplying.

Cancer cells can also change (mutate), which allows them to circumvent the actions of the immune system. Immunotherapy is a treatment that assists the body's own immune system to fight cancer. It does this by boosting the immune system to enable it to work more effectively or by removing barriers to the immune system attacking the cancer cells. Most commonly it assists the T cells to recognise and fight the cancer cells.

Immunotherapy can be administered orally, intravenously, topically and intravesically. It is administered in cycles, with a period of treatment followed by a period of rest. The main types of immunotherapy are treatments using monoclonal antibodies, nonspecific immunotherapies and cancer vaccines. The table below outlines the types of immunotherapy.

Type of Immunotherapy	Pronunciation	Definition
monoclonal antibodies	mon-oh-CLO-nal an-tee-bod-eez	Monoclonal antibodies are produced in a laboratory in a similar way to how the body naturally produces antibodies, as outlined in Chapter 7 Lymphatic and Immune Systems. When the body detects a harmful substance that causes disease, an antibody is produced to fight the cancer by targeting the cancer cells to alter their growth. Monoclonal antibodies can be designed to change the cancer cells in a number of ways, including by: attaching to the cancer cell to flag to the immune system to destroy the cell; slowing the growth of the cell by blocking the parts that assist growth; carrying medication directly to the cancer cells; and using the antibodies to deliver radiotherapy to the cancer cells without damaging the healthy cells.
nonspecific immunotherapies	non-spe-SIF-ik im-YOON-oh-THER-a-peez	Nonspecific immunotherapies are usually given in conjunction with chemotherapy and radiotherapy. This treatment uses cytokines, which are proteins produced by leucocytes that control the immune response, to assist the immune system to destroy the cancer cells. The cytokines in this form of immunotherapy are produced in a laboratory and include interferons (which slow cell growth), interleukins (which increase production of leucocytes and antibodies) and haematopoietic growth factors (which counteract the effects of chemotherapy).
cancer vaccine	can-ser vak-seen	Cancer vaccines trigger the immune system to detect cancer cells. They can be prophylactic, preventing the cancer cells developing, or therapeutic, stimulating the immune system to fight existing cancer cells.

Exercises

EXERCISE 19.1: MATCH WORD ELEMENTS AND MEANINGS

Match the prefix, suffix or combining form in Column A with its meaning from Column B.

Column A	Answer	Column B
1. blast/o		A. white
2. rhabd/o		B. knowledge
3. chondr/o		C. hard
4. meta-		D. tumour
5. astr/o		E. nipple-shaped projection
6. tele-		F. ill, unpleasant, bad
7. leuc/o		G. genetic change
8. -plasia		H. cold
9. onc/o		I. more
10. cauter/o		J. fibres

Column A	Answer	Column B
11. scirrh/o		K. treatment
12. pleio-		L. embryonic or developing cell
13. mut/a		M. formation, development, growth
14. cry/o		N. change, beyond
15. brachy-		O. rod-shaped, striated (skeletal)
16. papill/o		P. cartilage
17. fibr/o		Q. distant, end, far, complete
18. -therapy		R. star
19. gnos/o		S. short
20. cac/o		T. heat, burn

EXERCISE 19.2: CIRCLE THE CORRECT SPELLING

Circle the correctly spelled medical term from the options provided.

proggnosis	prognosis	prognossis	prognosys
metastatic	metsastatic	metastic	metaststatic
newrofibroma	neurophibroma	newrophibroma	neurofibroma
enaplastic	anaplasstic	anaplastic	anplastic
adeenocarcinoma	adenocarcinoma	adenocarcnoma	adencarcinoma
cackecksia	cachecsia	cachexia	caccexia
scirhoid	scirrhiod	scirhiod	scirrhoid
sarocoma	sarcoma	sarkoma	sarcooma
carcinogenesis	carcinogenisis	carsinogenesis	carcinogenisis
onkologist	onkolgist	oncologist	oncolgist

EXERCISE 19.3: WORD ANALYSIS AND MEANING

Break up the medical terms below into their component parts (prefixes, suffixes, combining forms). Provide the meaning for each word element and each term as a whole.

Example:

astrocytoma

astr/o = star

cyt/o = cell

-oma = tumour

Meaning = a tumour with star-shaped cells

1. retinoblastoma _____

_____

2. chemotherapy _____

_____

3. pleomorphic _____

4. dysplasia _____

_____

5. immunosuppression _____

_____

6. osteochondroma _____

_____

7. brachytherapy _____

_____

8. neoplasm _____

_____

9. oncogenesis _____

_____

10. myeloma _____

_____

EXERCISE 19.4: EXPAND THE ABBREVIATIONS

Expand the abbreviations to form correct medical terms.

Abbreviation	Expanded Abbreviation
ABC	
ABMT	
ALL	
BM	
Bx	
Ca	
CLL	
DCIS	
FAP	
FOBT	
GIST	
LMP	

Abbreviation	Expanded Abbreviation
NED	
NK	
PET	
RAD	
SNB	
SPECT	
TCC	
TNM	

EXERCISE 19.5: APPLYING MEDICAL TERMINOLOGY

Fill in each blank with the correct medical term.

1. An _____ tumour is said to be pre-invasive and 'in place' or still in the organ of origin.

2. Cancer cells that are anaplastic are also called _____.

3. A _____ tumour consists of cells that range from well differentiated to undifferentiated.

4. A tumour that has spread to another part of the body is said to have _____.

5. Tumour cells that closely resemble the normal cells are called _____.

6. How quickly or how aggressively a tumour grows is known as the _____ of the tumour.

7. _____ tumours are normally well defined with regular cell boundaries and a surrounding capsule.

8. A tumour is also known as a _____, meaning new growth.

9. A _____ site is the location where the tumour first started.

10. The _____ of a cancer relates to the size of the tumour and the spread through the body.

EXERCISE 19.6: PRONUNCIATION AND COMPREHENSION

Read the following paragraphs aloud to practise your pronunciation. Using your textbook and a medical dictionary, find the meanings of the underlined medical terms.

This 48-year-old man initially presented to University Hospital for investigation of 12 months of lower back pain and <u>bilateral</u> leg weakness. An <u>intrathecal contrast computed tomography</u> (CT) scan of the spine and a <u>myelogram</u> showed a destructive <u>lytic</u> lesion involving T11 and T12 (<u>thoracic vertebrae</u> 11 and 12) with associated <u>cord compression</u> at T11.

He underwent a <u>thoracic decompression</u> via a <u>thoracotomy</u> under general anaesthetic (ASA = 3NE), and <u>histopathology</u> revealed secondary <u>adenocarcinoma</u> in the spine. The primary site was never identified. He had deep <u>x-ray radiation therapy</u> (<u>orthovoltage</u>, 1 field) to that region and went on to have 30G in 10 fractions over 2 weeks. His in-hospital stay was uncomplicated and his leg weakness and <u>paraesthesia</u> gradually began to resolve.

EXERCISE 19.7: CROSSWORD PUZZLE

Complete the puzzle by providing the medical term for each of the clues below.

ACROSS

1. Removal of internal organs (12)
5. Freezing a lesion to destroy the tissue (11)
7. Grading system for prostate cancer (7, 6)
9. Drugs that are derived from plants and which halt the process of mitosis (16)
10. Breaking up radiation dosages into smaller doses (13)

DOWN

2. Drugs that increase tumour sensitivity to x-rays (16)
3. Destruction of tissue using electric currents (20)
4. Cancers composed of more than one type of neoplastic tissue (5, 5)
6. Medical term for secondary site cancer (10)
8. X-ray image of the breast (9)

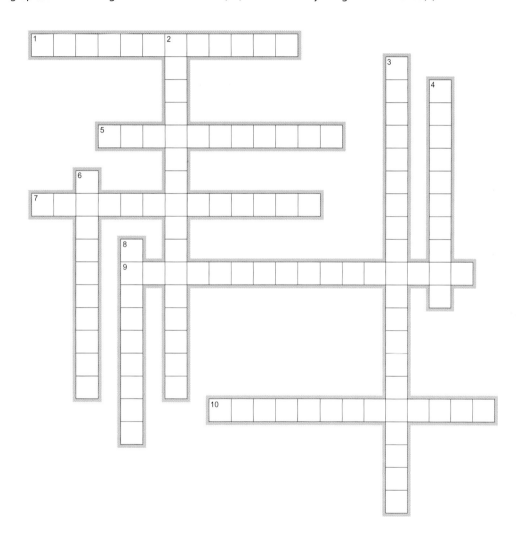

EXERCISE 19.8: ANAGRAMS

Work out each medical term from the jumbled letters below. Then, using the letters in brackets, determine the medical term that matches the description given.

1. glnmnatai	__ __ __ __ (__) __ __ __ __	another word for cancerous
2. sbopiy	(__) __ __ __ __ __	removal of tissue for pathological examination
3. oamnead	__ __ __ (__) __ __ __	a tumour in a gland
4. mirsnisoe	__ (__) __ __ __ __ __ __ __	disappearance of the clinical signs and symptoms of a malignant disease
5. lmoaanme	__ __ __ __ (__) __ __ __	a malignant neoplasm that originates in the skin
6. svniivae	(__) __ __ __ __ __ __ __	a tumour that spreads into surrounding tissue

Rearrange the letters in brackets to form a word that means 'a non-malignant tumour'.

__ __ __ __ __ __

EXERCISE 19.9: DISCHARGE SUMMARY ANALYSIS

Read the discharge summary below and answer the questions.

UNIVERSITY HOSPITAL DISCHARGE SUMMARY	**UR number:** 454647
	Name: Alice Green
	Address: 15 First Street, Picton
	Date of birth: 26/3/1944
	Sex: F
	Nominated primary healthcare provider: Dr Gemma Hudson

Episode details	Discharge details
Consultant: Dr Patrick	**Status:** Home
Registrar: Dr Andrews	**Date of discharge:** 26/1/2020
Unit: General medical	
Admission source: Emergency department	
Date of admission: 21/1/2020	

Reason for admission / Presenting problems:

Mrs Green described a troublesome cough for 2–3 weeks, which had been dry and associated with some exertional dyspnoea. She had suffered more fatigue than normal. She had also noticed some subcutaneous non-tender skin nodules over her abdomen and back.

Principal diagnosis: Adenocarcinoma of colon with bronchial secondaries

Comorbidities:	
Previous medical history:	
Infiltrating ductal Ca of the breast diagnosed in 1995 – mastectomy and postoperative radiotherapy. Adenocarcinoma colon in August 2013 – right hemicolectomy.	
Clinical synopsis:	
On examination, she was not distressed. She was haemodynamically stable. Auscultation of the chest revealed decreased air entry at the left base with a monophonic wheeze. There was no hepatosplenomegaly. A number of small subcutaneous nodules were noted, particularly over the abdomen.	
Mrs Green had a bronchoscopy performed on the 22.1.2020 under IV sedation (ASA = 3NE). This revealed an overt endobronchial tumour in the left main bronchus with marked extrinsic compression. There was almost 95% occlusion of the bronchus, with some distal collapse. Bronchial washings revealed the presence of adenocarcinoma cells. She was reviewed by Dr Patrick, who felt that chemotherapy would benefit her. She was commenced on a regime of IV CMF, having her first course (2 hours × 2 days) in hospital.	
Complications: Nil	
Clinical interventions: Bronchoscopy	
Diagnostic interventions:	
FBC: Hb. 12.2; platelets 261; WCC 4.65; ESR 5; coag profile – normal.	
Electrolytes: Normal	
Liver function tests: Normal	
Medications at discharge:	
Dexamethasone – 4 mg q.i.d.	
Ceased medications:	
Allergies: Nil	
Alerts: Nil	
Arranged services:	
Recommendations: IV CMF	
Information to patient/relevant parties:	
To be followed up in OPD.	
Authorising clinician: Dr Andrews	
Document recipients:	
Patient and LMO: Dr Gemma Hudson	

1. **Expand the following abbreviations as found in the discharge summary above.**

   Ca

   CMF

   FBC

   IV

   q.i.d.

   WCC

2.　**What is the meaning of haemodynamically stable?**

3.　**What is meant by the term bronchial washings and why are they performed?**

4.　**What is meant by the term monophonic wheeze?**

5.　**Based on the information in the summary, how did the clinicians know the secondary cancer in the lungs was a metastasis from the colorectal cancer and not the breast cancer?**

CHAPTER 20

Infectious and Parasitic Diseases

Contents

OBJECTIVES 475

INTRODUCTION 476

NEW WORD ELEMENTS 476

    Combining forms 476

    Prefixes 476

    Suffixes 476

VOCABULARY 477

ABBREVIATIONS 477

TYPES OF INFECTIONS 478

    Viruses 478

    Bacteria 478

    Parasites 478

    Mycoses 478

    Opportunistic infection 478

    Modes of transmission 478

    Outbreaks of disease, disease
control and monitoring 479

PATHOLOGICAL DESCRIPTIONS
OF SOME SPECIFIC INFECTIOUS
AND PARASITIC DISEASES 481

    Vaccine-preventable diseases 482

    Vector-borne diseases 484

    Other infectious and parasitic
diseases 485

TESTS AND PROCEDURES 485

EXERCISES 488

Objectives

After completing this chapter you should be able to:

1. state the meanings of the word elements related to infectious and parasitic diseases

2. build words using the word elements associated with infectious and parasitic diseases

3. recognise, pronounce and effectively use medical terms associated with infectious and parasitic diseases

4. expand abbreviations related to infectious and parasitic diseases

5. describe the different types of infections and modes of transmission

6. describe how outbreaks of disease, disease control and monitoring are managed in Australia

7. describe common pathological conditions associated with infectious and parasitic diseases

8. describe common laboratory tests and diagnostic and surgical procedures associated with infectious and parasitic diseases

9. apply what you have learned by interpreting medical terminology in practice.

Demonstrate your knowledge of infectious and parasitic diseases by completing the relevant exercises at the end of this chapter.

INTRODUCTION

Infectious diseases are also known as contagious, transmissible or communicable diseases. This chapter includes the study of infective and parasitic agents that cause illness and the body's response to invasion by them. These agents include bacteria, viruses, fungi, parasites and protozoa, which are spread by a variety of methods including physical contact, contaminated food, body fluids, objects, airborne inhalation or through vector organisms.

NEW WORD ELEMENTS

Here are some word elements related to infectious and parasitic diseases. To reinforce your learning, write the meanings of the medical terms in the spaces provided. Use the Glossary of medical terms on page 561 to help you work out the meanings. You may also need to check the meaning in a medical dictionary, but make an attempt yourself first.

Combining forms

Combining Form	Meaning	Medical Term	Meaning of Medical Term
bacill/o	bacillus, rod-shaped bacterium	bacilluria	
bacteri/o	bacteria	bacteriolytic	
bi/o	life	biological	
cocc/o	coccus, berry-shaped bacterium	coccogenous	
fung/i	fungus, mushroom	fungicide	
fung/o		antifungal	
helminth/o	worm	helminthiasis	
myc/o	fungus, mould	mycotoxicosis	
path/o	disease	pathogen	
protozo/o	protozoa	protozoiasis	
septic/o	infection	septicaemia	
staphyl/o	bunch of grapes, cluster	staphylococcus	
strept/o	twisted	streptococcaemia	
tox/o	poison, toxin	mycotoxin	
vir/o	virus	enteroviral	

Prefixes

Prefix	Meaning	Medical Term	Meaning of Medical Term
anti-	against	antibiotic	
crypto-	hidden	cryptococcosis	
micro-	small	microbiology	
retro-	backwards, behind	retroviral	

Suffixes

Suffix	Meaning	Medical Term	Meaning of Medical Term
-aemia	condition of blood	viraemia	
-al	pertaining to	antibacterial	
-cide	killing, agent that kills	bacteriocide	
-coccus	berry-shaped bacteria	pneumococcus	
-form	having the form of	fungiform	

Table continued

Suffix	Meaning	Medical Term	Meaning of Medical Term
-itis	inflammation	bronchitis	
-logy	study of	parasitology	
-sepsis	infection	asepsis	

VOCABULARY

The following list provides many of the medical terms used for the first time in this chapter. Pronunciations are provided with each term. As you read the rest of the chapter, make sure you identify each of these terms and understand their meanings.

Term	Pronunciation
bacteria	bak-TEER-ee-a
bronchoscopy	bron-KOS-kop-ee
chest x-ray	chest EKS-ray
dengue fever	DEN-gee FEE-va
ELISA test	e-LYZ-a test
erythrocyte sedimentation rate	e-REETH-roh-syt sed-ee-men-TAY-shun rayt
immunisation	im-yoon-eye-ZAY-shun
lumbar (spinal) puncture	LUM-bah PUNK-cha
malaria	mal-AIR-ee-ah
meningococcal disease	men-in-joh-KOK-al diz-eez
mycoses	my-KOH-seez
parasite	pa-ra-syt
pertussis	per-TUSS-is
pneumococcal vaccination	nyoo-moh-KOK-al vak-sin-AY-shun
rapid strep test	RAP-id strep test
Ross River fever	ross RIV-ah FEE-va
rotavirus	ROH-ta VY-rus
septicaemia	sep-ti-SEE-me-ah
tuberculin test	too-BERK-yoo-lin test
urea breath test	yoo-ree-a breth test
vaccination	vak-sin-AY-shun
virus	VY-rus

ABBREVIATIONS

The following abbreviations are commonly used in the Australian healthcare environment. Because some abbreviations can have more than one meaning, check the context in which the abbreviation is used before assigning a meaning to it.

Abbreviation	Definition
ADT	adult diphtheria tetanus vaccine
AFB	acid fast bacilli
AIDS	acquired immunodeficiency syndrome
BSE	bovine spongiform encephalopathy
C&S	culture and sensitivity
CJD	Creutzfeldt-Jakob disease
CMV	cytomegalovirus
COVID-19	coronavirus disease
CSF	cerebrospinal fluid
DTP	diphtheria tetanus pertussis vaccine
EBV	Epstein-Barr virus
EIA	enzyme immunoassay
ELISA	enzyme-linked immunosorbent assay
ESR	erythrocyte sedimentation rate
HAV, HBV, HCV, HDV, HEV	hepatitis A virus, hepatitis B virus, hepatitis C virus, hepatitis D virus, hepatitis E virus
Hib	*Haemophilus influenzae* type b
HIV	human immunodeficiency virus
HPV	human papillomavirus
HSV	herpes simplex virus
IgA, IgD, IgE, IgG, IgM	classes of immunoglobulins, Immunoglobulin A, D, E, G, M
LP	lumbar puncture
MERS-CoV	Middle East respiratory syndrome coronavirus
MMR	measles-mumps-rubella vaccine
MMRV	measles-mumps-rubella-varicella vaccine
MRSA	methicillin (or multiple)-resistant *Staphylococcus aureus*
PCP	*Pneumocystis* pneumonia
PCR	polymerase chain reaction
SARS	severe acute respiratory syndrome
STI/STD	sexually transmitted infection / sexually transmitted disease
TB	tuberculosis

TYPES OF INFECTIONS

Viruses

Viruses are microscopic biological agents that enter the body from the environment or from another person via the nose, mouth or any breaks in the skin and will then find a cell to infect. For example, the influenza virus will target cells in the respiratory system and norovirus will target cells in the digestive tract. Viruses cannot grow or reproduce on their own but need to enter a host cell and take over the cell to help them multiply. The virus causes its host cell to rapidly produce large numbers of identical copies of the original virus. A virus consists of genes that carry genetic information and a protein layer that protects the genes. Some viruses also have a layer of surrounding fat that protects them when they are not enclosed in a host cell.

Viruses are responsible for many of the everyday diseases humans experience such as the common cold, influenza and certain 'childhood' diseases such as varicella zoster (chickenpox), rubeola (measles) and mumps. Viral infections, although they cause disease, are generally eradicated by the body's immune response. This immune reaction may grant subsequent lifetime immunity to the host that is specific to that virus.

Antibiotics have no effect on viruses. Some antiviral drugs have been developed to treat serious viral infections, such as human immunodeficiency virus (HIV) disease. These act by inhibiting the development of the virus, rather than killing it. Vaccines act to stimulate the body's immune response and can therefore provide lifelong immunity to some viral infections.

Bacteria

Bacteria are single-celled organisms that, unlike viruses, have the ability to divide and replicate by themselves. Some bacteria are harmful and cause disease, but many are useful. In humans, some bacteria, such as those in the gastrointestinal tract that assist with digestion, are necessary for maintaining health, but others cause diseases such as food poisoning, gonorrhoea, gastritis, meningitis, pneumonia and a variety of infections in other body sites. Antibiotics are agents that can successfully treat many forms of bacterial infection. However, breeds of antibiotic-resistant bacterial strains have now emerged. Vaccination may also prevent many bacterial diseases.

Parasites

In humans, parasitic diseases are caused by protozoa and helminths (worms), resulting in conditions such as malaria, amoebic dysentery, toxoplasmosis, scabies and lice. Parasites and their human hosts have a symbiotic relationship whereby the parasite benefits at the expense of the host. Parasites cannot live alone, requiring a host to provide them with nourishment. Human parasites are divided into endoparasites (e.g. tapeworm), which cause infection inside the body, and ectoparasites (e.g. scabies), which cause infection superficially within the skin.

Mycoses

A mycosis is a disease caused by a fungal infection. In humans, mycoses are classified according to the type and extent of tissue colonised. For example, **superficial mycoses** (affecting skin and hair), **cutaneous mycoses** (extending into the epidermis), **subcutaneous mycoses** (affecting the dermis, subcutaneous tissues, muscle and fascia) and **systemic mycoses** (such as primary mycoses arising in a specific body tissue but that spread to other parts of the body). Mycoses are treated with topical or systemic agents, depending on the site of infection.

Opportunistic infection

An opportunistic infection refers to any infection caused by a microorganism such as a bacterium, virus, protozoa or fungus that does not infect a healthy person but may affect a person whose resistance is low or whose immune system is compromised by an unrelated disease. Those at risk include people living with HIV, those receiving chemotherapy and patients receiving immunosuppressive drugs after an organ transplant.

Modes of transmission

For an infection to be spread from one person to another, there needs to be a chain of infection. The chain has these three components:

- a susceptible host
- a biological agent sufficient to cause disease
- a mode of transmission.

The way that a disease is transmitted depends on the organism that causes it – some diseases have more than one possible way of being transmitted. The most common methods for spreading a disease are:

- direct contact and physical transfer of microorganisms from an infected person to a healthy one
- indirect contact whereby a person is infected from contact with a surface on which there are living microorganisms
- droplet contact, which occurs when a person sneezes, coughs or talks, releasing droplets containing microorganisms that make contact with another person's eyes, nose or mouth
- airborne transmission, when dust containing microorganisms or residue from evaporated droplets remains suspended in the air and is inhaled

- faecal–oral transmission, which occurs as microorganisms enter the body through ingesting contaminated food or water or where bacteria or viruses present in the faeces of an infected person pass into the mouth of another person, generally due to inadequate hygiene practices
- vector-borne transmission, whereby animals such as mosquitoes, flies, mites, fleas, ticks, rats or dogs transmit disease through biting, spreading faeces or depositing microorganisms on the host's body.

Outbreaks of disease, disease control and monitoring

The occurrence of cases of a disease in excess of what would normally be expected in a community or geographical area or over a specific time period is called a disease outbreak. A disease outbreak confined to a specific population group is called an epidemic, whereas an outbreak that spreads across the world is called a pandemic. An outbreak may last for only a few days or weeks or may be longer term and persist for several years. An outbreak may also be said to occur if:

- a single case of a communicable disease that has been absent for a long time from a population reappears
- a bacteria or virus not previously diagnosed in a community or area is identified
- a disease that has been previously unknown appears.

Globally, information is generally collected by local agencies such as health clinics, national ministries or departments of health, non-governmental organisations and other individuals involved in managing the outbreak. A local response may be initiated or the reports may be collated, analysed and assessed by disease specialists in the World Health Organization (WHO) regional offices or headquarters. Reports produced by WHO cover all the surveillance information required to release a warning of a communicable disease outbreak, including a description of where the disease is known to have been identified, how widespread it is, and what control measures are in place and whether these are adequate.

The Office of Health Protection in the Australian Government Department of Health has issued guidelines about assessing an infectious disease outbreak. These include identifying:

- the time the outbreak began
- the total number of cases and unaffected people to calculate the proportion of people affected
- symptoms and duration of illness
- type of outbreak setting

- what mode of transmission is implicated
- results of any laboratory tests that may have been done.

This information can be used to develop an epidemic curve to:

- determine how the disease is being spread
- review symptoms and the duration of illness to create a case definition to assist with identifying and counting further infections
- provide information for future review and prevention purposes, including the type of outbreak setting, characteristics of cases and the attack rate of illness.

In Australia, each state and territory health department has a unit responsible for maintaining statewide communicable disease monitoring and surveillance systems. These units also analyse and report on communicable disease trends, including vaccination rates, maintain data quality and management procedures, and conduct and disseminate collaborative research within and between their jurisdictions. The departments also collect notifications of communicable diseases under their respective public health legislations. In 2007 the *National Health Security Act 2007* (National Health Security Act, No. 174) was passed to provide a legislative basis for exchanging health information, including personal information, between jurisdictions and the Commonwealth of Australia. The Act provides the basis for the National Notifiable Diseases Surveillance System, which includes diseases that must be reported at the time of diagnosis. The following infectious and parasitic diseases are included:

Blood-borne diseases

Hepatitis (not elsewhere classified)
Hepatitis B (newly acquired)
Hepatitis B (unspecified)
Hepatitis C (newly acquired)
Hepatitis C (unspecified)
Hepatitis D

Gastrointestinal diseases

Botulism
Campylobacteriosis
Cryptosporidiosis
Haemolytic uraemic syndrome
Hepatitis A
Hepatitis E
Listeriosis
Salmonellosis
STEC/VTEC (Shiga toxin/verotoxin-producing *Escherichia coli*)
Shigellosis
Typhoid fever

Other bacterial infections
Legionellosis
Leprosy
Meningococcal disease (invasive)
Tuberculosis

Quarantinable diseases
Cholera
Highly pathogenic avian influenza (human)
Plague
Rabies
Severe acute respiratory syndrome (SARS)
Smallpox
Viral haemorrhagic fever (not elsewhere classified)
Yellow fever

Sexually transmissible infections
Chlamydial infection
Donovanosis
Gonococcal infection
Syphilis – congenital
Syphilis < 2 years
Syphilis > 2 years or unspecified duration

Vaccine-preventable diseases
Diphtheria
Haemophilus influenzae type b
Influenza (laboratory-confirmed)
Measles
Mumps
Pertussis
Pneumococcal disease (invasive)
Poliovirus infection
Rotavirus
Rubella
Rubella congenital
Tetanus
Varicella zoster (chickenpox)
Varicella zoster (shingles)
Varicella zoster (unspecified)

Vector-borne diseases
Barmah Forest virus infection
Chikungunya virus infection
Dengue virus infection
Flavivirus infection (unspecified)
Japanese encephalitis virus infection
Kunjin virus infection
Malaria
Murray Valley encephalitis virus infection
Ross River virus infection

Zoonoses
Anthrax
Australian bat lyssavirus
Brucellosis
Leptospirosis
Lyssavirus (not elsewhere classified)
Ornithosis (otherwise known as psittacosis)
Q fever
Tularaemia

Listed human diseases
Human influenza in humans with pandemic potential
Middle East respiratory syndrome coronavirus (otherwise known as MERS-CoV)
Plague
Severe acute respiratory syndrome (otherwise known as SARS)
Smallpox
Viral haemorrhagic fevers
Yellow fever

Diseases under national surveillance performed by surveillance bodies other than the Department of Health
Creutzfeldt-Jakob disease (CJD)
Variant Creutzfeldt-Jakob disease (vCJD)
Human immunodeficiency virus (HIV)

Reference: http://www.health.gov.au/internet/main/publishing.nsf/Content/cda-surveil-nndss-casedefs-distype.htm

The Australian Government established the National Immunisation Program in 1997 as a strategy to increase the rate of immunisation coverage. As part of this program, the Australian Immunisation Register is used to record the vaccinations given to people of all ages in Australia. Free vaccinations are given according to the National Immunisation Program Schedule, which specifies the series of immunisations to be given at specific times from birth through to adulthood.

Monitoring of other specific infectious diseases is also undertaken through initiatives such as the Australian Gonococcal Surveillance Programme, Australian Meningococcal Surveillance Programme, Australian Paediatric Surveillance Unit, Australian National Creutzfeldt-Jakob Disease Registry, HIV and AIDS surveillance, poliomyelitis surveillance, gastroenteritis surveillance, Laboratory Virology and Serology Reporting Scheme, the OzFoodNet collection for food-borne disease surveillance.

In New Zealand, both local and national authorities undertake notifiable disease surveillance activities. The Institute of Environmental Science and Research Ltd operates under contract to the New Zealand Ministry of Health for national public health surveillance efforts. The institute operates the national notifiable disease surveillance database, EpiSurv, on behalf of the

Ministry of Health. EpiSurv collects notifiable disease information on a real-time basis from the public health services, including case demographics, clinical features and risk factors. In New Zealand, the following infectious diseases are notifiable.

Notifiable infectious diseases under the *Health Act 1956*

INFECTIOUS DISEASES NOTIFIABLE TO A MEDICAL OFFICER OF HEALTH AND LOCAL AUTHORITY

Acute gastroenteritis
Campylobacteriosis
Cholera
Cryptosporidiosis
Giardiasis
Hepatitis A
Legionellosis
Listeriosis
Meningoencephalitis – primary amoebic
Salmonellosis
Shigellosis
Typhoid and paratyphoid fever
Yersiniosis

INFECTIOUS DISEASES NOTIFIABLE TO MEDICAL OFFICER OF HEALTH

Anthrax
Arboviral diseases
Brucellosis
Creutzfeldt-Jakob disease and other spongiform encephalopathies
Cronobacter species
Diphtheria
Haemophilus influenzae b
Hepatitis B
Hepatitis C
Hepatitis (viral) – not otherwise specified
Highly pathogenic avian influenza (including HPAI subtype H5N1)
Hydatid disease
Invasive pneumococcal disease
Leprosy
Leptospirosis
Malaria
Measles
Middle East respiratory syndrome coronavirus (MERS-CoV)
Mumps
Neisseria meningitidis invasive disease
Non-seasonal influenza (capable of being transmitted between human beings)
Pertussis
Plague
Poliomyelitis
Q fever
Rabies and other lyssaviruses
Rheumatic fever
Rickettsial diseases
Rubella
Severe acute respiratory syndrome (SARS)
Tetanus
Tuberculosis (all forms)
Veratoxin-producing or Shiga-toxin producing *Escherichia coli*
Viral haemorrhagic fevers
Yellow fever

INFECTIOUS DISEASES NOTIFIABLE TO A MEDICAL OFFICER OF HEALTH WITHOUT IDENTIFYING INFORMATION OF THE PATIENT OR DECEASED PERSON

Acquired immunodeficiency syndrome (AIDS)
Gonorrhoeal infection
Human immunodeficiency virus (HIV) infection
Syphilis

Reference: https://www.health.govt.nz/our-work/diseases-and-conditions/notifiable-diseases

PATHOLOGICAL DESCRIPTIONS OF SOME SPECIFIC INFECTIOUS AND PARASITIC DISEASES

The following section provides a list of common diseases and pathological conditions relevant to infectious and parasitic diseases. There are many infectious and parasitic diseases that occur in Australia and New Zealand. Some are common (influenza, sexually transmitted infections, hepatitis), while some occur infrequently (HIV/AIDS, Hendra virus, lyssavirus) but are still important, particularly from an epidemiological perspective. Infections that are specific to a particular body system have been discussed in the relevant body system chapter. The infections that are discussed below are more systemic in manifestation; that is, they affect the body as a whole rather than one particular organ. Not all infections or parasitic diseases have been included, only the more commonly occurring ones.

Vaccine-preventable diseases

Term	Pronunciation	Definition
diphtheria	dif-thee-ree-a	Diphtheria is caused by the bacteria *Corynebacterium diphtheria* or *Corynebacterium ulcerans*. There are four different types: classical respiratory diphtheria, laryngeal diphtheria, nasal diphtheria and cutaneous diphtheria. The bacteria release a toxin that most commonly infects the upper airways and may cause a membrane consisting of bacteria, dead cells from the mucous membranes and fibrin to block the larynx. Myocarditis and peripheral neuropathy may also be present in severe cases. Vaccination has been extremely effective at reducing the number of cases of diphtheria in Australia and New Zealand.
pertussis	per-TUSS-is	Pertussis is an upper respiratory infection caused by the *Bordetella pertussis* bacteria. It is transmitted through droplet infection and is highly contagious. Initially, pertussis presents with symptoms like the common cold but after a few days, results in uncontrollable coughing and dyspnoea. It is often called whooping cough – named after the sound made when the patient tries to breathe. A vaccine against pertussis has been widely available for several decades so the infection was rarely seen. However, in recent years there has been an increase in the incidence of the disease, possibly due to fewer babies being immunised because parents think the disease no longer exists. There is also a school of thought that suggests the immunity can wear off. Pertussis used to mainly affect babies and young children but is now more commonly seen among adolescents and adults. Older patients normally make a full recovery from the disease, but pertussis can cause pneumonia, encephalopathy, seizures and even death in babies and infants.
rotavirus	ROH-ta vy-rus	Rotavirus is the most common cause of viral gastroenteritis worldwide. It is transmitted by the oral–faecal route. Symptoms include vomiting, watery diarrhoea, fever and abdominal pain. It can lead to dehydration and ultimately death if hydration is not maintained. Dehydration from rotavirus kills more than 600,000 children each year, mostly in developing countries where it is very difficult to treat. Proper handwashing after toileting is the most useful measure to prevent spread of the virus. Because rotavirus is a viral infection, antibiotics are not used as a treatment. Rehydration may be necessary if dehydration has occurred. A vaccine that is highly effective in preventing the disease is now available.
rubella (German measles)	roo-BEL-a	This previously common childhood illness is caused by a rubella viral infection. Now less common because of routine vaccinations, rubella is also known as German measles because the disease was first described by German doctors in the mid-18th century. Rubella causes an erythematous rash, low-grade fever, joint pain, headaches and conjunctivitis and is spread by airborne droplet emission. It generally disappears within a few days. However, in pregnant women, there is a risk of transplacental spread, with serious consequences for an unborn baby. The effects include cardiac, cerebral, ophthalmic and auditory congenital anomalies, prematurity, low birth weight, and neonatal thrombocytopenia, anaemia and hepatitis.
rubeola (measles)	roo-bee-O-la	Rubeola or measles is a highly contagious viral infection that is relatively rare now because of vaccination programs, although it has also suffered a resurgence in recent years. Its symptoms include an itchy macropapular rash (Fig. 20.1), fever, symptoms of a cold, photophobia and conjunctivitis. The virus is spread through contaminated droplets in the air. In most patients, measles is an uncomplicated infection, but pneumonia, ear infection, bronchitis or encephalitis are possible consequences.

Table continued

Term	Pronunciation	Definition
		Figure 20.1 Measles (Zitelli & Davis 2007) 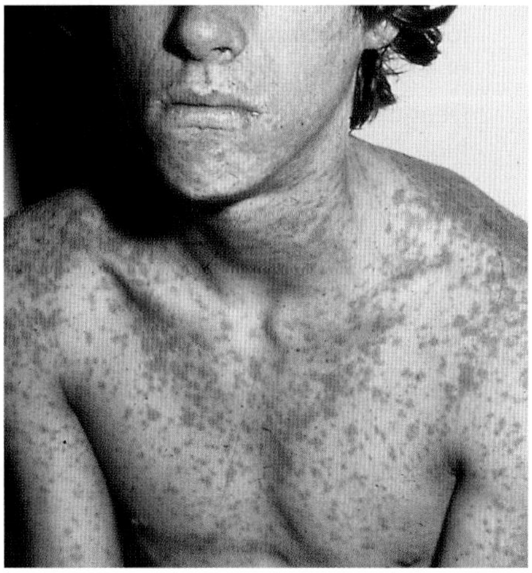
varicella zoster (chickenpox)	va-ree-SEL-a zos-ta	Varicella zoster or chickenpox is a highly contagious viral disease spread through the air from coughing or sneezing or direct contact with the lesions on an infected person. It consists of an itchy vesicular rash (Fig. 20.2), which can become pock marks if scratched, with other symptoms including fever, malaise, myalgia, headache and sore throat. A vaccine is available. In most patients, the disease is minor and self-limiting; however, the virus may lie dormant in the nerve cells and cause a late complication called herpes zoster or **shingles** when it reactivates decades after the initial episode of chickenpox. Shingles causes an intense pain and tingling or burning at the site of infected nerves followed by a red blistering rash. The pain of shingles can be severe and is called **post-herpetic neuralgia** if it persists after the rash has disappeared. There is no cure for shingles, but antiviral medication taken early can alleviate symptoms. A vaccine to prevent shingles is now available. **Figure 20.2 Chickenpox** (Callen 2000) 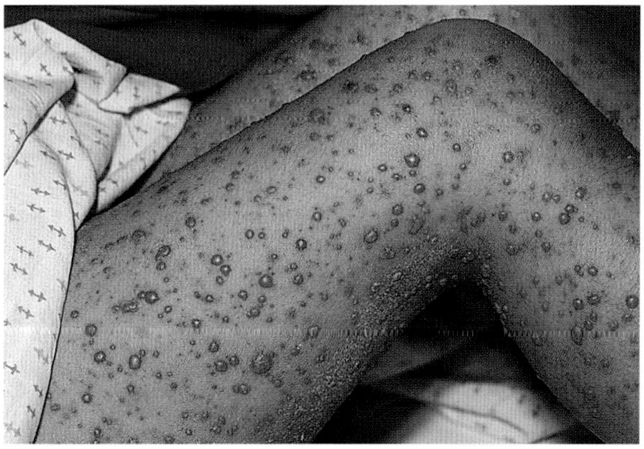

Vector-borne diseases

Term	Pronunciation	Definition
Barmah Forest virus	BAH-mah fo-rest VY-rus	Barmah Forest virus is spread via mosquitoes, particularly in warm, wet environments. Australia is the only country in the world in which this virus has been identified. It causes fever, chills, headache and muscle pain; swelling of joints with stiffness and pain; a rash, usually on the trunk or limbs; and a feeling of lethargy and weakness.
dengue	den-gee	Dengue is caused by a virus transmitted by mosquitoes. Symptoms include high fever, severe headaches, lymphadenopathy, myalgia, arthralgia and a characteristic rash. The acute phase of the illness lasts between 1 and 2 weeks. **Dengue haemorrhagic fever** is a severe variant of the virus that involves abdominal pain, haemorrhage and circulatory failure. Because dengue is viral in aetiology, there is no specific treatment. Any treatment given is to relieve symptoms. Dengue is prevalent in tropical and subtropical regions. In Australia, the distribution of the dengue-carrying mosquito is currently limited to North Queensland. Eradication of the mosquitoes is the best form of prevention.
malaria	mal-air-ee-a	Malaria is a parasitic disease that is passed from human to human by the bite of infected Anopheles mosquitoes. The parasites mature in the liver then enter the bloodstream, where they infect erythrocytes. Symptoms include high fevers, chills, flu-like symptoms, severe headaches and anaemia caused by the destruction of the erythrocytes. Splenomegaly and hepatomegaly are often present.
		Falciparum malaria is a severe variant of the infection characterised by cerebral inflammation, haemolytic anaemia, haemolysis, kidney and liver failure, meningitis, pulmonary oedema and splenorrhexis. It is potentially fatal.
		Malaria is prevalent in tropical and subtropical regions. Because treatment options are limited, it is important to prevent infection in the first place. Various drugs such as doxycycline, chloroquine and mefloquine are used to prevent infection. However, they should be used in conjunction with strategies such as wearing protective clothing, applying insect repellent and using mosquito nets and screens.
Ross River fever	ross RIV-a FEE-va	Ross River fever is a mosquito-borne viral infection transmitted through mosquito bites. The Ross River virus usually lives in native mammals, rodents and horses. These animals act as natural reservoirs for the virus. When a female mosquito bites an infected animal, she picks up the virus. If the mosquito then bites a human, the virus is passed into the bloodstream.
		Symptoms include polyarthritis, arthralgia, myalgia, fever, headache, fatigue and a rash on the trunk and limbs. Incubation period is between 3 and 21 days. There is no specific treatment, so it is important to prevent infection in the first place by avoiding mosquito bites, wearing protective clothing and using insect repellent. Analgesics, anti-inflammatories or antipyretics may help lessen the severity of symptoms. Symptoms will eventually subside but relapses of polyarthritis, arthralgia and fatigue are common. Ross River fever is endemic to Australia.

Other infectious and parasitic diseases

Term	Pronunciation	Definition
septicaemia	sep-ti-SEE-me-ah	Septicaemia is a bacterial infection of the blood, also known as sepsis or blood poisoning. Septicaemia is a serious, life-threatening infection that can worsen rapidly.
		It is usually caused by infection with *Escherichia coli (E. coli), Pneumococcus, Klebsiella, Pseudomonas, Staphylococcus* or *Streptococcus*. The bacteria enter the bloodstream as a result of a previous infection, burn, infected wound or other break in the skin. Septicaemia is also linked to serious conditions such as osteomyelitis, meningitis and endocarditis.
		Symptoms include spiking fevers, chills, tachypnoea and tachycardia. The patient can deteriorate rapidly with shock, hypothermia, hypotension, oliguria and delirium. Septicaemia is a medical emergency requiring urgent hospital treatment such as intravenous antibiotics, oxygen and fluids to maintain blood pressure. If treatment is given early enough, the prognosis is good.
meningococcal disease	men-in-joh-KOK-al diz-eez	Meningococcal disease is a severe, life-threatening infection caused by the meningococcus (*Neisseria meningitides*) bacterium. These bacteria occur naturally in the population without causing illness. In a small percentage of people, a specific strain of the bacterium enters the bloodstream and causes meningococcal disease. The bacterium can then be transmitted to others through saliva or close, prolonged contact. Most at risk are children up to the age of 5 and teenagers and young adults aged 15–26.
		There are two main forms of meningococcal infection: meningococcal meningitis and meningococcal septicaemia. In meningococcal meningitis, infected meningeal fluid passes into the spinal cord, resulting in the symptoms of severe headache, stiff neck, fever, photophobia, drowsiness, confusion and the characteristic reddish-purple pinprick rash. Meningeal and cerebral oedema can result. Intravenous antibiotics need to be given urgently. Even with immediate treatment, patients may still lose their hearing, suffer permanent brain damage or die.
		Meningococcal septicaemia is even more serious. It affects the whole body; blood vessels can haemorrhage, and vital organs such as the heart, lungs and kidneys fail. Patients can die within a few hours. It is not uncommon for patients who survive to lose limbs due to gangrene.
		Both these infections are medical emergencies as meningococcal disease carries a high mortality rate if untreated. Therefore accurate, early diagnosis and treatment with antibiotics are essential.
		Vaccines have been developed for some strains of meningococcal disease. However, this does not protect against the B strain, which is the strain that currently causes most of the meningococcal disease.

TESTS AND PROCEDURES

The following section provides a list of common diagnostic tests and procedures and clinical interventions and surgical procedures that are undertaken for infectious and parasitic diseases.

Test/Procedure	Pronunciation	Definition
bronchoscopy	bron-KOS-kop-ee	Bronchoscopy is a procedure that allows for visual examination of the bronchi and for the sampling of tissue via biopsy or washings. The bronchoscope (either rigid or flexible) is inserted into the bronchi via the pharynx, larynx and trachea.
chest x-ray	chest EKS-ray	A chest x-ray involves taking radiographic images of two views of the chest. The first is in the coronal plane, which takes images from the anterior–posterior view or posterior–anterior view. The second is in the sagittal plane, taking a lateral view.
ELISA test	e-LY-za test	The enzyme-linked immunosorbent assay (ELISA) test is used to detect immune responses in the body. The test detects substances such as hormones, antigens and antibodies and is used to detect antibodies to HIV antigens that are of a specific molecular weight.
erythrocyte sedimentation rate (ESR)	e-REETH-roh-syt sed-ee-men-TAY-shun rayt	ESR is a measure to determine the rate at which erythrocytes settle out of plasma in a test tube. Venous blood is collected in an anticoagulant and allowed to stand in a vertical position. The sedimentation rate is a measure of the distance the erythrocytes have fallen in a given time period. In diseases such as infections, joint inflammation and tumours, which increase the immunoglobulin content of blood, the sedimentation rate is increased.
lumbar (spinal) puncture	LUM-bah PUNK-cha	A lumbar puncture is a procedure that involves inserting a needle between the vertebrae and into the dura mater surrounding the spinal cord to obtain a sample of cerebrospinal fluid for analysis. The spinal cord terminates by the level of the L2–L3 intervertebral space. Therefore a lumbar puncture is usually performed at or below the L3–L4 intervertebral space because there is less risk of injuring the spinal cord. A lumbar puncture may also be done to measure the pressure of cerebrospinal fluid or as a method for injecting medications or contrast material for a myelography.
polymerase chain reaction (PCR)	pol-ee-mer-aze cheyne ree-AK-shun	PCR tests are used to identify specific constituents in the DNA and RNA through creating and testing multiple copies of the genetic materials. A PCR test is used as a means of diagnosing certain genetic conditions, cancers and infections. It has particular value in testing for HIV disease because it can discriminate the presence of the virus in the DNA before antibodies appear in the blood. PCR tests are also used for genetic testing in the antenatal period and prior to assisted reproductive techniques. Because of its ability to create a definitive genetic fingerprint, it is also increasingly being used in forensic applications.
rapid strep test	RAP-id strep test	A rapid strep test is performed to determine if the cause of a sore throat is due to infection by group A streptococcus.
tuberculin test	too-BERK-yoo-lin test	A tuberculin test is also known as a Mantoux test and is done to identify infection (either old or current) by tuberculosis. It is performed by injecting tuberculin intradermally and measuring the skin response at 48 hours and 72 hours.
urea breath test	yoo-REE-a breth test	A urea breath test is performed to identify the presence of *Helicobacter pylori*. Carbon-labelled urea is swallowed and is metabolised by *H. pylori*, which produces labelled carbon dioxide. This is then absorbed into the bloodstream and can then be detected in the exhaled breath of affected people.
vaccination	vak-sin-AY-shun	**Vaccination** is the administration of a vaccine, usually by injection but can be orally, to produce an immune response to a specific disease in the body. **Immunisation** is the process of both receiving a vaccine and becoming immune to the disease as a result. The vaccine stimulates the immune system so it can recognise the organism causing the disease and grant protection from future infection from that specific organism. The terms vaccination and immunisation are often, incorrectly, used interchangeably. They mean quite different things and should not be confused. Vaccinations do not always create immunity despite being designed to do so. There are many different types of vaccinations available. Some are discussed in the following section.

Table continued

Test/Procedure	Pronunciation	Definition
– diphtheria, tetanus, pertussis vaccination	dip-thee-ree-ah, tet-a-nes, per-TUS-is vak-sin-AY-shun	This is a combination vaccine for all three conditions. It is administered in five doses at 2, 4, 6 and 18 months of age, with a booster at 4 years of age. Vaccination against these conditions is also recommended for parents, grandparents and close family members if not recently immunised against pertussis.
– hepatitis A & B vaccination	hep-a-TY-tis A & B vak-sin-AY-shun	Hepatitis A vaccine is made from killed hepatitis A virus which, when administered, causes the immune system to produce antibodies. Two doses over a 6-month period are required. Hepatitis B vaccine contains a protein that stimulates the production of antibodies. Three doses over a 6-month period are required. A combination vaccine for both types is available that is administered in three doses over a 6-month period.
– human papilloma virus vaccination	hyoo-man pap-e-LOH-ma vy-rus vak-sin-AY-shun	The HPV vaccine was developed to protect against nine types of HPV, which account for 90% of all HPV-related cancers of the cervix, anus, vulva, vagina, penis and throat. In Australia the vaccine is offered through schools to both males and females. If the person is under 14 years old, they are given two injections 6–12 months apart. If the person is over 15 years or didn't receive the injections 6 months apart, they are given three injections with the doses administered at 0, 2 and 6 months.
– influenza vaccination	in-floo-EN-za vak-sin-AY-shun	Influenza vaccination is required on an annual basis because influenza viruses have the ability to mutate or change their surface structure. The vaccine contains a small amount of inactivated virus that then allows for the production of antibodies.
– measles, mumps, rubella and varicella vaccination	MEE-silz, mumps, roo-BEL-ah and va-ree-SEL-ah vak-si-NAY-shun	Measles, mumps, rubella and varicella vaccination is given as a combination injection at 18 months of age. The vaccine contains small amounts of live virus. It is considered 99% successful in preventing measles, mumps, German measles and chickenpox.
– meningococcal vaccination	men-in-ja-KOK-al vak-si-NAY-shun	In Australia, there are five types of meningococcal bacteria that are commonly found: A, B, C, W and Y. There is no one vaccine that can protect against all five types, so more than one vaccination is required. Vaccination against meningococcal B may be given from 6 weeks of age, and vaccination against meningococcal ACWY may be given from 2 months of age. Vaccination is recommended for babies, young children and adolescents.
– pneumococcal vaccination	nyoo-moh-KOK-al vak-si-NAY-shun	Pneumococcal vaccination is administered to prevent respiratory infection due to *Streptococcus pneumoniae* bacterium. The vaccine provides protection against 23 of the 80 known pneumococci bacteria by stimulating the production of antibodies.
– polio vaccination	poh-lee-oh vak-si-NAY-shun	Although Australia has been free of polio since 2000 it is still recommended that children are vaccinated against this disease. This is due to the possibility of it being brought into the country due to immigration or contracted during travel. Polio vaccine may be given on its own or is often included with the diphtheria, tetanus and pertussis vaccination.
– shingles vaccination	SHING-gulz vak-si-NAY-shun	The shingles vaccine is given by injection. Because shingles is predominantly a condition that arises in old age, the vaccine is provided free of charge for adults aged 65 years or older in New Zealand or 70 years or older in Australia. Anyone over the age of 50 years may still be vaccinated but will have to pay for the vaccine if they have not reached the threshold age. The vaccine may be given to younger patients who have had shingles as a protection against post-herpetic neuralgia and as a treatment to reduce acute and chronic zoster-associated pain.

Exercises

EXERCISE 20.1: MATCH WORD ELEMENTS AND MEANINGS

Match the prefix, suffix or combining form in Column A with its meaning from Column B.

Column A	Answer	Column B
1. bacill/o		A. life
2. -cide		B. infection (2)
3. bi/o		C. poison, toxin
4. cocc/o		D. inflammation
5. crypto-		E. virus
6. fung/i		F. backwards, behind
7. helminth/o		G. bacillus, rod-shaped bacterium
8. myc/o		H. coccus, berry-shaped bacterium
9. path/o		I. having the form of
10. protozo/o		J. against
11. septic/o		K. twisted
12. staphyl/o		L. killing
13. strept/o		M. worm
14. tox/o		N. hidden
15. vir/o		O. fungus (1)
16. -sepsis		P. disease
17. -itis		Q. fungus (2)
18. -form		R. bunch of grapes, cluster
19. anti-		S. protozoa
20. retro-		T. infection (1)

EXERCISE 20.2: WORD ELEMENTS AND WORD BUILDING

Using the following table of word elements, build a medical term for each then provide the meaning for that term.

Word Element	Build a Medical Term	Provide the Meaning
anti-		
bacill/o		
bi/o		
-cide		
cocc/o		
crypt/o		

Word Element	Build a Medical Term	Provide the Meaning
-form		
fung/i		
helminth/o		
-itis		
myc/o		
path/o		
protozo/o		
retro-		
-sepsis		
septic/o		
staphyl/o		
strept/o		
tox/o		
vir/o		

EXERCISE 20.3: BUILDING MEDICAL TERMS

Complete the medical terms below using the correct word elements.

1. _____ itis is an inflammation of the nose.

2. _____ itis is an inflammation of the ear.

3. _____ itis is an inflammation of the stomach.

4. _____ itis is an inflammation of the liver.

5. _____ itis is an inflammation of the tongue.

6. _____ itis is an inflammation of the skin.

7. _____ itis is an inflammation of a joint.

8. _____ itis is an inflammation of the gums.

9. _____ itis is an inflammation of the gallbladder.

10. _____ itis is an inflammation of the urinary bladder.

11. _____ itis is an inflammation of the vagina.

12. _____ itis is an inflammation of the glans penis.

13. _____ itis is an inflammation of the large intestine.

14. _____ itis is an inflammation of the appendix.

15. _____ itis is an inflammation of the mouth.

16. _____ itis is an inflammation of the thyroid gland.

17. _____ itis is an inflammation of the oesophagus.

18. _____ itis is an inflammation of the sac surrounding the heart.

19. _____ itis is an inflammation of the bronchi.

20. _____ itis is an inflammation of the brain.

EXERCISE 20.4: EXPAND THE ABBREVIATIONS

Expand the abbreviations to form correct medical terms.

Abbreviation	Expanded Abbreviation
ADT	
AIDS	
BSE	
CJD	
CMV	
C&S	
CSF	
DTP	
EBV	
EIA	
ELISA	
HBV	
HiB	
HIV	
HPV	
HSV	

Abbreviation	Expanded Abbreviation
IgA	
LP	
MMR	
MRSA	
PCP	
STI/STD	
TB	

EXERCISE 20.5: VOCABULARY BUILDING

Provide the medical term for each of the definitions below.

1. One who specialises in the study of bacteria: _____

2. Condition of blood infection: _____

3. Pertaining to killing bacteria: _____

4. Pertaining to bacteria in the urine: _____

5. Condition of virus in the blood: _____

6. Abnormal condition of a fungus: _____

7. The study of small life: _____

8. Virus that infects the nose: _____

9. The study of parasites: _____

10. (An agent that) kills a fungus: _____

EXERCISE 20.6: PRONUNCIATION AND COMPREHENSION

Read the following paragraphs aloud to practise your pronunciation. Using your textbook and a medical dictionary, find the meanings of the underlined medical terms.

Rob Nelson is a 21-year-old male who presented to hospital with a 5-day history of fevers, arthralgia, pharyngitis, irritability, photophobia and mild nuchal rigidity. There was no underlying confusion and the patient had previously been well.

Examination demonstrated a mild neck stiffness and photophobia. He appeared quite dehydrated. There were no other examination features of note. Baseline investigations included lumbar puncture, which showed mild elevation of white cells and a pressure of 21 centimetres. Gram stain and subsequent bacteriology were negative. Baseline biochemistry and haematology were unremarkable.

The patient was assessed as having viral meningitis and was treated symptomatically with analgesics and intravenous rehydration. The patient improved over a period of 2 days and was discharged home on 3-12-2020.

EXERCISE 20.7: CROSSWORD PUZZLE

Complete the puzzle by providing the medical term for each of the clues below.

ACROSS

3. A virus transmitted from bats to horses to people (6, 5)
4. A parasite that causes infection inside the body (12)
5. A disease-producing organism (8)
7. Also called German measles (7)
9. A mosquito-borne viral infection that lives in native mammals, rodents and horses (4, 5, 5)
10. A procedure to protect against specific diseases (12)

DOWN

1. A bacterial infection caused by *Neisseria meningitidis* bacterium (13, 7)
2. Means 'without infection' (7)
6. The most common cause of viral gastroenteritis (9)
8. Another name for a worm (8)

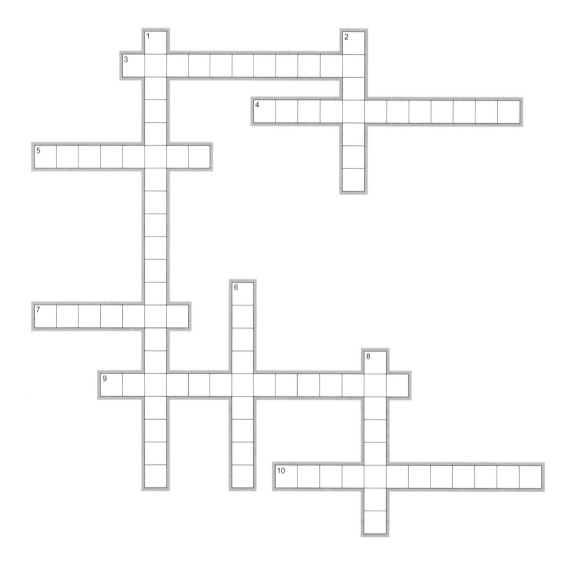

EXERCISE 20.8: DISCHARGE SUMMARY ANALYSIS

Read the discharge summary below and answer the questions.

UNIVERSITY HOSPITAL DISCHARGE SUMMARY	**UR number:** 010203
	Name: Edith Jackson
	Address: 17a Milperra Court, Huttons Beach
	Date of birth: 19 February 1934
	Sex: F
	Nominated primary healthcare provider:
	Dr Fiona Mitchell

Episode details	**Discharge details**
Consultant: Dr David Dunstan	**Status:** Deceased
Registrar: Dr Bruce Robert	**Date of discharge:** 15 September 2020
Unit: Medical	
Admission source: Emergency department	
Date of admission: 13 September 2020	

Reason for admission / Presenting problems:

Severe hypotension, lethargy and sepsis

Principal diagnosis: Sepsis

Comorbidities:

Persistent pneumothorax and left pleural effusion secondary to metastatic breast cancer in her lung; ICC in situ

Acute renal failure

Previous medical history:

Breast Ca Dx 2009

Clinical synopsis:

BIBA with severe hypotension, lethargy and sepsis. Readmission to hospital after recently being discharged following the elective insertion of an ICC for a left pleural effusion secondary to metastatic breast cancer in her lung. On admission her blood pressure was 60 systolic, her ICC mucky. She had a persisting pneumothorax on chest x-ray and signs of ARF.

She was started on gentamicin, vancomycin and dobutamine but despite these measures remained profoundly hypotensive and unwell with oliguria and a deteriorating conscious state over the next 24 hours. She died in the early hours of 15 September 2020. Why she became septic and deteriorated so rapidly is uncertain, though it may have been related to her ICC site.

Complications:

Creatinine 0.22, coagulopathy and toxic changes in her WBCs.

Clinical interventions:

Diagnostic interventions:

Chest x-ray

Medications at discharge:

At time of death – gentamicin, vancomycin and dobutamine

Ceased medications:

Allergies:

Alerts:

Arranged services:

Recommendations:

Information to patient/relevant parties:

Authorising clinician:

Document recipients:

LMO

1. Expand the following abbreviations as found in the discharge summary above.

    BIBA

    ICC

    WBC

    ARF

    Ca

    Dx

2. What is sepsis?

3. Explain in lay terms what metastatic breast cancer in the lungs means?

4. What are the symptoms of a pneumothorax?

5. What is an ICC and what does it treat?

CHAPTER 21

Radiology and Nuclear Medicine

Contents

OBJECTIVES	495
INTRODUCTION	496
NEW WORD ELEMENTS	496
Combining forms	496
Prefixes	496
Suffixes	497
VOCABULARY	497
ABBREVIATIONS	497
RADIOLOGY	498
Characteristics of x-rays	498
Diagnostic techniques	499
Positioning	501
NUCLEAR MEDICINE	502
Nuclear medicine techniques	504
RADIOTHERAPY	505
Radiotherapy techniques	505
EXERCISES	506

Objectives

After completing this chapter you should be able to:

1. state the meanings of the word elements related to radiology and nuclear medicine

2. build words using the word elements associated with radiology and nuclear medicine

3. recognise, pronounce and effectively use medical terms associated with radiology and nuclear medicine

4. expand abbreviations related to radiology and nuclear medicine

5. describe the different types of imaging technologies that are currently in use and their application in the diagnosis and treatment of disease and injury

6. apply what you have learned by interpreting medical terminology in practice.

Demonstrate your knowledge of radiology and nuclear medicine by completing the exercises at the end of this chapter

INTRODUCTION

Radiology is the medical specialty that incorporates the study of the technology of imaging and its application to diagnosing and treating injury and disease in the body. In broad terms, there are two fields of radiology. **Diagnostic radiology** uses a range of imaging technologies such as radiography, ultrasound, fluoroscopy, tomography and magnetic resonance imaging to diagnose injury and disease. Doctors who specialise in this area are called **radiologists**. **Therapeutic radiology** uses radiation to treat diseases such as cancer. **Radiotherapists** are responsible for planning and delivering radiotherapy treatments, generally under the direction of **radiation oncologists**.

Nuclear medicine is the medical specialty that uses radioactive substances (radioisotopes) to both diagnose and treat injury and disease. Doctors who specialise in this area are called **nuclear medicine physicians**.

This chapter looks at the different imaging technologies that are currently in use.

NEW WORD ELEMENTS

Here are some word elements related to radiology and nuclear medicine. To reinforce your learning, write the meanings of the medical terms in the spaces provided. Use the Glossary of medical terms on page 561 to help you work out the meanings. You may also need to check the meaning in a medical dictionary, but make an attempt yourself first.

Combining forms

Combining Form	Meaning	Medical Term	Meaning of Medical Term
anter/o	front	anteroposterior	
cinemat/o	movement	roentgenocinematography	
dist/o	away, far, distant	distal	
fluor/o	fluorescent, luminous	fluoroscopy	
later/o	side	lateral	
medi/o	middle	mediolateral	
proxim/o	near, nearest	proximal	
radi/o	x-ray, radius	radiotherapist	
roentgen/o	x-rays	roentgenocardiogram	
scint/i	sparkling, flash of light	scintigraph	
scintill/o		scintillation detector	
son/o	sound	sonographer	
therapeut/o	treatment	therapeutic	
therm/o	heat	thermography	
tom/o	slice, section, cut	tomogram	
top/o	place, location	radioisotope	

Prefixes

Prefix	Meaning	Medical Term	Meaning of Medical Term
brachy-	short	brachytherapy	
cine-	movement	cineangiogram	
echo-	reflected, repeated sound	echocardiogram	
iso-	equal, same	isothermal	
ultra-	beyond, excess	ultrasonogram	

Suffixes

Suffix	Meaning	Medical Term	Meaning of Medical Term
-gram	record, writing	venogram	
-graph	product of recording	angiograph	
-graphy	process of recording	radiography	
-ist	one who specialises in	radiologist	
-lucent	shine	radiolucent	
-opaque	obscure	radio-opaque	

VOCABULARY

The following list provides many of the medical terms used for the first time in this chapter. Pronunciations are provided with each term. As you read the rest of the chapter, make sure you identify each of these terms and understand their meanings.

Term	Pronunciation
absorptiometry	ab-sawp-she-OH-me-tree
brachytherapy	bray-kee-THER-a-pee
cineradiography	sin-ee-ray-dee-OG-raf-ee
computed tomography	kom-PYOO-ted tom-OG-raf-ee
contrast media	kon-trahst MEE-dee-ah
external beam therapy	ek-stern-al beem THER-a-pee
fluoroscope	FLOO-roh-scope
gamma camera	GAM-a KAM-ra
half-life	hahf lyf
in vitro	in VIT-troh
in vivo	in VEE-voh
ionising radiation	eye-on-eye-zing ray-dee-AY-shun
magnetic resonance imaging	mag-NET-ik rez-on-ans IM-a-jing
multiple gated acquisition scan	mul-ti-pul gayt-ed ak-wi-SI-shun skan
myocardial perfusion scan	my-oh-KAH-dee-al per-fyoo-chun ckan
nuclear medicine	NYOO-klee-a MED-i-sin
photon	foh-ton
positron emission tomography	POZ-i-tron e-MISH-un to-MOG-ra-fee
projection radiography	proh-JEK-shun ray-dee-OG-ra-fee
radioactive iodine (^{131}I) therapy	ray-dee-oh-ak-TIV eye-oh-dyne ^{131}I THER-a-pee

Table continued

Term	Pronunciation
radioactivity	ray-dee-oh-ak-TIV-ee-tee
radionuclide	ray-dee-oh-NYOO-klyd
radio-opaque	ray-dee-oh-PAYK
radiopharmaceutical	ray-dee-oh-fah-ma-SYOO-tik-al
radiotracer	ray-dee-oh-TRAY-sa
scintigraphy	sin-TIG-ra-fee
single-photon emission computed tomography	sing-gel FOH-ton e-MISH-un kom-PYOO-ted tom-OG-raf-ee
systemic radioisotope therapy	sis-TEM-ik ray-dee-oh-EYE-so-tope THER-a-pee
tagging	TAG-ing
thallium scan	thal-ee-um skan
tracer study	TRAY-sa STUD-ee
transducer probe	tranz-DYOO-sa prohb
ultrasound	UL-tra-sownd
uptake	UP-tayk

ABBREVIATIONS

The following abbreviations are commonly used in the Australian healthcare environment. Because some abbreviations can have more than one meaning, check the context in which the abbreviation is used before assigning a meaning to it.

Abbreviation	Definition
^{131}I	radioactive iodine
3DCRT	three-dimensional conformal radiation therapy
^{67}**Ga**	radioactive gallium
µCi	microcuries

Table continued

Abbreviation	Definition
AP	anteroposterior
Ba	barium
BE	barium enema
BMD scan	bone mineral density scan
CT	computed tomography
CAT	computed axial tomography
Ci	curies
CTCA	CT coronary angiography
CTG	cardiotocography
CVC	central venous catheter
CXR	chest x-ray
DEXA	dual energy x-ray absorptiometry
DSA	digital subtraction angiography
DXT	deep x-ray therapy
ECG	electrocardiogram
FNA	fine-needle aspiration
Gy	gray
ICCM	iodine-containing contrast medium
IVP	intravenous pyelogram
IMRT	intensity-modulated radiation therapy
mCi	millicuries
MIBI scan	sestamibi scan
MRI	magnetic resonance imaging
MUGA	multiple gated acquisition scan
NT scan	nuchal translucency scan
PA	posteroanterior
PET scan	positron emission tomography scan
PICC	peripherally inserted central venous catheter
rad/RAD	radiation
	radiation absorbed dose
	roentgen absorbed dose
RAI	radioactive iodine
RAIU	radioactive iodine uptake
SIRT	selective internal radiation therapy
SIS	saline infusion sonohysterography
SPECT	single photon emission computed tomography
SRS	stereotactic radiosurgery
SRT	stereotactic radiotherapy
U/S	ultrasound
VQ scan	ventilation–perfusion scan
XR	x-ray

RADIOLOGY

Characteristics of x-rays

Wilhelm Conrad Roentgen, a scientist from Germany, identified x-rays in 1895. X-rays are a very low dose of ionising radiation that has very high levels of wave-like forms of electromagnetic energy carried by particles called photons. In fact, the dose of radiation from an x-ray is far less than the naturally occurring background radiation dose that people are exposed to every day. This specific form of ionising radiation allows the invisible x-ray to go through the body to create an image of the internal structures. X-ray-sensitive film or an x-ray plate is put on one side of the body, and x-rays are beamed through. The process is called projection radiography. The x-rays travel in straight lines, and the beam of the x-rays moves away from its source. The first structures the beam encounters appear exaggerated in size compared with those nearer to the x-ray plate. The image is produced because the x-ray beam is absorbed differently by different structures or body parts. Bone, having a very dense atomic structure, absorbs a high percentage of the x-ray beam (and appears light grey on the resultant image), while soft tissues, having a lower density of atoms, absorb less (and appear dark grey on the image). Because there are many structures of differing densities in the body, these create the image (Fig. 21.1).

Figure 21.1 X-ray machine and chest x-ray

(Ballinger & Frank 2003; LaFleur Brooks 2005)

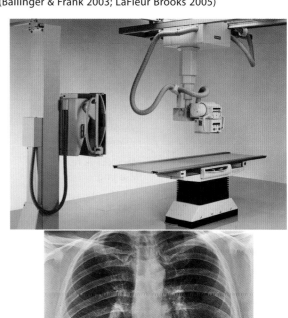

Diagnostic techniques

In a normal x-ray image, soft tissue shows up less clearly than bones. However, there are processes that can provide a clearer view of soft tissue and blood vessels. To create the clearer image, a contrast medium is injected or swallowed into the body. Contrast media are liquids that absorb x-rays more efficiently than the surrounding tissue and therefore block or limit the ability of x-rays to pass through. As a result, blood vessels, organs and other body tissue that temporarily contain the contrast change their appearance on x-ray or CT images. For x-rays of the digestive and endocrine systems, the patient swallows a contrast medium mixture that generally contains barium or iodine. Alternatively, it may be administered into the rectum via an enema. For examining the blood vessels, the contrast medium is injected into the bloodstream. **Fluoroscopy** is a procedure whereby a fluoroscope is used with a contrast medium. A fluoroscope is an instrument with a flat screen that has chemicals on its surface. When x-rays or other forms of radiation pass through the body onto this fluorescent screen, a moving x-ray image is produced and can be used to track the passage of the contrast medium through the body system under investigation or to create a video image of the functioning of the organs being assessed.

Another method used for diagnosis is **cineradiography**, which integrates cinematography, fluoroscopy and radiography processes. This technique involves creating a moving picture of the images that are displayed on a fluorescent screen. Body structures can be highlighted using an injected radio-opaque medium.

Another form of radiographic technique is a **dual energy x-ray absorptiometry** or DEXA, used to assess bone density. This is generally used for osteoporosis testing, and the amount of calcium in the bones (generally the head of the femur, lumbar spine or calcaneum) is assessed. The dose of radiation used in DEXA scans is very low, much lower than more common x-ray examinations.

A **computed tomography** (CT) scan is a method of using x-rays to take radiographic images in very fine slices through all or a specific part of the body. The slices can be less than 1 mm thick. The slices can be used to reconstruct cross-sectional images of the whole body or used to review the specific structures or parts of the body that require investigation. An iodine-containing contrast medium may be used to better display certain blood vessels and organs (Fig. 21.2).

Another radiology technique uses sound waves in a process known as an **ultrasound**. This involves using a machine that transmits high-frequency pulses of sound from a transducer probe. The sound waves pass into the body until they encounter an edge between different types of tissue (e.g. between fluid and soft tissue, soft tissue and bone). Some of the sound waves get reflected back to the probe, and others continue until they reach another boundary and then bounce back. The probe is connected to a computer that calculates the distance from the probe to the tissue or organ using the speed of sound in the tissue and the time that the sound waves take to return. These allow the computer to show the distances and intensities of the echoes on a screen, forming two-dimensional and,

Figure 21.2 **CT scanner and scans through different body regions**

A. CT scanner; **B.** A CT scanner has an x-ray source that rotates around electronic detectors

(photo copyright Mlanovic/Photos.com; Caldermeyer & Buckwalter 1999)

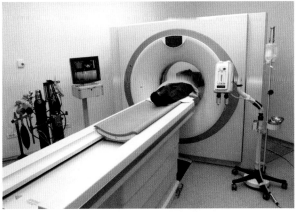

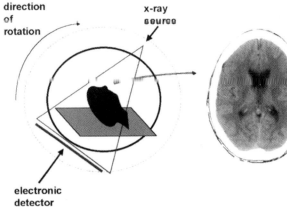

A

B

Continued

Figure 21.2 CT scanner and scans through different body regions (cont'd)

C. Scans of different levels of the body. The level of the scan is indicated on the figure of the body. The bar below the figure indicates the gradient of structure density as represented by black (least dense, such as air) and white (most dense, such as bone). Parts of the body with the greatest density are shown as white (bone) and those that have least density are dark (air).

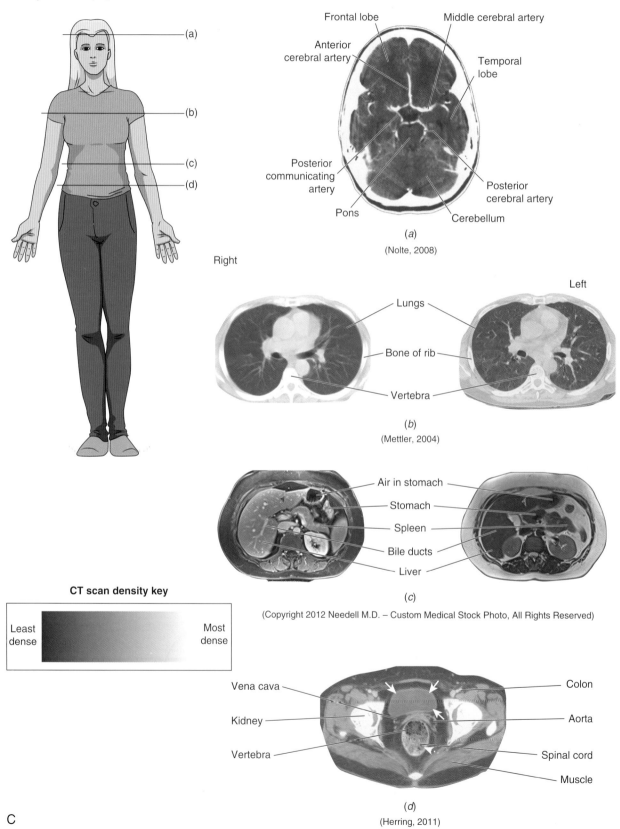

(a)
(Nolte, 2008)

(b)
(Mettler, 2004)

(c)
(Copyright 2012 Needell M.D. – Custom Medical Stock Photo, All Rights Reserved)

(d)
(Herring, 2011)

C

more recently, three- and four-dimensional images (Fig. 21.3).

Magnetic resonance imaging, or MRI, is a scanning procedure that uses magnetic fields and radiofrequency pulses, and not radiation, to gather signals from the body. The body's soft tissue contains water molecules that contain microscopic substances called protons. The magnetic field created by the MRI machine magnetises the protons, causing them to send out an echo in reaction to the MRI scan's radio waves. These echoes are detected by a radio antenna, and an image or data is created from them by a computer (Fig. 21.4). An MRI is generally used to obtain more specific detail after other tests such as an x-ray or ultrasound indicate a problem. Because of the use of magnetism in the MRI, this type of test is used cautiously for patients with certain forms of metallic implant such as surgical clips, staples, stents or prostheses. Some specific MRI tests are conducted using a contrast medium. For example, a stress perfusion MRI is used for assessing the blood supply to the heart. The contrast dye is injected to assess the functioning of the heart at rest and under stress or exercise. The MRI shows the areas of the heart muscle that have a good blood supply, while areas that have less efficient blood supply do not show up as well on the images with the contrast.

Positioning

The positioning of the patient when a radiology test is done is essential to ensure a clear image of the body structures being investigated. The general positions, or views, are posteroanterior (PA), anteroposterior (AP), lateral and oblique.

The most common type of x-ray, that of the chest, is taken in a posterior to anterior or PA position, with the x-rays being beamed from the back of the patient to the x-ray plate positioned in front. However, in patients too ill to stand, an anterior to posterior or AP film may be done with the patient in a supine position; that is, the x-rays are beamed from the front to the back of the patient as they are lying face up. Magnification of images changes according to the distance between the x-ray source and the patient, and a more divergent x-ray beam may be required to cover the same anatomical field depending on the patient's position and relative positioning of body structures. For example, in an AP projection the heart appears larger than it actually is because it is further from the detector. The x-ray beam is also more divergent because its source is nearer to the patient.

A lateral view is obtained in a similar fashion as the PA view, with the patient standing or lying with both arms raised but the x-ray taken from the side. Generally, though not always, the patient's left side is against the x-ray plate so that the right side is magnified. The lateral position is named according to the side of the patient closest to the film.

An oblique view x-ray is taken with the rays at an angle to any of the planes of the body. The patient is generally lying on their side with a rotated body position. These x-rays are generally described by the side of the body and body surface closest to the x-ray film. Therefore a 'right anterior oblique' position is when the patient's right side is closest to the film and the central x-ray has travelled on an angle from a posterior to an anterior surface.

Figure 21.3 Ultrasound scanner and 3D and 4D scans of fetus in final trimester

(Ballinger & Frank 2003; Hoath & Mauro 2015)

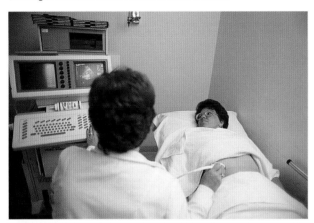

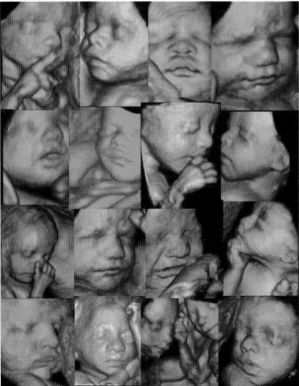

Figure 21.4 MRI scanner and scan of lumbar spine with herniated disc identified by arrow
A. Magnetic resonance scanner; **B.** Sagittal scan of the lumber spine with herniated disc (arrow)

(Driscoll & Lane 2007; LaFleur Brooks 2005)

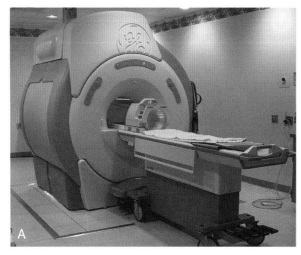
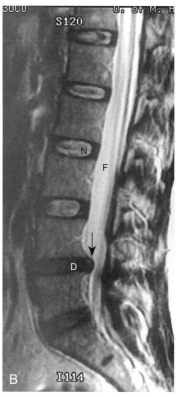

NUCLEAR MEDICINE

Nuclear medicine is a branch of medical imaging that uses small amounts of radioactive material called radioactive isotopes (or radionuclides) to diagnose and treat diseases such as cancer, heart disease and thyroid conditions. Radionuclides are combined with other organic compounds to form radiopharmaceuticals. These radiopharmaceuticals are administered by injection, orally or inhaled as a gas. The organic compound transports the radiopharmaceutical to its target organ where it passes through or accumulates and emits gamma rays. The radiation emitted by these radiopharmaceuticals is captured by a gamma camera, a positron emission tomography (PET) scanner and/ or a probe (Fig. 21.5). In conjunction with computer technology, the amount of radiopharmaceutical absorbed is measured. Images showing both the structure and function of organs and tissues are produced. Nuclear medicine procedures primarily demonstrate physiological functioning rather than the anatomical imaging shown by techniques such as CT scans or MRI.

As well as diagnostic techniques, nuclear medicine also includes therapeutic procedures. The beginning of nuclear medicine can be traced back to the discovery of artificially produced radioisotopes by Frédéric Joliot-Curie and Irène Joliot-Curie in 1934. The first time nuclear medicine was used as a clinical treatment was in 1946 when a patient's thyroid cancer was exposed to radioactive iodine, reducing the size of the tumour. As knowledge about radionuclides, radioactivity and the use of radionuclides to trace biochemical processes has increased, the use of nuclear medicine as a specialty has grown.

When used for therapeutic purposes, the radioactive agent is taken up by, and destroys, the targeted tissue. An example is radioactive iodine (^{131}I) therapy, which uses small amounts of radioactive material to treat cancer and other medical conditions affecting the thyroid gland.

Development of the first PET scanner revolutionised diagnosis and treatment practices. Similarly, the nuclear medicine technique called a single-photon emission computed tomography (SPECT) scan, which combines use of a CT scan and a radioactive tracer, has enabled

Figure 21.5 Nuclear medicine scanner and PET-CT examination of a patient with carcinoma of the lung

The primary tumour is seen on both the PET image and CT scan (white arrows), and there is a metastatic lymph node in the mediastinum (broken white arrows). There is also increased uptake on the PET image in the liver, kidneys and stomach, with very high uptake in the bladder (curved white arrow) due to urinary excretion of isotope.

(Ballinger & Frank 2003; Waldman & Campbell 2011)

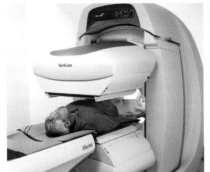
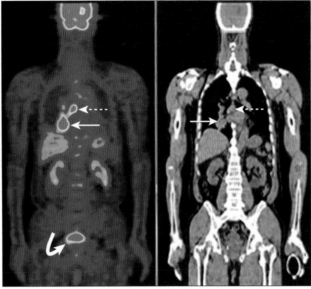

demonstration of blood flow to various body tissues and organs.

The most recently developed therapeutic technique is radioimmunotherapy, which is a combination of radiation therapy and immunotherapy most commonly used to treat lymphomas. As discussed in more detail in Chapter 19 Oncology, radioimmunotherapy involves monoclonal antibodies. These are antibodies made in a laboratory that are designed to specifically target a certain antigen such as one found on some cancer cells. Once attached to the antigen, the antibodies then recruit the body's own immune system to inhibit the ability of the cancer antigens to grow and metastasise, operating in a way that is similar to the body's own ability to fight infections. The advantage of this form of treatment is that it focusses on the specific target on the cancer cells, producing a minimal effect on normal cells.

To be able to understand nuclear medicine procedures, it is important to become familiar with some terms that are used, as defined in the following table.

Term	Description
half-life	Radiopharmaceuticals are used in the field of nuclear medicine as tracers in diagnosing and treating many diseases including various neoplasms, and in assessing the functioning of various organs including the heart, thyroid, lungs, liver, gallbladder, kidneys, skeleton and the blood. Tracers attach to body substances, and how the body handles and distributes these differs when there is disease present in the organ or body system under study. The amount of the radiopharmaceutical given to a patient must be enough to obtain the required information before it decays. The time that it takes to decay is described using the radioisotope's half-life. The half-life is the time it takes a radioisotope to lose 50% (half) of its activity through radioactive decay. The longer the half-life, the slower the isotope decays.

Table continued

Term	Description
in vitro	In vitro refers to the examination of a substance in an artificial environment such as in a test tube. For example, a radioimmunoassay is an in vitro test in which very small quantities of hormones, drugs and other substances in blood and urine can be measured using particular antibodies or antigens to which radioactive tracers have been attached. Since the patient does not receive the radioactive material, there is no exposure to the dose of radiation.
in vivo	In vivo refers to radiological images taken within a living human body.
radioactive	A radioactive substance is one that has a spontaneous emission of a stream of high-speed particles or electromagnetic radiation from its interior as it decays.
radionuclide	A radionuclide is another name for a radioactive isotope. Radionuclides occur naturally but can also be artificially produced. They spontaneously decay, emitting radiation as they do. The most common radioisotope used in diagnosis is technetium-99m (^{99m}Tc).
radio-opaque	Radio-opaque refers to the property of not being transparent to x-rays or other forms of radiation. For example, bones are relatively radio-opaque and therefore show as white areas on an x-ray because they stop the passage of the x-rays.
radiopharmaceuticals	Radiopharmaceuticals are radioactive chemicals or drugs that contain a radiotracer such as a radionuclide. They are used for both diagnostic and treatment purposes. Following the passage of the chemical in the body is called **tagging**. Some examples of radiopharmaceuticals include iodine-123 (^{123}I), which is used to diagnose thyroid disease and renal function, and iodine-131 (^{131}I), which is used to treat thyroid cancer and hyperthyroidism.
radiotracer	A radiotracer is a radioactive substance that is injected, inhaled or swallowed to identify diseased tissue. The absorption of a radiotracer is called the **uptake**. A **tracer study** is a procedure that follows the passage of the radiotracer around the body.

Nuclear medicine techniques

There are many nuclear medicine imaging procedures that provide information about nearly every body system. Some of the more commonly performed procedures are outlined below.

Term	Description
scintigraphy	Scintigraphy is a diagnostic nuclear medicine test in which radioisotopes are injected into the body. The emitted radiation is captured by a gamma camera (also called a scintillation counter) to create 2D images called scintigrams.
single-photon emission computed tomography (SPECT)	SPECT is a 3D tomographic technique that can view organs from many different angles. It uses gamma camera data from many projections that can be reconstructed in different planes. The camera builds a computer-enhanced image from the radiation source. Metabolic and physiological functions of organs such as the brain, heart, liver, spleen and bones are commonly studied using SPECT. It is a more sensitive and specific procedure than a PET scan.
positron emission tomography (PET)	PET is a technique that creates images by computer analysis after a radionuclide has been injected into the body and accumulates in the target tissue. As it decays, it emits a positron, which is detected by the PET camera. The most important clinical role of PET is in oncology, with fluorine-18 (^{18}F) as the tracer. PET has proven to be the most accurate, noninvasive method of detecting and evaluating the behaviour of many cancers. It is also commonly used in cardiac and brain imaging for conditions such as Parkinson's disease, epilepsy and some dementias.

SPECT/CT, PET/CT and PET/MRI are technologies that combine molecular and anatomic imaging. Nuclear medicine is effective at identifying molecular and physiological information but is not as effective at obtaining anatomic information. These combined technologies have solved this problem. Nuclear medicine images can be superimposed on CT or MRI to produce more detailed views. These views allow the information from two different studies to be combined and interpreted as one image. SPECT/CT and PET/CT units that are able to perform both imaging studies are available, providing higher quality information and more accurate diagnoses. |

Table continued

Term	Description
cardiac nuclear medicine	Cardiac nuclear medicine is commonly used to diagnose coronary artery disease and cardiomyopathy. The most frequently performed cardiac nuclear medicine procedure is a **myocardial perfusion scan**, which allows visualisation of the blood flow patterns to the heart walls. A **thallium scan**, using the radionuclide thallium-201 (^{201}TI), is used in cardiac nuclear medicine and to detect tumours. A **multiple gated acquisition scan** (MUGA scan) is a noninvasive procedure that assesses cardiac function. A MUGA scan is performed by attaching ^{99m}Tc to erythrocytes and injecting them into the patient's bloodstream. The patient is then placed under a gamma camera, which can detect the low-level radiation being emitted by the technetium-labelled erythrocytes. The scan produces a moving image of the beating heart and the heart chambers.
radioactive iodine (^{131}I) therapy	Radioactive iodine (^{131}I) therapy is a nuclear medicine treatment for hyperthyroidism. Hyperthyroidism can be caused by Graves' disease, or by overactive nodules within the gland itself. When a small dose of ^{131}I is swallowed, it is absorbed into the bloodstream in the gastrointestinal tract and concentrated from the blood by the thyroid gland. It then begins destroying the thyroid gland's cells. Radioactive iodine ^{131}I may also be used to treat thyroid cancer.

RADIOTHERAPY

Radiotherapy is the use of radiation to treat diseases such as cancer by destroying cancerous cells through exposure to high-dose radiation. The radiation may be delivered by a machine (external-beam radiation therapy), from radioactive material placed in the body near cancer cells (brachytherapy) or by radioactive isotopes that are ingested or injected (systemic radioisotope therapy).

Radiotherapy techniques

Term	Description
external beam radiotherapy	External beam radiotherapy involves delivering a beam of high-energy radiation to a tumour. The radiation beam is directed through the skin to the tumour and the surrounding tissue to destroy cancer cells. Beams are generated by a linear accelerator, external to the patient. The size and shape of the beam, and how it is directed at the tumour, is carefully calculated so the tumour is effectively treated but damage to the normal tissue surrounding the cancer cells is minimised.
brachytherapy	Brachytherapy (internal radiation therapy) is a form of radiation therapy in which the radiation source, commonly gold seeds, is precisely implanted in direct contact with the tumour. This differs from most radiation treatments, which use radiation beams from an x-ray machine external to the body. Brachytherapy gives a high radiation dose to the actual tumour while reducing the radiation exposure to the surrounding healthy tissues. *Brachy-* means short. Brachytherapy is radiation therapy given at a short distance. Brachytherapy is commonly used as an effective treatment for cervical, prostate, breast and head and neck cancers.
systemic radioisotope therapy	Systemic radioisotope therapy uses radioactive substances, such as radioactive iodine, that travel in the bloodstream to destroy cancer cells or other targeted tissue. An example of this is radioactive iodine (^{131}I) therapy, which was discussed in the previous section.

Exercises

EXERCISE 21.1: MATCH WORD ELEMENTS AND MEANINGS

Match the prefix, suffix or combining form in Column A with its meaning from Column B.

Column A	Answer	Column B
1. anter/o		A. process of recording
2. brachy-		B. away, far, distant
3. cine-		C. side
4. cinemat/o		D. middle
5. dist/o		E. sound
6. echo-		F. obscure
7. fluor/o		G. sparkling, flash of light
8. -gram		H. front
9. -graph		I. near, nearest
10. -graphy		J. x-rays
11. iso-		K. record, writing
12. -ist		L. short
13. later/o		M. slice, section, cut
14. -lucent		N. beyond, excess
15. medi/o		O. treatment
16. -opaque		P. movement (1)
17. proxim/o		Q. product of recording
18. radi/o		R. reflected, repeated sound
19. roentgen/o		S. place, location
20. scint/i		T. shine
21. son/o		U. fluorescent, luminous
22. therapeut/o		V. movement (2)
23. therm/o		W. equal, same
24. tom/o		X. one who specialises in
25. top/o		Y. x-ray, radius
26. ultra-		Z. heat

EXERCISE 21.2: CIRCLE THE CORRECT SPELLING

Select the correctly spelled medical term from the options provided.

veinogram	venogram	venegram	veinagram
radioloocent	radioloosent	radiolucent	radiolusent
yoorography	urrography	urografy	urography
radionuclide	radionooclide	radionucleide	radionucyde
radiofarmaceutical	radiopharmiceutical	radiopharmaceutical	radiofarmiceutical
thalium	thaliem	thalleum	thallium
brachytherapy	brachitherapy	brachatherapy	brachietherapy
telatherapy	telotherapy	teletherapy	telletherapy
nouclear	nuclear	nooclear	nucleer
scintigraphy	sintigraphy	cintigraphy	scintography

EXERCISE 21.3: IDENTIFY THE COMBINING FORMS AND MEANING OF MEDICAL TERMS

Select the combining form from each of the medical terms below, then define each term.

Medical Term	Combining Form	Meaning of Medical Term
cineradiography		
mammogram		
angiography		
ultrasonography		
cardiotocography		
radiopharmaceutical		
fluoroscope		
tomogram		
echocardiogram		
isothermic		

EXERCISE 21.4: EXPAND THE ABBREVIATIONS

Expand the abbreviations to form correct medical terms.

Abbreviation	Expanded Abbreviation
AP	
Ba	

Abbreviation	Expanded Abbreviation
BE	
BMD scan	
CT	
CTCA	
CTG	
CXR	
DEXA	
DSA	
DXT	
IVP	
MIBI scan	
MRI	
MUGA	
PET scan	
SPECT	
SRS	
U/S	
XR	

EXERCISE 21.5: MATCH THE PROCEDURE WITH ITS MEANING

Match the procedure in Column A with its meaning from Column B.

Column A	Answer	Column B
1. brachytherapy		A. ultrasound technique for observing the heart
2. radioimmunotherapy		B. x-ray examination of the bile ducts using a contrast dye
3. thallium scan		C. x-ray of the rectum after infusion of barium sulphate
4. MUGA scan		D. another term for an x-ray
5. cholangiography		E. measurement of bone density
6. cholecystography		F. imaging technique that uses sound waves
7. barium enema		G. radiotherapy in which the source of radiation is placed close to the tumour

Column A	Answer	Column B
8. MRI		H. nuclear medicine procedure that assesses cardiac function
9. dual energy x-ray absorptiometry		I. x-ray examination of the gallbladder using a contrast dye
10. ultrasound		J. a form of radiation therapy combined with monoclonal antibody therapy
11. echocardiography		K. nuclear imaging technique that uses ^{201}Tl
12. roentgenogram		L. an imaging technique that uses electromagnetic radiation

EXERCISE 21.6: VOCABULARY BUILDING

Provide the medical term for each of the definitions below.

1. _____ are radioactive chemicals or drugs that contain a radiotracer such as a radionuclide.

2. Radionuclides are also known as _____.

3. The absorption of a radiotracer is called the _____.

4. A _____ scan is a method of using x-rays to take radiographic images in very fine slices through all or a specific part of the body.

5. The branch of medical imaging that uses small amounts of radioactive material called radioactive isotopes in the diagnosis and treatment of diseases is _____.

6. A _____ allows visualisation of the blood flow patterns to the heart walls.

7. _____ is a nuclear medicine treatment for hyperthyroidism.

8. Using radiation to treat diseases such as cancer by destroying cancerous cells through exposure to high-dose radiation is _____.

9. _____is the medical specialty that incorporates the study of the technology of imaging and its application to diagnosing and treating injury and disease in the body.

10. Following the passage of a radiopharmaceutical in the body is called _____.

EXERCISE 21.7: PRONUNCIATION AND COMPREHENSION

Read the following paragraphs aloud to practise your pronunciation. Using your textbook and a medical dictionary, find the meanings of the underlined medical terms.

The nuclear myocardial scan is an imaging study to identify myocardial ischaemia. Another diagnostic technique is to use stress echocardiography, and this is more common because it is more readily available.

A different technology involves assessing underline{myocardial perfusion} and function using underline{positron emission tomography} imaging. The cost of the technology has decreased, and as positron-emitting underline{radiopharmaceuticals} have become more available, it has become more common. Newer underline{gamma cameras} have the potential to offer similar benefits to PET technology but use the less costly ^{99m}Tc-based radiopharmaceuticals.

Currently, nuclear myocardial scans include both perfusion and underline{gated wall motion images}. Coronary artery blood flow is assessed, and the scans used to accurately determine the underline{left ventricular ejection fraction}, the underline{end-systolic volume of the left ventricle} and wall thickening.

EXERCISE 21.8: CROSSWORD PUZZLE

Complete the puzzle by providing the medical term for each of the clues below.

ACROSS

2. A radioisotope used in cardiac nuclear medicine (8)
8. A person who takes x-rays (12)
9. The original name for an x-ray (8)
10. The abbreviation for magnetic resonance imaging (3)

DOWN

1. An instrument that projects an x-ray image onto a fluorescent screen (11)
3. Absorption of a radioisotope into tissue (6)
4. Use of sound waves to image internal structures of the body (10, 7)
5. A substance that allows x-rays to penetrate (11)
6. The abbreviation for single-photon emission computed tomography (5)
7. Rays emitted by radioactive substances (5, 4)

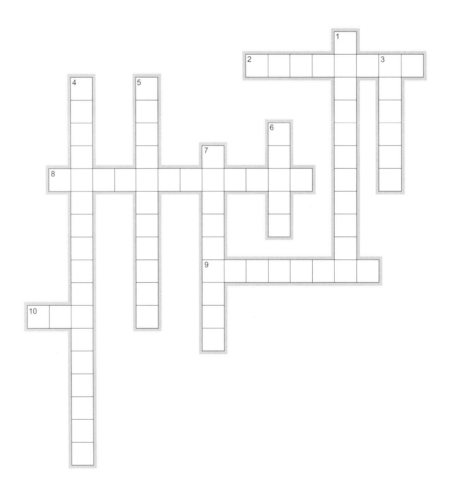

EXERCISE 21.9: DISCHARGE LETTER ANALYSIS

Read the discharge letter below and answer the questions.

UNIVERSITY HOSPITAL
DEPARTMENT OF RADIOLOGY AND NUCLEAR MEDICINE

25 October 2020
Dr Hazel Bishop
Healthcare Family Practice
Augusta Place
Nelson Harbour

Dear Dr Bishop

Thank you for referring **Mr Bruce Dunstan, D.O.B. 14 October 1944** to University Hospital for a total body scan to assess extent of bone metastases from his prostate cancer, which was diagnosed in September 2020. This study is compared with the 22-09-20 scan, which was performed just after original diagnosis.

This procedure was performed on 24 October 2020.

Following the intravenous administration of 27.4 mCi of ^{99m}Tc MDP, bone scintigraphy was performed with image acquisition of the axial and appendicular skeleton occurring at 3 hours post injection.

FINDINGS:

There is persistent left hydronephrosis, which has increased since the last exam. There is mild right collecting system dilatation.

The bilateral rib lesions seen on the last exam have not changed. Intense increased uptake involving the lower cervical and upper thoracic spine on the last exam appears to be less obvious at this time. Abnormal uptake at T12 and L1 appears to be stable. Abnormal sacral uptake is still present and appears to be covering a larger area than on the last exam. There is persistent abnormal uptake involving the right femoral neck and intertrochanteric region without a significant change. Abnormal uptake within the inferior ischiopubic rami is present, and this appears to be more obvious than on the last exam, particularly on the right side.

SUMMARY:

1. Increasing left hydronephrosis.
2. Decreased density of abnormal uptake involving the thoracic spine in comparison with the last exam.
3. Stable metastases in the thoracolumbar region.
4. Increased size of a large sacral metastasis.
5. Left iliac, right femoral neck and intertrochanteric metastases are all unchanged from the previous scan.
6. Bilateral inferior ischiopubic rami metastases are larger than before.

Due to the increase in metastatic disease, it is suggested that Mr Dunstan have a SPECT scan to locate any small lesions in the spine. He has been given an appointment to return for this scan in 1 week. I shall forward the SPECT report to you then.

Yours sincerely
Dr John Campbell
Nuclear Medicine Registrar
University Hospital

1. Mr Dunstan was given 27.4 mCi of ⁹⁹ᵐTc MDP. What does this mean?

_____

_____

_____

2. A bone scintigraphy was performed on Mr Dunstan. What is that procedure?

_____

_____

_____

3. Why were the images not taken for 3 hours after the radioisotope was injected?

_____

_____

_____

4. Mr Dunstan was referred for a SPECT scan. What is that procedure?

_____

_____

_____

5. Why was it important for Mr Dunstan to have a SPECT performed?

_____

_____

_____

CHAPTER 22

Pharmacology

Contents

OBJECTIVES   **513**

INTRODUCTION   **514**

NEW WORD ELEMENTS   **514**

    Combining forms   **514**

    Prefixes   **515**

    Suffixes   **515**

ABBREVIATIONS   **515**

GLOSSARY OF COMMONLY USED
PHARMACOLOGICAL TERMS   **516**

HOW DRUGS ARE NAMED   **518**

REGULATION AND REGISTRATION
OF MEDICATIONS IN AUSTRALIA
AND NEW ZEALAND   **518**

ADMINISTRATION OF DRUGS   **519**

TERMINOLOGY OF DRUG
ACTION   **520**

DRUG CLASSES   **521**

ANAESTHESIA   **522**

ASA (AMERICAN SOCIETY OF
ANESTHESIOLOGISTS) PHYSICAL
STATUS CLASSIFICATION   **522**

EXERCISES   **523**

Objectives

After completing this chapter you should be able to:

1. state the meanings of the word elements related to pharmacology

2. build words using the word elements associated with pharmacology

3. recognise, pronounce and effectively use medical terms associated with pharmacology

4. expand abbreviations related to pharmacology

5. describe how drugs are named, regulated and registered in Australia and New Zealand

6. describe how drugs are administered, the classes of drugs and drug toxicity

7. apply what you have learned by interpreting medical terminology in practice.

Demonstrate your knowledge of pharmacology by completing the exercises at the end of this chapter.

INTRODUCTION

Pharmacology is the science and study of the preparation, properties, nature, uses and actions of drugs. It is important to note that the term *drug* is used in this chapter to mean a substance, either natural or chemical, that is used in the diagnosis, treatment or prevention of disease. It includes any medicinal substance that is prescribed by a healthcare practitioner, available for purchase over the counter or obtained from other sources such as online or illegally.

Because medicinal substances are commonly used and available in society, many terms used in this chapter will be familiar to you.

NEW WORD ELEMENTS

Here are some word elements related to pharmacology. To reinforce your learning, write the meanings of the medical terms in the spaces provided. Use the Glossary of medical terms on page 561 to help you work out the meanings. You may also need to check the meaning in a medical dictionary, but make an attempt yourself first.

Combining forms

Combining Form	Meaning	Medical Term	Meaning of Medical Term
aer/o	air, gas	aerotherapy	
aesthes/o	feeling, sensation	anaesthesia	
algesi/o	pain	analgesic	
bacteri/o	bacteria	antibacterial	
bronch/o	bronchus	bronchodilator	
chem/o	drug, chemical	chemotherapeutic	
cutane/o	skin	subcutaneous	
derm/o	skin	transdermal	
emet/o	vomiting	emetic	
erg/o	work	synergy	
hist/o	tissue	histamine	
hypn/o	sleep	narcohypnosis	
iatr/o	physician, medicine, treatment	iatrogenic	
lingu/o	tongue	sublingual	
myc/o	mould, fungus	antimycobacterial	
narc/o	stupor	pseudonarcotic	
or/o	mouth	orolingual	
pharmac/o	drug	pharmacologist	
prurit/o	itching	antipruritic	
pyret/o	heat, fire, burning, fever	antipyretic	
rect/o	rectum	rectal	
thec/o	sheath	intrathecal	
top/o	place, location	topical	
tox/o	poison, toxin	toxin	
toxic/o		toxicology	
vas/o	vessel, ductus (vas) deferens, duct	vasoconstrictor	
ven/o	vein	intravenous	
vit/o	life	vitamin	

Prefixes

Prefix	Meaning	Medical Term	Meaning of Medical Term
ana-	up, towards, apart	anaphylaxis	
anti-	against	antibiotic	
contra-	against	contraceptive	
intra-	within, into	intrauterine	
par	aside, beyond, apart from, other than, near, against	parenteral	
syn-	together, with	synergism	

Suffixes

Suffix	Meaning	Medical Term	Meaning of Medical Term
-al	type of medicinal drug *(these suffixes usually mean pertaining to but have a different meaning in pharmacology)*	antifungal	
-ic		antispasmodic	
-ive		antihypertensive	
-tic		embolytic	
-ase	enzyme	amylase	
-cide	killing, agent that kills	protozoacide	
-gen	producing, originating, causing	trypsinogen	
-lytic	drug that breaks down	mucolytic	
-ose	type of sugar	glucose	
-phylaxis	protection	prophylaxis	
-sol	solution	aerosol	

ABBREVIATIONS

The following abbreviations are commonly used in the Australian healthcare environment. Because some abbreviations can have more than one meaning, check the context in which the abbreviation is used before assigning a meaning to it. Many of the definitions provided are the Latin terminology, with the English equivalent meaning.

Abbreviation	Definition
a.c.	*ante cibum*, before meals
ad. lib	*ad libitum*, freely as desired
alt. dieb.	*alternis diebus*, every other day
aq.	*aqua*, water
b.d.	*bis die*, twice a day
b.i.d.	*bis in die*, twice a day
AMH	Australian Medicines Handbook
b.i.n.	*bis in nocte*, two times a night
cap., caps.	*capsula*, capsule

Table continued

Abbreviation	Definition
g	*gramme*, gram(s)
gtt(s)	*gutta(e)*, drop(s)
h.	*hora*, hour
IM	intramuscular
IV	intravenous
L	litre(s)
mane	*mane*, in the morning
mcg	microgram(s)
mg	milligram(s)
MIMS	Monthly Index of Medical Specialties
mL	millilitre(s)
mmol	millimole(s)
NBM	nil by mouth
noct.	*nocte*, at night
n.p.o.	*nil per os*, nothing by mouth
PBS	Pharmaceutical Benefits Scheme

Table continued

Abbreviation	Definition
p.c.	*post cibum*, after meals
PCA	patient-controlled analgesia
p.o.	*per os*, by mouth
p.r.n.	*pro re nata*, as required
q.4h.	*quaque 4 hora*, every four hours
q.6h.	*quaque 6 hora*, every six hours
q.d.	*quaque die*, every day
q.d.s.	*quater die sumendus*, four times a day
q.h.s.	*quaque hora somni*, every night at bedtime
q.i.d.	*quater in die*, four times a day
q.a.m.	*quaque die ante meridiem*, every morning (every day before noon)
q.n.	*quaque nocte*, every night

Table continued

Abbreviation	Definition
Rx	symbol for prescription or treatment
stat.	*statum*, immediately
tab.	*tabletta*, tablet
t.d.s.	*ter die sumendum*, three times a day
TGA	Therapeutic Goods Administration
t.i.d.	*ter in die*, three times a day

GLOSSARY OF COMMONLY USED PHARMACOLOGICAL TERMS

The following table contains some common terms that are used in the specialty of pharmacology. Some terms may have a more specific meaning in the language of pharmacology than in normal English usage.

Pharmacological Term	Description
adverse effect or reaction	An adverse reaction is any unintended and unpredictable reaction to a drug that is administered in the correct dose by the proper route. The reaction generally results from drug toxicity, patient idiosyncrasies or hypersensitivity reactions caused by the drug itself, or by ingredients added during manufacture, such as preservatives or flavourings. Some drug reactions may occur in everyone, whereas others occur only in susceptible patients.
allergic reaction	An allergic reaction results from a chemical reaction within the body that produces an allergic response to a medication. It is an immunological reaction that only occurs after re-exposure to the specific drug. The first time the drug is taken the immune system is stimulated. The next time the drug is taken, an immune response that produces antibodies and histamine occurs. The intensity of the reaction may range from mild urticaria to anaphylaxis.
anaphylactic reaction (anaphylaxis)	Anaphylaxis is an extreme allergic reaction characterised by wheezing, coughing, dyspnoea, chills, diaphoresis, pruritic urticaria, agitation, flushing, palpitations and cardiovascular collapse. This is a medical emergency and is potentially life threatening.
antagonism	Antagonism occurs when the combined effect of two or more drugs is less than the sum of the effects produced by each agent separately.
bioavailability	Bioavailability refers to the amount of active drug that reaches its target site(s) after administration by any route. The amount of drug absorbed is a measure of the ability of the formulation to deliver the drug to the sites of drug action to produce its expected pharmacodynamic and therapeutic effects.
bioequivalence	Bioequivalence provides a means of comparing generic brand name drugs or similar drugs from different suppliers, different batches or different sources for equivalence. Bioequivalent drugs must have the same active ingredient(s) in the same dosage so they produce the same therapeutic effect.
chemotherapy	Chemotherapy refers to the treatment of diseases using chemical agents or drugs that are selectively toxic.
cold chain	The maintenance of proper vaccine temperatures during storage, transport and handling to preserve the potency of the vaccine. The safe temperature range is between +2°C and +8°C.

Table continued

Pharmacological Term	Description
compliance	Compliance means the extent to which a patient agrees to and follows a prescribed treatment regimen. Poor compliance will potentially result in a negative outcome for the patient.
contraindication	A contraindication is a factor or situation that makes the administration of a drug inadvisable and potentially harmful to the patient. For example, a previous allergic reaction to a drug would be a contraindication to prescribing the drug again.
dependence	Dependence is a physical or psychological state in which a person needs a particular drug or substance to function normally. If the drug is stopped suddenly the person will display withdrawal symptoms. Dependence may be psychological or physiological.
dose	Dose refers to a quantity of drug administered to a patient at a given time and in a particular way.
efficacy	Efficacy is the effectiveness of a drug in producing the required effect.
idiosyncratic response	An idiosyncratic response refers to an abnormal or unusual response to a drug that is unique to the individual who exhibits it.
pharmacist	A pharmacist is a person qualified to dispense drugs.
pharmacodynamics	Pharmacodynamics is the science and study of the biological effects of drugs on the body and how those effects are produced.
pharmacokinetics	Pharmacokinetics is the science and study of how drugs are absorbed, distributed, used and excreted by the body.
pharmacology	Pharmacology is the science and study of the preparation, properties, nature, uses and actions of drugs.
pharmacotherapy	Pharmacotherapy refers to the science and study of the use of drugs in diagnosing, preventing and treating disease.
pharmacy	Pharmacy is the science of preparing, compounding and dispensing drugs. The term is also used to describe the retail or hospital outlet where drugs and other products are produced, packaged or sold, commonly known in Australia and New Zealand as a chemist.
placebo	A placebo is a drug with no actual relevant pharmacological action but that is effective because of the power of suggestion on the recipient. In some people, the act of taking a drug is enough to elicit a response in the body.
side effect	Side effects are the unwanted effects of a drug that are not part of its desired therapeutic effect. With increasing doses of a drug, the intensity or the frequency of the side effect is increased.
synergy	Synergy occurs when the combined effect of two or more drugs administered together is greater than the sum of each individual drug acting independently.
tolerance	Tolerance is the term for the need for increased amounts of a drug in order to achieve the required effect. Conversely, tolerance also refers to the diminished effect of a drug with continued use of the same amount.
toxicity	Toxicity refers to a reaction to a drug that is serious and potentially life threatening to the patient. Toxicity is related to the level of the drug in the bloodstream. It may be due to an overdose of medication, cumulative build-up of the drug in the body over time or the inability of the patient's body to excrete the drug. Toxic effects may be idiosyncratic or allergic in nature or may be an extreme extension of the therapeutic effect of the specific drug produced by overdosing.
toxicology	Toxicology is the study of the harmful effects of drugs and chemicals on the body and the amount (dose) required for the desired effect to occur.

HOW DRUGS ARE NAMED

Naming a drug is a complex procedure. Each drug will have multiple names. Coming up with these names can be difficult because the names cannot be similar to those of any other drug, as the potential for medication errors is increased if names sound or look similar. All drugs have a chemical name and a generic name, and most will also have a brand or trade name.

Initially, new drugs are protected by patents and are manufactured by only one company. The patent period allows the drug manufacturers to recover what it cost them for research and to develop the drug. After the patent period ends (and this can be many years), other companies may sell their own versions of the drug. The drug may then be sold as a generic product or with other brand names.

The **chemical name** is a scientific name based on the chemical structure of the drug. It is the chemical formula for the drug. This name is usually long, complex and unpronounceable and is almost never used to identify the drug for clinical or marketing purposes.

The **generic name** is the name used to identify a drug both officially and scientifically during its clinical lifetime. It is also known as its International Nonproprietary Name or INN. An INN is allocated by the World Health Organization to allow for unique identification of each drug. The INN is a specific name that is globally recognised and is public property.

The **brand name** or **trade name** is the name that a drug is marketed and sold under. The drug company that owns the drug patent also creates (and owns) its brand name. When the patent period has expired, other drug companies may sell the drug using their own brand name. Therefore, a drug may have several brand names.

The following table shows the different names for some commonly prescribed or used medications.

Chemical Name	Generic Name	Brand Names
9-chloro-2-methyl-6-phenyl-2,5-diazabicyclo[5.4.0] undeca-5,8,10,12-tetraen-3-one	diazepam	Valium, Valpam, Antenex, Ducene
(±)-N-methyl-3-phenyl-3[(α,α,α-trifluoro-p-tolyl) oxy] propylamine hydrochloride	fluoxetine hydrochloride	Prozac, Auscap, Lovan
2-(4-isobutylphenyl) propionic acid	ibuprofen	Advil, Bugesic, Herron Blue, Nurofen

The Australian Government's Brand Substitution Policy allows pharmacists to substitute bioequivalent generic drugs without seeking advice from the prescribing clinician, unless otherwise indicated on the prescription. These generic drugs must, by law, contain the same active ingredient as the brand name drug and undergo the same strict quality controls. However, the inactive ingredients that give the drug its colour, taste, shape, texture or smell may be quite different. The price of these drugs to the consumer may also differ substantially. The Australian Government, through the Pharmaceutical Benefits Scheme, subsidises up to the price of the cheapest brand. If a pharmacist dispenses a more expensive brand, the consumer pays the difference in price.

REGULATION AND REGISTRATION OF MEDICATIONS IN AUSTRALIA AND NEW ZEALAND

Drug companies selling medicines in Australia are regulated by the Therapeutic Goods Administration (TGA), which is part of the Australian Department of Health. In New Zealand the equivalent body is Medsafe, the Medicines and Medical Devices Safety Authority. The TGA is responsible for administering the provisions of the *Therapeutic Goods Act 1989* to provide a national framework for regulating therapeutic goods in Australia so as to ensure the quality, safety and efficacy of medicines and the quality, safety and performance of medical devices. The TGA regulates the availability and provision of:

* medicines that are prescribed by a doctor or dentist
* medicines that are available from a pharmacy but only from behind the counter
* medicines that are available in the general display shelves in a pharmacy
* medicines that can be purchased from supermarkets
* complementary medicines, including vitamins and herbal and traditional medicines
* medical devices, ranging from simple equipment and materials such as bandages to complex technologies such as heart pacemakers
* devices that are used to test for diseases or conditions
* vaccines, blood products and other biological substances.

The TGA also regulates the way these products are manufactured and advertised. It carries out a range of assessment and monitoring activities to ensure therapeutic goods available in Australia are of an acceptable standard. At the same time the TGA aims to ensure the Australian community has access, within a reasonable time, to therapeutic advances. More information about the TGA is available at www.tga.gov.au.

In Australia all therapeutic goods must be entered on the Australian Register of Therapeutic Goods (ARTG) before they can be supplied. The ARTG is a computerised database of information about therapeutic goods for human use approved for supply in, or export from, Australia. Two useful references for medical practitioners and other clinicians are MIMS (Monthly Index of Medical Specialities) (www.mimsonline.com.au) and the Australian Medicines Handbook (https://amhonline.amh.net.au). These are drug and product information references accessible in print, electronically and online. They contain detailed information about drug usage (e.g. dosage), adverse reactions and drug interactions. As a result of the Trans-Tasman Mutual Recognition Arrangement (June 1997), New Zealand registers all therapeutic goods on the ARTG and has an equivalent drug reference known as MIMS New Zealand (www.mims.co.nz).

ADMINISTRATION OF DRUGS

The most important aspects for all health professionals to consider when administering a drug to a patient are to make sure they have the correct person, route, dose, medication and time.

There are various ways a substance may be introduced into the body, and these are collectively called routes of administration. Although referring to the path the active substance takes from the point of application to the location where it has its target effect, the route is generally classified by the application location, as outlined in the following table.

Route of Administration	Description
oral	Medications are taken by mouth in pill, capsule or liquid form and are absorbed into the body through the digestive system. For oral drugs, the rate of absorption is generally slow.
enteral	Medications are delivered directly to the gastrointestinal tract via a gastric feeding tube or gastrostomy.

Table continued

Route of Administration	Description
mucosal	Medications are delivered through the nose or inhaled through the mouth and are absorbed through the nasal mucosa or bronchioles. Oral transmucosal administration involves tablets placed under the tongue (sublingual) or inside the cheek (buccal). These mucosal surfaces are rich in blood supply, providing for rapid movement of the drug to the systemic circulation. Vaginal administration of a medication is also considered mucosal.
parenteral	Administration of a substance via a syringe by injecting it directly into a vein (intravenous; Fig. 22.1), muscle (intramuscular), artery (intra-arterial), bone marrow (intraosseous), abdominal cavity (intraperitoneal), heart (intracardiac) or into the tissue beneath the skin (subcutaneous) (Fig. 22.2). Although the speed of absorption of the substance varies, this route is generally faster than oral administration and is therefore preferred when more complete and faster absorption of a drug is needed.
percutaneous	Direct absorption of the substance through the skin for either local or systemic effects. For example, some hormone replacements are administered by transdermal patches that are absorbed slowly and regularly by the bloodstream through the skin.
rectal (enteric)	Administration of a substance through the rectum via a suppository or a solution mixed with a fluid such as water with absorption by the lower digestive tract.
topical	Direct application of the drug onto a defined area of the body requiring treatment such as local anaesthetic onto the skin, eye drops onto the conjunctiva or ear drops into the external or middle ear.

Figure 22.1 Intravenous infusion
(Sorrentino 2008)

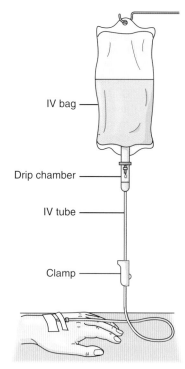

IV bag

Drip chamber

IV tube

Clamp

Figure 22.2 Angles of insertion for injections
(Bonewit-West 2008)

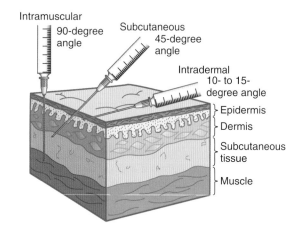

Intramuscular
90-degree angle

Subcutaneous
45-degree angle

Intradermal
10- to 15-degree angle

Epidermis

Dermis

Subcutaneous tissue

Muscle

TERMINOLOGY OF DRUG ACTION

Medications are usually classified by their actions – that is, the means by which a substance causes a desired effect. With few exceptions, drugs act on target proteins such as enzymes, carriers, ion channels and receptors. The primary effect of a drug is the desired therapeutic effect. Secondary effects are all other effects besides the desired effect, and these may be either beneficial or detrimental. The choice of drug depends on any changes it causes in normal metabolic processes and any abnormalities that may be present. Each substance introduced into the body follows one or more of these processes over time: liberation, absorption, distribution, metabolism and excretion.

Liberation refers to drugs administered orally whereby the active element of a tablet, capsule or pill is released and is absorbed by the gastrointestinal tract.

Absorption refers to the uptake of the agent from its site of administration into the circulatory system. Both liberation and absorption are affected by the solvent effect of the coating of the tablet or capsule, by the solubility of the drug, by its acidity or alkalinity and by its concentration. Aspects relating to the patient, such as the current disease state, interactions with food or other drugs, blood flow and absorbing surface, are also relevant.

Distribution of a drug or substance refers to the rate of perfusion or passage of a fluid through the vessels of the organ that it is targeting, the collection of the drug in body tissues and the ability of the substance to cross natural barriers or membranes such as the blood–brain barrier or placenta.

Metabolism is the process by which the body breaks down and converts a medication into an active chemical substance that is generally more easily absorbed for use by the body. The liver is the primary site of drug metabolism where enzymes chemically change components of a drug into substances known as metabolites. Metabolites are then joined to other substances for uptake into the systemic circulation, excretion through the lungs or bodily fluids (e.g. saliva, sweat, breast milk and urine) or through reabsorption by the intestines.

Excretion of unused substances and their metabolites is important so that they do not adversely affect the body's normal metabolism. This is mainly the role of the kidneys and the gastrointestinal system, which eliminate the waste products via the urine and faeces. The lungs also play a role in excreting gases, and the skin excretes through sweating.

All drugs target particular body sites and their mechanism of action is through receptor interactions or non-receptor mechanisms. Importantly, individual classes of drug only combine with certain targets, and conversely, individual targets recognise only particular classes of drug. However, not all drugs are specific in their actions. A **receptor interaction** occurs when the drug interacts with molecular components of the organ it is targeting. The interaction between a drug and the binding site of the receptor depends on the 'fit' of the two molecules, acting like a key and a lock. This interaction between the drug and the organ receptor causes an alteration to the organ's function, which hopefully produces the desired therapeutic effect. **Non-receptor** mechanisms do not act in this way but may change the actions of enzymes, or change some of the body's physical processes (e.g. creating more urine), changing normal metabolic processes or altering the permeability of a cell membrane.

The way a drug acts is a result of the **dose–response relationship**. The relationship between the amount of a drug given and the response seen depends on a variety of factors including: the individual rate of absorption, metabolism and elimination of the drug; the site of action of the drug in the body; and the presence of other drugs or disease. Generally, a patient's response to a drug increases in direct proportion to increases in the dose. When higher doses of the drug are given, the amount of change in response to an increase in the dose gradually decreases until a plateau is reached, such that no further increase in the response is noted. Doctors try to prescribe a dose that is the lowest that shows a therapeutic effect – in other words, a favourable effect – before the patient begins to demonstrate any adverse effect. Over time, drug tolerance may occur. This happens when a person's reaction to a drug reduces even though the dose or concentration given is the same. This means that larger doses are required to achieve the same effect.

The dose–response relationship may be affected by another drug the person is taking. This is called a drug–drug interaction. This may be additive (where the action of a combination of drugs provides an effect that is equal to the sum of each individual drug effect) or synergistic (where the action of two or more drugs given together is greater than the sum of each individual drug effect). Drug action may also be altered by food, beverages or supplements the person is consuming (drug–nutrient interaction), by another disease the person has (drug–disease interaction) or by genetics, the age, gender or weight of the patient. A placebo effect may also alter the patient's response to a substance. The term placebo is Latin for 'I will please' and refers to any medical treatment that is inactive or inert or any substance without any actual therapeutic agent. The patient who believes the placebo is a medication may experience alleviation of their symptoms.

DRUG CLASSES

Drugs may be classified or grouped according to the way the drug is used to treat a condition or by the chemical type of the active ingredient. Listed below are common drug class groupings. Note that some drugs can be grouped into more than one class.

Class of Drug	Description
analgesics	Analgesics are a class of drug that relieves pain. They include mild, narcotic (opioid) and non-steroidal anti-inflammatory drugs.
anaesthetics	Anaesthetics are drugs that, when administered, can result in complete or partial loss of sensation/feeling or consciousness. Anaesthesia can be administered so that it affects the whole body (general) or be limited to a region (regional) or site (local, topical). See the Anaesthesia section in this chapter for more detail.
antibiotics and antivirals	Antibiotic and antiviral drugs can destroy or hinder the development of a living organism or virus. They include antifungals, antituberculars, antivirals, cephalosporins, erythromycins, penicillins, quinolines, sulfonamides and tetracyclines.
anticoagulants	Anticoagulants are a class of drug that stops or slows down the clotting process in blood.
anticonvulsants	Anticonvulsants are drugs administered to prevent seizures.
antidepressants	Antidepressants are a class of drugs used to relieve mood disorders such as depression.
antihistamines	Antihistamines block the effects of histamine when released during an allergic reaction.
cardiovascular	Cardiovascular drugs are used to treat conditions of the heart such as hypertension, angina, myocardial infarction, congestive heart failure and arrhythmias. They include angiotensin converting enzyme (ACE) inhibitors, beta-blockers, calcium antagonists, cholesterol-lowering drugs, diuretics, angiotensin II receptor antagonists and antiarrhythmics.
endocrine	Endocrine drugs perform the functions of hormones that generally occur naturally in the body. They include androgen, anti-androgen, oestrogen, anti-oestrogen, aromatase inhibitor, glucocorticoid, progestin, SORM (selective oestrogen receptor modulator) and thyroid hormone.

Table continued

Class of Drug	Description
gastrointestinal	Gastrointestinal drugs are used to alleviate gastrointestinal symptoms, rather than act as a cure for gastrointestinal disease. They include antacid, antidiarrhoeal, antinauseant, anti-ulcer, anti-GORD and cathartic drugs.
hypoglycaemics	Hypoglycaemic drugs are used to treat diabetes mellitus.
respiratory	Respiratory drugs are used to treat respiratory disorders such as emphysema, asthma, bronchitis and bronchospasm. They include bronchodilators, leucotriene modifiers, steroid-inhalers and intravenous or oral steroids.
sedative-hypnotics	Sedative-hypnotics cause central nervous system depression.
stimulants	Stimulants are drugs that temporarily induce improvement in physical or mental function such as increasing alertness or wakefulness.
tranquillisers	Tranquillisers are administered to create calm in an anxious or agitated person.
vaccines	Vaccines are antigenic substances prepared from a weakened or attenuated form of an agent that causes a disease or from an artificial substitute. They produce immunity from the disease in the patient by causing the body to produce antibodies. They can be administered by injection, orally or by aerosol. Vaccines can prevent a disease from occurring in the first place and also decrease the risk of complications and risk of transmitting the disease in a population.
vitamins	Vitamins are organic compounds that can be isolated from plant or animal sources and provided through diet or dietary substances.

ANAESTHESIA

Anaesthesia means to be without sensation. Anaesthesia can be:

- **General** – agents administered intravenously or via inhalation, resulting in reversible unconsciousness, analgesia, muscle relaxation and depression of reflexes. This physical state then allows for invasive surgeries to be performed.
- **Regional** – anaesthetic agents injected to a specific region to block a group of nerves. Types of regional anaesthesia include spinal, epidural and nerve block.
- **Local and topical** – application of an anaesthetic agent to a small area of the body either via injection or onto the surface of the skin. The resulting loss of sensation allows for minor procedures such as removal of teeth or skin lesions to be performed.

ASA (AMERICAN SOCIETY OF ANESTHESIOLOGISTS) PHYSICAL STATUS CLASSIFICATION

The ASA Physical Status Classification is a system for determining the fitness of a person prior to surgery. As part of an anaesthetic work-up, an anaesthetist will identify the patient's surgical risk, with the score representing the risk level. The score should generally appear on the anaesthetic form or record. The classes are:

ASA Physical Status 1 – a normal healthy patient

ASA Physical Status 2 – a patient with mild systemic disease

ASA Physical Status 3 – a patient with severe systemic disease

ASA Physical Status 4 – a patient with severe systemic disease that is a constant threat to life

ASA Physical Status 5 – a moribund patient who is not expected to survive without the operation

ASA Physical Status 6 – a declared brain-dead patient whose organs are being removed for donor purposes.

A second character is added to the score to indicate if the surgery that is to be performed is an emergency or planned procedure. An 'E' recorded with the score indicates that the surgery being performed is considered an emergency procedure.

Note that the 'American Society of Anesthesiologists' has been spelled using the American spelling because it is the name of the organisation.

Exercises

EXERCISE 22.1: WORD ELEMENT MEANINGS AND WORD BUILDING

Define each word element below, then use the element correctly in a medical term.

Word Element	Meaning	Medical Term
aer/o		
aesthes/o		
algesi/o		
ana-		
anti-		
bacteri/o		
-cide		
contra-		
cutane/o		
emet/o		
hypn/o		
lingu/o		
-lytic		
narc/o		
-phylaxis		
thec/o		
top/o		
ven/o		

EXERCISE 22.2: IDENTIFY THE COMBINING FORMS AND MEANING OF MEDICAL TERMS

Select the combining form from each of the medical terms below, then define each term.

Medical Term	Combining Forms	Meaning of Term
pharmacologist		
toxicology		
antipruritic		
chemotherapy		
bronchospasm		
antihistamine		
iatrogenic		
mycotoxic		
antipyretic		
intradermal		

EXERCISE 22.3: MATCH THE ROUTE OF ADMINISTRATION WITH THE DEFINITION

Match the route of administration in Column A with its meaning from Column B.

Column A	Answer	Column B
1. topical		A. via the digestive system (e.g. rectal suppository)
2. transdermal		B. into the abdominal cavity
3. otic		C. into a vein
4. ophthalmic		D. into the spinal canal
5. enteral		E. through the skin
6. intra-articular		F. into a muscle
7. subcutaneous		G. through the mucosa under the tongue
8. intramuscular		H. into the ear
9. intrathecal		I. under the skin
10. intravenous		J. into the mouth
11. oral		K. into the eye
12. sublingual		L. direct application to a specific body part
13. intraperitoneal		M. into a joint

EXERCISE 22.4: MATCH THE DRUG ACTION WITH THE DRUG TYPE

Match the drug action in Column A with the drug type from Column B.

Column A	Answer	Column B
1. drug that relieves pain		A. antiemetic
2. drug that induces a loss of feeling or sensation		B. tranquilliser
3. drug that relieves mood disorders		C. bronchodilator
4. drug that blocks the effect of an allergic reaction		D. antihypertensive
5. drug that induces sleep		E. antidepressant
6. drug that opens the airways		F. anticoagulant
7. drug that lowers blood pressure		G. hypoglycaemic
8. drug that increases urine output		H. anticonvulsant
9. drug that lowers blood cholesterol		I. analgesic
10. drug that reduces glucose levels		J. antibiotic
11. drug that stops vomiting		K. sedative
12. drug that stops blood from clotting		L. anaesthetic
13. drug that prevents seizures		M. diuretic
14. drug that reduces anxiety levels		N. antihistamine
15. drug that treats bacterial infections		O. antihyperlipidaemic

EXERCISE 22.5: EXPAND THE ABBREVIATIONS

Expand the abbreviations or provide their English translation to form correct medical terms.

Abbreviation	Expanded Abbreviation or English Translation
PCA	
p.c.	
g	
b.i.d.	
q.n.	
NBM	
gtt	
MIMS	
p.r.n.	
q.4h.	
q.6h.	

Abbreviation	Expanded Abbreviation or English Translation
q.d.	
q.i.d.	
stat.	
tab.	
t.i.d.	
Rx	
q.a.m.	
mcg	
IM	

EXERCISE 22.6: APPLYING MEDICAL TERMINOLOGY

Fill in each blank below with the correct medical term.

1. An _____ is any unintended and unpredictable reaction to a drug that is administered in the correct dose by the proper route.

2. An _____ results from a chemical reaction within the body that produces an allergic response to a medication.

3. _____ is an extreme allergic reaction characterised by wheezing, coughing, dyspnoea, chills, diaphoresis, pruritic urticaria, agitation, flushing, palpitations and cardiovascular collapse.

4. An _____ refers to an abnormal or unusual response to a drug that is unique to the individual who exhibits it.

5. A _____ is a drug with no actual relevant pharmacological action but that is effective because of the power of suggestion on the recipient.

6. _____ refers to a reaction to a drug that is serious and potentially life threatening to the patient.

7. _____ are the unwanted effects of a drug that are not part of its desired therapeutic effect.

8. The way a drug acts is a result of the _____.

9. _____ is the process by which the body breaks down and converts a medication into an active chemical substance that is generally more easily absorbed for use by the body.

10. _____ is a physical or psychological state in which a person needs a particular drug or substance to function normally.

EXERCISE 22.7: BUILDING MEDICAL TERMS

Complete the medical terms below using the correct word elements.

1. A pharma_____ is a person qualified to dispense drugs.

2. Pharma_____ refers to the science and study of the use of drugs in the diagnosis, prevention and treatment of disease.

3. Pharma_____ is the science and study of how drugs are absorbed, distributed, used and excreted by the body.

4. Pharma_____ is the science and study of the biological effects of drugs on the body and how those effects are produced.

5. Pharma_____ is the science of preparing, compounding and dispensing drugs.

EXERCISE 22.8: PRONUNCIATION AND COMPREHENSION

Read the following paragraphs aloud to practise your pronunciation. Using your textbook and a medical dictionary, find the meanings of the underlined medical terms.

The patient was examined on arrival by the emergency department doctor after being found at home by a family member with a suspected <u>drug overdose</u>. A <u>urine toxicology screen</u> was performed and was positive for both <u>cocaine</u> and <u>opiates</u>. It was noted that he had decreased breath sounds in both lungs with associated <u>dyspnoea</u>.

The patient remained under observation in ED. After 2 hours his condition started to deteriorate. It was determined the patient was in <u>respiratory arrest</u> and <u>asystolic</u>. <u>Cardiopulmonary resuscitation</u> was commenced but was not successful and the patient died 3 hours after arrival at ED.

An <u>autopsy</u> was performed. Relevant findings included a needle puncture with <u>ecchymosis</u> in the left forearm, <u>left ventricular hypertrophy</u> and <u>congestion</u> in the lung <u>parenchyma</u>, liver and kidneys. <u>Blood toxicology studies</u> were negative for <u>codeine</u>, <u>morphine</u> and cocaine but were positive for benzoylecgonine, a cocaine <u>metabolite</u>. The coroner listed the cause of death as <u>cocaine intoxication</u>.

EXERCISE 22.9: CROSSWORD PUZZLE

Complete the puzzle by providing the medical term for each of the clues below.

ACROSS

3. The amount of drug given to a patient (4)
4. Drug index that clinicians use for information about prescribing drugs (4)
6. A factor that makes the administration of a drug inadvisable (16)
8. The science of preparing, compounding and dispensing drugs (8)
9. This injection is given under the skin (12)

DOWN

1. This drug is given to stop itching (12)
2. This drug is given to prevent pregnancy (13)
5. This person specialises in the study of drugs (14)
7. Administration of a drug into a vein (11)
8. This drug is given for protection (11)

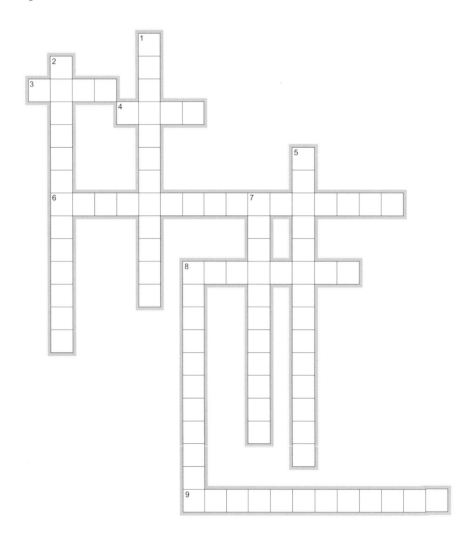

EXERCISE 22.10: INTERPRET THE PRESCRIPTION

Provide an explanation of each prescription below.

Example:
Mirtazapine 30 mg q.n. = 1 × 30 mg tablet every night

Drug and Dosage Instructions	Translated Dosage Instructions
Zovirax 400 mg t.d.s.	
Aropax 20 mg q.a.m.	
Warfarin 5 mg noct.	
Tagamet 400 mg b.d.	
Temazapam 10 mg q.h.s.	
Efudix cream 5% 20 g q.d.	
Ventolin 100 mcg 1–2 inhalations q.i.d.	
Pethidine hydrochloride IMI 50 mg q.d.s.	
Flagyl 400 mg b.d. a.c.	
Ibuprofen 200 mg p.r.n. up to 6 tabs. q.d.	

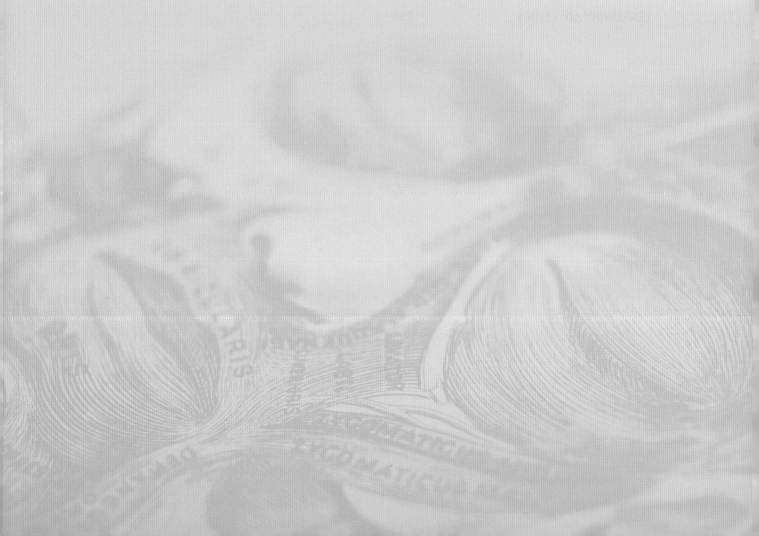

MODULE 5

Special Applications

CHAPTER 23

Complementary and Alternative Therapies

Contents

OBJECTIVES   532

INTRODUCTION   533

COMPLEMENTARY MEDICINES   533

COMPLEMENTARY THERAPIES   534

GLOSSARY OF TERMS   534

Objectives

The objective of this chapter is to provide a glossary of terms related to complementary and alternative therapies. It is not expected that you will remember all these terms. This glossary is provided as a reference tool to use if required.

INTRODUCTION

Traditional medicine is the term used to describe the sum total of knowledge, skills and practice of holistic care for diagnosing sickness, maintaining health and treating physical or mental disease, based on indigenous theories, beliefs and experiences handed down from generation to generation (WHO International Standard Terminologies on Traditional Medicine in the Western Pacific Region, 2009). Since the Declaration of Alma-Ata mentioned the role of traditional practitioners in primary health care in 1978, more attention has been given to traditional medicine. Almost three decades later, at the Fifty-ninth World Health Assembly of the World Health Organization in Geneva in 2006, the 192 member states were encouraged to integrate traditional medicine into their public health systems and to promote harmonisation with modern Western medicine. With the development of the 11th revision of the International Classification of Diseases (ICD), a chapter relating to traditional medicine disorders and patterns specifically for ancient Chinese medicine, commonly used in China, Japan and Korea, has been included for the first time. This initiative allows for the standardised measurement, counting, analysis and monitoring of traditional medicine use over time in the same way as has been possible for so-called Western medicine since the initial development of the ICD (World Health Organization, 2018; https://icd.who.int/en/). When a form of traditional medicine is taken up by other people outside its indigenous origins, it is often termed alternative or complementary medicine.

COMPLEMENTARY MEDICINES

In Australia, the Therapeutic Goods Administration (TGA) is responsible for guaranteeing that therapeutic goods available in Australia are safe and fit for purpose. The TGA is part of the Australian Government Department of Health. The definition of therapeutic goods is broad and includes over-the-counter medications, prescription medicines and complementary medicines, as well as medical devices, vaccines, blood products and surgical implants. Products that claim medicinal benefits and that contain herbs, vitamins and minerals, including nutritional supplements, homoeopathic medicines and certain aromatherapy products, are called 'complementary medicines' in Australia. These are regulated in the same way as 'traditional' medicines under the *Therapeutic Goods Act 1989*. Australia employs a risk-based method of legislating medicines, incorporating two tiers of regulation for all medicines, including complementary medicines:

- Lower risk medicines that contain preapproved, low-risk ingredients and make limited health benefit claims may be listed on the Australian Register of Therapeutic Goods (ARTG).
- Higher risk medicines must be registered on the ARTG. Prior to registration, the quality, safety and effectiveness of the medicine must be evaluated.

Complementary medicines encompass traditional medicines, including traditional Chinese medicines, Ayurvedic medicines and Australian indigenous medicines. Complementary medicines may also be called 'alternative', 'natural' or 'holistic' medicines.

Complementary medicines are regulated through the Therapeutic Goods Act and accompanying Therapeutic Goods Regulations 1990. These two pieces of legislation define what a complementary medicine is and specify the active ingredients that may be used in such medicines. One or more specific active ingredients may be included in a complementary medicine, and each must have a designated identity and an accepted traditional use. This means that the designated active ingredient must have a well-documented use, according to the experience of many traditional healthcare practitioners over an extended period, and there must be common and accepted procedures for its preparation, application and dosage.

The ARTG is a database comprising details of all therapeutic goods that are imported into, supplied in, or exported from Australia. The TGA maintains the register. It is a legal requirement that, unless specifically exempt or excluded, all therapeutic goods are included on the ARTG prior to their supply. In order to be included on the ARTG, an application must be lodged by a sponsor for those goods. Applications for complementary medicines to be included on the ARTG must follow the Australian Regulatory Guidelines for Complementary Medicines, which were initially developed in 2001 and are regularly updated to:

- provide necessary details to assist sponsors of complementary medicines to understand and adhere to obligations under therapeutic goods legislation
- ensure that applications for inclusion on the register for complementary medicines include necessary details to cover regulatory requirements to facilitate timely processing
- improve understanding and acceptance of the processes whereby complementary medicines are registered on the ARTG.

However, it is important to know that while complementary medicines are assessed for the safety and quality of their ingredients under Australian law, how well they work is not always measured.

COMPLEMENTARY THERAPIES

In addition to complementary medicines, there are several complementary therapies practised in Australia. State governments are responsible for regulating complementary therapists and practitioners, meaning that the laws that encompass them differ from state to state. This means that the complementary therapy industry is largely self-regulated. However, many therapists are associated with a professional association, requiring that they maintain standards of care. Membership is often voluntary, which means there is no legal obligation to affiliate with an association.

The exceptions to self-regulation are those practising Aboriginal and Torres Strait Islander remedies, Chinese medicine, chiropractic and osteopathy, which are formally managed under the National Registration and Accreditation Scheme implemented by the Australian Health Practitioner Regulation Agency (AHPRA). AHPRA supports the National Health Practitioner boards, which are responsible for setting the standards and policies that all registered health practitioners must meet.

Complementary therapies supplement conventional medical treatment, while alternative therapies are those that offer alternatives to conventional diagnosis and treatment. When used in combination with conventional medicine, these forms of treatments are known as integrative medicine. Such therapies include acupuncture, aromatherapy, Ayurvedic medicine, Chinese medicine, chiropractic, herbal medicine, homoeopathy, hypnotherapy, iridology, kinesiology, massage, meditation, naturopathy, nutritional medicine, osteopathy, reflexology, shiatsu, spiritual healing and yoga.

GLOSSARY OF TERMS

Therapy	Meaning
acupuncture	Acupuncture involves inserting small needles into various points in the body ('acupoints') to stimulate nerve impulses. Acupoints are locations in the body where nerves, muscles and connective tissue are stimulated. This increases blood flow to the area and triggers the action of the body's natural painkillers. Traditionally a Chinese form of medicine, and commonly practised in China, Japan, Korea and other Eastern countries, acupuncture has as its foundation the belief in 'qi' or vital energy, which travels around the body along 'meridians' that the acupuncture points influence. Acupuncture also has a place in Western medicine, although how it works from a scientific perspective is not clear. It is suggested that it works by balancing vital energy or possibly by having a neurological effect. Herbs, electricity, magnets and lasers may also be used in combination with the needles. Acupuncture is principally used for pain relief.
aromatherapy	Aromatherapy uses aromatic essential oils to enhance wellbeing. A mix of specific essential oils, which are the extracts from fragrant plants, is designed to create a therapeutic response in an individual and to encourage feelings of psychological and physical wellbeing. Essential oils may be applied by local application, massage, inhalation or immersion in water.
Ayurvedic medicine	A form of therapy originating in India, the central belief behind Ayurvedic medicine is that illness is caused by an imbalance of the physical body and the three vital energies, or 'doshas', which are made up of combinations of five elements, namely earth, water, fire, air and ether. The practice aims at balancing these doshas to increase life energy. Ayurveda includes a range of treatments including yoga, massage, acupuncture and herbal medicine.
Chinese traditional medicine	The idea that underpins traditional Chinese medicine is that the body consists of a dynamic energy system. Therefore, the intention of Chinese traditional medicine is to maintain or restore harmony in the body and to balance the two types of energy (yin and yang) using acupuncture, herbal medicines, massage, Tai Chi and the practice of Qigong. Qigong involves aligning breath, physical activity and awareness for mental, spiritual and body health, as well as stimulating a person's potential.

Table continued

Therapy	Meaning
chiropractic	Chiropractic focuses on the association between the structure of the body (mainly the spine) and its function. Chiropractors manipulate (or adjust) the spine to address problems in nerves, bones and muscles. Although there are various pieces of equipment used by chiropractors, most of the manipulation is done manually.
Feldenkrais method	The Feldenkrais method of therapy, developed by Dr Moshe Feldenkrais, is designed to improve movement through lessons designed to train the body to move with minimum effort. The lessons focus on improved posture, breathing techniques, movement coordination and balance.
herbal medicine	Herbal remedies are medications made from plants and plant extracts. They are used to treat diseases and maintain good health.
homeopathy	Homeopathic medicine claims to treat diseases by promoting the body's own defence mechanisms and healing responses through ingestion of specially prepared, highly diluted preparations intended to encourage the body to heal itself. Homeopathy uses the 'law of similars', whereby homeopathy practitioners believe that substances that produce sickness in a healthy person can be used to treat similar symptoms in a sick person. The National Health and Medical Research Council (NHMRC) states that there are no health conditions for which there is reliable evidence that homeopathy is effective (see: https://www.nhmrc.gov.au/about-us/resources/homeopathy).
hypnotherapy	Hypnotherapy uses the process of suggestion while the patient is in a 'trance' or hypnotic state to alter unwanted behaviours. While the person is under hypnosis, the body and conscious mind are in a relaxed state and the subconscious mind is alert and open to suggestion. A suggestion that is within the patient's normal belief system is made by the therapist, aimed at changing the behaviour or reaction of the patient to a particular scenario or issue. It is commonly used for changing habits such as smoking or as treatment to relieve stress or anxiety.
iridology	Iridology is the process of examining the patterns, colours and other characteristics of the iris to determine information about a person's health. Iris charts are used to identify which parts of the body relate to different sections of the iris, providing a 'window' into the body systems.
kinesiology	Kinesiology is the study of movement by addressing muscular activity, anatomy and the physiology and mechanics of body part movement. Kinesiologists treat a variety of disorders including allergies, muscle complaints and nervous disorders through biofeedback to identify what is causing 'imbalances' in the body.
lymphatic drainage therapy	Lymphatic drainage therapy involves a therapist massaging lymph nodes and other points of the body to help lymph fluid move through the body. The belief is that the lymphatic drainage will lead to a healthier body because lymphatic blockages will be reduced.
massage	Massage involves soothing muscles and soft tissues to aid in relaxation. Different types of massage can help to treat various problems such as back pain, anxiety and hypertension. There are many forms of massage including aromatherapy massage, massage for babies, reflexology, shiatsu massage, remedial massage, sports massage, deep tissue massage and relaxation massage.
meditation	Meditation is a state of consciousness that involves eliminating all external distractions by focusing on a sound, a breath, a thought or symbol, leading to a state of relaxation. The technique can be used for spiritual growth, healing, improving concentration and stress management.
music therapy	Music therapy is a form of adjunct psychotherapy that aims to assist people to attain and maintain health and wellbeing through the tailored use of music. Music therapy addresses a variety of objectives such as socialisation, communication and relaxation through a range of techniques such as instrument playing, singing and improvisation.
naturopathy	Naturopathy is the name given to a variety of traditional healing methods aimed at producing holistic or whole-body health care. Such methods include nutrition, herbal medicine, homoeopathy and massage.

Table continued

Therapy	Meaning
nutritional medicine	Nutritional medicine is the study of food, its nutrients and how diet affects health and wellbeing. It uses the belief that nutrition has an important role in nearly every medical problem. Concentrating on existing nutritional imbalances and adopting a healthy diet are believed to provide relief of symptoms. Nutritional medicine uses foods and individual nutritional supplements for medicinal and therapeutic effects.
osteopathy	Osteopaths treat patients by manipulating the soft tissues and stretching and manoeuvring of bones and muscles to encourage mobility and maintain structural balance. The tenet of this form of medicine is that a healthy body relies on a structurally sound musculoskeletal system.
Pilates	The Pilates method of exercise is aimed at building flexibility, strength, endurance and coordination in the legs, abdomen, arms and back. Through using exercises and equipment designed to isolate and develop specific muscles, enhanced body awareness and movement and improvements in body alignment and breathing are achieved.
reflexology	Reflexology operates on the premise that a system of zones and reflex areas of the body are reflected in the feet and hands. The basis of this form of therapy is that through applying pressure to a specific part of the feet or hands, circulation is improved, tension is released and overall functioning is improved.
reiki	Reiki is a technique developed in Japan, aimed at reducing stress and promoting relaxation and healing, administered by the 'laying of hand'. It is based on the tenet that there is a 'life force energy' flowing through us and if this energy is high then there is a greater likelihood of being happy and well.
shiatsu	Shiatsu is a Japanese healing technique involving the principles of anatomy, physiology and pathology. The name comes from the Japanese word for 'finger pressure', although the technique involves applying pressure to various parts of the body through the thumbs, palms, elbows, knees and feet. A shiatsu therapist aims to balance the body's energy system by promoting the flow of 'chi' (or energy) through the body's pathways or meridians and the internal organs. Imbalance, caused by too little or too much chi, can cause various problems, depending on which meridians are affected. The assumption is that the body can heal itself, with the therapist supporting naturally occurring processes.
spiritual healing	Spiritual healing is a general term used for healing encouraged through the use of energy, prana, chi or light. The premise of this form of treatment is that emotional, mental and physical healing occurs without the need for any medicines or remedies. An example of spiritual healing is chakra balancing. The chakra or energy may become stressed or blocked, causing a negative effect on the organs in that region of the body and contributing to negative emotional states such as depression and anxiety. The practitioner works to channel energy and light through the chakras until they are clear.
yoga	Yoga is a physical, mental and spiritual discipline that focuses on consciousness, breathing mechanisms, posture and body musculature aimed at physical and mental wellbeing.

CHAPTER 24

Public Health, Epidemiology and Research Terms

Contents

OBJECTIVES   537

INTRODUCTION   538

GLOSSARY OF TERMS   538

Objectives

The objective of this chapter is to provide a glossary of terms related to public health, epidemiology and research. It is not expected that you will remember all these terms. This glossary is provided as a reference tool to use if required.

INTRODUCTION

Public health is the organised response by society to protecting and promoting health, and to preventing illness, injury and disability. It involves structuring efforts and informing choices made by communities and individuals about their health. Public health incorporates the interdisciplinary approaches of epidemiology and research and informs actions undertaken by health services. Epidemiology is the study of the distribution and causes of disease and illness at the population level and the application of this study to help control health problems. Public health research includes population health surveillance, monitoring health information, measurement of burden of disease, population-based surveys, biostatistics, spatial analysis, evaluation of health interventions/outcomes and mapping of infrastructure, health facilities and boundaries.

GLOSSARY OF TERMS

Term	Definition
advocacy	Advocacy is the process used by a group or individuals to influence public policy and resource allocation within political, economic and social systems.
bias	Bias in the statistical perspective relates to sampling or testing error caused by systematically favouring some outcomes over others.
blinding	Blinding is a process used in clinical trials to prevent bias. One or more of the people involved in the trial are not told if an individual participant is part of the control group or the case or treatment group. In a **single-blind trial**, the participant does not know their status, and in a **double-blind trial** neither the subject nor the researchers know.
body mass index (BMI)	BMI is a proxy measure used to calculate the total amount of body fat. It is calculated by mass (kilograms)/height (metres^2).
bulk-billing	Bulk-billing is when a health professional accepts the Medicare Benefits Schedule benefit as full payment for a service. See Medicare Benefits Schedule below.
burden of disease	The burden of disease is a measurement designed to summarise the effect of various diseases and injuries on the population under study. It is a mechanism to assess the degree of loss of good health and early death due to various diseases and injuries. To estimate the burden of disease, two common measures are used: • the number of years of life a person loses as a consequence of dying early due to a disease • the number of years of life a person lives with a disability that has been caused by a disease. When added together, these two measures allow the calculation of disability-adjusted life-years (DALYs), which are further described below.
case control study	A case control study design is used in epidemiology to compare subjects who have a disease or condition (cases) with people who are similar in characteristics but who do not have the disease or condition (controls). Factors that are more common among the cases may be considered as possible risk factors for the disease being investigated.
climate change	Climate change refers to lasting and significant change in the statistical distribution of weather patterns over a specified time period.
clinical trial	A clinical trial is a type of scientific research study performed to evaluate the effectiveness and safety of drugs, medical devices and procedures by monitoring their effects on human subjects. A **phase I trial** determines the safety of the drug, device or procedure, how it works and how well it is tolerated by testing it on a small number of healthy volunteers. A **phase II trial** determines the safety and efficacy of the drug, device or procedure by testing it on a small number of patients who have the disease being studied. A **phase III trial** determines whether the drug, device or procedure shows clinical benefit in treating the disease(s) for which safety and efficacy was demonstrated in phase II clinical trials. These trials also determine the nature and likelihood of any side effects by testing on a large number of patients who have the disease being studied. A **phase IV trial** is performed after the drug, device or procedure has been approved to treat a particular disease. The phase IV trials compare the new treatment to a wider range of existing therapies to determine where it is best used and also to investigate the drug, device or procedure in the normal clinical setting of the disease.

Table continued

Term	Definition
clinical trial (research) coordinator	A clinical trial coordinator is the person responsible for the administration and operational activities of a clinical trial. The coordinator acts as the liaison between subjects, researchers and trial sponsors/funders.
cluster	A cluster is a group of cases of a particular disease (e.g. cases of a specific type of cancer) in a specific time and place that may or may not be greater than normal. Investigations of disease clusters are used to confirm cases, determine whether they represent an unusual disease occurrence and identify possible causes or contributing environmental factors.
cohort	A cohort is a group of subjects sharing a common characteristic such as ethnicity or age that is followed prospectively in an epidemiological study, with data being collected from the group at set times.
confounding variable	A confounding variable is an extra factor, the presence of which affects the variables being studied so that the results obtained may not reflect the actual relationship between the variables under investigation.
control group	A control group of subjects in a clinical trial receives a placebo and not the treatment being investigated. The group is used to compare with a group of cases that have similar characteristics to help determine any random effects not associated with the treatment.
crossover study	A crossover study is a type of clinical trial in which the subjects receive both the placebo and the treatment in a random order. With this type of study, every participant serves as their own control.
cross-sectional study	A cross-sectional study is a descriptive study that measures the prevalence of health outcomes or determinants of health, or both, in a population at a specific point in time. Cross-sectional studies can be thought of as providing a 'snapshot' of the frequency and characteristics of a disease in a population at a point in time.
database	A database is a collection of data, stored electronically, that is organised so it can easily be accessed, managed and updated. Specific pieces of data can be quickly located and used.
Declaration of Alma-Ata	The Alma-Ata Declaration of 1978 was a major milestone in the field of public health, identifying primary health care as the key to attaining the goal of Health for All. The declaration stated that health is a state of complete physical, mental and social wellbeing, and not merely the absence of disease or infirmity, and should be considered a fundamental human right. The attainment of the highest possible level of health is a fundamental international goal that requires the action of many other social and economic sectors in addition to the health sector.
Declaration of Helsinki	The Declaration of Helsinki was a statement of ethical principles developed by the World Medical Association in 1964 as a guide to clinicians and other researchers involved in research with human subjects, human material or identifiable data.
demographic data	Demographic data is statistical data that describes a population. Common types of demographic data are gender, age, ethnicity, employment status and location.
determinants of health	The determinants of health are the social, economic, physical, environmental and personal factors that influence the health status of individuals or populations.
disability-adjusted life-years (DALYs)	DALYs are health measures that calculate the sum of years of productive life lost due to disability. One DALY is generally considered one year of 'healthy' life lost. By summing DALYs across a population, the burden of disease can be calculated.
ecology	Ecology is the study of the relationship organisms have with their environment.
effect size	An effect size is a descriptive measure of the strength of a relationship between two statistical variables. The estimated magnitude of a relationship measures the relationship without a statement about whether the apparent relationship in the data reflects a true relationship in the population.
eligibility	Eligibility refers to a set of criteria that subjects must comply with before they are able to participate in a research study or clinical trial.
endemic	An endemic disease is one that is confined to a specific geographic location.
environmental determinants of health	Environmental factors, such as physical, chemical and microbiological factors, are those that impact on the health of an individual or population but over which the individual or population has no control.

Table continued

Term	Definition
environmental health	The health of the environment can influence the physical and mental health of humans. Environmental health refers to the study of aspects of health that are determined by physical, chemical and microbiological agents in the environment. Some of the known issues relating to the environment that have a bearing on human health include the impact of pollution and air quality, chemical safety, noise pollution, water and sanitation. Climate change is also beginning to cause health effects due to increasing temperatures, more common extreme weather events, changes in the geographic spread of vectors carrying some infectious diseases and changes to ecosystems affecting natural resources.
epidemic	An epidemic is the widespread occurrence of a disease in a defined location or among members of a population.
epidemiology	Epidemiology is the study of diseases in a population, including describing disease patterns and identifying the causes of diseases.
ethics	Ethics involves consideration of moral issues through personal reflection. Ethics is concerned with what is good for individuals and society as a whole.
evaluation	Evaluation is a process of determining the worth of something, generally against a set of criteria or standards.
evidence-based medicine (EBM)	EBM involves using the best available evidence to inform clinical decision making in the context of a particular patient.
evidence-based practice (EBP)	EBP involves using evidence (research, data, information) to inform decision making to adopt best practice processes.
exclusion criteria	Exclusion criteria are criteria that, if met, will eliminate a potential subject from participating in a research study or clinical trial.
experimental study	An experimental study is a type of research design that uses manipulation and controlled testing to understand causal processes. The researcher manipulates one or more variables and controls and measures any change in other variables.
genetic modification	Genetic modification involves direct human manipulation using biotechnology to alter the genetic make-up of an organism such as a plant or animal.
genetics	Genetics is the study of genes, heredity and how characteristics are passed from parent to child.
genome	A genome represents the entire genetic information of an individual – the complete DNA sequence.
healthcare claim	A healthcare claim is a request for payment that a patient or healthcare provider submits to an insurer for reimbursement for items or services for which the patient has private health cover or insurance.
health education	Health education is any combination of learning experiences designed to help individuals and communities improve their health by increasing their knowledge or influencing their attitudes.
health promotion	Health promotion is the process of enabling people to understand and increase control over, and therefore to improve, their health.
human wellbeing	Human wellbeing is a state of complete physical, mental and social health.
hypothesis	A hypothesis is a tentative explanation for an observation, phenomenon or scientific problem that can be tested by further investigation. It is a specific, testable prediction about what is expected to happen in a research study.
incidence	Incidence is defined as the number of new cases of a disease occurring during a specified time period. It is one of the measures of the health status of a population. An incidence rate is the number of new cases of the disease occurring in a specific time period divided by the size of the population at risk of becoming a case during that period.
informed consent	Informed consent is a legal requirement to ensure a subject knows and understands all the risks involved in a specific treatment or study. The elements of informed consent include informing the patient of the nature of the treatment, possible alternative treatments and the potential risks and benefits of the treatment and of refusing treatment. For informed consent to be considered valid, the patient must be mentally competent to give consent and the consent must be given voluntarily.

Table continued

Term	Definition
intersectoral partnering	Intersectoral partnering refers to collaboration between two or more sectors of society (business, government, civil society) to undertake intergovernmental/agency initiatives on an issue. This process allows for a more sustainable approach to development activities.
local hospital networks (LHNs)	LHNs have been established by the Australian Government. They are groups of hospitals or one individual hospital located in a specific geographical area or region. LHNs aim to ensure the hospital services that are required in the jurisdiction are provided.
longitudinal study	A longitudinal study is a research study that involves repeated observations and measurements of the same subjects over a period of time – often many decades.
Medicare	Medicare is Australia's national public health insurance scheme that provides free or subsidised health care for all Australians. It makes public hospital care freely available and allows for benefits to be paid for health care services and medicines prescribed through the Medicare Benefits and Pharmaceutical Benefits schemes. Australians contribute to Medicare through their income tax.
Medicare Benefits Schedule (MBS)	The benefit a patient receives from Medicare is based on a schedule of fees for medical services, known as the MBS. This schedule of fees is set by the Australian Government and covers the standard fee for a range of consultations, procedures and tests. The schedule fee is the amount the government considers appropriate for one of these services. Australians registered for Medicare can claim 100% of this fee as a rebate for general practice services and 85% for non-GP services from Medicare when the services are not provided in a hospital. For services provided in a private hospital, Medicare will rebate 75% of the schedule fee. However, a provider of a health service also may charge a patient a cost above the schedule fee, meaning the patient must pay the 'gap' between the government's reimbursement and the fee charged.
meta-analysis	A meta-analysis is a process of combining relevant research studies using appropriate statistical methods to allow for a precise estimate of treatment effect.
metadata	Metadata is data about data and supports understanding and accurate interpretation of data by providing extra detail about it (such as the origin of the data, how the data is collected and descriptions of the data elements). This helps turn the data into meaningful information. Metadata can be descriptive, structural, administrative, reference and statistical.
morbidity	Morbidity refers to a state of illness in an individual or rate of illness in a population.
mortality	Mortality refers to death in an individual or rate of death in a population.
Nuremberg code	The Nuremberg code is a code of ethics, principles and standards for human medical research outlined by the Nuremberg War Crimes Tribunal in 1947 following disclosure of the infamous Nazi experiments conducted during World War II.
Organisation for Economic Co-operation and Development (OECD)	The OECD is an intergovernmental organisation comprising 34 nations that are tasked with promoting policies aimed at improving the economic and social wellbeing of member and non-member states.
Ottawa Charter	The Ottawa Charter is the name of an international agreement signed at the First International Conference on Health Promotion, organised by the World Health Organization (WHO) and held in Ottawa, Canada, in 1986. It launched a series of actions among international organisations, national governments and local communities to achieve the goal of 'Health for All' by the year 2000 and beyond. The charter identifies the prerequisites for health, methods to achieve health promotion through advocacy, enabling and mediation, as well as five key action areas: • Building healthy public policy. • Creating supportive environments. • Strengthening community action. • Developing personal skills. • Re-orientating healthcare services towards prevention of illness and promotion of health.
outbreak	An outbreak is the sudden increase in the incidence of a disease in greater numbers than expected. In certain populations, one new case may be considered an outbreak if the disease has not previously been present in the population or has been absent for a long time.

Table continued

Term	Definition
outcome	The outcome is the result or consequence of a program or plan in terms of success or failure.
pandemic	A pandemic is a global outbreak of a specific disease.
parallel study design	A parallel study design is used where subjects are randomly assigned to one of two treatment groups. One group receives only treatment 'A' for the entire study, while the other group receives only treatment 'B'.
participant (subject)	A participant or subject is a human volunteer who agrees to be a part of a research study or clinical trial.
Pharmaceutical Benefits Scheme (PBS)	The PBS is part of the Australian Government's National Medicines Policy, aimed at providing timely, reliable and affordable access to necessary medicines for all Australians. It facilitates optimal health outcomes within an appropriate economic framework. Under the PBS, the government subsidises the cost of medicines for most medical conditions.
pilot study	A pilot study is a small study designed to conduct a preliminary analysis and gather information prior to a larger study in order to improve the latter's quality and efficiency. A pilot study can reveal problems with the design of the proposed study. These can then be addressed before time and resources are expended on a large-scale study.
plan	A plan is a statement of a set of activities that will be undertaken to achieve a specified outcome.
policy	A policy is a principle or rule to guide decision making and help meet outcomes.
population health	Population health is the study of health and disease in the community through addressing differences and improving health by means of priority health approaches.
prevalence	Prevalence refers to the total number of cases of a disease in a population at a specified point in time. It is affected by both the incidence and the duration of the disease in the population.
primary (1°) health care	A primary healthcare clinician is generally the first point of contact in the health system. A primary healthcare clinician may be a doctor (usually a general practitioner), a dentist, nurse, allied health professional or a pharmacist. Primary healthcare settings include general practice, community or allied health centres, outpatient or emergency services in a health facility or Aboriginal Community Controlled Health Services. Primary healthcare services also provide health promotion and disease prevention activities and health education. Depending on the patient's condition, they may be referred on to secondary or tertiary care for further assistance.
Primary Health Networks (PHNs)	PHNs aim to increase the efficiency and effectiveness of medical services for patients and to improve coordination of care by facilitating integrated care services. PHNs operate directly with general practitioners and other primary healthcare providers, secondary care providers and hospitals to facilitate improved outcomes for patients. The priorities for PHNs are mental health, Aboriginal and Torres Strait Islander health, population health, health workforce, eHealth and aged care. PHNs have been operational in Australia since mid-2015.
principal investigator	The principal investigator is the person responsible for the management, conduct and integrity of a research study or clinical trial.
probability	Probability refers to patterns that occur in random events. It is used to determine statistically how likely it is that a particular event will occur where the result cannot be predicted in advance. For example, probability may refer to the likelihood that 'heads' will be displayed a certain number of times when a coin is flipped 10 times.
program	A program is a bringing together of people, equipment and funding to carry out a set of activities to meet health objectives.
prospective study	A prospective study is a study in which the subjects are identified and then followed forward in time. They are exposed to longitudinal observation over time, with results being collected at regular intervals.
protocol	A protocol is a detailed written outline of a research study that ensures the study is properly conducted for the right purposes. A research protocol should include the aims/objectives, hypotheses, calculation of sample size, criteria for eligibility, methodology, study schedule and costings.

Table continued

Term	Definition
public health	Public health refers to the organised response by society to protect and promote health and to prevent illness, injury and disability.
quality-adjusted life-years (QALYs)	QALYs are an approach for estimating quality of life used in economic evaluations to determine the extent of benefits gained from different interventions in terms of health-related quality of life and survival. One QALY is equal to 1 year of life in perfect health. The calculation of a QALY is undertaken by estimating the years of life remaining for a patient following a particular treatment or intervention and weighting each year with a quality of life score that ranges on a scale from zero (death) to 1 (perfect health), with some states considered worse than death having a negative score. A QALY often measures a person's ability to perform the activities of daily life, free from pain and mental disturbance.
random sample	A random sample is a sample from a population in which every person in the population has an equal chance of being selected for the study.
randomisation	Randomisation is the process of using an element of chance to allocate subjects to receive one or other of the alternative treatments being investigated in a research study or clinical trial.
randomised controlled trial	A randomised controlled trial is a study design in which investigators examine two or more clinical interventions in a cohort of subjects who are allocated at random (using chance alone) to receive one of the interventions.
rate	A rate refers to the mathematical relationship between the numerator (number of deaths, cases of disease, disabilities, services, etc.) and denominator (population at risk), based on a specific time period. Rates allow comparisons between populations and different time periods.
registry	A registry is a facility that collects, analyses and reports data on various diseases and health problems (e.g. a cancer registry). It is a system of ongoing registration of all cases of a disease or health condition in a defined population and is a mechanism for surveillance of disease. Registries are population-based, hospital-based or special purpose.
research	Research refers to scientific enquiry or investigation designed to develop or contribute to a body of knowledge.
retrospective study	A retrospective study uses historical information – usually from medical records, surveys and interviews with patients – to learn what factors may be associated with the disease under investigation. The study generally compares two groups of people: those with the disease (cases) and a very similar group of people who do not have the disease (controls).
risk–benefit ratio	A risk benefit ratio was outlined in Principle 16 of the Declaration of Helsinki and highlights the need for careful assessment of predictable risks and burdens when compared with the foreseeable benefits on the human subjects and others.
risk factor	Risk factors are personal behaviours, lifestyle characteristics or environmental exposures (e.g. cigarette smoking, excessive alcohol consumption) that are known to be associated with negative health outcomes. The presence of a risk factor gives an increased probability that the negative health outcome will occur, but it is not necessarily a causal factor.
risk management	Risk management is the process of identifying potential risks, assessing the likelihood and impact of the risks and determining alternative actions or mitigation strategies.
sample size	A sample size is the number of subjects chosen from a population to be part of a research study or clinical trial. The actual number is expressed as $n =$.
secondary (2°) health care	Contact with patients that is not provided in a primary care setting (e.g. general practice, community care, outpatient or emergency services) is generally termed secondary health care. Secondary care includes 'acute care' such as the services generally provided in a healthcare facility (e.g. a hospital) or by a specialist clinician (e.g. a psychiatrist or physiotherapist) but not necessarily in a hospital. In Australia, a referral from a primary care clinician is required to access secondary care services.
social capital	Social capital refers to the resources that are created as a result of networks, relationships and reciprocity.
social cohesion	Social cohesion describes the connections and relationships between individuals, groups and societal units. It is the glue that holds communities together.

Table continued

Term	Definition
sponsor	A sponsor is the individual, organisation, company or agency that initiates and takes responsibility for a research study or clinical trial but who does not actually conduct the investigation. The sponsor may also provide funding for the study.
strategies	Strategies are the methods applied to move from a current state to a desired state to achieve a desired outcome.
surveillance	Surveillance refers to the ongoing systematic collection, recording, analysis, interpretation and timely dissemination of health-related information that reflects the health status of a community or population, identifies any problems that require action, and is used to control disease. Epidemiological surveillance is essential for planning, implementing and evaluating public health programs.
sustainable development	Sustainable development is defined as development that meets the needs of the present without compromising the ability of future generations to meet their own needs.
Sustainable Development Goals (SDGs)	The SDGs are a set of 17 universal goals, targets and indicators that United Nations member states are using to frame development agendas over the period 2015–2030. They build on the eight Millennium Development Goals that the United Nations developed in 2000. The SDGs are to (as quoted from the UN website): 1. End poverty in all its forms everywhere. 2. End hunger, achieve food security and improved nutrition, and promote sustainable agriculture. 3. Ensure healthy lives and promote well-being for all at all ages. 4. Ensure inclusive and equitable quality education and promote lifelong learning opportunities for all. 5. Achieve gender equality and empower all women and girls. 6. Ensure availability and sustainable management of water and sanitation for all. 7. Ensure access to affordable, reliable, sustainable and modern energy for all. 8. Promote sustained, inclusive and sustainable economic growth, full and productive employment, and decent work for all. 9. Build resilient infrastructure, promote inclusive and sustainable industrialization, and foster innovation. 10. Reduce inequality within and among countries. 11. Make cities and human settlements inclusive, safe, resilient and sustainable. 12. Ensure sustainable consumption and production patterns. 13. Take urgent action to combat climate change and its impacts. 14. Conserve and sustainably use the oceans, seas and marine resources for sustainable development. 15. Protect, restore and promote sustainable use of terrestrial ecosystems, sustainably manage forests, combat desertification and halt and reverse land degradation, and halt biodiversity loss. 16. Promote peaceful and inclusive societies for sustainable development, provide access to justice for all and build effective, accountable and inclusive institutions at all levels. 17. Strengthen the means of implementation and revitalize the global partnership for sustainable development. Reference: https://www.un.org/sustainabledevelopment/
target group	The target group is the group of people the message from a program aims to reach or influence.
tertiary (3°) care	Tertiary care is highly specialised health care, normally provided to inpatients in a hospital setting following referral from a primary or secondary health clinician. Tertiary health care generally includes very complex medical or surgical procedures.

Table continued

Term	Definition
Universal Health Coverage (UHC)	UHC refers to the international program of work aimed at ensuring all people and communities have access to appropriate and effective health services at a cost that is affordable. There are three aims of UHC: equity in access to health care for all persons; quality of care that improves health; and protection against financial vulnerability as a result of needing health care. UHC supports the World Health Organization mandate that specifies health as a fundamental human right and relates to the Alma Ata Declaration of Health for All. UHC also supports all the health-related Sustainable Development Goals.
variable	A variable is a quantity, attribute, phenomenon or event that may take on a set of values. In a research study, it is the data item for which values need to be obtained. Variables are generally referred to as dependent or independent. The independent variable is generally the variable that signifies the value being manipulated, controlled or changed, and the dependent variable is the observed response to the independent variable being manipulated. In other words, the value of the dependent variable depends on that of the independent variable. In statistical terms, the independent variable is generally characterised as x and the dependent variable as y.
years of potential life lost (YPLL)	YPLL is a measure of the years of life lost due to a particular cause of death as a proportion of the total YPLLs lost due to premature mortality in the population.

Word element glossary

a- no, not, without, absence of

ab- away from

abdomin/o abdomen

-able capable of, having ability to

abort/o premature expulsion of fetus

abrupt/o broken away from

-ac pertaining to

acanth/o thorny, spiny

acet/o vinegar

acetabul/o acetabulum

achill/o Achilles tendon

acid/o acid

acous/o hearing

-acousia hearing (condition of)

acro- extremities

acromi/o shoulder

-acusis hearing

ad- towards

aden/o gland

adenoid/o adenoids

adhesi/o adhesion

adip/o fat

adnex/o bound to, conjoined

adren/o adrenal glands

adrenal/o adrenal glands

-aemia blood (condition of)

aer/o air, gas

aesthes/o feeling, sensation

aesthesi/o feeling, sensation

-aesthesia feeling, sensation (condition of)

aeti/o cause

af- to, towards, near

ag- to, towards, near

agglutin/o clumping, gluing, sticking together

-ago abnormal condition, disease

-agon assemble, gather together

agora- marketplace, open space

-aise comfort, ease

-al pertaining to, drug action

alb/o white

albin/o white

albumin/o albumin

algesi/o pain

-algesia pain (condition of)

-algia pain (condition of)

aliment/o food or nutritive material

all/o other, different

alopec/o baldness

alveol/o alveolus, air sac

ambi- both sides

ambly/o dull, dim

ambulat/o to walk

-amine nitrogen compound

amni/o amnion, amniotic fluid

amnion/o amnion, fetal membrane

-amnios amnion, amniotic fluid

amyl/o starch

-an pertaining to, characteristic of

an- *(used when combining form starts with a vowel)* no, not, without, absence of

an/o anus

ana- up, towards, apart

andr/o male

aneurysm/o aneurysm

angi/o vessel

angin/o choking

aniso- unequal, asymmetrical, dissimilar

ankyl/o crooked, bent, stiff

-ant characteristic of

ante- before, forward

anter/o front

anthrac/o black, coal

anthrop/o man, human

anti- against

antr/o antrum, maxillary sinus

anxi/o uneasy, distressed

aort/o aorta

ap- to, towards, near

ap/o away from, detached, derived from

-apheresis remove, carry away

aphth/o ulcer

apic/o apex

aponeur/o aponeurosis

appendic/o appendix

aqu/i water

aqu/o water

aqua- water

aque/o water

-ar pertaining to

arachn/o spider

arc/o bow, arc

-arche beginning, first

areol/o small open space

arter/o artery

arteri/o artery

arteriol/o arteriole

arthr/o joint

articul/o joint

-ary pertaining to, connected with

-ase enzyme

-asia state of, condition

-asis state of, condition

-asthenia weakness (condition of)

astr/o star

-ate use, subject to

atel/o imperfect, incomplete

ather/o fatty plaque

-ation process, action, condition

-atresia closure, occlusion, absence of opening

atri/o atrium

audi/o hearing

audit/o hearing

aur/i ear

aur/o ear

-aural ear (pertaining to)

auricul/o ear

auscult/o listen

auto- self

ax/o axis, main stem

axill/o armpit

azot/o nitrogen, urea

bacill/o bacillus, rod-shaped bacterium

bacteri/o bacteria

balan/o glans penis

bar/o weight, pressure

bartholin/o Bartholin's gland

bas/o base, basis

batho- deep

bathy- deep

bi- two, twice, double

bi/o life

bifid/o split, cleft into two parts

bil/i gall, bile

bilirubin/o bile pigment

bin- two, twice, double

bis- two, twice, double

-blast embryonic or developing cell

blast/o embryonic, developing cell

-blastoma immature tumour

blephar/o eyelid

bol/o ball

borborygm/o rumbling sound

brachi/o arm

brachy- short

brady- slow

brevi- short

bromidr/o stench, smell of sweat

bronch/i bronchus

bronch/o bronchus

bronchiol/o bronchiole

bront/o thunder

brux/o grind

bucc/o cheek

burs/o bursa

cac/o ill, unpleasant, bad, abnormal

caec/o caecum

calc/i calcium

calc/o calcium

calcane/o calcaneus

calcin/o calcium

calcul/o stone

cali/o cup, calyx

calic/o cup, calyx

calor/i heat

cancer/o cancer

canth/o canthus, corner of eye

capill/o capillary

capit/o head

capn/o carbon dioxide

-capnia carbon dioxide (condition of)

capsul/o capsule

carb/o carbon dioxide

carb/o carbon

carcin/o cancerous, malignant

cardi/o heart

-cardia heart (condition of)

cari/o decay, rot

carp/o carpal

cata- down, lower

cathart/o cleansing, purging

caud/o tail, downward

caus/o burn, burning

caust/o burn, burning

cauter/o heat, burn

-cele hernia, protrusion

cellul/o cell

-centesis surgical puncture to remove fluid

centi- hundred

centr/i centre

centr/o centre

cephal/o head

cer/o wax

cerebell/o cerebellum

cerebr/o cerebrum, brain

cerumin/o wax

cervic/o neck, cervix uteri

-chalasis slackening, loosening

cheil/o lip

cheir/o hand

chem/o drug, chemical

chemic/o drug, chemical

-chezia defecation, elimination of waste products

chir/o hand

chlor/o green

chol/e gall, bile

cholangi/o bile duct

cholecyst/o gallbladder

choledoch/o common bile duct

cholesterol/o cholesterol

chondr/o cartilage

chore/o dance, jerky movement

chori/o chorion

chorion/o chorion

choroid/o choroid

chrom/o colour

chromat/o colour

chron/o time

chym/o to pour

cib/o meal

-cide killing, agent that kills

cili/o hair-like projections

cine- movement

cinemat/o movement

circum- around, about

cirrh/o orange, yellow

cis/o to cut

-cision cutting

-clasis break

-clast break

claustr/o barrier, enclosed

clavic/o clavicle

clavicul/o clavicle

cleid/o clavicle

clon/o turmoil

-clysis irrigating, washing

co- with, together

coagul/o clotting

cocc/i coccus, berry-shaped bacterium

cocc/o coccus, berry-shaped bacterium

-coccus berry-shaped bacterium

coccyg/o coccyx

cochle/o cochlea

coel- coel/o cavity

coeli/o abdomen

coit/o coming together

col/o colon, large intestine

colon/o colon, large intestine

colp/o vagina

column/o pillar

com- with, together

comat/o coma

con- together, with

condyl/o condyle

coni/o dust

conjunctiv/o conjunctiva

-constriction narrowing

contra- against

copr/o faeces, obscenity

cor/o pupil of the eye

core/o pupil of the eye

-coria pupils (condition of)

corne/o cornea

coron/o heart

cortic/o cortex, outer layer of organ

cost/o ribs

cox/o hip, hip joint

crani/o cranium, skull

crepit/o crackling

crepitat/o crackling

crin/o secrete

-crine secrete

-crit separate

cry/o cold

crypto- hidden

cubit/o elbow

culd/o cul-de-sac

-cule small

cune/i wedge-shaped

-cusis hearing

cut/i skin

cutane/o skin

cyan/o blue

cycl/o ciliary body of the eye, circular, recurring

cyes/i pregnancy

cyes/o pregnancy

-cyesis pregnancy

cyst/o bladder, cyst, sac

cyt/o cell

-cyte cell

-cytosis abnormal condition of cells

dacry/o tears, tear duct, lacrimal sac

dacryocyst/o lacrimal sac

dactyl/o finger, toe

de- removal of, away from, loss of, lack of, less

deci- ten

dehisc/o burst open, split

dem/o people

demi- half

dendr/o tree, branches

dent/i teeth

dent/o teeth

dentin/o dentine of tooth

derm/o skin

-derma skin

dermat/o skin

-desis to bind, surgical fixation, fusion

dextro- right side

di- double, twice

dia- through, across

-dialysis separate

diaphor/o profuse sweating

diaphragmat/o diaphragm

digit/o finger, toe

-dilation widening, stretching

dipl/o double

dips/o thirst

dis- reversal, separation, duplication

disc/o intervertebral disc

dist/o away, far, distant

diverticul/o diverticulum, blind pouch

doch/o duct

dors/o back (of body)

dorsi- back

duct/o to lead, tube to carry

duoden/o duodenum

dupl/i double

dur/o dura mater

dynam/o force, power of movement

-dynia pain (condition of)

dys- bad, painful, difficult

-eal pertaining to

ec- out, outside

echo- reflected, repeated sound

ect- out, outside, outer part

-ectasia expansion, dilatation, stretching out

-ectasis expansion, dilatation, stretching out

ecto- out, outside

-ectomy excision, surgical removal

ectop/o displaced

ectro- congenital absence, miscarriage

electr/o electricity, electrical activity

electro- electricity, electrical activity

ellipt/o ellipse-shaped

em- *(used when combining form starts with a b, m or p)* in

-ema condition

embol/o embolism, plug

embry/o embryo, fetus

-emesis vomiting

emet/o vomiting

emmetr/o normally proportioned

en- in

encephal/o brain

endo- within, inside, inner

endometri/o endometrium

-ent person, agent

enter/o intestine (usually small)

eosin/o red, dawn, rosy

epi- above, upon, on

epididym/o epididymis

epiglott/o epiglottis

episi/o vulva

epitheli/o epithelium

equi- equal, equality

equin/o horse

-er one who

erg/o work

erot/o sexual love

eruct/o belch forth

erythem/o red

erythemat/o red

erythr/o red

-esis abnormal state, condition

eso- inward, within

eu- good, normal

eury- broad, wide

ex- outward, outside

exo- outward, outside

-externa external

extra- outside

exud/o to sweat out

faci/o face

faec/o faeces

fasci/o fascia (a band)

febr/o fever

femor/o femur

fer/o carry, bear

-ferent carrying

-ferous bearing, carrying, producing

ferr/o iron

fet/o fetus

fibr/o fibre

fibrill/o muscular twitching

fibrin/o fibrinogen

fibros/o fibrous connective tissue

fibul/o fibula

fil/o thread

fimbri/o fringe

fiss/o crack

fissur/o crack

fistul/o tube, pipe

-flect bend

flex/o bend

fluor/o fluorescent, luminous

foc/o focus

follicul/o small sac, follicle

foramin/o opening

fore- before, in front of

-form having the form of

foss/o depression

front/o front, forehead

fund/o base or bottom of an organ

fung/i fungus, mushroom

fung/o fungus, mushroom

furc/o branching

galact/o milk

gangli/o ganglion, knot

gastr/o stomach

-gen producing, originating, causing

gen/o producing, originating, causing

-genesis pertaining to formation, producing

geni/o chin

-genic pertaining to formation, producing

genicul/o knee

genit/o genitals, reproductive organs

-genous arising from, produced by, producing

ger/i old age, aged

ger/o old age, aged

geront/o old age, aged

geus/o sense of taste

gingiv/o gums

glauc/o grey

gli/o glue

-globin protein

-globulin protein

glomerul/o glomerulus

gloss/o tongue

glott/o back of tongue

gluc/o glucose, sugar, sweet(ness)

glyc/o glucose, sugar, sweet(ness)

glycogen/o glycogen, animal starch, glucose

glycos/o glucose, sugar, sweet(ness)

gnath/o jaw

gnos/o knowledge

-gnosis knowledge, judgment

gon/o seed, semen, knee

gonad/o gonads, sex glands (ovaries and testes)

-grade to go

-graft transplant of tissue

-gram record, writing

granul/o granules

-graph instrument for recording

-graphy process of recording

-gravida pregnancy

gyn/o woman, female

gynaec/o woman, female

-gyric pertaining to circular motion

haem/o blood

haemangi/o blood vessel

haemat/o blood

haemoglobin/o haemoglobin

halit/o breath

hallucin/o hallucination, to wander in the mind

hel/i sun

helc/o ulcer

helminth/o worm

hemi- half

hepat/o liver

hepatic/o hepatic bile duct

herni/o hernia

hetero- different

-hexia habit

hiat/o opening

hidr/o sweat

hist/o tissue

histi/o tissue

hol/o entire, whole

home/o same, alike

homo- same, alike

hormon/o hormone

humer/o humerus

hyal/o glass-like

hydr/o water

hydra- water

hygr/o moisture

hymen/o hymen

hyper- above, excessive

hypn/o sleep

hypo- below, under, deficient, less than normal

hyster/o uterus

-ia process, condition of

-iac pertaining to

-ial pertaining to

-iasis condition or state

iatr/o physician, medicine, treatment

-iatrics medical specialty

-iatry treatment by doctor, medical specialty

-ible able to be, capable of being

-ic pertaining to, drug action

-ical pertaining to

ichthy/o scaly, dry

-ician person associated with, specialist

-ictal seizure (pertaining to)

-icterus jaundice

idi/o self, unique to individual or organ

-igo attack, abnormal condition

-ile capable of, able

ile/o ileum, small intestine

ili/o ilium, hip

im- in, none, not

immun/o protection

in- in, none, not

-in made of, having the nature of, relating to

incud/o incus

-ine made of, having the nature of, relating to

infer/o below

infra- inferior to, below

infundibul/o funnel

inguin/o groin

insulin/o insulin

inter- between

intra- within, inside

intro- into, within, inwards

introit/o entrance, passage

intus- in, into

iod/o iodine

-ion action (condition resulting from)

-ior pertaining to

iri/o iris

irid/o iris

is/o equal, same

isch/o deficiency, blockage, hold back

ischi/o ischium

-ism state of

-ismus process, state, condition

iso- equal, same

-ist one who specialises in

-itis inflammation

-ity state, condition

-ium structure, tissue

-ive pertaining to, drug action

jejun/o jejunum

jugul/o throat, neck

juxta- adjoining, near

kal/i potassium

kary/o nucleus

kel/o growth, tumour

kerat/o hard, horny tissue, cornea

keratin/o keratin

ket/o ketone bodies

keton/o ketone bodies

kinesi/o movement, motion

-kinesia movement (condition of), motion (condition of)

-kinesis motion, movement

kinet/o movement, motion

klept/o steal

kyph/o humpback

labi/o lip

labyrinth/o labyrinth, inner ear

lacrim/o tear

lact/i milk

lact/o milk

lactat/o to secrete milk

-lalia disorder of speech

lamin/o lamina

lapar/o abdomen

laryng/o larynx, voice box

later/o side

lei/o smooth

leiomy/o smooth muscle

-lemma confining membrane, sheath

-lepsy seizure

lept/o thin, fine, slender

-leptic type of seizure

leuc/o white

leuk/o white *(used in Australia for the word leukaemia and derivative terms only)*

lex/o word, phrase

ligament/o ligament

-ligation tying off

lingu/o tongue

lip/o fat

-listhesis slip or slide

-lith stone, calculus

-lithiasis stones (abnormal condition of)

lith/o stone, calculus

lob/o lobe

loc/o place

log/o study of

-logy study of

lord/o curve, swayback

-lucent shine

lumb/o loins, lower back

lun/o moon

lute/o yellow, corpus luteum

lymph/o lymphoid tissue, lymph gland

-lysis separation, destruction, breakdown, dissolution

-lytic pertaining to destruction, drug that breaks down

macro- large

macul/o spot, blotch

mal- bad

malac/o soft, softening

-malacia condition of softening

malign/o bad, harmful, cancerous

malle/o malleus, hammer

malleol/o malleolus, little hammer

mamm/o breast

mammill/o nipple

man/o pressure

mandibul/o mandible, lower jaw

-mania state of mental disorder, frenzy

mast/o breast

mastoid/o mastoid process

maxill/o maxilla, upper jaw

meat/o meatus

medi/o middle

-media middle

mediastin/o mediastinum

medull/o inner part, medulla

mega- abnormally large

megal/o enlargement

-megaly enlargement

melan/o black

mellit/o honey

men/o menses, menstruation

mening/o meninges

meningi/o meninges

menisc/o meniscus, crescent

ment/o mind

mes/o middle, intermediate

meta- change, beyond

metacarp/o metacarpal

metatars/o metatarsal

-meter instrument used to measure, measurement

metr/o uterus

metri/o uterus

-metry process of measuring

mi/o smaller, less

micro- small

mid- middle

mono- one, single

-morph form, shape

morph/o form, shape

mort/o death

muc/o mucus

multi- many, much

muscul/o muscle

mut/a genetic change

my/o muscle

myc/o fungus, mould

mydr/o widen, enlarge

mydri/o dilation, widening

myel/o bone marrow, spinal cord

myocardi/o myocardium

myos/o muscle

myring/o eardrum, tympanic membrane

myx/o mucus

narc/o stupor, sleep

nas/o nose

nat/i birth

nat/o birth

-natal birth (pertaining to)

natr/o sodium

necr/o death, dead

nect/o connect, bind, tie together

neo- new

nephr/o kidney

neur/o nerve

neutr/o neutral

noct/i night

nod/o knot, swelling

norm/o rule, order

nos/o disease

nuch/o neck region

nucle/o nucleus

nulli- none

nutri/o nourishment

nyct/o night, darkness

nyctal/o night, darkness

o/o egg, ovum

obstetr/o midwife

occipit/o occiput

occlus/o shut, close up

occult/o hidden

ocul/o eye

odont/o teeth

-oedema swelling due to fluid

oesophag/o oesophagus

oestr/o oestrogen, female hormone

-oid derived from, resembling

-ole little, small

olecran/o olecranon

olfactor/o sense of smell

olig/o scanty, deficiency, few

-oma tumour, collection, mass, swelling

omphal/o umbilicus

onc/o tumour

-one hormone

onych/o nail

oo/o egg, ova

oophor/o ovary

-opaque obscure

ophthalm/o eye

-opia vision (condition of)

-opsia vision (condition of)

-opsy to view, process of viewing

opt/i eye, vision

opt/o eye, vision

optic/o eye, vision

-or person, agent

or/o mouth

orbit/o orbit of eye

orch/o testis, testicle

orchi/o testis, testicle

orchid/o testis, testicle

-orexia appetite (condition of)

orth/o straight, upright

-ory pertaining to

os- bone, mouth, orifice

-ose pertaining to, full of, sugar

-osis abnormal condition

osm/o sense of smell

-osmia sense of smell (condition of)

osphresi/o odour

oss/i bone

osse/o bone

ossicul/o ossicles

oste/o bone

ot/o ear

-otia ear (condition of)

-ous composed of, pertaining to, relating to

ov/i egg, ovum

ov/o egg, ovum

ovar/i ovary

ovari/o ovary

ovul/o egg, ovum

ox/i oxygen

ox/o oxygen

oxia oxygen (condition of)

oxy- quick, sharp

oz/o to smell, odour

pachy- thick

paed/o child

palae/o old, primitive

palat/o palate

palpat/o touch, feel, stroke

palpebr/o eyelid

palpit/o throbbing

pan- all, entire

pancreat/o pancreas

papill/o nipple-shaped projection

papul/o pimple

par- aside, beyond, apart from, other than, near, against

para- beside, near, alongside

-para to bear, bring forth

parathyr/o parathyroid gland

parathyroid/o parathyroid gland

-paresis slight, incomplete paralysis

pariet/o wall

parotid/o parotid gland

-parous to bear, bring forth

part/o bear, give birth to

-partum childbirth, labour

patell/o patella

path/o disease

-pathy disease process

-pause stopping

pect- chest, breast, thorax

pector/o chest

ped/o foot

pedicul/o lice

pelv/i pelvis

pelv/o pelvis

pen/i penis

-penia deficiency

-pepsia digestion (condition of)

pept- digestion

pept/o digestion

per through

percuss/o strike hard

peri- around, surrounding

perine/o perineum

peritone/o peritoneum

petr/o stone, rock

-pexis surgical fixation

-pexy fixation, put in place

phac/o lens of the eye

phae/o dusky, dark

phag/o eat, swallow

-phage eat, swallow

-phagia eat, swallow

phak/o lens of the eye

phalang/o phalanx

phall/o penis

pharmac/o drug

pharmaceutic/o drug

pharyng/o pharynx, throat

phas/o speech

-phasia speech

-pheresis removal

-phil affinity for, attraction to

phil/o attraction to, love

-philia attraction to

phim/o muzzle

phleb/o vein

phob/o fear, sensitivity

-phobia fear (condition of)

phon/o voice, sound

-phonia sound (condition of)

phor/o carry, bear

-phoresis movement in a specified way

-phoria feeling, emotional state

phot/o light

phren/o mind, diaphragm

phrenic/o diaphragm, mind, phrenic nerve

-phylaxis protection

-phyma swelling, tumour

phys/o gas, air

physi/o related to nature

-physis growth

phyt/o plant, fungus

pil/o resembling or composed of hair

pineal/o pineal gland

pituitar/o pituitary gland

placent/o placenta

-plakia condition of plaques

plan/o flat

plant/o sole of the foot

plas/o formation

-plasia formation, development, growth

-plasm growth, formation, substance

plasm/o formative substance, growth

plasma- plasma cell

-plasty surgical, plastic repair

-plegia paralysis (condition of)

pleio- more

pleo- more

pleur/o pleura

plex/o network of nerves

-plexy strike, paralyse

plic/o fold, ridge

pneum/o lungs, respiration, air

pneumat/o lungs, respiration, air

pneumon/o lungs, respiration, air

-pnoea breathing

pod/o foot

-poiesis formation of, production of

-poietin substance that forms

poikil/o varied, irregular

pol/o extreme

polio- grey matter

poly- many, much

polyp/o polyp

pont/o pons, bridge

poplit/o back of the knee

por/o passage, pore

port/o portal vein

post- after, behind

poster/o behind, back

posth/o prepuce, foreskin

-prandial meal

-praxia achieve, do

pre- before, in front of

presby/o old age

primi- first

pro- before, forward

proct/o anus, rectum

progest/o progesterone

prostat/o prostate gland

prote/o protein

proto- first

protozo/o protozoa

proxim/o near, nearest

prurit/o itching

pseudo- false

psych/o mind

-ptosis downward displacement, prolapse

ptyal/o saliva

-ptysis spitting

pub/o pubis

puerper/o childbirth

pulm/o lungs

pulmon/o lungs

pupill/o pupil

purpur/o purple

purul/o pus filled

py/o pus

pyel/o renal pelvis

pylor/o pylorus, pyloric sphincter

pyr/o fire, heat

pyret/o heat, fire, burning, fever

quadri- four

rachi/o spine

radi/o x-ray, radius

radic/o nerve root

radicul/o nerve root

re- back, again

rect/o rectum

ren/o kidney

reticul/o net-like

retin/o retina

retro- backwards, behind

rhabd/o rod-shaped, striated (skeletal)

rhabdomy/o striated muscle

rheumat/o watery flow

rhin/o nose

rhiz/o nerve root

rhonc/o snore

rhytid/o wrinkle, crease

roentgen/o x-ray

-rrhage bursting forth, excessive discharge or flow

-rrhagia bursting forth, excessive discharge or flow (condition of)

-rrhaphy suture

-rrhexis rupture

-rrhoea discharge, flow

rug/o wrinkle, ridge

sacr/o sacrum

salping/o fallopian tube, eustachian (auditory) tube

-salpinx uterine tube

sangui/o blood

sanguin/o blood

sapr/o dead or decaying

sarc/o flesh

scapul/o scapula

scat/o faeces

-schisis split

schist/o splitting, parting

schiz/o split

scint/i sparkling, flash of light

scintill/o sparkling, flash of light

scirrh/o hard

scler/o sclera, hardening

-sclerosis hardening (condition of)

scoli/o crooked, bent

-scope instrument to view

-scopy process of viewing

scot/o darkness

scrot/o scrotum, bag or pouch

seb/o sebum

sebace/o sebum

-section cut

secundi- second

semi- half

semin/i semen, seed

sen/i old

sensor/i sensation

-sepsis infection

sept/o septum

septic/o infection

sequester- sequestrum (portion of dead bone)

ser/o serum

sial/o saliva, salivary

sider/o iron

sigmoid/o sigmoid colon

silic/o glass

sinistr/o left side

sinus/o sinus, cavity

-sis state of

sit/o food

-sol solution

som/o body

somat/o body

somatic/o body

somn/i sleep

somn/o sleep

son/o sound

-spasm involuntary contraction

sperm/i spermatozoa, sperm

sperm/o spermatozoa, sperm

spermat/o spermatozoa, sperm

sphen/o wedge-shaped, sphenoid bone

spher/o globe, round

sphygm/o pulse

spin/o spine, thorn

spir/o breathe

splen/o spleen

spondyl/o vertebra

squam/o scale

-stalsis contraction

staped/o stapes, ossicle

stapedi/o stapes, ossicle

staphyl/o cluster, bunch of grapes

-stasis stop, control, stand still

-static pertaining to stopping, controlling or standing still

-staxis dripping (especially of blood)

stear/o fat

steat/o fat

sten/o narrow, constricted

-stenosis narrowing, stricture

stere/o three-dimensional

stern/o sternum

stert/o snoring

steth/o chest

sthen/o strength

-stitial pertaining to standing or positioned

stomat/o mouth

stom/o mouth

-stomy create surgical opening

strab/o squinting

strept/o twisted

striat/o stripe, groove

sub- under, below

sudor/o sweat

super- above, excessive

super/o above, excessive

-suppression to stop

supra- above, excessive

sym- together, with

syn- together, with

syncop/o cut short

synov/o synovial membrane, synovial fluid

synovi/o synovial membrane, synovial fluid

systol/o contraction

tachy- rapid, fast

tact/i touch

tal/o ankle

tars/o tarsal

tax/o order, coordination

-taxia order, coordination

tel/o distant, end, far, complete

tele- distant, end, far, complete

ten/o tendon

tend/o tendon

tendin/o tendon

terat/o monster, malformed

test/i testis, testicle

test/o testis, testicle

testicul/o testis, testicle

tetan/o rigid, tense, tetanus

tetra- four

thalam/o thalamus

thalass/o sea

thanat/o death

the/o to place

thec/o sheath

thel/o nipple

therapeut/o treatment

-therapy treatment

therm/o heat

-thermy heat

thorac/o thorax, chest

-thorax pleural cavity, chest

thromb/o clot

thym/o thymus gland

-thymia mind (condition of), emotion

-thymic mind, emotion

thyr/o a shield, thyroid gland

thyroid/o a shield, thyroid gland

tibi/o tibia

-tic pertaining to, drug action

till/o pluck, pull

toc/o childbirth, labour

-tocia childbirth (condition of), labour (condition of)

tom/o slice, section, cut

-tome instrument to cut

-tomy incision, cut into

ton/o tone, tension, pressure

tonsill/o tonsils

top/o place, location

tort/i twisted

tox/o poison, toxin

toxic/o poison, toxin

trache/o trachea

trachel/o neck, uterine cervix

trans- across, through, over

-tresia opening, perforation

tri- three

trich/i hair

trich/o hair

trigon/o trigone (base of the bladder)

-tripsy to crush

troph/o nourishment, development

-trophic nourishment (pertaining to), stimulation (pertaining to)

-trophin stimulating the effect of (a hormone)

-trophy development, nourishment

-tropia to turn

-tropic affinity for

trop/o turn, change, reaction

tuss/i cough

tympan/o eardrum, tympanic membrane

-ula small

-ule little, small

uln/o ulna

ultra- beyond, excess

-ulum small

-ulus small

-um structure, tissue, thing

umbilic/o umbilicus, navel

un- not, opposite of, release from

ungu/o nail

uni- one

ur/o urine, urinary tract, urea

urat/o urates

-urea compound containing urea

-uresis excrete urine, urinate

ureter/o ureter

urethr/o urethra

-uria urination, urine condition, presence of substance in urine

urin/o urine

urticar/i hives, rash

-us thing, structure

uter/o uterus

uve/o uvea, vascular layer of eye

uvul/o uvula, little grape

vag/o vagus nerve

vagin/o vagina

valv/o valve

valvul/o valve

varic/o swollen, twisted vein

vas/o ductus (vas) deferens, vessel, duct

vascul/o vessel

vect/o carry

ven/i vein

ven/o vein

vener/o sexual intercourse

ventr/o front, belly side

ventricul/o ventricle

venul/o venule, small vein

verm/i worm

-version to turn

vertebr/o vertebra, spinal column

vesic/o urinary bladder, blister

vesicul/o seminal vesicle

vestibul/o vestibule

vibr/o vibration

vir/o virus

viril/o masculine

visc/o sticky

viscer/o internal organs

vit/o life

vitre/o glassy

viv/i life

vol/o volume, palm or sole

vulv/o vulva

xanth/o yellow

xen/o foreign, strange

xer/o dry

xiph/i xiphoid process, sword

xiph/o xiphoid process, sword

-y process, condition

zo/o animal life

zyg/o union, fusion, joined

zygomat/o zygomatic arch, cheekbone

Glossary of medical terms

abdomen abdomin/o, celi/o, coeli/o, lapar/o

ability to -able

able -ile

able to be -ible

abnormal cac/o

abnormal condition -ago, -igo, -osis

abnormal condition of cells -cytosis

abnormal state -esis

abnormally large mega-

about circum-

above epi-, hyper-, super-, super/o, supra-

absence of a-, an- (*used when combining form starts with a vowel*)

absence of opening -atresia

acetabulum acetabul/o

achieve -praxia

Achilles tendon achill/o

acid acid/o

across dia-, trans-, -ation

action (condition resulting from) -ion

adenoids adenoid/o

adhesion adhesi/o

adjoining juxta-

adrenal glands adren/o, adrenal/o

affinity for -tropic, -phil

after post-

again re-

against anti-, par-, contra-

aged ger/i, ger/o, geront/o

agent -or, -ent

agent that kills -cide

air aer/o, phys/o, pneum/o, pneumat/o, pneumon/o

air sac alveol/o

albumin albumin/o

alike home/o, homo-

all pan-

alongside para-

alveolus alveol/o

amnion amni/o, amnion/o, -amnios

amniotic fluid amni/o, -amnios

aneurysm aneurysm/o

animal life zo/o

animal starch glycogen/o

ankle tal/o

antrum antr/o

anus an/o, proct/o

anxious anxi/o

aorta aort/o

apart ana-

apart from par-

apex apic/o

aponeurosis aponeur/o

appendix appendic/o

appetite (condition of) -orexia

arc arc/o

arising from -genous

arm brachi/o

armpit axill/o

around circum-, peri-

arteriole arteriol/o

artery arter/o, arteri/o

aside par-

assemble -agon

asymmetrical aniso-

atrium atri/o

attack -igo

attraction to -phil, phil/o, -philia

away dist/o

away from ab-, ap/o, de-

axis ax/o

bacillus bacill/o

back dorsi-, poster/o, re-

back (of body) dors/o

back of tongue glott/o

backwards retro-

bacteria bacteri/o

bad cac/o, dys-, mal-, malign/o

bag or pouch scrot/o

baldness alopec/o

ball bol/o

barrier claustr/o

Bartholin's gland bartholin/o

base, basis bas/o

base or bottom of an organ fund/o

bear phor/o, part/o, fer/o, -para, -parous

bearing -ferous

before ante-, fore-, pre-, pro-

beginning -arche

behind post-, poster/o, retro-

belch forth eruct/o

belly side ventr/o

below hypo-, infer/o, infra-, sub-

bend -flect, flex/o

bent scoli/o, ankyl/o

berry-shaped bacterium -coccus, cocc/i, cocc/o

beside para-

between inter-

beyond meta-, par-, ultra-

bile bil/i, chol/e

bile duct cholangi/o

bile pigment bilirubin/o

bind nect/o, -desis

birth -partum, nat/o, nat/i

birth (pertaining to) -natal

black anthrac/o, melan/o

blind pouch divertul/o

blister vesic/o

blockage isch/o

blood haem/o, haemat/o, sangui/o, sanguin/o

blood (condition of) -aemia

blood vessel haemangi/o

blotch macul/o

blue cyan/o

body som/o, somat/o, somatic/o

bone os-, oss/i, osse/o, oste/o

bone marrow myel/o

both sides ambi-

bound to adnex/o

bow arc/o

brain cerebr/o, encephal/o

branches dendr/o

branching furc/o

break -clasis, -clast

breakdown -lysis

breast mamm/o, mast/o, pect-

breath halit/o

breathe spir/o

breathing -pnoea

bridge pont/o

bring forth -para, -parous

broad eury-

broken away from abrupt/o

bronchiole bronchiol/o

bronchus bronch/o, bronch/i

bunch of grapes staphyl/o

burn caus/o, caust/o, cauter/o

burning caus/o, caust/o, pyret/o

bursa burs/o

burst open dehisc/o

bursting forth -rrhage

bursting forth (condition of) -rrhagia

caecum caec/o

calcaneus calcane/o

calcium calc/i, calc/o, calcin/o

calculus -lith, lith/o

calyx cali/o, calic/o

cancer cancer/o

cancerous carcin/o, malign/o

canthus canth/o

capable of -able, -ile

capable of being -ible

capillary capill/o

capsule capsul/o

carbon carb/o

carbon dioxide capn/o, carb/o

carbon dioxide (condition of) -capnia

carpal carp/o

carry phor/o, vect/o, fer/o

carry away -apheresis

carrying -ferent, -ferous

cartilage chondr/o

cause aeti/o

causing -gen, gen/o

cavity sinus/o, coel/o

cell cyt/o, cellul/o, -cyte

centre centr/o, centr/i

cerebellum cerebell/o

cerebrum cerebr/o

cervix uteri cervic/o

change meta-, trop/o

characteristic of -an, -ant

cheek bucc/o

cheekbone zygomat/o

chemical chem/o, chemic/o

chest pect-, pector/o, steth/o, thorac/o, -thorax

child paed/o

childbirth puerper/o, toc/o, -partum

childbirth (condition of) -tocia

chin geni/o

choking angin/o

cholesterol cholesterol/o

chorion chori/o, chorion/o, choroid/o

choroid choroid/o

ciliary body of the eye cycl/o

circular cycl/o

clavicle clavic/o, clavicul/o, cleid/o

cleansing cathart/o

cleft into two parts bifid/o

close up occlus/o

closure -atresia

clot thromb/o

clotting coagul/o

clumping agglutin/o

cluster staphyl/o

coal anthrac/o

coccyx coccyg/o

cochlea cochle/o

cold cry/o

colon col/o, colon/o

colour chrom/o, chromat/o

coma comat/o

comfort -aise

coming together coit/o

common bile duct choledoch/o

complete tel/o, tele-

composed of -ous

compound containing urea -urea

condition -asia, -asis, -ation, -cina, -ia, -iasis, -ismus, -ity, -y

condition of -esis

condyle condyl/o

confining membrane -lemma

congenital absence ectro-

conjoined adnex/o

conjunctiva conjunctiv/o

connect nect/o

connected with -ary

constricted sten/o

contraction -stalsis, systol/o

control -stasis

controlling (pertaining to) -static

coordination tax/o, -taxia

cornea kerat/o, corne/o

corner of eye canth/o

corpus luteum lute/o

cortex cortic/o

cough tuss/i

crack fiss/o, fissur/o

crackling crepit/o, crepitat/o

cranium crani/o

crease rhytid/o

create surgical opening -stomy

crescent menisc/o

crooked ankyl/o, scoli/o

crush -tripsy

cul-de-sac culd/o

cup cali/o, calic/o

curve lord/o

cut cis/o, -section, tom/o

cut into -tomy

cut short syncop/o

cutting -cision

cyst cyst/o

dance, jerky movement chore/o

dark phae/o

darkness nyct/o, nyctal/o, scot/o

dawn eosin/o

dead necr/o

dead or decaying sapr/o

death mort/o, necr/o, thanat/o

decay cari/o

deep batho-, bathy-

defecation -chezia

deficiency isch/o, olig/o, -penia

deficient hypo-

dentine of tooth dentin/o

depression foss/o

derived from ap/o, -oid

destruction -lysis

detached ap/o

developing cell -blast, blast/o

development -plasia, troph/o, -trophy

diaphragm diaphragmat/o, phren/o, phrenic/o

different all/o, hetero-, dys-

digestion pept-

digestion (condition of) pept/o, -pepsia

dilatation -ectasia, -ectasis

dilation mydri/o

dim ambly/o

discharge -rrhoea

disease -ago, nos/o, path/o

disease process -pathy

disorder of speech -lalia

displaced ectop/o

dissimilar aniso-

dissolution -lysis

distant dist/o, tel/o, tele-

distressed anxi/o

diverticulum diverticul/o

do -praxia

double bi-, bin-, bis-, di-, dipl/o, dupl/i

down cata-

downward caud/o

downward displacement -ptosis

dripping (especially of blood) -staxis

drug chem/o, chemic/o, pharmac/o, pharmaceutic/o

drug action -al, -ic, -ive, -tic

drug that breaks down -lytic

dry ichthy/o, xer/o

duct doch/o, vas/o, ambly/o

ductus (vas) deferens vas/o

duodenum duoden/o

duplication dis-

dura mater dur/o

dusky phae/o

dust coni/o

ear aur/i, aur/o, auricul/o, ot/o

ear (condition of) -otia

ear (pertaining to) -aural

eardrum myring/o, tympan/o

ease -aise

eat phag/o, -phage, -phagia

egg oo/o, ov/i, ov/o, ovul/o

elbow cubit/o

electrical activity electr/o, electro-

electricity electr/o, electro-

elimination of waste products -chezia

ellipse-shaped ellipt/o

embolism embol/o

embryo embry/o

embryonic, developing cell -blast, blast/o

emotion -thymia, -thymic

emotional state -phoria

enclosed claustr/o

end tel/o, tele-

endometrium endometri/o

enlarge mydr/o

enlargement megal/o, -megaly

entire hol/o, pan-

entrance introit/o

enzyme -ase

epididymis epididym/o

epiglottis epiglott/o

epithelium epitheli/o

equal is/o, iso-, equi-

eustachian (auditory) tube salping/o

excess ultra-

excessive hyper-, super-, super/o, supra-

excessive discharge or flow -rrhage

excessive discharge or flow (condition of) -rrhagia

excision ectomy

excrete urine -uresis

expansion -ectasia, -ectasis

external -externa

extreme pol/o

extremities acro-

eye ocul/o, ophthalm/o, opt/i, opt/o, optic/o

eye (vascular layer) uve/o

eyelid blephar/o, palpebr/o

face faci/o

faeces faec/o, copr/o, scat/o

fallopian tube salping/o

false pseudo-

far dist/o, tel/o, tele-

fascia (a band) fasci/o

fast tachy-

fat adip/o, lip/o, stear/o, steat/o

fatty plaque ather/o

fear phob/o

fear (condition of) -phobia

feel palpat/o

feeling aesthes/o, aesthesi/o, -phoria

feeling (condition of) -aesthesia

female gynaec/o, gyn/o, oestr/o

femur femor/o

fetal membrane amnion/o

fetus embry/o, fet/o

fever febr/o, pyret/o

few olig/o

fibre fibr/o

fibrinogen fibrin/o

fibrous connective tissue fibros/o

fibula fibul/o

fine lept/o

finger digit/o, dactyl/o

fire pyr/o, pyret/o

first -arche, primi-, proto-

fixation -pexy

flash of light scint/i, scintill/o

flat plan/o

flesh sarc/o

flow -rrhoea

fluorescent fluor/o

focus foc/o

fold plic/o

follicle follicul/o

food sit/o

food or nutritive material aliment/o

foot ped/o, pod/o

force dynam/o

forehead front/o

foreign xen/o

foreskin posth/o

form -morph, morph/o

formation plas/o, -plasia, -plasm

formation (pertaining to) -genesis, -genic

formation of -poiesis

formative plasm/o

forwards ante-, pro-

four quadri-, tetra-

frenzy -mania

fringe fimbri/o

front anter/o, front/o

front (belly side) ventr/o

full of -ose

fungus fung/i, fung/o, myc/o, phyt/o

funnel infundibul/o

fusion -desis, zyg/o

gall chol/e, bil/i

gallbladder cholecyst/o

ganglion gangli/o

gas aer/o, phys/o

gather together -agon

genetic change mut/a

genitals genit/o

give birth to part/o

gland aden/o

glans penis balan/o

glass, glass-like, glassy silic/o, hyal/o, vitre/o

globe spher/o

glucose gluc/o, glyc/o, glycos/o, glycogen/o

glomerulus glomerul/o

glue gli/o

gluing agglutin/o

glycogen glycogen/o

go -grade

gonads gonad/o

good eu-

granules granul/o

green chlor/o

grey glauc/o

grey matter polio-

grind brux/o

groin inguin/o

groove striat/o

growth kel/o, -physis, -plasia, -plasm, plasm/o

gums gingiv/o

habit -hexia

haemoglobin haemoglobin/o

hair trich/o, trich/i

hair-like projections cili/o

half demi-, hemi-, semi-

hallucination hallucin/o

hammer malle/o

hand cheir/o, chir/o

hard kerat/o, scirrh/o

hardening scler/o, -sclerosis

harmful malign/o

having the form of -form

having the nature of -in, -ine

head cephal/o, capit/o

hearing acous/o, -acusis, audi/o, audit/o, -cusis

hearing (condition of) -acousia

heart cardi/o, coron/o

heart (condition of) -cardia

heat cauter/o, calor/i, pyr/o, pyret/o, therm/o, -thermy

hepatic bile duct hepatic/o

hernia -cele, herni/o

hidden crypto-, occult/o

hip, hip joint ili/o, cox/o

hives urticar/i

hold back isch/o

hollow celi/o

honey mellit/o

hormone hormon/o, -one

horny tissue kerat/o

horse equin/o

human anthrop/o

humerus humer/o

humpback kyph/o

hundred centi-

hymen hymen/o

ileum ile/o

ilium ili/o

ill cac/o

immature tumour -blastoma

imperfect atel/o

in intus-, in-, im-, en-, em- (*used when combining form starts with a b, m or p*)

in front of fore-, pre-

incision -tomy

incomplete atel/o

incus incud/o

infection -sepsis, septic/o

inferior to infra-

inflammation -itis

inner endo-

inner ear labyrinth/o

inner part medull/o

inside endo-, intra-

instrument for recording -graph

instrument to cut -tome

instrument to view -scope

instrument used to measure meter

insulin insulin/o

intermediate mes/o

internal organs viscer/o

intervertebral disc disc/o

intestine enter/o

into intro-, intus-

involuntary contraction -spasm

inward eso-, intro-

iodine iod/o

iris iri/o, irid/o

iron ferr/o, sider/o

irregular poikil/o

irrigating -clysis

ischium ischi/o

itching prurit/o

jaundice -icterus

jaw gnath/o

jaw, lower mandibul/o

jaw, upper maxill/o

jejunum jejun/o

joined zyg/o

joint arthr/o, articul/o

judgment -gnosis

keratin keratin/o

ketone bodies ket/o, keton/o

kidney nephr/o, ren/o

killing -cide

knee gon/o, genicul/o

knee (back of) poplit/o

knot gangli/o, nod/o

knowledge gnos/o, -gnosis

labour -partum, toc/o

labour (condition of) -tocia

labyrinth labyrinth/o

lacrimal sac dacryocyst/o

lack of de-

lamina lamin/o

large macro-

large intestine col/o, colon/o

larynx laryng/o

lead duct/o

left side sinistr/o

lens of the eye phac/o, phak/o

less mi/o, de-

less than normal hypo-

lice pedicul/o

life bi/o, vit/o, viv/i

ligament ligament/o

light phot/o

lip cheil/o, labi/o

listen auscult/o

little ole, ule

little grape uvul/o

little hammer malleol/o

liver hepat/o

lobe lob/o

location top/o

loins lumb/o

loosening -chalasis

loss of de-

love phil/o

lower back lumb/o

lower jaw mandibul/o

luminous fluor/o

lungs pneum/o, pneumat/o, pneumon/o, pulm/o, pulmon/o

lymph gland lymph/o

lymphoid tissue lymph/o

made of -in, -ine

main stem ax/o

male andr/o

malformed terat/o

malignant carcin/o

malleolus malleol/o

malleus malle/o

man anthrop/o

mandible mandibul/o

many multi-, poly-

marketplace agora-

masculine viril/o

mastoid process mastoid/o

maxilla maxill/o

maxillary sinus antr/o

meal cib/o, -prandial

measurement -meter

meatus meat/o

mediastinum mediastin/o

medical specialty -iatrics, -iatry

medicine iatr/o

medulla medull/o

meninges mening/o, meningi/o

meniscus menisc/o

menses men/o

menstruation men/o

metacarpal metacarp/o

metatarsal metatars/o

middle medi/o, -media, mes/o, mid-

midwife obstetr/o

milk galact/o, lact/o, lact/i

mind ment/o, phren/o, phrenic/o, psych/o, -thymic

mind (condition of) -thymia

miscarriage ectro-

moisture hygr/o

monster terat/o

moon lun/o

more pleio-, pleo-

motion kinesi/o, -kinesis, kinet/o

motion (condition of) -kinesia

mould myc/o

mouth or/o, os-, stomat/o

movement cine-, cinemat/o, kinesi/o, -kinesis, kinet/o

movement (condition of) -kinesia

movement (power of) dynam/o

movement in a specified way -phoresis

much multi-, poly-

mucus muc/o, myx/o

muscle muscul/o, my/o, myos/o

muscular twitching fibrill/o

mushroom fung/i, fung/o

muzzle phim/o

myocardium myocardi/o

nail onych/o, ungu/o

narrow sten/o

narrowing -constriction, -stenosis

nature (related to) physi/o

navel umbilic/o

near proxim/o, af-, ag-, ap-, juxta-, par-, para-

neck cervic/o, jugul/o, trachel/o

neck region nuch/o

nerve neur/o

nerve root radic/o, radicul/o, rhiz/o

net-like reticul/o

network of nerves plex/o

neutral neutr/o

new neo-

night noct/i, nyct/o, nyctal/o

nipple mammill/o, thel/o

nipple-shaped projection papill/o

nitrogen azot/o

nitrogen compound -amine

no a-, an- (*used when combining form starts with a vowel*)

none im-, in-, nulli-

normal eu-

normally proportioned emmetr/o

nose rhin/o, nas/o

not a-, an- (*used when combining form starts with a vowel*), im-, in-, un-

nourishment nutri/o, troph/o, -trophy

nourishment (pertaining to) -trophic

nucleus kary/o, nucle/o

obscenity copr/o

obscure -opaque

occiput occipit/o

occlusion -atresia

odour osphresi/o, oz/o

oesophagus oesophag/o

oestrogen oestr/o

old palae/o, sen/i

old age ger/i, ger/o, geront/o, presby/o

olecranon olecran/o

on epi-

one mono-, uni-

one who -er

one who specialises in -ist

open space agora-

opening foramin/o, hiat/o, -tresia

opposite of un-

orange cirrh/o

orbit of eye orbit/o

order norm/o, tax/o, -taxia

orifice os-

originating -gen, gen/o

ossicle staped/o, stapedi/o, ossicul/o

other all/o

other than par-

out ec-, ect-, ecto-

outer layer of organ cortic/o

outer part ec-, ect-, ecto-, ex-, exo-, extra-

outward ex-, exo-

ova oo/o

ovary oophor/o, ovar/i, ovari/o

over trans-

ovum o/o, ov/i, ov/o, ovul/o

oxygen ox/o, ox/i

oxygen (condition of) -oxia

pain algesi/o

pain (condition of) -algesia, -algia, -dynia

painful dys-

palate palat/o

palm of hand vol/o

pancreas pancreat/o

paralyse -plexy

paralysis (condition of) -plegia

paralysis, incomplete -paresis

parathyroid gland parathyr/o, parathyroid/o

parotid gland parotid/o

parting schist/o

passage introit/o, por/o

patella patell/o

pelvis pelv/o, pelv/i

pelvis (kidney) pyel/o

penis phall/o, pen/i

people dem/o

perforation -tresia

perineum perine/o

peritoneum peritone/o

person -ent, -or

person associated with -ician

pertaining to -ac, -al, -an, -ar, -ary, -eal, -iac, -ial, -ic, -ior, -ive, -ory, -ose, -ous, -tic

pertaining to circular motion -gyric

pertaining to destruction -lytic

phalanx phalang/o

pharynx pharyng/o

phrenic nerve phrenic/o

physician iatr/o

pillar column/o

pimple papul/o

pineal gland pineal/o

pipe fistul/o

pituitary gland pituitar/o

place loc/o, top/o, the/o

placenta placent/o

plant phyt/o

plaques (condition of) -plakia

plasma cell plasma-

plastic repair -plasty

pleura pleur/o

pleural cavity -thorax

pluck till/o

plug embol/o

poison tox/o, toxic/o

polyp polyp/o

pons pont/o

pore por/o

portal vein port/o

potassium kal/i

pour chym/o

pregnancy cyes/i, cyes/o, -cyesis, -gravida

premature expulsion of fetus abort/o

prepuce posth/o

presence of substance in urine -uria

pressure bar/o, man/o, ton/o

primitive palae/o

process -ation, -ia, -ismus, -y

process of measuring -metry

process of recording -graphy

process of viewing -opsy, -scopy

produced by -genous

producing -ferous, -gen, gen/o

producing (pertaining to) -genesis, -genic

product of recording -graph

production of -poiesis

profuse sweating diaphor/o

progesterone progest/o

prolapse -ptosis

prostate gland prostat/o

protection immun/o, -phylaxis

protein prote/o, -globin, -globulin

protozoa protozo/o

protrusion -cele

pubis pub/o

pull till/o

pulse sphygm/o

pupil pupill/o

pupil of the eye cor/o, core/o

pupils (condition of) -coria

purging cathart/o

purple purpur/o

pus py/o

pus-filled purul/o

put in place -pexy

pylorus, pyloric sphincter pylor/o

quick oxy-

radius radi/o

rapid tachy-

rash urticar/i

reaction trop/o

record -gram

rectum proct/o, rect/o

recurring cycl/o

red erythr/o, eosin/o, erythem/o, erythemat/o

reflected, repeated sound echo-

relating to -in, -ine, ous

release from un-

remove -apheresis, -pheresis

removal of de-

renal pelvis pyel/o

reproductive organs genit/o

resembling -oid

resembling or composed of hair pil/o

respiration pneum/o, pneumat/o, pneumon/o

retina retin/o

reversal dis-

reversing de-

ribs cost/o

ridge plic/o, rug/o

right side dextro-

rigid tetan/o

rock petr/o

rod-shaped rhabd/o

rod-shaped bacterium bacill/o

rosy eosin/o

rot cari/o

round spher/o

rule norm/o

rumbling sound borborygm/o

rupture -rrhexis

sac cyst/o

sacrum sacr/o

saliva ptyal/o, sial/o

salivary sial/o

same home/o, homo-, is/o, iso-, equis-

scale squam/o

scaly ichthy/o

scanty olig/o

scapula scapul/o

sclera scler/o

scrotum scrot/o

sea thalass/o

sebum seb/o, sebace/o

second secundi-

secrete crin/o, -crine

secrete milk lactat/o

section tom/o

seed semin/i

seen gon/o

seizure -lepsy

seizure (pertaining to) -ictal

self auto-, idi/o

semen gon/o, semin/i

seminal vesicle vesicul/o

sensation aesthes/o, aesthesi/o, sensor/i

sensation (condition of) -aesthesia

sense of smell olfactor/o, osm/o, oz/o

sense of smell (condition of) -osmia

sense of taste geus/o

sensitivity phob/o

separate -crit, -dialysis

separation dis-, -lysis

septum sept/o

sequestrum (portion of dead bone) sequester-

serum ser/o

sex glands (ovaries and testes) gonad/o

sexual intercourse vener/o

sexual love erot/o

shape -morph, morph/o

sharp oxy-

sheath -lemma, thec/o

shield thyr/o, thyroid/o

shine -lucent

short brachy-, brevi-

shoulder acromi/o

shut occlus/o

side later/o

sigmoid colon sigmoid/o

single mono-

sinus sinus/o

skin derm/o, dermat/o, -derma, cutane/o, cut/i

skull crani/o

slackening -chalasis

sleep hypn/o, narc/o, somn/o, somn/i

slender lept/o

slice tom/o

slight paralysis -paresis

slip or slide -listhesis

slow brady-

small micro-, -cule, -ole, -ula, -ule, -ulum, -ulus

small intestine ile/o

small open space areol/o

small sac follicul/o

small vein venul/o

smaller mi/o

smell of sweat bromidr/o

smooth lei/o

smooth muscle leiomy/o

snore, snoring rhonc/o, stert/o

sodium natr/o

soft malac/o

softening (condition of) -malacia, malac/o

sole of foot vol/o, plant/o

solution -sol

sound phon/o, son/o

sound (condition of) -phonia

sparkling scint/i, scintill/o

specialist -ician, -ist

speech phas/o, -phasia

sperm, spermatozoa sperm/o, sperm/i, spermat/o

sphenoid bone sphen/o

spider arachn/o

spinal column vertebr/o

spinal cord myel/o

spine rachi/o, spin/o

spiny acanth/o

spitting -ptysis

spleen splen/o

split bifid/o, dehisc/o, -schisis, schiz/o

splitting schist/o

spot macul/o

squinting strab/o

stand still -stasis

standing or positioned (pertaining to) -stitial

standing still (pertaining to) -static

stapes staped/o, stapedi/o

star astr/o

starch amyl/o

state -iasis, -ismus, -ity

state of -asia, -asis, -ism, -sis

state of mental disorder -mania

steal klept/o

stench bromidr/o

sternum stern/o

sticking together agglutin/o

sticky visc/o

stiff ankyl/o

stimulating the effect of (a hormone) -trophin

stimulation (pertaining to) -trophic

stomach gastr/o

stone calcul/o, -lith, lith/o, petr/o

stones (abnormal condition of) -lithiasis

stop -stasis, -suppression

stopping -pause

stopping (pertaining to) -static

straight orth/o

strange xen/o

strength sthen/o

stretching -dilation

stretching out -ectasia, -ectasis

striated rhabd/o

striated muscle rhabdomy/o

stricture -stenosis

strike -plexy

strike hard percuss/o

stripe striat/o

stroke palpat/o

structure -ium, -um, -us

study of log/o, -logy

stupor narc/o

subject to -ate

substance -plasm, plasm/o

substance that forms -poietin

sugar gluc/o, glyc/o, glycos/o, -ose

sun hel/i

surgical fixation -desis, -pexis

surgical puncture to remove fluid -centesis

surgical removal -ectomy

surgical repair -plasty

surrounding peri-

suture -rrhaphy

swallow phag/o, -phage, -phagia

swayback lord/o

sweat exud/o, hidr/o, sudor/o

swelling nod/o, -phyma,

swelling due to fluid -oedema

swollen vein varic/o

sword xiph/o, xiph/i

synovial fluid synov/o, synovi/o

synovial membrane synov/o, synovi/o

tail caud/o

tarsal tars/o

tear lacrim/o

tears, tear duct dacry/o

teeth dent/o, dent/i, odont/o

ten deci-

tendon ten/o, tend/o, tendin/o

tense tetan/o

tension ton/o

testicle orch/o, orchi/o, orchid/o, test/i, test/o, testicul/o

testis orch/o, orchi/o, orchid/o, test/i, test/o, testicul/o

tetanus tetan/o

thalamus thalam/o

thick pachy-

thin lept/o

thing -um, -us

thirst dips/o

thorax pect-, thorac/o

thorn spin/o

thorny acanth/o

thread fil/o

three tri-

three-dimensional stere/o

throat jugul/o, pharyng/o

throbbing palpit/o

through dia-, per-, trans-

thunder bront/o

thymus gland thym/o

thyroid gland thyr/o, thyroid/o

tibia tibi/o

tie together nect/o

time chron/o

tissue hist/o, histi/o, -ium, -um

to af-, ag-, ap-

toe digit/o, dactyl/o

together co-, com-, con-, sym-, syn-

tone ton/o

tongue gloss/o, lingu/o

tonsils tonsill/o

touch palpat/o, tact/i

towards ad-, ap-, af-, ag-, ana-

toxin tox/o, toxic/o

trachea trache/o

transplant of tissue -graft

treatment iatr/o, therapeut/o, -therapy

treatment by doctor -iatry

tree dendr/o

trigone (base of the bladder) trigon/o

tube fistul/o

tube to carry duct/o

tumour -oma, onc/o, kel/o, -phyma

turmoil clon/o

turn -tropia, trop/o -version

twice bi-, bin-, bis-, di-

twisted strept/o, tort/i

twisted vein varic/o

two bi-, bin-, bis-

tying off -ligation

tympanic membrane myring/o, tympan/o

type of seizure -leptic

ulcer aphth/o, helc/o

ulna uln/o

umbilicus omphal/o, umbilic/o

under hypo-, sub-

uneasy anxi/o

unequal aniso-

union zyg/o

unique to individual or organ idi/o

unpleasant cac/o

up ana-

upon epi-

upright orth/o

urates urat/o

urea azot/o, ur/o

ureter ureter/o

urethra urethr/o

urinary bladder cyst/o, vesic/o

urinary tract ur/o

urinate -uresis

urination -uria

urine ur/o, urin/o

urine (condition of) uria

use -ate

uterine cervix cervic/o, trachel/o

uterine tube -salpinx

uterus hyster/o, metr/o, metri/o, uter/o

uvea uve/o

uvula uvul/o

vagina colp/o, vagin/o

vagus nerve vag/o

valve valv/o, valvul/o

varied poikil/o

vas deferens vas/o

vein phleb/o, ven/o, ven/i

ventricle ventricul/o

venule venul/o

vertebra spondyl/o, vertebr/o

vessel angi/o, vas/o, vascul/o

vestibule vestibul/o

vibration vibr/o

view -opsy

vinegar acet/o

virus vir/o

vision opt/i, opt/o, optic/o

vision (condition of) -opia, -opsia

voice phon/o

voice box laryng/o

volume vol/o

vomiting -emesis, emet/o

vulva episi/o, vulv/o

walk ambulat/o

wall pariet/o

wander in the mind hallucin/o

washing -clysis

water aqu/i, aqu/o, aqua-, aque/o, hydr/o, hydra-

watery flow rheumat/o

wax cer/o, cerumin/o

weakness (condition of) -asthenia

wedge-shaped sphen/o, cune/i

weight bar/o

white alb/o, albin/o, leuc/o, leuk/o (*used in Australia for the word leukaemia and derivative terms only*)

whole hol/o

wide eury-

widen mydr/o

widening -dilation, mydri/o

with co-, com-, con-, sym-, syn-

within endo-, eso-, intra-, intro-

without a-, an- (*used when combining form starts with a vowel*)

woman gyn/o, gynaec/o

word, phrase lex/o

work erg/o

worm helminth/o, verm/i

wrinkle rhytid/o, rug/o

writing -gram

xiphoid process xiph/o, xiph/i

x-ray radi/o, roentgen/o

yellow cirrh/o, lute/o, xanth/o

zygomatic arch zygomat/o

Specific word elements

WORD ELEMENTS RELATED TO TIME AND PLACE

ante-, pro- before, forward

co-, com-, con-, sym-, syn- together, with

fore-, pre- before, in front of

-gen, gen/o originating, producing, causing

meta- beyond, change

noct/i night

nyct/o night, darkness

par- beyond, aside, apart from, other than, near, against

post- after, behind

primi-, proto-, -arche first

tel/o, tele- distant, end, far, complete

ultra- beyond, excess

WORD ELEMENTS DESCRIBING DIRECTION AND POSITION IN RELATION TO OTHER PARTS

ab- away from

ad- toward

af-, ag-, ap- to, towards, near

ana- up, towards, apart

ap/o away from, detached, derived from

de- away from, removal of, lack of, less

dextro- right side

dia- through, across

ec-, ect-, ecto- out, outside

endo- within, inside, inner

epi- above, upon, on

hyper- above, excessive

hypo- below, under, deficient, less than normal

in-, im- in, none, not

infra- inferior to, below

inter- between

intra- within, inside

juxta- adjoining, near

medi/o, mes/o middle

para- beside, near, alongside

peri- around, surrounding

retro- behind, backward

sinistr/o left side

sub- under, below

supra- above, excessive

trans- across, through, over

WORD ELEMENTS DESCRIBING NUMBER AND QUANTITY

ambi- both sides

bi- two, twice, double

dipl/o, dupl/i double

**equi-,
iso-** equal, same

hemi- half

hol/o whole, entire

mono- one, single

multi- many, much

nulli- none

olig/o scanty, deficiency, few

pan- all, entire

pleo- more

poly- many, much

quadri- four

semi- half

tetra- four

tri- three

uni- one

WORD ELEMENTS RELATING TO SIZE AND AMOUNT

aniso- unequal, asymmetrical, dissimilar

brachy- short

-cule small

lept/o thin, fine, slender

macro- large

mega- abnormally large

micro- small

-ole little, small
olig/o scanty, few, deficiency

WORD ELEMENTS DENOTING COLOUR

albin/o, alb/o white
chlor/o green
chrom/o, chromat/o colour
cirrh/o orange, yellow
cyan/o blue
eosin/o red, dawn, rosy
erythr/o, erythem/o, erythemat/o red
leuc/o, leuk/o white
melan/o black
xanth/o yellow

WORD ELEMENTS RELATING TO BODY PARTS

aden/o gland
angi/o (blood) vessel
aort/o aorta
arteri/o, arter/o artery
balan/o glans penis
blephar/o eyelid
brachi/o arm
cardi/o heart
carp/o carpal, wrist
cephal/o head
cheil/o lip
cheir/o, chir/o hand
cholecyst/o gallbladder
colp/o vagina
cor/o, core/o pupil (of the eye)
crani/o cranium, skull
cyst/o sac, urinary bladder, cyst
dactyl/o finger, toe
-derma, derm/o, dermat/o skin
encephal/o brain
enter/o intestine (usually small)
epididym/o epididymis

epiglott/o epiglottis
episi/o vulva
gastr/o stomach
gloss/o, glott/o tongue
gnath/o jaw
gon/o knee, seed, semen
haem/o, haemat/o blood
hepat/o liver
hepatic/o hepatic bile duct
hyster/o, metr/o uterus
kerat/o hard, horny tissue, cornea
lapar/o abdomen
laryng/o larynx, voice box
lip/o fat
mast/o breast
my/o muscle
myel/o bone marrow, spinal cord
nephr/o kidney
neur/o nerve
odont/o teeth
omphal/o umbilicus
onych/o nail
oo/o eggs, ova
oophor/o ovary
ophthalm/o eye
orch/o, orchi/o, orchid/o testis
oste/o bone
ot/o ear
pector/o chest
ped/o foot
pelv/i, pelv/o pelvis
pen/i penis
periton/o peritoneum
phac/o, phak/o lens of the eye
phall/o penis
pharyng/o pharynx, throat
phleb/o vein
pleur/o pleura
pneum/o, pneumat/o, pneumon/o lungs, respiration, air
psych/o mind

pyel/o renal pelvis

rhin/o nose

salping/o fallopian tubes, eustachian (auditory) tube

som/o, somat/o, somatic/o body

steth/o chest

stomat/o mouth

thel/o nipple

thorac/o thorax, chest

thromb/o clot

trache/o trachea

trachel/o neck, uterine cervix

trich/o hair

ur/o urine, urinary tract, urea

ureter/o ureter

urethr/o urethra

WORD ELEMENTS PROVIDING DESCRIPTION

ankyl/o crooked, bent, stiff

bar/o weight, pressure

brachy-, brevi- short

brady- slow

cac/o ill, unpleasant, bad, abnormal

cry/o cold

dys- bad, painful, difficult

eu- good, normal

eury- broad, wide

gyn/o, gynaec/o woman, female

iso- equal, same

macro- large

mal- bad

malac/o soft, softening

-malacia condition of softening

mega- abnormally large

megal/o enlargement

micro- small

mort/o, necr/o dead, death

neo- new

oestr/o oestrogen, female hormone

orth/o upright, straight

oxy- quick, sharp

pachy- thick

plan/o flat

poikil/o irregular, varied

pseudo- false

-sclerosis hardening

sten/o narrow, constricted

tachy- rapid, fast

viril/o masculine

Normal reference values for haematological testing

These reference values and results have been taken from *Mosby's Dictionary of Medicine, Nursing & Health Professions* (revised 3rd Australian and New Zealand edition) by Harris, Nagy and Vardaxis (editors).

Over time, changes in tests, techniques and equipment may occur. Value ranges may also vary between different pathology laboratories. Therefore values quoted in the reference values listed here may also change over time, so caution should be used when using the material contained here.

There are two main systems of measurement for reporting of haematological results: conventional units and the International System of Units, better known as SI units. In the reference values listed here, other than for a few exceptions, SI unit ranges are provided because this is the system normally used for scientific and technical reporting. SI units are absolute counts, not percentages.

Some common measurement abbreviations found in these reference values are listed in the following column.

fL	femtolitre (equivalent of one cubic micrometre (μm))
g/L	grams per litre
IU	international unit
kPa	kilopascal
L	litre
mg	milligram
mg/L	milligrams per litre
mL	millilitre
mm	millimetre
mmHg	millimetres of mercury
mmol/L	millimoles per litre
ng/mL	nanograms per litre
nmol/L	nanomoles per litre
pg	picogram
pmol/L	picomoles per litre
s	seconds
U/L	units per litre
μg/L	micrograms per litre
μmol/L	micromoles per litre

NORMAL REFERENCE VALUES TABLE

Reference intervals for haematology	
Test	**SI units**
Alkaline phosphatase, leucocyte	Total score 14–100
Cell counts	
Erythrocytes	
Males	$4.5–6.5 \times 10^{12}$/L
Females	$3.4–5.8 \times 10^{12}$/L
Children (varies with age)	$4.5–5.1 \times 10^{12}$/L
Leucocytes, total	$4.0–11.0 \times 10^{9}$/L
Leucocytes, differential counts	
Myelocytes	0/L
Neutrophils	$2.0–7.5 \times 10^{9}$/L
Lymphocytes	$1.5–4.0 \times 10^{9}$/L
Monocytes	$0.2–0.8 \times 10^{9}$/L
Eosinophils	$0.04–0.4 \times 10^{9}$/L
Basophils	$< 0.2 \times 10^{9}$/L
Platelets	$150–400 \times 10^{9}$/L
Reticulocytes	$25–75 \times 10^{9}$/L (0.2%–2.0% of erythrocytes)

Table continued

Test	SI units
Coagulation tests	
Anti-Factor Xa Sampling time: 3–4 hours post injection	0.5–1.2 Anti-Xa IU/mL
Bleeding time (template)	2.75–8.0 min
Coagulation time (glass tube)	5–15 min
D-dimer	< 0.5 mg/L
Factor VIII and other coagulation factors	0.5–1.5 of normal
Fibrin split products	< 10 mg/L
Fibrinogen	2.0–4.0 g/L
International normalised ratio (INR) (conventional units used in Australia)	Conventional 0.9–1.1 (normal)
Partial thromboplastin time, activated (aPTT)	Conventional 25.0–41.0 s
Prothrombin time (PT)	Conventional 12.0–14.0 s
Coombs' test	
Direct	Negative
Indirect	Negative
C-reactive protein (CRP)	< 5 mg/L
Corpuscular values of erythrocytes	
Mean corpuscular haemoglobin (MCH)	26–34 pg/cell
Mean corpuscular volume (MCV)	80–100 fL
Mean corpuscular haemoglobin concentration (MCHC)	320–360 g/L
Haptoglobin	0.20–1.65 g/L
Haematocrit (packed cell volume)	
Males	0.40–0.54
Females	0.37–0.47
Newborns	0.49–0.54
Children (varies with age)	0.35–0.49
Haemoglobin (conventional units used in Australia)	
Males	Conventional 130–180 g/L; SI 8.1–11.2 mmol/L
Females	Conventional 115–165 g/L; SI 7.4–9.9 mmol/L
Newborns	Conventional 165–195 g/L; SI 10.2–12.1 mmol/L
Children (varies with age)	Conventional 112–165 g/L; SI 7.0–10.2 mmol/L
Haemoglobin, fetal	< 0.01 of total
Haemoglobin A_{1c}	0.03–0.05 of total
Haemoglobin A_2	0.015–0.03 of total
Haemoglobin, plasma	0.0–3.2 μmol/L
Methaemoglobin	19–80 μmol/L
Sedimentation rate (ESR)	
Males	17–50 years: 1–10 mm/hour 51–70 years: < 14 mm/hour > 70 years: < 30 mm/hour
Females	17–50 years: 3–19 mm/hour 51–70 years: < 20 mm/hour > 70 years: < 35 mm/hour

Reference intervals* for clinical chemistry (blood, serum, plasma)

Analyte	SI units
Acetoacetate plus acetone	
Qualitative	Negative
Quantitative	30–200 µmol/L
Acid phosphatase, serum (thymolphthalein monophosphate substrate)	0.1–0.6 U/L
Alanine aminotransferase (ALT) serum (previously SGPT)	1–45 U/L
Albumin, serum	32–45 g/L
Aldolase, serum	0.0–7.0 U/L
Aldosterone, plasma	
Standing	140–830 pmol/L
Recumbent	80–275 pmol/L
Alkaline phosphatase (ALP), serum	
Adult (non-pregnant)	25–100 U/L
Adolescent	100–500 U/L
Child	70–350 U/L
Neonate	50–300 U/L
Ammonia nitrogen, plasma	10–50 µmol/L
Amylase, serum	25–125 U/L
Anion gap, serum, calculated	8–16 mmol/L
Apolipoprotein A1 (apo A1)	1.0–1.8 g/L
Apolipoprotein B (apo B)	Ideally < 0.9 g/L
Ascorbic acid, blood	23–85 µmol/L
Aspartate aminotransferase (AST) serum (previously SGOT)	1–40 U/L
Base excess, arterial blood, calculated	0 +/– 2 mmol/L
Beta-carotene, serum	1.1–8.6 µmol/L
Bicarbonate	
Arterial blood	22–26 mmol/L
Venous blood	23–27 mmol/L
Bile acids, serum	0.8–7.6 µmol/L
Bilirubin, serum	
Conjugated	1.7–9.0 µmol/L
Total	5.1–19.0 µmol/L
Calcium, serum	2.1–2.6 mmol/L
Calcium, ionised, serum	1.16–1.30 mmol/L
Carbon dioxide, total, serum or plasma	24–31 mmol/L
Carbon dioxide tension (Pco_2), blood	4.6–6 kPa
Chloride, serum or plasma	95–110 mmol/L
Cholesterol, serum or ethylenediaminetetraacetic acid (EDTA) plasma	
Desirable range total (fasting)	< 4 mmol/L
Low-density lipoprotein (LDL) cholesterol	< 2.5 mmol/L
High-density lipoprotein (HDL) cholesterol	> 1.0 mmol/L
LDL/HDL ratio	< 4.5

Table continued

Analyte	SI units
Copper	11–22 µmol/L
Corticotrophin (ACTH), plasma, 8 AM	2–18 pmol/L
Cortisol, plasma	
8 AM	170–630 nmol/L
4 PM	80–410 nmol/L
10 PM	< 50% of 8 AM value
C-peptide	Fasting 0.8–0.9 µg/L
Creatine, serum	
Males	15–40 µmol/L
Females	25–70 µmol/L
Creatine kinase (CK), serum	
Males	60–220 U/L
Females	30–180 U/L
Creatine kinase MB isoenzyme, serum	< 5% of total CK activity < 5.0 ng/mL by immunoassay or > 12 U/L
Creatinine, serum	
Males	0.06–0.12 mmol/L or 60–120 µmol/L
Females	0.05–0.11 mmol/L or 50–110 µmol/L
Estimated glomerular filtration rate (eGFR)	Normal > 90 mL/min/1.73 m^2
Ferritin, serum	
Males	30–300 µg/L
Females	15–200 µg/L
Fibrinogen, plasma	2.0–4.0 g/L
Folate, serum	6.8–45 nmol/L
Erythrocytes	360–1400 nmol/L
Follicle-stimulating hormone (FSH), plasma	
Males	4–25 U/L
Females, premenopausal	4–30 U/L
Females, postmenopausal	40–250 U/L
Gamma-glutamyltransferase (GGT), serum	
Males	< 50 U/L
Females	< 30 U/L
Gastrin, fasting, serum	0–100 ng/L
Glucose, fasting, plasma or serum	3.0–7.8 mmol/L
Glycosylated haemoglobin (HbA1c)	
Non diabetics	< 6.0%
Diabetics	< 7%
Growth hormone (hGH), plasma, adult, fasting	0–6 µg/L
Haptoglobin, serum	0.20–1.65 gm/L
Iron, serum	10–30 µmol/L
Iron binding capacity, serum	
Total	45–73 µmol/L
Saturation	0.20–055

Table continued

Analyte	SI units
Lactate	
Venous whole blood	0.6–2.2 mmol/L
Arterial whole blood	0.6–1.7 mmol/L
Lactate dehydrogenase (LD or LDH), serum	110–280 U/L
Lipase, serum	10–140 U/L
Luteinising hormone (LH), serum	
Males	1–9 U/L
Females	
Follicular phase	2–10 U/L
Midcycle peak	15–65 U/L
Luteal phase	1–12 U/L
Postmenopausal	12–65 U/L
Magnesium serum	0.8–1.0 mmol/L
Oestradiol-17 beta, adult	
Males	35–240 pmol/L
Females	
Follicular	110–370 pmol/L
Ovulatory	730–1470 pmol/L
Luteal	180–510 pmol/L
Osmolality	285–295 mOsm/kg
Oxygen tension (partial pressure of oxygen in blood)	
Arterial blood (PaO$_2$)	10.6–13.3 kPa (age and altitude dependent)
Venous blood (PvO$_2$)	3.3–5.3 kPa
Saturation (SaO$_2$)	95–98%
pH	
Arterial blood	7.35–7.45
Venous blood	7.32–7.43
Phosphate, inorganic, serum	
Adult	0.8–1.75 mmol/L
Child	0–1 year 1.4–2.4 mmol/L
	2–10 years 1.0–2.0 mmol/L
Potassium	
Serum	3.8–5.0 mmol/L
Plasma	3.4–4.5 mmol/L
Progesterone, serum, adult	
Males	0.0–1.3 mmol/L
Females	
Follicular phase	0.3–4.8 mmol/L
Luteal phase	8.0–89.0 mmol/L
Prolactin, serum	
Males	1.0–15.0 µmol/L
Females	1.0–20.0 µmol/L

Table continued

Analyte	SI units
Protein, serum, electrophoresis	60–80 g/L
Albumin	35–55 g/L
Globulins	
Alpha$_1$	2.0–4.0 g/L
Alpha$_2$	5.0–9.0 g/L
Beta	6.0–11.0 g/L
Gamma	7.0–17.0 g/L
Pyruvate, blood	0.03–0.10 mmol/L
Rheumatoid factor	0.0–30.0 kIU/L
Sodium, serum or plasma	135–145 mmol/L
Testosterone, plasma	
Males, adult	10.4–41.6 nmol/L
Females, adult	0.7–2.6 nmol/L
Pregnant women	1.4–6.9 nmol/L
Thyroglobulin	3.42 µg/L
Thyrotrophin (hTSH), serum	
Both genders	0.1–5.0 mIU/L
Gestation (0–13 weeks)	< 0.03–3.0 mIU/L
Thyroxine (FT$_4$), free, serum	9–27 pmol/L
Thyroxine (T$_4$), serum	58–154 nmol/L
Thyroxine-binding globulin (TBG)	15.0–34.0 mg/L
Transferrin	15–45%
Triglycerides, serum, 12-hour fast	< 2 mmol/L or 0.4–1.5 g/L
Free Triiodothyronine (FT$_3$)	2.5–6.0 pmol/L
Triiodothyronine (T$_3$), serum	1.1–2.9 nmol/L
Triiodothyronine uptake, resin (T$_3$RU)	0.25–0.38
Urate	
Males	0.2–0.45 mmol/L
Females	0.15–0.40 mmol/L
Urea, serum or plasma	3.0–8.0 mmol/L
Urea nitrogen, serum or plasma	8.0–16.4 mmol/L
Viscosity, serum	1.4–1.8 × water
Vitamin A, serum	0.70–2.80 µmol/L
Vitamin B$_{12}$, serum	133–664 pmol/L
Zinc	9–16 µmol/L
Reference values may vary, depending on the method and sample source used.	

Abbreviations

1°, 2°, 3° primary (first degree), secondary (second degree), tertiary (third degree)

¹³¹I radioactive iodine

3DCRT three-dimensional conformal radiation therapy

⁶⁷Ga radioactive gallium

A&E accident and emergency department

AAA abdominal aortic aneurysm

Ab antibody

ABC advanced breast cancer

ABCDE asymmetry (shape), border (irregularity), colour (variation within lesion), diameter (> 6 mm), evolving (changes in size, shape or colour over time) – characteristics associated with skin cancer

ABGs arterial blood gases

ABMT autologous bone marrow transplant

ABO three main blood types, type A, type B, type O

AC anterior chamber

a.c. *ante cibum*, before meals

acc accommodation

ACE inhibitors angiotensin-converting enzyme inhibitors

ACG angle closure glaucoma

ACL anterior cruciate ligament

ACS acute coronary syndrome

ACTH adrenocorticotrophic hormone

AD *auris dextra* (right ear)

AD Alzheimer's disease

ad. lib. *ad libitum*, freely as wanted

AD(H)D attention-deficit (hyperactivity) disorder

ADH antidiuretic hormone

adj adjuvant therapy

ADL activities of daily living

ADT adult diphtheria tetanus vaccine

AF atrial fibrillation

AFB acid fast bacilli

AFP alpha fetoprotein

Ag antigen

AI aortic insufficiency

AI aromatase inhibitor

AI artificial insemination

AIDS acquired immunodeficiency syndrome

AKA above knee amputation

AL, AS *auris laeva, auris sinistral* (left ear)

ALL acute lymphocytic leukaemia, acute lymphoblastic leukaemia

alt. dieb. *alternus diebus*, on alternative days

AMI acute myocardial infarction

AML acute monocytic leukaemia, acute myelocytic leukaemia, acute myeloblastic leukaemia, or acute myeloid leukaemia

AMML acute myelomonocytic leukaemia

ANS autonomic nervous system

AOM acute otitis media

AP anteroposterior

APH antepartum haemorrhage

aq. *aqua*, water

AR aortic regurgitation

ARDS acute/adult respiratory distress syndrome

ARF acute respiratory failure

ARF acute renal failure

ARM artificial rupture of membranes

ARMD age-related macular degeneration

ART assisted reproductive treatment/technology

AS aortic stenosis

ASA American Society of Anesthesiologists physical classification system

ASC anterior subcapsular cataract

ASD atrial septal defect

ASD autism spectrum disorder

AST aspartate aminotransferase

ATN acute tubular necrosis

AU, a.u. *aures unitas, auris uterque* (both ears)

aur *auris* (the ear)

AV, A V atrioventricular

B-cells beta cells

Ba barium

BAER brainstem auditory evoked response

BBA born before arrival

BBB bundle branch block

BCC basal cell carcinoma

b.d. *bis die*, twice a day

BE barium enema

BERA brainstem evoked response audiometry

BF breastfeeding

BIBA brought in by ambulance

b.i.d. *bis in die*, twice a day

b.i.n. *bis in nocte*, two times at night

BKA below knee amputation

BM bone marrow

BMD scan bone mineral density scan

BMI body mass index

BMT bone marrow transplant

BNO bladder neck obstruction

BNO bowels not open

BP blood pressure

BPD bronchopulmonary dysplasia

BPH benign prostatic hypertrophy

bpm beats per minute

BRCA1 breast cancer 1

BRCA2 breast cancer 2

BS breath sounds

BSE breast self-examination

BSE bovine spongiform encephalopathy

BSM bilateral suction myringotomy

BUN blood urea nitrogen

Bx biopsy

C cervical — there are 7 cervical vertebrae: C1–C7

C&S culture and sensitivity

C1–C7 cervical vertebrae 1–7

Ca calcium

Ca cancer, carcinoma

CA chronological age

CABG coronary artery bypass graft

CACG chronic angle closure glaucoma

CAD coronary artery disease

CAL chronic airways limitation

cap., caps *capsula*, capsule

CAPD continuous ambulatory peritoneal dialysis

CAT computed axial tomography

CBT cognitive behaviour therapy

CCF congestive cardiac failure

CCPD continuous cycling peritoneal dialysis

CCS classical caesarean section

CCU coronary care unit

CE cataract extraction

CF cystic fibrosis

CHD congestive heart disease

CHD congenital heart disease

chemo chemotherapy

CHF congestive heart failure

Ci curies

CIN cervical intraepithelial neoplasia

CIS carcinoma in situ

CJD Creutzfeldt-Jakob disease

CKD chronic kidney disease

CLL chronic lymphocytic leukaemia

CMF cyclophosphamide, methotrexate and fluorouracil

CML chronic myelogenous leukaemia, chronic myeloid leukaemia, chronic myelocytic leukaemia

CMML chronic myelomonocytic leukaemia

CMV cytomegalovirus

CNS central nervous system

CO$_2$ carbon dioxide

CoA coarctation of aorta

COAD chronic obstructive airways disease

COLD chronic obstructive lung disease

COPD chronic obstructive pulmonary disease

COVID-19 coronavirus disease

CPAP continuous positive airways pressure

CPD cephalopelvic disproportion

CPR cardiopulmonary resuscitation

CRF chronic renal failure

CSF cerebrospinal fluid

CT, CAT computed tomography, computed axial tomography

CTCA computed tomography coronary angiography

CTG cardiotocograph

cTn1 cardiac troponin 1

CTS carpal tunnel syndrome

CVA cerebrovascular accident

CVC central venous catheter

CVD cardiovascular disease, cerebrovascular disease

CVP central venous pressure

CVS chorionic villus sampling

cx cervix

CXR chest x-ray

D&C dilation (dilatation) and curettage

D&V diarrhoea and vomiting

DCIS ductal carcinoma in situ

DEXA dual energy x-ray absorptiometry

DI diabetes insipidus

DIC disseminated intravascular coagulation or coagulopathy

diff. differential count (white blood cells)

DJD degenerative joint disease

DM diabetes mellitus

DMARD disease-modifying antirheumatic drugs

DMD Duchenne's muscular dystrophy

DOA dead on arrival

DOE dyspnoea on exertion

DOTS directly observed treatment, short course

DRE digital rectal examination

DSA digital subtraction angiography

DSM-5 (R) *Diagnostic and Statistical Manual of Mental Disorders* (American Psychiatric Association, 5th edition, 2013)

DT delirium tremens

DTP diphtheria tetanus pertussis vaccine

DUB dysfunctional uterine bleeding

DVT deep venous thrombosis

Dx diagnosis

DXT deep x-ray therapy

EAC external auditory canal

EBM expressed breast milk

EBV Epstein-Barr virus

ECC extracorporeal circulation

ECC external cardiac compression

ECCE extracapsular cataract extraction

ECG electrocardiogram

echo echocardiography

ECT electroconvulsive therapy

ECV external cephalic version

ED erectile dysfunction

ED emergency department

EDC estimated date of confinement

EDD estimated date of delivery

EEG electroencephalogram

EF ejection fraction

EIA enzyme immunoassay

ELISA enzyme-linked immunosorbent assay

EMG electromyogram

ENT ear, nose and throat

EOM extraocular movements

EPO erythropoietin

ERA evoked response audiometry

ERCP endoscopic retrograde cholangiopancreatography

ESR erythrocyte sedimentation rate

ESRD end-stage renal disease

ESWL extracorporeal shock wave lithotripsy

ET eustachian tube

ETOH ethanol (or alcohol)

ETT exercise tolerance test

ETT endotracheal tube

FAP familial adenomatous polyposis

FBC full blood count

FBG fasting blood glucose

FBS fasting blood sugar

Fe iron

FEV$_1$ forced expiratory volume in 1 second

FH fundal height

FHR fetal heart rate

FHx family history

FIGO International Federation of Gynecology and Obstetrics

FIT faecal immunochemical test

FNA fine-needle aspiration

FNA(B) fine-needle aspiration (biopsy)

FOBT faecal occult blood test

FS frozen section

FSH follicle-stimulating hormone

FTP failure to progress

FVC forced vital capacity

fx fracture

G gravida

g *gramme*, gram(s)

GA general anaesthetic

GAD generalised anxiety disorder

GCS Glasgow Coma Score

GCS Glasgow Coma Scale

GFR glomerular filtration rate

GH growth hormone

GIST gastrointestinal stromal tumour

GI(T) gastrointestinal (tract)

GnRH gonadotrophin-releasing hormone

GORD gastro-oesophageal reflux disease

GTT glucose tolerance test

gtt(s) *gutt(e)*, a drop(s)

GVH graft-versus-host

GVHD graft-versus-host disease

Gy gray

gyn/gynae gynaecology

h *hora*, hour

HAART highly active antiretroviral therapy

HAV, HBV, HCV, HDV, HEV hepatitis A virus, hepatitis B virus, hepatitis C virus, hepatitis D virus, hepatitis E virus

Hb, Hgb haemoglobin

hCG human chorionic gonadotrophin

Hct haematocrit

HDL high-density lipoproteins

HDN haemolytic disease of the newborn

HELLP haemolysis, elevated liver enzymes, low platelets

HER2 human epidermal growth factor receptor

Hib *Haemophilus influenza* type b

HIE hypoxic ischaemic encephalopathy

HIV human immunodeficiency virus

HLA human leucocytic antigen

HMD hyaline membrane disease

HPV human papillomavirus

HR heart rate

HRT hormone replacement therapy

HSV herpes simplex virus

H/T, HTN hypertension

HVS high vaginal swab

Hx history

I & D incision and drainage

IBD inflammatory bowel disease

IBS irritable bowel syndrome

ICC intercostal catheter

ICCE intracapsular cataract extraction

ICCM iodine-containing contrast medium

ICD implantable cardioverter defibrillator

ICP intracranial pressure

ICSI intracytoplasmic sperm injection

ICU intensive care unit

IDC indwelling catheter

IDDM insulin-dependent diabetes mellitus

iFOBT immunochemical faecal occult blood test

IgA, IgD, IgE, IgG, IgM immunoglobulin A, D, E, G, M

IM intramuscular

IM infectious mononucleosis

IMRT intensity modulated radiation therapy

IOFB intraocular foreign body

IOL intraocular lens

IOL induction of labour

IOP intraocular pressure

IQ intelligence quotient

ITP immune (idiopathic) thrombocytopenia purpura

IUCD intrauterine contraceptive device

IUD intrauterine device

IUD intrauterine death

IUGR intrauterine growth retardation

IUI intrauterine insemination

IV intravenous

IVF in-vitro fertilisation

IVP intravenous pyelogram

Ix investigation

JVP jugular venous pressure

KUB kidneys, ureters, bladder

L lumbar — there are five lumbar vertebrae, L1–L5

L litre(s)

L1–L5 lumbar vertebrae 1–5

L&D labour and delivery

LA local anaesthetic

LA left atrium

LASIK laser-assisted in situ keratomileusis

LBBB left bundle branch block

LBW low birthweight

LDL low-density lipoproteins

LEEP loop electrosurgical excision procedure

LFT(s) liver function test(s)

LGA large for gestational age

LH luteinising hormone

LHN Local Health Network

LIF left iliac fossa

LLETZ large loop excision of transformation zone

LLL left lower lobe (of lung)

LLQ left lower quadrant

LMO local medical officer

LMP last menstrual period

LMP low malignant potential

LMWH low molecular weight heparin

LOC loss of consciousness

LP lumbar puncture

LUL left upper lobe (of lung)

LUQ left upper quadrant

L(U)SCS lower (uterine) segment caesarean section

LV left ventricle

LVAD left ventricular assist device

LVH left ventricular hypertrophy

MA mental age

mane *mane*, in the morning

MAOI monoamine oxidase inhibitor

MBS Medicare Benefits Schedule

mcg microgram(s)

MCH mean corpuscular haemoglobin

MCHC mean corpuscular haemoglobin concentration or count

mCi millicuries

MCU micturating cystourethrogram

MCV mean corpuscular volume

MDD major depressive disorder

MERS-CoV Middle East respiratory syndrome coronavirus

mets metastases

mg milligram(s)

MHx medical history

MI myocardial infarction

MIBI scan sestamibi scan

MIDCAB minimally invasive direct coronary artery bypass

MIMS Monthly Index of Medical Specialties

mL millilitre(s)

mmHg millimetres of mercury

mmol millimole(s)

MMPI Minnesota Multiphasic Personality Inventory

MMR measles, mumps and rubella vaccine

MMSE Mini-Mental State Examination

MOAB monoclonal antibody

mono monocyte

MR mitral regurgitation

MRI magnetic resonance imaging

MROP manual removal of placenta

MRSA methicillin-resistant *Staphylococcus aureus*

MS multiple sclerosis

MSE Mental State Examination

MSH melanocyte stimulating hormone

MSQ Mental Status Questionnaire

MSU midstream urine

MSUCS midstream urine culture and sensitivity

MUGA multiple gated acquisition scan

MVP mitral valve prolapse

MVP mean venous pressure

N nitrogen

N&V nausea and vomiting

NBM nil by mouth

NEC necrotising enterocolitis

NED no evidence of disease

NG nasogastric

NGU non-gonococcal urethritis

NHL non-Hodgkin lymphoma

NIDDM non-insulin-dependent diabetes mellitus

NIHL noise-induced hearing loss

NK natural killer (cells)

NMSC non-melanoma skin cancer

NND neonatal death

NNJ neonatal jaundice

noct. *nocte*, at night

NOF neck of femur

n.p.o. *nil per os*, nothing by mouth

NSAID non-steroidal anti-inflammatory drug

NSR normal sinus rhythm

NSTEMI non-ST-elevation myocardial infarction

NSU non-specific urethritis

NT scan nuchal translucency scan

NVD normal vaginal/vertex delivery

O&G obstetrics and gynaecology

O$_2$ oxygen

OA osteoarthritis

OA occipitoanterior

OCD obsessive-compulsive disorder

OCP oral contraceptive pill

OD *oculus dexter* (right eye)

OD overdose

OE otitis externa

O/E on examination

OGD oesophagogastroduodenoscopy

OM otitis media

OME otitis media with effusion

OP occipito posterior

OPD outpatient department

ORIF open reduction and internal fixation (of fracture)

OS *oculus sinister* (left eye)

OT operating theatre

OT occipito transverse

OU *oculus uterque* (both eyes)

P para (the outcome of previous pregnancies)

PA posteroanterior

PAC premature atrial contraction

Pap smear Papanicolaou smear

PBS Pharmaceutical Benefits Scheme

p.c. *post cibum*, after meals

PCA patient-controlled analgesia

PCI percutaneous coronary intervention

PCP *Pneumocystis* pneumonia

PCR polymerase chain reaction

PD peritoneal dialysis

PDA patent ductus arteriosus

PE pulmonary embolism

PE physical examination

PE tube pressure-equalising tube

PEARL pupils equal and reactive to light

PEARLA pupils equal and reactive to light and accommodation

PEG tube percutaneous endoscopic gastrostomy tube

PEJ tube percutaneous endoscopic jejunostomy tube

PET positron emission tomography

PET pre-eclamptic toxaemia

PFR peak flow rate

pH a measure of acidity

phaco phacoemulsification

PHN Primary Health Network

PHx past history, personal history

PICC peripherally inserted central catheter

PID pelvic inflammatory disease

PIH pregnancy-induced hypertension

PKD polycystic kidney disease

PKU phenylketonuria

PMHx past medical history

PMN polymorphonuclear neutrophil

PMNL, poly polymorphonuclear leucocyte

PMS premenstrual syndrome

PND paroxysmal nocturnal dyspnoea

PNS peripheral nervous system

p.o. *per os*, by mouth

POAG primary open angle glaucoma

POC products of conception

(P)OP (persistent) occipito posterior

POP plaster of Paris

PPH postpartum haemorrhage

PR per rectum

p.r.n. *pro re nata*, as required

PPROM persistent premature rupture of membranes

PROM premature rupture of membranes

PSA prostate-specific antigen

PSHx past surgical history

PT prothrombin time

PTCA percutaneous transluminal coronary angioplasty

PTHC percutaneous transhepatic cholangiography

PTSD post-traumatic stress disorder

PTT partial thromboplastin time

PUD peptic ulcer disease

PUJ pelviureteric junction

PUL percutaneous ultrasonic lithotripsy

PUVA psoralen and ultraviolet A therapy

PVC premature ventricular contraction

PVD peripheral vascular disease

q.4h. *quaque 4 hora*, every four hours

q.6h. *quaque 6 hora*, every six hours

q.d. *quaque die*, every day

q.d.s. *quaque die sumendus*, four times a day

q.h.s. *quaque mora somni*, every night at bed time

q.i.d. *quater in die*, four times a day

q.a.m. *quaque die ante meridiem*, every morning

q.n. *quaque nocte*, every night

RA rheumatoid arthritis

RA right atrium

RAD radiation absorbed dose, roentgen absorbed dose

rad radiation

RAIU radioactive iodine uptake

RBBB right bundle branch block

RBC red blood cell, red blood count

RCC red cell count

RDS respiratory distress syndrome

REM rapid eye movement

RFA radiofrequency ablation

RIF right iliac fossa

RLL right lower lobe (of lung)

RLQ right lower quadrant

RMO resident medical officer

ROM range of movement

ROP retinopathy of prematurity

RP, RPG retrograde pyelogram

RPOC retained products of conception

RPR rapid plasma reagin (test for syphilis)

RR respiratory rate

RUL right upper lobe (of lung)

RUQ right upper quadrant

RV right ventricle

Rx symbol for prescription or treatment

S sacral

S1–S5 sacral vertebrae 1–5

SA, S-A sinoatrial

SAD seasonal affective disorder

SARS severe acute respiratory syndrome

SC subcutaneous

SCC squamous cell carcinoma

SCN special care nursery

SGA small for gestational age

SIADH syndrome of inappropriate antidiuretic hormone

SIDS sudden infant death syndrome

SIRT selective internal radiation therapy

SIS saline infusion sonohysterography

SLE systemic lupus erythematosus

SLE slit lamp examination

SMA sequential multiple analysis

SNB sentinel node biopsy

SNHL sensorineural hearing loss

SOB shortness of breath

SOBOE shortness of breath on exertion

SOM serous otitis media

SPECT single-photon emission computed tomography

SPF sunscreen protective factor

SROM spontaneous rupture of membranes

SRS stereotactic radiosurgery

SRT stereotactic radiotherapy

SSM superficial spreading melanoma

SSNHL sudden sensorineural hearing loss

SSRI selective serotonin reuptake inhibitor

stat. *statum*, immediately

STD sexually transmitted disease

STEMI ST-elevation myocardial infarction

STI sexually transmitted infection

SUD substance abuse disorder

SUDI sudden unexpected death in infancy

SVD spontaneous vaginal delivery

SHx surgical history

T thoracic

T-cells lymphocytes, matured in thymus

T&A tonsils and adenoids, tonsillectomy and adenoidectomy

T1–T12 thoracic vertebrae 1–12

T4, T8 T-cell lymphocytes

tab. *tabletta*, tablet

TAH total abdominal hysterectomy

TAHBSO total abdominal hysterectomy with bilateral salpingo-oophorectomy

TB tuberculosis

TBI traumatic brain injury

TBSA total body surface area

TCC transitional cell carcinoma

t.d.s. *ter die sumendum*, three times a day

TENS transcutaneous electrical nerve stimulation

TFTs thyroid function tests

TGA Therapeutic Goods Administration

THR total hip replacement

TIA transient ischaemic attack

t.i.d. *ter in die*, three times a day

TKR total knee replacement

TM tympanic membrane

TMJ temporomandibular joint

TMR transmyocardial revascularisation

TNM tumour, node, metastasis

TOE trans-oesophageal echocardiography

TOL trial of labour

TOP termination of pregnancy

TORP total ossicular replacement prosthesis

tPA, TPA tissue plasminogen activator

TPN total parenteral nutrition

TRAM flap transverse rectus abdominis myocutaneous flap

TRH thyrotrophin-releasing hormone

TRUS transrectal ultrasound

TSH thyroid-stimulating hormone

TSS toxic shock syndrome

TTN transient tachypnoea of newborn

TULIP transurethral ultrasound-guided laser-induced prostatectomy

TUNA transurethral needle ablation

TURP transurethral resection of the prostate

TVH total vaginal hysterectomy

U/S ultrasound

UA unstable angina

UA, U/A urinalysis

UACR urine albumin/creatinine ratio

Ung. *ungentum*, ointment

URTI upper respiratory tract infection

UTI urinary tract infection

UV ultraviolet

VA visual acuity

VAIN vaginal intraepithelial neoplasia

VBAC vaginal birth after caesarean

VCU(G) voiding cystourethrogram

VD venereal disease

VDRL venereal disease research laboratory

VE vaginal examination

VE vacuum extraction

VF ventricular fibrillation

VF visual field

VIN vulvar intraepithelial neoplasia

VMO visiting medical officer

VQ scan ventilation-perfusion scan

VSD ventricular septal defect

VT ventricular tachycardia

VV varicose vein

WAIS Wechsler adult intelligence scale

WBC white blood cell

WCC white cell count

WISC(-R) Wechsler intelligence scale for children (revised)

XR x-ray

♂ symbol for male

♀ symbol for female

↑ symbol meaning increase

↓ symbol meaning decrease

Ψ symbol for psychiatry/psychology

ΨRx symbol for psychotherapy

\# symbol for fracture

Dx symbol for diagnosis

Ix symbol for investigation

Rx symbol for prescription or treatment

μ**Ci** microcuries

Answer Guide

CHAPTER 1: BASIC WORD STRUCTURE

Exercise 1.1: WORD ANALYSIS

1. **therm / o / graph / ic**
   WR CV WR S
   (CF)

2. **gastr / o / enter / itis**
   WR CV WR S
   (CF)

3. **bronch / o / scopy**
   WR CV S
   (CF)

4. **an / aesthes / ia**
   P WR S

5. **angi / o / gram**
   WR CV S
   (CF)

6. **lapar / o / tomy**
   WR CV S
   (CF)

7. **blephar / o / plasty**
   WR CV S
   (CF)

8. **ather / o / sclerosis**
   WR CV S
   (CF)

9. **hepat / o / megaly**
   WR CV S
   (CF)

10. **col / o / stomy**
    WR CV S
    (CF)

Exercise 1.2: IDENTIFYING PREFIXES

1. a / pnoea; a- = no, not, without, absence of; meaning = absence of breathing
2. ante / flexion; ante- = before, forward; meaning = to bend or lean forward
3. post / menopausal; post- = after, behind; meaning = pertaining to after menopause
4. super / numerary; super- = above, excessive; meaning = pertaining to excessive number
5. hemi / gastrectomy; hemi- = half; meaning = surgical excision of half of the stomach
6. trans / urethral; trans- = across, through, over; meaning = pertaining to through the urethra
7. hypo / calcaemia; hypo- = below, under, deficient, less than normal; meaning = condition of less than normal calcium in the blood
8. epi / dermal; epi- = above, upon, on; meaning = pertaining to the top layer of the skin
9. dys / phagia; dys- = bad, painful, difficult; meaning = condition of difficulty swallowing
10. peri / cardium; peri- = around, surrounding; meaning = tissue surrounding the heart

Exercise 1.3: IDENTIFYING SUFFIXES

1. arthr / algia; -algia = pain; meaning = pain in joint
2. cholecyst / itis; -itis = inflammation; meaning = inflammation of gallbladder
3. carcin / oid; -oid = derived from, resembling; meaning = derived from, resembling cancer
4. cranio/ tomy; -tomy = incision, cut into; meaning = incision, cut into skull, cranium
5. osteo / genic; -genic = pertaining to formation, producing; meaning = pertaining to formation, producing bone

6. hyperglyc / aemia; -aemia = condition of blood; meaning = condition of excessive sugar in blood
7. cysto / scopy; -scopy = process of viewing; meaning = process of viewing urinary bladder
8. gastro / scope; -scope = instrument to view; meaning = instrument to view stomach
9. rhino / plasty; -plasty = surgical, plastic repair; meaning = surgical, plastic repair of nose
10. haematolog / ist; -ist = one who specialises in; meaning = one who specialises in the study of blood

Exercise 1.4: WORD ROOTS AND COMBINING FORMS

1. d
2. a
3. d
4. a
5. d
6. b
7. a
8. a
9. c
10. a
11. a
12. b
13. a
14. d
15. a

Exercise 1.5: WORD BUILDING

1. electrocardiogram
2. syndactyly
3. enteralgia
4. bradycardia
5. thermometer
6. oliguria
7. cystoscope
8. hypoglycaemia
9. dermatitis
10. haematology
11. hepatosis
12. anaemia
13. encephalopathy
14. enterectomy
15. epigastric
16. endocardium
17. cephalic
18. gastralgia
19. hypodermic (subcutaneous)
20. uraemia

Exercise 1.6: CROSSWORD PUZZLE

ACROSS
4. combining form
7. prefix
8. word root
9. suffix
10. dermal

DOWN
1. latin
2. combining vowel
3. hysterotomy
5. medical terminology
6. diarrhoea

CHAPTER 2: BUILDING A MEDICAL VOCABULARY

Exercise 2.1: SPELLING

1. c. arteriosclerosis
2. b. tonsillectomy
3. b. intramuscular
4. c. ileostomy
5. c. uraemia
6. a. antenatal
7. b. cystography
8. c. abdominocentesis
9. a. hemigastrectomy
10. c. axillary

Exercise 2.2: SPELLING AND CONTEXT

Medical term	Meaning	Medical term	Meaning
haematuria	condition of blood in urine	uraemia	condition of urea in blood
ilium	part of hip bone	ileum	part of small intestine
ureter	tube that carries urine from kidney to bladder	urethra	tube that carries urine from bladder to exterior

Medical term	Meaning	Medical term	Meaning
stomatitis	inflammation of mouth	infected stoma site	infection of artificial opening
poliomyelitis	inflammation of grey matter (of central nervous system)	osteomyelitis	inflammation of bone and bone marrow

Exercise 2.3: FORMING PLURALS AND SINGULAR TERMS

Medical term singular	Medical term plural
bacterium	bacteria
calyx	calyces
phalanx	phalanges
calculus	calculi
ecchymosis	ecchymoses
chalazion	chalazia
sinus	sinuses

Medical term plural	Medical term singular
spermatozoa	spermatozoon
ova	ovum
varices	varix
metastases	metastasis
ganglia	ganglion
epididymides	epididymis
rhonchi	rhonchus
vertebrae	vertebra

Exercise 2.4: EPONYMS – WHAT AM I?

1. A type of catheter inserted into the bladder to drain urine
2. A type of neurological disorder
3. A chart used in testing eyesight
4. A unilateral paralysis of the facial nerve
5. A break in the distal radius
6. A degenerative brain disease
7. First test given to a newborn
8. Acute bacterial pneumonia
9. A form of red-green colour blindness
10. A gynaecological screening test

Exercise 2.5: PRONUNCIATION AND COMPREHENSION

No answer provided – self-directed study.

Exercise 2.6: ANAGRAMS

1. dysp(h)agia
2. a(b)duct
3. ep(o)nym
4. (A)lzheimer's
5. il(i)um
6. Cow(p)ers

PHOBIA

Exercise 2.7: CROSSWORD PUZZLE

ACROSS
3. Down syndrome
6. Nissen fundoplication
8. Cushing's syndrome
9. Crohn's disease

DOWN
1. Bartholin's gland
2. Parkinson's disease
4. Shirodkar's suture
5. Penrose drain
7. Burkitt's lymphoma

CHAPTER 3: THE HUMAN BODY

Exercise 3.1: LABEL THE DIAGRAMS

1. right hypochondriac region
2. epigastric region
3. right lumbar region
4. right inguinal (iliac) region
5. left hypochondriac region
6. umbilical region
7. left lumbar region
8. left inguinal (iliac) region
9. hypogastric region

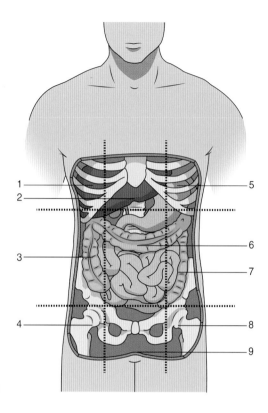

Figure 3.8
Regions of the abdomen

1. frontal plane or coronal plane
2. midsagittal plane
3. transverse plane

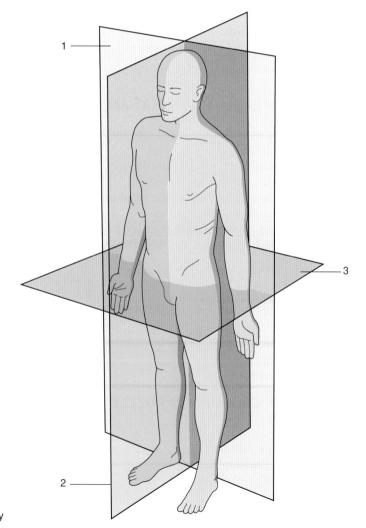

Figure 3.9
Planes of the body

1. superior
2. inferior
3. posterior/dorsal – back
4. proximal
5. distal
6. median line
7. medial   lateral
8. anterior/ventral – front
9. superficial
10. deep

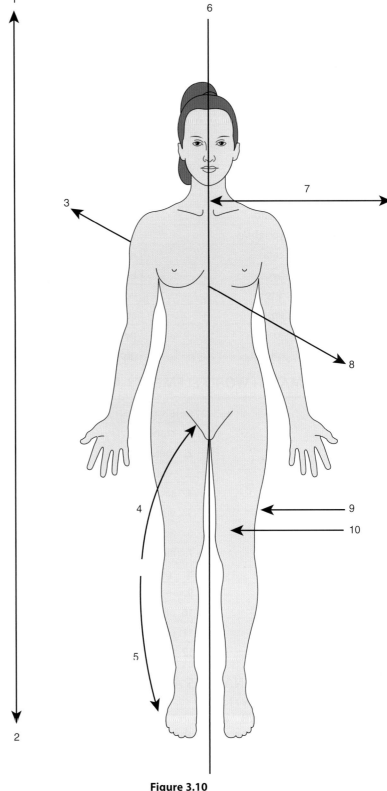

Figure 3.10
Anatomical directions

Exercise 3.2: WORD ELEMENT MEANINGS AND WORD BUILDING

No answer provided for the medical term – refer to your dictionary for the correct spelling.

Word element	Meaning
anter/o	front
coccyg/o	coccyx
cervic/o	neck, cervix uteri
cyt/o	cell
hist/o	tissue
inguin/o	groin
proxim/o	near
thel/o	nipple
vertebr/o	vertebra
cata-	down
hypo-	below, under, deficient, less than normal
inter-	between
epi-	above, upon, on
-ose	pertaining to, full of, sugar
-plasm	growth, formation, substance

Exercise 3.3: MATCH WORD ELEMENTS AND MEANINGS

Column A	Answer
1. crani/o	J
2. meta-	K
3. -eal	E
4. sacr/o	L
5. viscer/o	G
6. adip/o	I
7. ili/o	A
8. -plasia	C
9. -ectomy	D
10. umbilic/o	F
11. ov/o	B
12. kary/o	H

Exercise 3.4: WORD ANALYSIS AND MEANING

1. **abdomin / o / pelv / ic**
   WR CV WR S
   Meaning: pertaining to the abdomen and pelvis

2. **poster / o / later / al**
   WR CV WR S
   Meaning: pertaining to the back and sides

3. **thorac / ic**
   WR S
   Meaning: pertaining to the chest

4. **hypo / gastr / ic**
   P WR S
   Meaning: pertaining to below the stomach

5. **vertebr / al**
   WR S
   Meaning: pertaining to the vertebrae/spinal column

6. **inguin / al**
   WR S
   Meaning: pertaining to the groin

7. **pleur / al**
   WR S
   Meaning: pertaining to the pleura

8. **crani / o / tomy**
   WR CV S
   Meaning: incision into the skull

Exercise 3.5: VOCABULARY BUILDING

1. frontal or coronal
2. abdominal
3. connective
4. distal
5. supine
6. thoracic
7. adipose
8. sacrum
9. craniectomy
10. nucleus

Exercise 3.6: BUILDING MEDICAL TERMS

1. hypochondriac
2. spinal
3. epithelial
4. intervertebral
5. ventral
6. superior

Exercise 3.7: EXPAND THE ABBREVIATIONS

Abbreviation	Expanded abbreviation
RUQ	right upper quadrant
C1	first cervical vertebra
LUQ	left upper quadrant
T12–L1	space between 12th thoracic vertebra and 1st lumbar vertebra
LLQ	left lower quadrant
DNA	deoxyribonucleic acid
RLQ	right lower quadrant
AP	anteroposterior

Exercise 3.8: APPLYING MEDICAL TERMINOLOGY

1. superior or proximal
2. midsagittal
3. lateral
4. medial
5. superior
6. distal
7. transverse
8. coronal or frontal
9. external
10. inferior

Exercise 3.9: APPLYING MEDICAL TERMINOLOGY

cell, tissue, organ, body system

Exercise 3.10: PRONUNCIATION AND COMPREHENSION

No answer provided – self-directed study.

Exercise 3.11: CROSSWORD PUZZLE

ACROSS
4. prone
5. coronal
8. intervertebral

DOWN
1. superior
2. pelvic
3. cell
6. anatomy
7. gene

Exercise 3.12: ANAGRAMS

1. med(i)al
2. (v)entral
3. peri(t)oneum
4. lar(y)nx
5. (c)hondroma
6. org(a)ns
CAVITY

CHAPTER 4: MUSCULOSKELETAL SYSTEM

Exercise 4.1: LABEL THE DIAGRAMS

1. frontal bone
2. nasal bone
3. zygomatic bone
4. sternum
5. ribs
6. vertebral column
7. coxal (hip) bone
8. ilium
9. sacrum
10. coccyx
11. greater trochanter of femur
12. pubis
13. ischium
14. orbit
15. maxilla
16. mandible
17. clavicle
18. manubrium
19. scapula
20. costal cartilage
21. xiphoid process
22. humerus
23. radius
24. ulna
25. carpal bones
26. metacarpal bones
27. phalanges
28. femur
29. patella
30. tibia
31. fibula
32. tarsal bones
33. metatarsal bones
34. phalanges
35. axial skeleton
36. appendicular skeleton

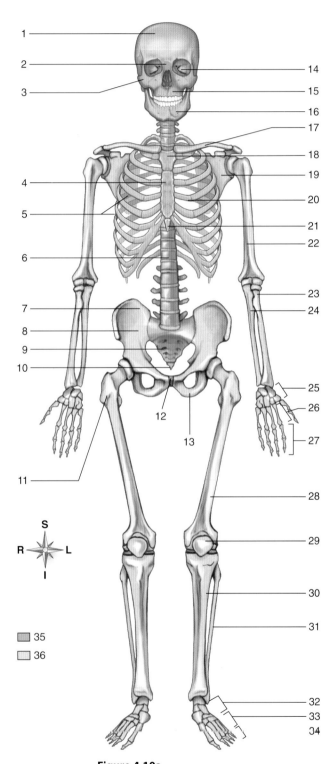

Figure 4.10a
Anterior view of the skeleton

1. clavicle
2. acromion
3. scapula
4. ribs
5. humerus
6. ulna
7. radius
8. sacrum
9. coccyx
10. ischium
11. parietal bone
12. occipital bone
13. cervical vertebrae (7)
14. thoracic vertebrae (12)
15. lumbar vertebrae (5)
16. coxal (hip) bone
17. carpal bones
18. metacarpal bones
19. phalanges
20. femur
21. tibia
22. fibula
23. tarsal bones
24. phalanges
25. metatarsal bones
26. calcaneus

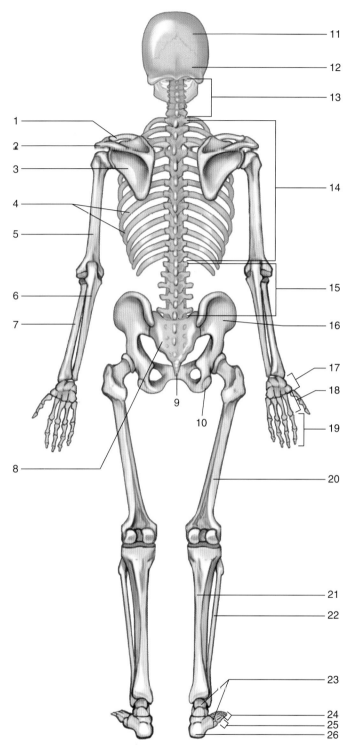

Figure 4.10b
Posterior view of the skeleton

Exercise 4.2: WORD ANALYSIS AND MEANING

1. cost/o = ribs; vertebr/o = vertebra, spinal column; -al = pertaining to; meaning = pertaining to the ribs and spinal column
2. arthr/o = joint; -scopy = process of viewing; meaning = process of viewing a joint
3. oste/o = bones; -genic = pertaining to formation; meaning = pertaining to formation of bones
4. burs/o = bursa; -itis = inflammation; meaning = inflammation of bursa
5. menisc/o = meniscus; -ectomy = excision, surgical removal; meaning = excision, surgical removal of meniscus
6. poly = many, much; myos/o = muscle; -itis = inflammation; meaning = inflammation of many muscles
7. inter = between; vertebr/o = vertebra, spinal column; -al = pertaining to; meaning = pertaining to between the vertebrae
8. fibr/o = fibre; my/o = muscle; -algia = pain; meaning = pain in muscle fibre
9. dys- = bad, painful, difficult; kinesia = pertaining to movement, motion; meaning = pertaining to bad, painful or difficult movement
10. lord/o = curve, sway back; -osis = abnormal condition; meaning = abnormal condition of sway back

Exercise 4.3: MATCH WORD ELEMENTS AND MEANINGS

Column A	Answer
1. spondyl/o	D
2. -listhesis	E
3. scoli/o	G
4. lei/o	I
5. -desis	C
6. articul/o	B
7. rhabd/o	F
8. cleid/o	A
9. tort/i	L
10. lumb/o	K
11. -stenosis	H
12. -asthenia	J

Exercise 4.4: MATCH MEDICAL TERMS AND MEANINGS

Column A	Answer
1. metatarsals	B
2. radius	K
3. occipital bone	G
4. fibula	H
5. patella	A
6. Ischium	J
7. femur	C
8. calcaneus	L
9. zygoma	F
10. sternum	D
11. mandible	E
12. ethmoid	I

Exercise 4.5: EXPAND THE ABBREVIATIONS

Abbreviation	Expanded abbreviation
ACL	anterior cruciate ligament
CT scan	computed tomography scan
CTS	carpal tunnel syndrome
MRI	magnetic resonance imaging
NOF	neck of femur
NSAID	non-steroidal anti-inflammatory drug
OA	osteoarthritis
ORIF	open reduction internal fixation
T1–T12	thoracic vertebrae 1–12
TKR	total knee replacement

Exercise 4.6: APPLYING MEDICAL TERMINOLOGY

1. d
2. d
3. c
4. d
5. b

6. c
7. a
8. c
9. b
10. d

Exercise 4.7: CORRECT THE SPELLING AND IDENTIFY THE INCORRECT TERMS

1. atrofy = atrophy; authopedic = orthopaedic
2. spondilosis = spondylosis; vertebrae = vertebra; lumber = lumbar; saccrum = sacrum
3. bylateral carple tunnel syndrome = bilateral carpal tunnel syndrome; compress = decompress; middle = median
4. arteritis = arthritis; prosthotic = prosthetic
5. spinal = spiral

Exercise 4.8: PRONUNCIATION AND COMPREHENSION

No answer provided – self-directed study.

Exercise 4.9: CROSSWORD PUZZLE

ACROSS
2. rotator cuff syndrome
4. fracture
5. cartilage
8. ossification
9. polymyositis
10. fibrous

DOWN
1. striated
3. aponeurosis
6. arthritis
7. scoliosis

Exercise 4.10: ANAGRAMS

1. ligamen(t)
2. myalg(i)a
3. (s)ubluxation
4. flex(i)on
5. m(a)ndible

6. clavi(c)le
7. fas(c)ia
8. (a)bduction
SCIATICA

Exercise 4.11: DISCHARGE SUMMARY ANALYSIS

1. GA = general anaesthetic; ORIF = open reduction internal fixation; IV = intravenous; Dx = diagnosis; # = fracture

2. A non-union of a fracture is the failure of the broken bones to unite in the time expected for a particular type of fracture in a specific bone. In other words, a non-union of a fracture is one that has failed to heal after several months. This should not be confused with a malunion of a fracture, which is a bone that has healed in a deformed position, causing significant impairment and loss of function or that may be cosmetically unacceptable.

3. An autologous bone graft is a procedure in which missing bone is replaced with bone harvested from the patient's own body (auto = self) and used to repair bone fractures. The harvested bone provides a framework for new bone to grow on. The bone for grafting is often harvested from the iliac crest.

4. The brachial plexus is a network of nerves that originate near the neck and shoulder and conduct signals from the spinal cord, to the shoulder, arm and hand. Brachial plexus injuries are caused by damage to these nerves. The nerves are fragile and can easily be injured by stretching when the head and neck are forced away from the shoulder. This can occur in a motorcycle accident, as happened to Mr Brown.

5. A hypersensitivity reaction is also called an allergic reaction. It occurs when a foreign substance such as pollen, dust or a medication (in this case, cloxacillin) enters the body. When the body senses the foreign substance (called an antigen), the immune system is triggered. It sets off an allergic response that can range from mild symptoms such as urticaria to a life-threatening anaphylactic reaction. These reactions may occur within seconds or minutes, especially if the body has been exposed to the allergen previously and has been 'sensitised'.

CHAPTER 5: INTEGUMENTARY SYSTEM

Exercise 5.1: LABEL THE DIAGRAM

1. epidermis
2. dermis
3. subcutaneous fat
4. nerve
5. muscle
6. sebaceous gland
7. upper vascular plexus
8. hair follicle
9. sweat gland
10. lower vascular plexus

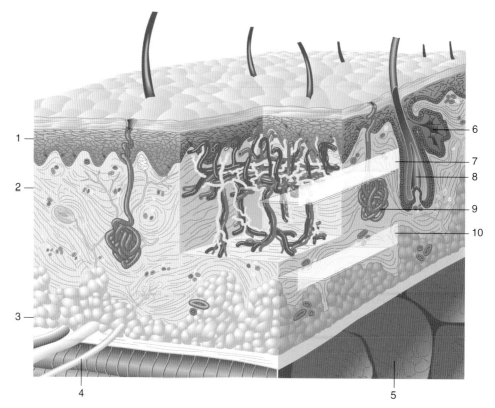

Figure 5.14
Structure of the skin

Exercise 5.2: WORD ANALYSIS AND MEANING

1. sub- = under, below; ungu/o = nail; -al = pertaining to; meaning = pertaining to under the nail
2. blephar/o = eyelid; -plasty = surgical, plastic repair; meaning = surgical, plastic repair of eyelid
3. onych/o = nail; myc/o = fungus; -osis = abnormal condition; meaning = abnormal condition of fungus in the nails
4. dermat/o = skin; fibr/o = fibres; -oma = tumour; meaning = tumour of skin fibres
5. xanth/o = yellow; -derma = skin; meaning = skin that is yellow
6. trich/o = hair; phyt/o = plant, fungus; -osis = abnormal condition; meaning = abnormal condition of fungus in hair
7. hidr/o = sweat; aden/o = gland; -itis = inflammation; meaning = inflammation of sweat gland
8. albin/o = white; -ism = state of; meaning = state of white
9. xen/o = foreign, strange; -graft = transplant of tissue; meaning = transplant of tissue that is foreign
10. rhytid/o = wrinkle, crease; -ectomy = excision, surgical removal; meaning = excision of wrinkle

Exercise 5.3: MATCH WORD ELEMENTS AND MEANINGS

Column A	Answer
1. pachy-	G
2. pil/o	I
3. erythem/o	F
4. -trophy	A
5. cutane/o	B
6. diaphor/o	J
7. acanth/o	H
8. intra-	D
9. -plasty	C
10. -tropic	E

Exercise 5.4: MATCH MEDICAL TERMS AND MEANINGS

Column A	Answer
1. alopecia	G
2. ecchymosis	C
3. icterus	J
4. keloid	E
5. melanoma	H
6. nodule	I
7. scleroderma	B
8. telangiectasia	F
9. urticaria	A
10. verruca	D

Exercise 5.5: VOCABULARY BUILDING

1. squamous cell carcinoma
2. dermatitis
3. keratosis
4. seborrhoea
5. electrocautery
6. allograft or homograft
7. anhidrosis
8. lipocyte
9. rhinophyma
10. xeroderma

Exercise 5.6: EXPAND THE ABBREVIATIONS

Abbreviation	Expanded abbreviation
ABCDE	asymmetry, border, colour, diameter, evolving
BCC	basal cell carcinoma
Bx	biopsy
FS	frozen section
I&D	incision and drainage
PUVA	psoralen and ultraviolet A (therapy)
SCC	squamous cell carcinoma
SLE	systemic lupus erythematosus
SPF	sunscreen protection factor
UV	ultraviolet

Exercise 5.7: APPLYING MEDICAL TERMINOLOGY

1. c
2. c
3. c
4. b
5. c

6. c
7. a
8. a
9. c
10. d

Exercise 5.8: VOCABULARY BUILDING

No answer provided – self-directed study. Refer to medical dictionary for meaning of terms.

Exercise 5.9: CROSSWORD PUZZLE

ACROSS
2. sweat gland
6. melanoma
8. graft
10. eccrine gland

DOWN
1. vitiligo
3. dermis
4. rosacea
5. sebum
7. acne
9. flap

Exercise 5.10: ANAGRAMS

1. kcloi(d)
2. sebu(m)
3. ulce(r)
4. eryth(e)ma

5. alopcc(i)a
6. psoriasi(s)
DERMIS

Exercise 5.11: DISCHARGE SUMMARY ANALYSIS

1. SCC – squamous cell carcinoma; LA – local anaesthetic; ASA – American Society of Anesthesiologists; LMO = local medical officer
2. This procedure is indicated for removing an invasive SCC on the lip, particularly if it involves the vermillion border. A wedge-shaped section of tissue is removed and then the deficit is repaired. This type of excision allows for complete removal of the tumour and a better repair.
3. This refers to the shape of the repair to the lower lip after the lesion has been removed. Various geometrical shapes (usually described by a letter such as y, v, m) of skin can be used to fill in the defects left after the excision of a skin cancer. These are commonly used on the face to give better cosmetic results.

4. This means that all the SCC was removed and the edge of the lesion that was excised did not contain tumour.

5. These terms refer to the histologic grade of the tumour. They describe how different the cells are from normal cells. Well-differentiated SCC cells closely resemble the cells of origin, while poorly differentiated SCC cells are difficult to recognise as to their cell of origin. If a tumour is described as poorly differentiated, it has a poorer prognosis and is more likely to spread throughout the body.

CHAPTER 6: HAEMATOLOGY

Exercise 6.1: LABEL THE DIAGRAM

1. monocyte
2. eosinophil
3. plasma
4. erythrocyte
5. neutrophil
6. lymphocyte
7. basophil
8. platelet
9. leucocyte

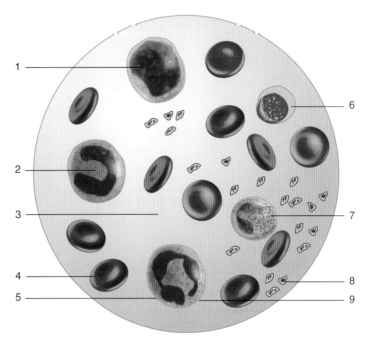

Figure 6.7
Blood smear

Exercise 6.2: WORD ELEMENT MEANINGS AND WORD BUILDING

No answer provided for the medical term – refer to your dictionary for the correct spelling.

Word element	Meaning
chrom/o	colour
erythr/o	red
haem/o	blood
leuc/o	white
mono-	one, single
myel/o	bone marrow, spinal cord
phag/o	eat, swallow
phleb/o	vein
pan-	all, entire
poly-	many, much
-aemia	condition of blood
-blast	embryonic or developing cell
-penia	deficiency
-philia	attraction for
-rrhage	bursting forth, excessive discharge or flow

Exercise 6.3: MATCH WORD ELEMENTS AND MEANINGS

Column A	Answer
1. cyt/o	J
2. -globin	E
3. macro-	K
4. poikil/o	A
5. -stasis	B
6. -rrhexis	C
7. -crit	L
8. micro-	G
9. -apheresis	D
10. -genesis	I
11. sangu/i	F
12. kary/o	H

Exercise 6.4: VOCABULARY BUILDING

1. leucocyte
2. erythrocytopenia
3. haematopoiesis
4. thrombocyte
5. splenomegaly
6. neutropenia

Exercise 6.5: WORD ANALYSIS AND MEANING

1. splen / o / rrhexis; meaning = rupture of the spleen
2. poly / cyt / haem / ia; meaning = condition of many blood cells (usually refers to erythrocytes)
3. erythr /o / blast / osis; meaning = abnormal condition of embryonic red cells
4. phleb / o / tomy; meaning = incision into vein
5. haem / o / chromat / osis; meaning = abnormal condition of blood colour
6. leuc / o / penia; meaning = deficiency of white (blood cells)
7. haem / o / lysis; meaning = breakdown of blood
8. an / aem / ia; meaning = without blood

Exercise 6.6: VOCABULARY BUILDING

1. anisocytosis
2. haemorrhage
3. haematoma
4. hypercalcaemia
5. hyperkalaemia
6. haematopoiesis
7. acidosis
8. haemostasis
9. blastocyte
10. poikilocytosis

Exercise 6.7: EXPAND THE ABBREVIATIONS AND MATCH WITH THE MEANING

Column A	Expanded abbreviation	Match
1. AML	acute monocytic, myelocytic, myeloblastic or myeloid leukaemia	H
2. FBC	full blood count	D
3. EBV	Epstein-Barr virus	F
4. RCC	red cell count	J
5. PT	prothrombin time	A
6. ITP	immune or idiopathic thrombocytopenia purpura	B
7. Hb	haemoglobin	C
8. ESR	erythrocyte sedimentation rate	I

Column A	Expanded abbreviation	Match
9. GVH	graft versus host	E
10. IgA	immunoglobulin A	G

Exercise 6.8: VOCABULARY BUILDING

1. plasma
2. haemoglobin
3. anacmia
4. platelets
5. phagocytosis
6. red cell count
7. transfusion
8. ncutrophils
9. white cell
10. pernicious

Exercise 6.9: PRONUNCIATION AND COMPREHENSION

No answer provided – self-directed study.

Exercise 6.10: ANAGRAMS

1. cyto(l)ogy
2. (s)ideropenia
3. pl(a)telet
4. baso(p)hil
5. (m)yeloid
6. hep(a)rin

PLASMA

Exercise 6.11: CROSSWORD PUZZLE

ACROSS
4. eosinophil
5. purpura
9. neutropenia
10. haemophilia
11. bilirubin
12. serum

DOWN
1. haemoglobin
2. apheresis
3. leucocyte
6. monocyte
7. septicaemia
8. anisocytosis

Exercise 6.12: APPLYING MEDICAL TERMINOLOGY

1. A, B, O, AB
2. Universal donor – Blood group O negative; Universal recipient – Blood group AB positive
3. Any

Exercise 6.13: MATCH THE ANAEMIA TYPE WITH THE DESCRIPTION

Column A	Answer
1. aplastic anaemia	D
2. haemolytic anaemia	E
3. haemorrhagic anaemia	A
4. sickle cell anaemia	C
5. thalassaemia	B

Exercise 6.14: DISCHARGE SUMMARY ANALYSIS

1. GI = gastrointestinal; GORD = gastro-oesophageal reflux disease; COAD = chronic obstructive airways disease; LV = left ventricle; Creat = creatinine; Hb = haemoglobin; Na = sodium; Ix = investigations; MI = myocardial infarction; LVH = left ventricular hypertrophy
2. Mrs Swifte was tired and fatigued and was diagnosed with anaemia with low iron levels due to a chronic blood loss. She was given a blood transfusion to increase the amount of iron in her blood.
3. Mrs Swifte had a chest x-ray because of her COAD/asthma with emphysema and exertional dyspnoea.
4. This means she is not interested in receiving any other tests or treatments.
5. End-stage kidney disease.

CHAPTER 7: LYMPHATIC AND IMMUNE SYSTEMS

Exercise 7.1: LABEL THE DIAGRAM

1. tonsils
2. cervical lymph node
3. right lymphatic duct
4. superficial cubital (supratrochlear) lymph nodes
5. aggregated lymphoid nodules (Peyer's patches)
6. red bone marrow
7. entrance of thoracic duct into subclavian vein
8. thymus gland
9. axillary lymph node
10. thoracic duct
11. spleen
12. cisterna chyli
13. inguinal lymph node

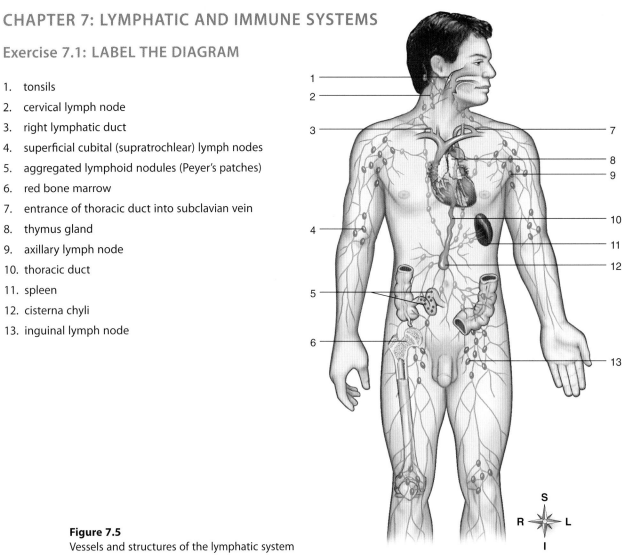

Figure 7.5
Vessels and structures of the lymphatic system

Exercise 7.2: WORD ELEMENT MEANINGS AND WORD BUILDING

No answer provided for the medical term – refer to your dictionary for the correct spelling.

Word element	Meaning
aden/o	gland
agglutin/o	clumping, gluing
angi/o	vessel
axill/o	armpit
inguin/o	groin
phag/o	swallow, eat
plas/o	formation
tox/o	poison, toxin
ana-	up, towards, apart
mono-	one
-blast	embryonic or developing cell
-genic	pertaining to formation, producing
-oid	derived from, resembling
-pathy	disease process
-phylaxis	protection

Exercise 7.3: MATCH WORD ELEMENTS AND MEANINGS

Column A	Answer
1. -poiesis	D
2. anti-	J
3. auto-	H
4. -stitial	I
5. cervic/o	K
6. -cyte	B
7. inter-	E
8. reticul/o	L
9. thym/o	A
10. retro-	C
11. -globin	G
12. immun/o	F

Exercise 7.4: WORD ANALYSIS AND MEANING

1. immunotherapy
   immun / o / therapy
     WR CV   S
   Meaning: treatment (to) protect

2. phagocytosis
   phag / o / cyt / osis
     WR CV WR S
   Meaning: abnormal condition of cells that eat

3. cytotoxic
   cyt / o / tox / ic
     WR CV WR S
   Meaning: pertaining to cells that are poisonous

4. lymphangiography
   lymph / angi / o / graphy
     WR   WR CV   S
   Meaning: process of recording lymph vessels

5. axillary
   axill / ary
     WR S
   Meaning: pertaining to the armpit

6. intercellular
   inter / cellul / ar
      P   WR   S
   Meaning: pertaining to between cells

7. lymphoid
   lymph / oid
     WR   S
   Meaning: resembling or derived from lymph (tissue)

8. lymphadenopathy
   lymph / aden / o / pathy
     WR WR CV   S
   Meaning: disease process of lymph glands

9. leucopoiesis
   leuc / o / poiesis
     WR CV   S
   Meaning: production of white (blood cells)

10. retropharyngeal
    retro / pharyng / eal
       P   WR   S
    Meaning: pertaining to behind the throat

Exercise 7.5: CIRCLE THE CORRECT SPELLING

axillary
reticulocyte
thymectomy
mononucleosis

agglutination
pyogenic
immunoglobulin
interstitial

Exercise 7.6: EXPAND THE ABBREVIATIONS

Abbreviation	Expanded abbreviation
AIDS	acquired immunodeficiency syndrome
B-cells	type of lymphocyte that produces antibodies, formed in bone marrow
CMV	cytomegalovirus
ELISA	enzyme-linked immunosorbent assay
HAART	highly active antiretroviral therapy
HIV	human immunodeficiency virus
IgA	immunoglobulin A
MOAB	monoclonal antibody
NHL	non-Hodgkin lymphoma
NK cells	natural killer cells
PCP	*Pneumocystis* pneumonia
SLE	systemic lupus erythematosus
T4, T8	T-cell lymphocytes
T-cells	lymphocytes, matured in thymus

Exercise 7.7: MATCH STRUCTURE WITH FUNCTION

Column A	Answer
1. macrophages	G
2. lymph vessels	C
3. adenoids	B
4. lymph	F
5. thymus gland	A
6. spleen	D
7. lymph nodes	H
8. interstitial fluid	E

Exercise 7.8: CROSSWORD PUZZLE

ACROSS
5. macrophages
6. tonsils
9. interstitial fluid
10. adenoids

DOWN
1. lymphocytes
2. thymus gland
3. anaphylaxis
4. ELISA test
7. spleen
8. AIDS

Exercise 7.9: ANAGRAMS

1. splee(n)
2. toxi(n)s
3. all(e)rgy
4. (T) cells

5. (a)denoids
6. (i)nguinal
7. (g)land
ANTIGEN

Exercise 7.10: DISCHARGE SUMMARY ANALYSIS

1. AIDS = acquired immunodeficiency syndrome; CMV = cytomegalovirus; HIV = human immunodeficiency virus; IV = intravenous; OPD = outpatient department
2. No. In a gastroscopy the scope is inserted through the oral cavity, down the oesophagus into the stomach and often through to the duodenum. In a colonoscopy the scope is inserted through the anus, into the rectum and up into the large intestine.
3. Cytomegalovirus commonly affects people at some time during their life but rarely causes signs or symptoms. It is a member of the herpesvirus family. Those who develop symptoms may experience an illness resembling infectious mononucleosis and have fever, swollen glands and feel tired. People with a compromised immune system (such as HIV-positive patients or those receiving chemotherapy) may experience more serious illness involving fever, pneumonia and other symptoms.
4. Candidiasis; Cytomegalovirus
5. This means that the patient has been given a drug intravenously to calm them down during surgery. As part of the anaesthetic work-up, the anaesthetist will identify the patient's surgical risk. The ASA (American Society of Anesthesiologists) score represents the risk level. A level 3 identifies that the patient has severe systemic disease that limits activity, and the NE indicates that the surgery is non-emergency.

CHAPTER 8: ENDOCRINE SYSTEM

Exercise 8.1: LABEL THE DIAGRAM

1. pineal
2. hypothalamus
3. pituitary
4. parathyroids
5. thyroid
6. thymus
7. adrenals
8. pancreas (islets)
9. ovaries (female)
10. testes (male)

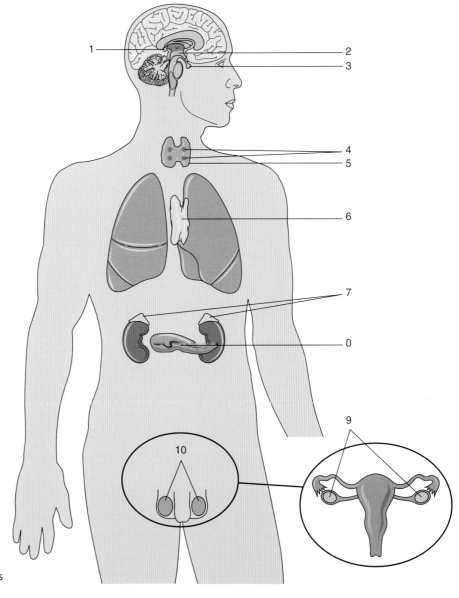

Figure 8.8
Endocrine glands

Exercise 8.2: WORD ANALYSIS AND MEANING

1. thyr/o = thyroid; chondr/o = cartilage; -tomy = incision into; meaning = incision into thyroid cartilage
2. acr/o = extremities; -megaly = enlargement; meaning = condition of enlargement of extremities
3. pancreat/o = pancreas; -tropic = affinity for; meaning = affinity for the pancreas
4. hyper- = above, excessive; natr/o = sodium; -aemia = condition of blood; meaning = condition of excess sodium in the blood
5. poly- = many, much; dips/o = thirst; -ia = condition of; meaning = condition of much thirst
6. poly- = many, much; ur/o = urine, urinary tract, urea; -ia = condition of; meaning = condition of much urine
7. endo- = within; crin/o = secrete; -logy = study of; meaning = study of secreting within (refers to glands that secrete within)
8. home/o = same, alike; -stasis = stop, control (stand still); meaning = stand still, the same (refers to the body's systems being in balance or staying the same)
9. keton/o = ketone bodies; ur/o = urine, urinary tract, urea; -ia = condition of; meaning = condition of ketone bodies in urine
10. phae/o = dusky, dark; chrom/o = colour; cyt/o = cell; -oma = tumour; tumour of dusky-coloured cells

Exercise 8.3: MATCH WORD ELEMENTS AND MEANINGS

Column A	Answer
1. endo-	H
2. oxy-	F
3. gonad/o	G
4. -crine	I
5. eu-	A
6. natr/o	J
7. andr/o	D
8. somat/o	B
9. -trophin	E
10. kal/i	C

Exercise 8.4: SPELLING AND MEANINGS

1. hirsutism – excessive hairiness in a female
2. thyrotoxicosis – also known as Graves' disease, an autoimmune disorder characterised by hyperthyroidism
3. hyperglycaemia – excessive glucose in the blood
4. pancreatectomy – surgical removal of the pancreas
5. cretinism – a congenital endocrine condition characterised by hypothyroidism
6. pituitary gland – an endocrine gland located near the base of the brain responsible for secretion of hormones associated with many vital functions
7. ketoacidosis – acidosis in association with an excess of ketones in the body
8. diabetes mellitus – a disorder characterised by a deficiency or absence of insulin secretion
9. goitre – enlargement of the thyroid gland
10. myxoedema – a form of advanced hypothyroidism in adults

Exercise 8.5: EXPAND THE ABBREVIATIONS

Abbreviation	Expanded abbreviation
ACTH	adrenocorticotrophic hormone
ADH	antidiuretic hormone
FBG	fasting blood glucose

Abbreviation	Expanded abbreviation
FSH	follicle stimulating hormone
GH	growth hormone
GTT	glucose tolerance test
HCG	human chorionic gonadotrophin
T1DM	type 1 diabetes mellitus
T2DM	type 2 diabetes mellitus
TSH	thyroid stimulating hormone

Exercise 8.6: APPLYING MEDICAL TERMINOLOGY

1. d
2. b
3. c
4. c
5. b
6. d
7. b
8. c
9. a
10. b
11. c
12. b
13. b
14. c
15. a

Exercise 8.7: MATCH TESTS, PROCEDURES AND MEANINGS

Column A	Answer
1. GTT	H
2. beta hCG	I
3. orchidectomy	E
4. cortisol test	F
5. thyroid scan	B
6. FBS	G
7. hypophysectomy	D
8. TRH test	A
9. radioimmunoassay	J
10. catecholamine analysis	C

Exercise 8.8: PRONUNCIATION AND COMPREHENSION

No answer provided – self-directed study.

Exercise 8.9: CROSSWORD PUZZLE

ACROSS
1. acromegaly
3. pancreas
4. myxoedema
6. endemic goitre
10. gigantism

DOWN
2. congenital hypothyroidism
5. hormone
7. insulin
8. dwarfism
9. peptoid

Exercise 8.10: ANAGRAMS

1. gigan(t)ism
2. acromegal(y)
3. (h)irsutism
4. glycosu(r)ia
5. (i)nsulin
6. g(o)itre
7. poly(d)ipsia
THYROID

Exercise 8.11: DISCHARGE SUMMARY ANALYSIS

1. LA = local anaesthetic; GA = general anaesthetic; OR = operating room; ug = microgram; FS = frozen section
2. Dysphagia is not a common symptom of Hashimoto's thyroiditis. The dysphagia is more likely to be due to Ms Scott's multinodular goitre, which causes a swelling in the neck and can make swallowing difficult for some patients.
3. Ms Scott would have had a chest x-ray for a couple of reasons. It is often performed as part of a preoperative work-up for patients. Ms Scott had also noted neck enlargement and dysphagia, so a chest x-ray would have been performed as part of the investigation for those two conditions to see if there was any lung disease that contributed to her symptoms.
4. 'Diffusely enlarged gland' means that the whole thyroid gland was enlarged. This is also described as goitre. 'Associated lymphadenopathy' means that the lymph glands related to the thyroid gland were enlarged.
5. Bleeding from an operative wound is a relatively frequent complication after surgery, despite precautionary techniques aimed at reducing such events. It may result in an early haematoma, which occurs within a couple of days of surgery. An early haematoma is an acute accumulation of fresh blood that causes a painful swelling. It is important to investigate and treat an early haematoma for two main reasons. There may be a vessel that is still bleeding internally. This needs to be located and stopped urgently. It can also lead to an infection, so this should be prevented. Ms Scott had her wound opened and the haematoma drained to stop the bleeding and prevent any infection from occurring.

CHAPTER 9: CARDIOVASCULAR SYSTEM

Exercise 9.1: LABEL THE DIAGRAM

1. superior vena cava (from upper body)
2. right pulmonary artery (to right lung)
3. right pulmonary veins (from right lung)
4. right atrium
5. right AV valve
6. inferior vena cava (from lower body)
7. pulmonary valve
8. right ventricle
9. aorta (to body)
10. aortic valve
11. left pulmonary artery (to left lung)
12. left pulmonary veins (from left lung)
13. left atrium
14. left AV valve
15. left ventricle

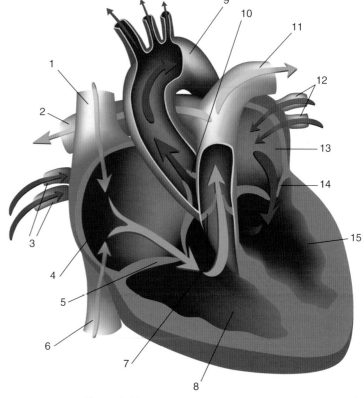

Figure 9.12
The pathway of blood through the heart

Exercise 9.2: MATCH WORD ELEMENTS AND MEANINGS

Column A	Answer
1. angi/o	K
2. tachy-	L
3. scler/o	G
4. arteri/o	P
5. cyan/o	T
6. echo-	S
7. pector/o	I
8. brachi/o	R
9. -stenosis	E
10. man/o	N
11. -meter	Q
12. phleb/o	B
13. -centesis	H
14. atri/o	A
15. trans-	J
16. sphygm/o	D
17. coron/o	M
18. embol/o	C
19. necr/o	O
20. brady-	F

Exercise 9.3: WORD ANALYSIS AND MEANING

1. vas/o = vessel, vas deferens, duct; -constriction = narrowing; meaning = narrowing of a vessel
2. hypo- = below, under, deficient, less than normal; vol/o = volume; -aemia = condition of blood; meaning = condition of blood where volume is less than normal
3. angi/o = vessel; -plasty = surgical, plastic repair; meaning = surgical, plastic repair of a vessel
4. ventricul/o = ventricle; -graphy = process of recording; meaning = process of recording the ventricle
5. pan- = all, entire; cyt/o = cell; -penia = deficiency; meaning deficiency of all cells
6. septic/o = infection; -aemia = condition of blood; meaning = condition of infection of blood
7. phleb/o = vein; -tomy = incision into; meaning = incision into vein
8. hypo- = below, under, deficient, less than normal; chrom/o = colour; -ic = pertaining to; micro- = small; cyt/o = cell; -ic = pertaining to; an- = no, not, without, absence of; -aemia = condition of blood; meaning = condition of no blood, cells that are small and less than normal colour
9. aneurysm/o = aneurysm; -rrhaphy = suture; suture of aneurysm
10. sphygm/o = pulse; man/o = pressure; -meter = instrument to measure; meaning = instrument to measure pressure of pulse

Exercise 9.4: VOCABULARY BUILDING

1. arrhythmia
2. cardiomegaly
3. aneurysm
4. atherosclerosis
5. echocardiography
6. endarterectomy
7. haemorrhage
8. hypoxia, hypoxaemia
9. pericarditis
10. cyanosis

Exercise 9.5: EXPAND THE ABBREVIATIONS

Abbreviation	Expanded abbreviation
AF	atrial fibrillation
AMI	acute myocardial infarction
BBB	bundle branch block
BP	blood pressure
CABG	coronary artery bypass graft
CAD	coronary artery disease
CCF	congestive cardiac failure
CCU	coronary care unit
CHD	congestive (or congenital) heart disease
CVP	central venous pressure
DVT	deep vein thrombosis
HDL	high density lipoproteins
LDL	low density lipoproteins
LV	left ventricle
NSTEMI	non-ST-elevation myocardial infarction
PDA	patent ductus arteriosus
PTCA	percutaneous transluminal coronary angioplasty
SOB	shortness of breath
TOE	trans-oesophageal echocardiography
VSD	ventricular septal defect

Exercise 9.6: APPLYING MEDICAL TERMINOLOGY

1. cardiologist
2. tachycardia
3. dextrocardia
4. cardiomegaly
5. cardiomyopathy
6. electrocardiogram
7. endocardium
8. cardiorrhexis
9. pericardioscopy
10. cardioplegia

Exercise 9.7: MATCH DRUG TYPE WITH USE

Column A	Answer
1. anticoagulant	C
2. antihyperlipidaemic	F
3. antiarrhythmic	G
4. thrombolytic	H
5. beta blocker	B
6. vasodilator	E
7. diuretic	A
8. vasoconstrictor	D

Exercise 9.8: APPLYING MEDICAL TERMINOLOGY

1. atrium
2. inferior vena cava
3. tricuspid or right atrioventricular
4. pulmonary
5. pulmonary
6. deoxygenated
7. atrium
8. pulmonary
9. oxygenated
10. ventricle
11. mitral, bicuspid or left atrioventricular
12. aortic
13. aorta

Exercise 9.9: PRONUNCIATION AND COMPREHENSION

No answer provided – self-directed study.

Exercise 9.10: CROSSWORD PUZZLE

ACROSS
3. sinoatrial node
4. pulmonary artery
5. right atrium
7. mitral valve prolapse
8. aorta
9. capillary

DOWN
1. aneurysm
2. vein
3. systemic artery
6. heart

Exercise 9.11: ANAGRAMS

1. vei(n)
2. (a)orta
3. i(n)farction
4. CAB(G)
5. myocard(i)um
6. ischaemi(a)
ANGINA

Exercise 9.12: DISCHARGE SUMMARY ANALYSIS

1. 40 mg nocte = 40 milligrams at night; b.d. = twice a day; q.d. = every day; q.i.d. = four times a day; t.d.s. = three times a day
2. This means that Mr Fredricks is not to have any surgery. He will be treated with the medications that are listed and will be monitored regularly.
3. Ischaemic cardiomyopathy refers to disease of the heart muscle due to inadequate oxygen delivery to the myocardium. The heart muscle tissue weakens, with a consequent deterioration of the function of the myocardium. The ischaemia usually results from some form of coronary artery disease. People with ischaemic cardiomyopathy are often at risk of arrhythmia or sudden cardiac death.
4. Mr Fredricks was given medication (aspirin and warfarin) to stop his blood from clotting and producing thrombi.
5. Auscultation is the process of listening to sounds arising within organs such as the heart and lungs using a stethoscope. It is an aid to diagnosis and treatment of many conditions. Normally the heart makes two sounds as it beats. Rarely, a third sound can be heard. The third heart sound is caused by rapid ventricular filling in early diastole. It is caused by vibration of the ventricular walls, resulting from the first rapid filling so it is heard just after the second sound. It is indicative of potential heart failure.

CHAPTER 10: RESPIRATORY SYSTEM

Exercise 10.1: LABEL THE DIAGRAM

1. upper respiratory tract
2. lower respiratory tract
3. bronchioles
4. nasal cavity
5. nasopharynx
6. oropharynx
7. laryngopharynx
8. pharynx
9. larynx
10. trachea
11. left and right primary bronchi
12. alveolar sac
13. bronchioles
14. capillary
15. alveolar duct
16. alveoli

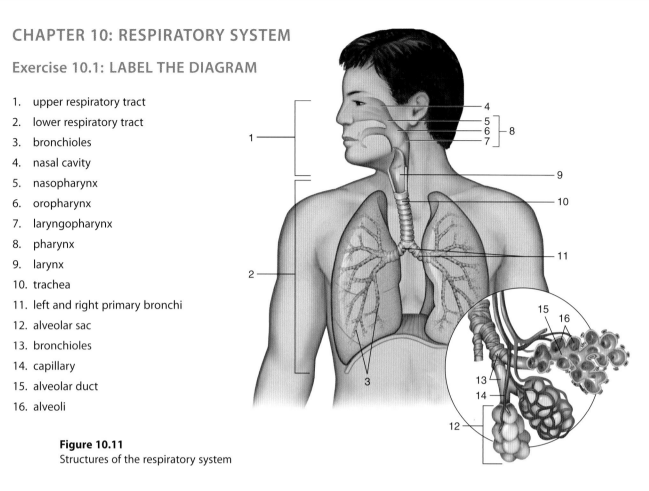

Figure 10.11
Structures of the respiratory system

Exercise 10.2: MATCH WORD ELEMENTS AND MEANINGS

Column A	Answer
1. -capnia	D
2. pneumat/o	H
3. -oxia	J
4. phren/o	A
5. steth/o	S
6. spir/o	P
7. -osmia	T
8. anthrac/o	B
9. pharyng/o	Q
10. coni/o	R
11. orth/o	M
12. dys-	E
13. rhin/o	C
14. -ectasis	F
15. -ptysis	L
16. tele-	O
17. cyan/o	G
18. sept/o	K
19. phon/o	N
20. lob/o	I

Exercise 10.3: WORD ANALYSIS AND MEANING

1. laryng/o = larynx, voice box; -eal = pertaining to; meaning – pertaining to the larynx
2. dys- = bad, painful, difficult; osm/o = sense of smell; -ia = process or condition; meaning = condition of a bad sense of smell
3. inter- = between; cost/o = ribs; -al = pertaining to; meaning = pertaining to between the ribs
4. a- = no, not, without, absence of; -pnoea = breathing; meaning = absence of breathing
5. thorac/o = thorax, chest; -scopy = process of viewing; meaning = process of viewing the chest
6. trache/o = trachea; -tomy = incision or cut into; meaning = incision into the trachea
7. pneum/o – lungs, respiration, air; -thorax – pleural cavity or chest; meaning – air in the pleural cavity
8. pleur/o = pleura; -itis = inflammation; meaning = inflammation of the pleura
9. hypo- = below, under, deficient, less than normal; capn/o = carbon dioxide; -ia = condition of; meaning = condition of deficient carbon dioxide
10. pleur/o = pleural; -al = pertaining to; em- = in; py/o = pus; -ema = condition; meaning = condition of pus in the pleural space

Exercise 10.4: VOCABULARY BUILDING

1. thoracoplasty
2. dyspnoea
3. tonsillectomy and adenoidectomy
4. hypoxia, hypoxaemia
5. laryngitis
6. pulmonary embolism
7. phrenoptosis
8. uvulopalatopharyngoplasty
9. hypercapnia
10. bronchospasm

Exercise 10.5: EXPAND THE ABBREVIATIONS

Abbreviation	Expanded abbreviation
ABGs	arterial blood gases
ARF	acute respiratory failure
BiPAP	bi-level positive airway pressure
BS	breath sounds
COAD	chronic obstructive airways disease
CPAP	continuous positive airways pressure
CXR	chest x-ray
CVS	continuous ventilatory support
DOE	dyspnoea on exertion
ETT	endotracheal tube
FEV$_1$	forced expiratory volume in 1 second
LUL	left upper lobe
O$_2$	oxygen
PCP	*Pneumocystis* pneumonia
PE	pulmonary embolism
RDS	respiratory distress syndrome
RLL	right lower lobe
SARS	severe acute respiratory syndrome
SOBOE	shortness of breath on exertion
T&A	tonsils and adenoids, tonsillectomy and adenoidectomy
TB	tuberculosis
URTI	upper respiratory tract infection

Exercise 10.6: MATCH MEDICAL TERMS WITH MEANINGS

Column A	Answer
1. dysphonia	G
2. bronchiectasis	H
3. status asthmaticus	P
4. laryngostomy	F
5. sinus actinomycosis	E
6. pleural effusion	O
7. hyperventilation	R
8. rhinolith	C
9. anosmia	A
10. anthracosis	I
11. pyopneumothorax	N
12. bradypnoea	M
13. hypercapnia	L
14. expectoration	K
15. lobectomy	J
16. pansinusitis	D
17. rhinorrhoea	B
18. haemoptysis	Q
19. thoracocentesis	T
20. Cheyne-Stokes respiration	S

Exercise 10.7: APPLYING MEDICAL TERMINOLOGY

1. c
2. d
3. b

4. b
5. c

Exercise 10.8: PRONUNCIATION AND COMPREHENSION

No answer provided – self-directed study.

Exercise 10.9: CROSSWORD PUZZLE

ACROSS
2. exhalation
5. pulmonary oedema
7. emphysema
8. cystic fibrosis
10. nose

DOWN
1. pneumoconiosis
3. alveoli
4. tracheostomy
6. visceral pleura
9. bronchitis

Exercise 10.10: ANAGRAMS

1. CO(A)D
2. b(r)onchi
3. pharyn(x)
4. lu(n)g

5. a(l)veoli
6. pleuris(y)
LARYNX

Exercise 10.11: DISCHARGE SUMMARY ANALYSIS

1. COAD = chronic obstructive airways disease; CXR = chest x-ray; ECG = electrocardiogram; JVP = jugular venous pressure; T2DM = type 2 diabetes mellitus; OPD = outpatient department; SCC = squamous cell carcinoma; SOB = shortness of breath

2. Kussmaul's sign is a rise in JVP on inspiration. It is seen in conditions in which right ventricular filling is limited by pericardial fluid. A positive Kussmaul's sign indicates constrictive pericarditis, restrictive cardiomyopathy or cardiac tamponade.

3. Lasix is a strong diuretic used to treat fluid retention in people with congestive heart failure, liver disease or a kidney disorder. It is also known as furosemide. Because she had not taken the Lasix for several days, Mrs Fox was exhibiting symptoms of fluid retention when she was admitted to hospital. She had oedema to her knees, marked shortness of breath and a raised JVP. These conditions disappeared after she started taking Lasix again.

4. *Haemophilus* is a genus of Gram-negative coccobacilli or rod-shaped bacteria commonly found in the respiratory tract. Under specific conditions it can cause infections such as bronchitis and influenza.

5. Atrial fibrillation (AF) is a type of heart arrhythmia characterised by tachycardia, palpitations, a fluttering heartbeat, irregular heartbeat, chest pains, dizziness and syncope. Treatment options include medication, surgery and defibrillation. An artificial pacemaker may be inserted to maintain regular heart rhythm. If not treated, complications may include stroke and heart attack.

CHAPTER 11: DIGESTIVE SYSTEM

Exercise 11.1: LABEL THE DIAGRAM

1. parotid gland
2. submandibular gland
3. pharynx
4. oesophagus
5. diaphragm
6. transverse colon
7. hepatic flexure
8. ascending colon
9. ileum
10. caecum
11. vermiform appendix
12. rectum
13. tongue
14. sublingual gland
15. larynx
16. trachea
17. liver
18. stomach
19. spleen
20. splenic flexure
21. descending colon
22. sigmoid colon
23. anal canal

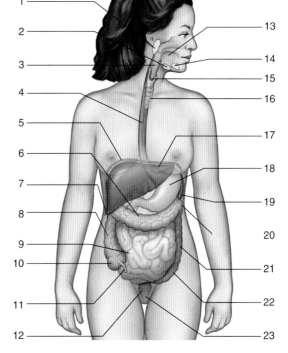

Figure 11.14a
Organs of the digestive system

1. hepatic duct
2. cystic duct
3. gallbladder
4. duodenum
5. pancreas
6. liver
7. stomach
8. spleen

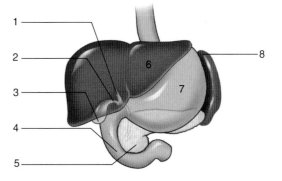

Figure 11.14b
The liver and stomach

Exercise 11.2: WORD ELEMENT MEANINGS AND WORD BUILDING

No answer provided for the medical term – refer to your dictionary for the correct spelling.

Meaning	Word element
anus	an/o
bile duct	cholangi/o
bile pigment	bilirubin/o
urinary bladder, sac	cyst/o
cheek	bucc/o
defecation, elimination of waste products	-chezia
digestion	-pepsia
eat, swallow	-phagia
enzyme	-ase
gall	chol/e
bile	bil/i
gallbladder	cholecyst/o
ileum	ile/o
lip	cheil/o or labi/o
meal	cib/o
orange/yellow	cirrh/o
small intestine	enter/o
starch	amyl/o
through, across	trans-, dia-
vomiting	-emesis

Exercise 11.3: MATCH MEDICAL TERMS AND MEANINGS

Column A	Answer
1. cholecystectomy	F
2. sublingual	N
3. steatolysis	A
4. jejunoileitis	Q
5. proctodynia	H
6. dyspepsia	O
7. cheiloplasty	R
8. splenomegaly	S
9. pharyngoscope	P
10. stomatitis	T
11. enterostomy	M
12. herniorrhaphy	B
13. colorectal	C
14. dysphagia	E
15. dentogingival	K
16. gastroscopy	L
17. protease	G
18. abdominocentesis	I
19. caecopexy	D
20. hyperemesis	J

Exercise 11.4: CIRCLE THE CORRECT SPELLING

diarrhoea   polydipsia
haemorrhoid   oesophagoscopy
cholecystitis   dysentery
intussusception   cirrhosis
parotitis   glucose

Exercise 11.5: EXPAND THE ABBREVIATIONS

Abbreviation	Expanded abbreviation
Ba	barium
b.i.d.	twice a day
BMI	body mass index
ERCP	endoscopic retrograde cholangiopancreatography
GORD	gastro-oesophageal reflux disease
IBD	inflammatory bowel disease
IBS	irritable bowel syndrome
LFTs	liver function tests
N&V	nausea and vomiting
NG	nasogastric
OGD	oesophagogastroduodenoscopy
PEJ tube	percutaneous endoscopic jejunostomy tube
PTHC	percutaneous transhepatic cholangiography
PUD	peptic ulcer disease
TPN	total parenteral nutrition

Exercise 11.6: VOCABULARY BUILDING

1. chyme
2. diverticulum
3. anal fissure
4. peristalsis
5. flatulence
6. oesophageal varices
7. colonic polyp
8. propulsion
9. saliva
10. defecation

Exercise 11.7: PRONUNCIATION AND COMPREHENSION

No answer provided – self-directed study.

Exercise 11.8: CROSSWORD PUZZLE

ACROSS
3. bolus
6. gastric banding
8. digestion
11. hepatitis

DOWN
1. cholecystectomy
2. liver function tests
4. colon
5. absorption
7. parotitis
9. tongue
10. saliva

Exercise 11.9: ANAGRAMS

1. liv(e)r
2. p(y)lorus
3. ileu(m)
4. dysp(h)agia
5. (c)aecum
CHYME

Exercise 11.10: DISCHARGE SUMMARY ANALYSIS

1. ED = emergency department; Hx = history of; LFTs = liver function tests; LMO = local medical officer; N&V = nausea and vomiting; NSAIDs = nonsteroidal anti-inflammatory drugs; RUQ = right upper quadrant; WCC = white cell count

2. The term acute abdomen denotes any sudden non-traumatic severe pain of unclear aetiology whose chief manifestation is in the abdominal area and for which urgent surgery may be necessary. An acute abdomen is one of the most common reasons for digestive system-related hospital admissions. The most common causes of acute abdomen are non-specific abdominal pain of which the cause is never identified, acute appendicitis, acute cholecystitis, peptic ulcers and biliary colic.

3. Yes, it does. Research over many years has identified that anyone who uses NSAIDs regularly is at risk of developing gastrointestinal problems such as peptic ulcers. The greatest risk is among people who require long-term use of very high-dose NSAIDs, especially patients with rheumatoid arthritis.

4. Most ulcers occur in the first layer of the inner lining of the stomach. If the ulcer is not treated, it can burn through the wall of the stomach (or other areas of the gastrointestinal tract), allowing digestive juices and food to leech into the abdominal cavity. Treatment generally requires immediate surgery.

5. Zantac (generic name ranitidine) belongs to a group of drugs called histamine-2 blockers. Zantac works by reducing the amount of acid produced in the stomach. It is used to treat and prevent ulcers in the stomach and intestines so would have been given to Ms Green to help her stomach heal and to prevent further ulcers developing.

CHAPTER 12: NERVOUS SYSTEM

Exercise 12.1: LABEL THE DIAGRAMS

1. hypothalamus
2. thalamus
3. diencephalon
4. cerebrum
5. pineal body
6. cerebellum
7. spinal cord
8. pyramid
9. medulla oblongata
10. pons
11. mid brain
12. brain stem
13. corpus callosum

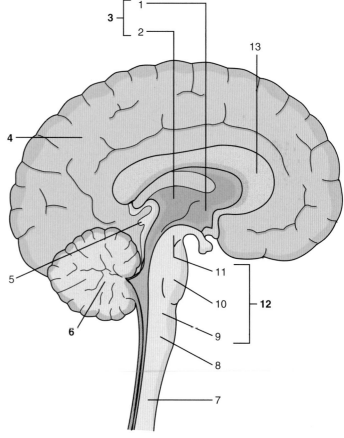

Figure 12.10
Major structures of the brain

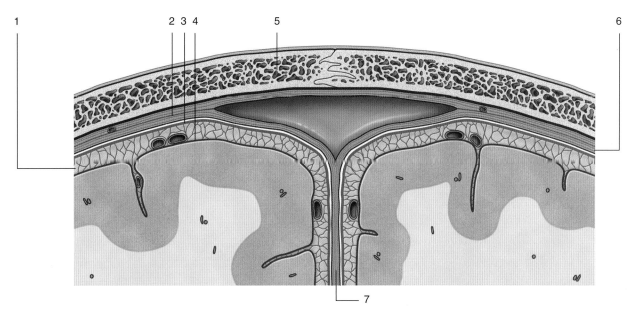

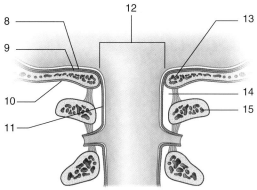

1. subarachnoid space

2. dura mater

3. arachnoid mater

4. pia mater

5. skull

6. subdural space

7. dural partition (falx cerebri)

8. meningeal layer of dura mater

9. periosteal layer of dura mater

10. periosteum

11. spinal dura mater

12. foramen magnum

13. skull

14. spinal extradural space

15. first cervical vertebra (C1)

Figure 12.11
The layers of the meninges

Exercise 12.2: PROVIDE THE WORD ELEMENTS

Meaning	Word element
burning	caus/o, cauter/o
cut short	syncop/o
electrical	electr/o
glue	gli/o
head	cephal/o
knowledge	gnos/o
nerve	neur/o
sound	echo-, phon/o, -phonia, son/o
star	astr/o
water	hydr/o, aqua-, aque/o, aqu/o, aqu/i

Exercise 12.3: WORD ELEMENT MEANINGS AND WORD BUILDING

No answer provided for the medical term – refer to your dictionary for the correct spelling.

Word element	Meaning
ment/o	mind
-praxia	achieve, to do
som/o	body
pont/o	pons, bridge
radicul/o	nerve root
-lepsy	seizure
-plegia	paralysis
thec/o	sheath
atel/o	incomplete, imperfect
gli/o	glue

Exercise 12.4: WORD ANALYSIS AND MEANING

1. an = no, not, without, absence of; encephal/o = brain; y = process, condition; meaning = condition of absence of the brain
2. crani/o = cranium, skull; -tomy = incision, cut into; meaning = incision into the skull
3. polio- = grey matter; encephal/o = brain; mening/o = meninges; myel/o = spinal cord; -itis = inflammation; meaning = inflammation of the grey matter of the brain, meninges and spinal cord
4. hemi = half; -plegia = condition of paralysis; meaning = condition of paralysis of half (the body)
5. astr/o = star; cyt/o = cell; -oma = tumour; meaning = tumour of star-shaped cells
6. radicul/o = nerve root; -itis = inflammation; meaning = inflammation of a nerve root
7. brady = slow; -kinesia = pertaining to movement, motion; meaning = pertaining to slow movement, motion
8. gli/o = glue; blast/o = embryonic or developing cell; -oma = tumour; meaning = tumour of embryonic or developing cells that have a glue-like consistency
9. hyper- = above, excessive; -aesthesia = feeling, sensation; meaning = feeling, sensation that is excessive
10. psych/o = mind; somat/o = body; -ic = pertaining to; meaning = pertaining to mind and body

Exercise 12.5: EXPAND THE ABBREVIATIONS

Abbreviation	Expanded abbreviation
CNS	central nervous system
CSF	cerebrospinal fluid
CVA	cerebrovascular accident
ECT	electroconvulsive therapy
EEG	electroencephalogram
GCS	Glasgow Coma Scale/Score
ICP	intracranial pressure
LP	lumbar puncture
MS	multiple sclerosis
PET	positron emission tomography
PNS	peripheral nervous system
REM	rapid eye movement
TBI	traumatic brain injury
TENS	transcutaneous electrical nerve stimulation
TIA	transient ischaemic attack

Exercise 12.6: MATCH MEDICAL TERMS AND MEANINGS

Column A	Answer
1. meningitis	F
2. ataxia	G
3. dementia	J
4. vertigo	B
5. aphasia	E
6. astrocytoma	C
7. apraxia	I
8. syncope	H
9. narcolepsy	A
10. palsy	D

Exercise 12.7: PRONUNCIATION AND COMPREHENSION

No answer provided – self-directed study.

Exercise 12.8: CROSSWORD PUZZLE

ACROSS
5. cerebellum
6. axon
7. pons
8. cerebrovascular accident
9. epilepsy

DOWN
1. hypothalamus
2. tegmentum
3. arachnoid membrane
4. migraine

Exercise 12.9: ANAGRAMS

1. gli(o)ma
2. syncop(e)
3. po(n)s
4. b(r)ain
5. ga(n)glion
6. cerebr(u)m

NEURON

Exercise 12.10: DISCHARGE SUMMARY ANALYSIS

1. MRI = magnetic resonance imaging; MS = multiple sclerosis; RPR = rapid plasma reagin; TFTs = thyroid function tests
2. The Hoffman's test is used to assess patients with symptoms of myelopathy. The test is done by quickly snapping or flicking the patient's middle fingernail. The test is positive for spinal cord compression when there is a reflexive response in the index finger, ring finger and/or thumb. Normally, there should be no reaction from the muscles in the thumb. A number of neurological conditions may elicit the Hoffman's response including cervical spondylitis, spinal cord compression, upper motor neuron disease and multiple sclerosis.
3. The test consists of stroking the outside sole of the foot from heel to toe with a pointed object. The normal response in adults and children is for the toes to reflex downwards. In babies and people with neurological disorders, there is downward flexion of the big toe and fanning outward of the toes. A positive Babinski's reflex is consistent with several neurological conditions including multiple sclerosis.
4. Her MS symptoms include tremor, weakness of her leg, spasticity in the right leg, difficulties with balance, tingling in her extremities, blurred vision, fatigue, malaise and loss of bladder control.
5. The use of magnetic resonance imaging (MRI) of the brain transformed the investigation, diagnosis and treatment of MS. Usually, MRI is the only imaging modality needed for imaging patients with MS, and it far surpasses all other tests with respect to its positive predictive value. MRI scans give detailed images of cross-sections of the brain. Multiple sclerosis lesions show up as paler areas on those images. From an MRI, the neurologist can identify that demyelination has occurred and also see where the lesions are.

CHAPTER 13: THE SENSES

Exercise 13.1: LABEL THE DIAGRAMS

1. cornea
2. lens
3. lacrimal caruncle
4. fibrous layer
5. vascular layer
6. inner layer
7. optic disc
8. central artery and vein
9. optic nerve
10. anterior chamber
11. pupil
12. iris
13. lower lid
14. ciliary body
15. suspensory ligament
16. retina
17. choroid
18. sclera
19. posterior chamber
20. macular
21. fovea centralis

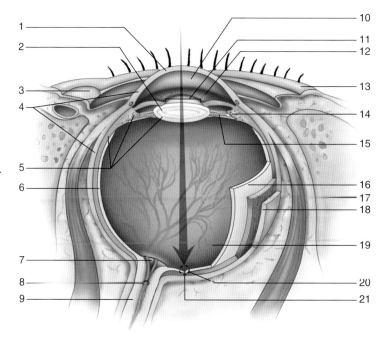

Figure 13.10
The eye

1. inner ear

2. middle ear

3. external ear

4. auricle (pinna)

5. external auditory (acoustic) meatus

6. temporal bone

7. tympanic membrane

8. semicircular canals

9. oval window

10. facial nerve

11. vestibular nerve

12. cochlear nerve

13. vestibulocochlear nerve

14. cochlea

15. vestibule

16. round window

17. auditory (eustachian) tube

18. malleus

19. incus

20. stapes

21. auditory ossicles

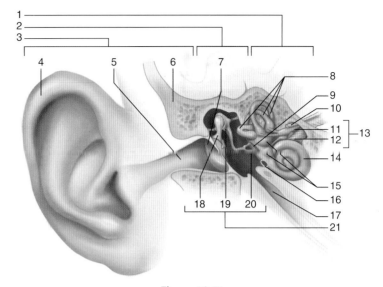

Figure 13.11
The ear

Exercise 13.2: MATCH WORD ELEMENTS AND MEANINGS

Column A	Answer
1. myring/o	E
2. aque/o	J
3. geus/o	H
4. ambly/o	M
5. malle/o	R
6. palpat/o	Q
7. dacry/o	O
8. acous/o	C
9. xer/o	T
10. corne/o	N
11. phac/o	I
12. glauc/o	D
13. osphresi/o	A
14. blephar/o	G
15. mydr/o	S
16. irid/o	B
17. staped/o	L
18. osm/o	F
19. scot/o	K
20. cerumin/o	P

Exercise 13.3: WORD ANALYSIS AND MEANING

1. oz/o = to smell, odour; stom/a = mouth; -ia = process, condition; meaning = condition of odour from the mouth
2. ot/o = ear; -sclerosis = hardening; meaning = hardening of the (bones in the middle) ear
3. hyper- = above, excessive; osphresi/o = odour; -ia = process, condition; meaning = condition of excessive odour
4. vestibul/o = vestibule; -tomy = incision, cut into; meaning = incision into the vestibule
5. aer/o = air, gas; ot/o = ear; -itis = inflammation; meaning = inflammation due to air (pressure) in the ear
6. dacry/o = tears, tear duct, lacrimal sac; aden/o = gland; -itis = inflammation; meaning = inflammation of the lacrimal gland
7. a- = no, not, without, absence of; sthen/o = strength; -opia = condition of vision; meaning = condition of vision with an absence of strength (of ocular ciliary muscles)
8. cerumin/o = wax; -osis = abnormal condition; meaning = abnormal condition of wax (in the ear)
9. an- = no, not, without, absence of; -acusis = hearing; meaning = no hearing
10. an- = no, not, without, absence of; osm/o = sense of smell; -ia = condition of; meaning = condition of no sense of smell

Exercise 13.4: VOCABULARY BUILDING

1. aphakia
2. aniscoria
3. blepharitis
4. exotropia
5. nyctopia
6. achromatopsia
7. otorhinolaryngologist
8. mastoidocentesis
9. otopyorrhoea
10. presbyopia

Exercise 13.5: EXPAND THE ABBREVIATIONS

Abbreviation	Expanded abbreviation
ACG	angle closure glaucoma
ARMD	age-related macular degeneration
ASC	anterior subcapsular cataract
BSM	bilateral suction myringotomy
EAC	external auditory canal
ENT	ear, nose and throat
IOFB	intraocular foreign body
IOL	intraocular lens
OM	otitis media
PE tube	pressure equalising tube
POAG	primary open angle glaucoma
REM	rapid eye movement
ROP	retinopathy of prematurity
SLE	slit lamp examination
SOM	serous otitis media
SSNHL	sudden sensorineural hearing loss
TM	tympanic membrane
TORP	total ossicular replacement prosthesis
VA	visual acuity
VF	visual field

Exercise 13.6: MATCH MEDICAL TERMS AND MEANINGS

Column A	Answer
1. retinopathy	J
2. anosmia	F
3. hypergeusia	D
4. hordeolum	C
5. conjunctivitis	I
6. presbycusis	E
7. blepharoptosis	H
8. umami	B
9. myopia	A
10. otorrhoea	G

Exercise 13.7: APPLYING MEDICAL TERMINOLOGY

1. d
2. c
3. b
4. d
5. d

6. c
7. a
8. d
9. d
10. b

Exercise 13.8: PRONUNCIATION AND COMPREHENSION

No answer provided – self-directed study.

Exercise 13.9: ANAGRAMS

1. enuc(l)eation
2. (s)clera
3. hyposmi(a)
4. kerato(m)alacia

5. facia(l)
6. a(u)diologist
7. oton(e)uralgia

MALLEUS

Exercise 13.10: CROSSWORD PUZZLE

ACROSS
2. vertigo
4. audiometry
6. nasendoscopy
8. cochlear
9. enucleation
10. astigmatism

DOWN
1. refraction
3. strabismus
5. labyrinthitis
7. deafness

Exercise 13.11: DISCHARGE SUMMARY ANALYSIS

1. 5 mg p.r.n. = 5 milligrams (of a drug, in this case Stemetil) *pro re nata* which means 'as required'; ALT = alanine transaminase; ECG = electrocardiogram; ENT = ear, nose and throat; FBC = full blood count; IV = intravenous; LFTs = liver function tests; THR = total hip replacement
2. Vestibular neuronitis is an ear disorder that involves inflammation, irritation and swelling of the inner ear. This interferes with the inner ear's function, resulting in several common symptoms, which are listed in the following answer. Vestibular neuronitis commonly occurs after otitis media or an upper respiratory infection. It is usually self-limiting and resolves within a few weeks. Treatment involves reducing symptoms such as vertigo. Viral labyrinthitis is a synonym for vestibular neuronitis, as is vestibular neuritis.

3. The most common symptoms are vertigo, nystagmus (difficulty focusing the eyes because of involuntary eye movements), dizziness, hearing loss in one ear, tinnitus, loss of balance, nausea and vomiting.

4. Ms Harris presented with dizziness, loss of hearing, nystagmus and vomiting.

5. Stemetil is an antiemetic or antinausea medication. Ms Harris was admitted with severe vomiting, so the Stemetil would have been prescribed to reduce that symptom.

CHAPTER 14: URINARY SYSTEM

Exercise 14.1: LABEL THE DIAGRAMS

1. adrenal gland
2. liver
3. twelfth rib
4. right kidney
5. ureter
6. urinary bladder
7. spleen
8. renal artery
9. renal vein
10. left kidney
11. abdominal aorta
12. inferior vena cava
13. common iliac artery and vein
14. urethra

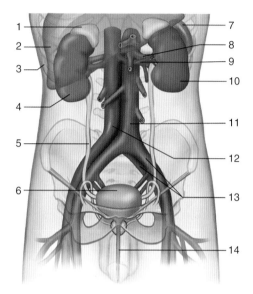

Figure 14.10
Urinary system and associated structures

1. interlobular arteries
2. renal column
3. renal sinus
4. hilum
5. renal pelvis
6. renal papilla of pyramid
7. ureter
8. capsule (fibrous)
9. cortex
10. minor calyces
11. major calyces
12. medullary pyramid
13. medulla

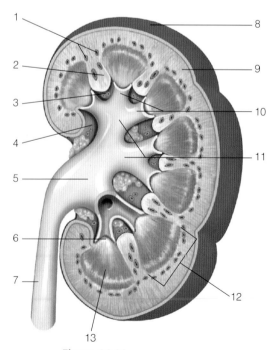

Figure 14.11
Internal structure of the kidney

Exercise 14.2: MATCH WORD ELEMENTS AND MEANINGS

Column A	Answer
1. trigon/o	E
2. pyel/o	G
3. meat/o	K
4. -cele	L
5. -clysis	N
6. cali/o	Q
7. urethr/o	A
8. kal/i	B
9. olig/o	O
10. dips/o	C
11. ur/o	T
12. -poietin	D
13. ket/o	H
14. nephr/o	I
15. -gram	S
16. -uresis	R
17. py/o	M
18. lith/o	F
19. poly-	P
20. azot/o	J

Exercise 14.3: WORD ANALYSIS AND MEANING

1. nephr/o = kidney; lith/o = stone, calculus; -tripsy = to crush; meaning = to crush kidney stones or calculus
2. cyst/o = sac, urinary bladder, cyst; -ectomy = excision, surgical removal; meaning = excision, surgical removal of the urinary bladder
3. glomerul/o = glomerulus; nephr/o = kidney; -itis = inflammation; meaning = inflammation of the glomerulus of the kidney
4. ureter/o – ureter; cyst/o – sac, urinary bladder, cyst; -stomy = create surgical opening; meaning = create surgical opening into the ureter and urinary bladder
5. haemat/o = blood; ur/o = urine, urinary tract, urea; -ia = condition of; meaning = condition of blood in the urine
6. poly- = many, much; dips/o = thirst; -ia = process, condition; meaning = condition of much thirst
7. pyel/o = pelvis of kidney; -graphy = process of recording; meaning = process of recording the pelvis of the kidney
8. ur/o = urine, urinary tract, urea; -logy = study of; meaning = study of the urinary tract
9. erythr/o = red; -poietin = substance that forms; meaning = substance that forms red (blood cells)
10. meat/o = meatus; -rrhaphy = suture; meaning = suture of the meatus

Exercise 14.4: VOCABULARY BUILDING

1. ureterocele
2. hyperkalaemia
3. ureteroenterostomy
4. vesicotomy (cystotomy)
5. nephroptosis
6. ketosis
7. cystogram
8. ureterectasis
9. suprarenal
10. urethrodynia

Exercise 14.5: MATCH THE ABBREVIATIONS AND MEANINGS

Column A	Answer
1. IVP	G
2. CRF	I
3. PKD	L
4. ESWL	K
5. UTI	R
6. BUN	S
7. ARF	M
8. GFR	N
9. BNO	E
10. ESRD	D
11. VCU(G)	C
12. ATN	F
13. CKD	B
14. PKU	H
15. CAPD	T
16. UA	J
17. C&S	P
18. PD	A
19. ADH	O
20. CCPD	Q

Exercise 14.6: VOCABULARY BUILDING

1. micturition, voiding, urination
2. urea
3. glycosuria
4. ketonuria, acetonuria
5. albuminuria, proteinuria
6. urologist
7. pyelogram
8. urinary catheterisation
9. lavage
10. nocturia
11. Nephroptosis is also known as a floating kidney. It refers to the downward movement of the kidney into the pelvis when the patient stands up. The cause is a congenital or traumatic weakness of the perirenal connective tissue which is supposed to hold the kidney in place.
12. Ureteral colic (also known as renal colic) is the severe pain that is felt as a calculus or kidney stone passes down the ureter.
13. Hydronephrosis is an accumulation of fluid in the kidney.
14. Nephrotic syndrome is a general term for a group of diseases affecting the glomeruli. It is characterised by severe oedema, excessive protein loss in the urine and decreased levels of albumin in the blood.
15. Ureterovesicoplasty is a surgical repair of the junction between the ureter and the urinary bladder. It is performed to prevent urinary reflux.

Exercise 14.7: APPLYING MEDICAL TERMINOLOGY

1. b
2. b
3. c
4. a
5. a

6. a
7. b
8. c
9. c
10. b

Exercise 14.8: PRONUNCIATION AND COMPREHENSION

No answer provided – self-directed study.

Exercise 14.9: CROSSWORD PUZZLE

ACROSS
1. nephroptosis
5. vesicoureteral reflux
6. filtration
8. tubular necrosis
9. renal failure

DOWN
2. hydroureter
3. kidney agenesis
4. pyelonephritis
7. cystocele

Exercises 14.10: ANAGRAMS

1. p(y)uria
2. ur(e)thra
3. voi(d)ing
4. (k)etosis

5. noctur(i)a
6. nephro(n)
KIDNEY

Exercise 14.11: DISCHARGE SUMMARY ANALYSIS

1. BP = blood pressure; IDC = indwelling catheter; T&As = tonsils and adenoids
2. Stress incontinence is an uncontrollable, involuntary loss of urine during physical exertions such as coughing, sneezing, laughing or exercise. Stress incontinence may occur as a result of weakened pelvic muscles that support the bladder and urethra or because of a malfunction of the urethral sphincter. It is often seen in women who have had multiple vaginal childbirths like Ms Mitchell.
3. A Pfannenstiel incision is a long horizontal lower abdominal incision made below the line of the pubic hair. It is sometimes called the bikini incision. It is preferred for cosmetic reasons. If properly placed, it is generally concealed by regrowth of pubic hair.
4. Residual urine is the urine left in the bladder after a person has urinated. It is important for the bladder to be fully emptied because residual urine greater than around 50 mL increases the potential for recurring urinary tract infections.
5. Ms Mitchell had the following procedures performed: urethral suspension, general anaesthetic, bladder ultrasound, urinary catheterisation and removal of catheter.

CHAPTER 15: MALE REPRODUCTIVE SYSTEM

Exercise 15.1: LABEL THE DIAGRAMS

1. seminal vesicle
2. ejaculatory duct
3. prostate gland
4. rectum
5. bulbourethral gland
6. anus
7. epididymis
8. testis
9. scrotum
10. ureter
11. urinary bladder
12. pubic symphysis
13. ductus (vas) deferens
14. urethra
15. penis
16. foreskin (prepuce)

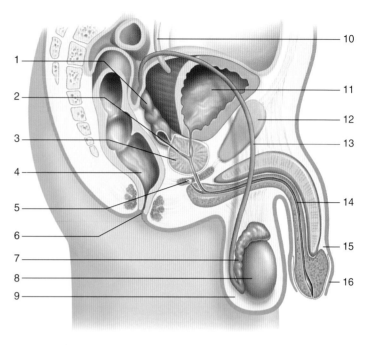

Figure 15.5a
Male reproductive organs and associated structures

1. pubic symphysis
2. urogenital triangle
3. anal triangle
4. ischial tuberosity
5. anus
6. coccyx

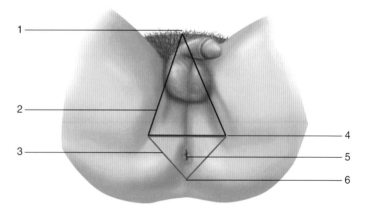

Figure 15.5b
External genitals of the male

Exercise 15.2: WORD ELEMENT MEANINGS AND WORD BUILDING

No answer provided for the medical term – refer to your dictionary for the correct spelling.

Word element	Meaning
andr/o	male
balan/o	glans penis
crypt/o	hidden
epididym/o	epididymis
fer/o	carry, bear
hydr/o	water
orch/o	testis, testicle
perine/o	perineum
phall/o	penis

Word element	Meaning
phim/o	muzzle
posth/o	prepuce, foreskin
prostat/o	prostate
semin/i	semen, seed
sperm/i	spermatozoa, sperm
terat/o	monster, malformed
test/i	testis, testicle
urethr/o	urethra
varic/o	swollen, twisted vein
vas/o	vessel, vas deferens, duct
vesicul/o	seminal vesicle

Exercise 15.3: VOCABULARY BUILDING

1. balanorrhoea
2. prostatomegaly, prostatic hypertrophy, prostatic hyperplasia
3. urethroplasty
4. spermatogenesis
5. vasoepididymostomy
6. epididymo-orchitis
7. spermaturia
8. intratesticular
9. orchidometer
10. spermatolysis
11. tumour of semen (this is the literal meaning but actually refers to a tumour of the testis)
12. suture of the ductus (vas) deferens
13. incision into the prostate gland and urinary bladder
14. excessive discharge or flow from the glans penis
15. surgical removal of the scrotum
16. incision into the seminal vesicle
17. pain in a testicle
18. inflammation of the penis
19. inflammation of the epididymis and testis
20. anastomosis of the ends of the ductus (vas) deferens after a vasectomy to attempt to restore function

Exercise 15.4: APPLYING MEDICAL TERMINOLOGY

1. b
2. b
3. c
4. d
5. b
6. a
7. b
8. a
9. b
10. c

Exercise 15.5: EXPAND THE ABBREVIATIONS

Abbreviation	Expanded abbreviation
BPH	benign prostatic hypertrophy
DRE	digital rectal examination
ED	erectile dysfunction
HPV	human papillomavirus
HSV	herpes simplex virus
NGU	non-gonococcal urethritis

Abbreviation	Expanded abbreviation
NSU	non-specific urethritis
PSA	prostate-specific antigen
RPR	rapid plasma reagin
STD	sexually transmitted disease
TRUS	transrectal ultrasound
TUNA	transurethral needle ablation
TUR(P)	transurethral resection (of prostate)
VD	venereal disease

Exercise 15.6: VOCABULARY BUILDING

1. anorchism
2. balanitis
3. paraphimosis
4. impotence
5. transrectal biopsy of the prostate gland
6. azoospermia
7. prostate gland
8. vasectomy
9. vasovasostomy
10. oligospermia

Exercise 15.7: MATCH MEDICAL TERMS AND MEANINGS

Column A	Answer
1. ejaculation	B
2. epididymis	D
3. hypospadias	G
4. orchiectomy	A
5. papilloma	C
6. prepuce	E
7. testicular torsion	H
8. varicocele	F

Exercise 15.8: PRONUNCIATION AND COMPREHENSION

No answer provided – self-directed study.

Exercise 15.9: CROSSWORD PUZZLE

ACROSS
4. balanitis
6. aspermia
7. psa test
8. varicocele

DOWN
1. phimosis
2. urethra
3. gynaecomastia
5. anorchism

Exercise 15.10: ANAGRAMS

1. peni(s)
2. pros(t)ate
3. impot(e)nce
4. ductu(s) deferens
5. ph(i)mosis
6. sperma(t)ozoa
TESTIS

Exercise 15.11: APPLYING MEDICAL TERMINOLOGY

1. bacterial prostatitis
2. digital rectal examination
3. epididymis
4. semen analysis
5. epispadias
6. circumcision
7. bulbourethral gland
8. ductus deferens

9. hydrocoele
10. paraphimosis
11. testosterone
12. gynaecomastia

13. priapism
14. prostate-specific antigen (PSA)
15. transurethral resection of the prostate (TURP)

Exercise 15.12: DISCHARGE SUMMARY ANALYSIS

1. TURP = transurethral resection of the prostate; ASA = American Society of Anesthesiologists; PSA = prostate-specific antigen; MI = myocardial infarction; DRE = digital rectal examination
2. The common signs and symptoms of prostate cancer that Mr Hendricks exhibited were poor urinary flow, frequency of urination, urinary hesitation, enlarged firm prostate and a raised PSA.
3. The Gleason score is a measurement of the severity of a prostate cancer, based on the appearance of the cancer cells when viewed pathologically. There are two parts to the score. Each patient is given a score from 1 to 5 for a primary grade and then a secondary grade. The Gleason score is the sum of the primary and secondary grades. As a result, the total score can be anything from a 2 (1 + 1) to a 10 (5 + 5). Scores from 2 to 4 are very low on the cancer aggression scale, while a score from 8 to 10 indicates that the cancer is highly aggressive. As a result, doctors can make predictions about a patient's prognosis based on the Gleason score.
4. Factors that will determine the type of treatment a patient is given include the age of the patient, the general health of the patient, the stage of disease at diagnosis, the level of PSA in the bloodstream, the Gleason score, the side effects of treatment and personal choice.
5. Options include active surveillance (watchful waiting), radiation therapy (external beam radiotherapy, brachytherapy with seeds and high dose rate brachytherapy), surgery (radical prostatectomy – open, laparoscopic or robotic), hormonal chemotherapy or HIFU (high-intensity focused ultrasound).
6. Mr Hendricks was able to pass urine (void) normally and he had good control over his ability to pass urine (continent).

CHAPTER 16: FEMALE REPRODUCTIVE SYSTEM

Exercise 16.1: LABEL THE DIAGRAM

1. fundus of uterus
2. body cavity of uterus
3. endometrium
4. myometrium
5. body of uterus
6. internal os of cervix
7. cervical canal
8. cervix of uterus
9. fornix of vagina
10. external os of vaginal cervix
11. isthmus of uterine tube
12. ovarian ligament
13. ampulla of uterine tube
14. infundibulum of uterine tube
15. infundibulopelvic ligament
16. fimbriae
17. ovary
18. broad ligament
19. uterine artery and vein
20. vagina

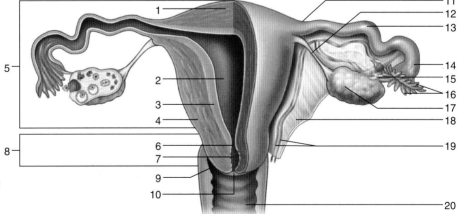

Figure 16.8
Pelvic female organs

Exercise 16.2: WORD ELEMENT MEANINGS AND WORD BUILDING

No answer provided for the medical term – refer to your dictionary for the correct spelling.

Word element	Meaning
colp/o	vagina
culd/o	cul-de-sac
endometri/o	endometrium
episi/o	vulva
fer/o	carry, bear
gynaec/o	woman, female
hyster/o	uterus
leiomy/o	smooth muscle
mamm/o	breast
mast/o	breast
men/o	menses, menstruation
metr/o	uterus
my/o	muscle
oophor/o	ovary
ov/i	egg, ovum
ovari/o	ovary
salping/o	fallopian tube, eustachian (auditory) tube
uter/o	uterus
vagin/o	vagina
vulv/o	vulva

Exercise 16.3: CIRCLE THE CORRECT SPELLING

menorrhagia

culdoscopy

myomectomy

salpingorrhaphy

oophorectomy

hysteroscopy

rectocele

hypomenorrhoea

endometriosis

fibromyoma

Exercise 16.4: WORD ANALYSIS AND MEANING

1. mast/o = breast; -ectomy = excision, surgical removal; meaning = surgical removal of breast
2. men/o = menses, menstruation; -arche = beginning, first; meaning = first menses
3. oligo- = scanty, deficiency, few; men/o = menses, menstruation; -rrhoea = discharge, flow; meaning = flow of menses that is scanty
4. o/o = egg, ovum; -blast = embryonic or developing cell; meaning = embryonic or developing cell (that forms an) ovum
5. cervic/o = neck, cervix uteri; -itis = inflammation; meaning = inflammation of the cervix uteri
6. hymen/o = hymen; -tomy = incision, cut into; meaning = incision into the hymen
7. hyster/o − uterus; -tomy − incision, cut into; meaning − incision into the uterus
8. mamm/o = breast; -gram = record, writing; meaning = record of the breast
9. metr/o = uterus; -ptosis = downward displacement, prolapsed; meaning = downward displacement, prolapse of uterus
10. uter/o = uterus; salping/o = fallopian tube, eustachian (auditory) tube; -graphy = process of recording; meaning = process of recording the uterus and fallopian tube (as this is the female reproductive system chapter)

Exercise 16.5: EXPAND THE ABBREVIATIONS

Abbreviation	Expanded abbreviation
BSE	breast self-examination
CIN	cervical intraepithelial neoplasia
CIS	carcinoma in situ
Cx	cervix
D&C	dilation (dilatation) and curettage
DUB	dysfunctional uterine bleeding
FSH	follicle stimulating hormone
HPV	human papillomavirus
HRT	hormone replacement therapy
IUD	intrauterine device
IVF	in vitro fertilisation
LEEP	loop electrosurgical excision procedure
LH	luteinising hormone
LMP	last menstrual period
PID	pelvic inflammatory disease
STI	sexually transmitted infection
TAH	total abdominal hysterectomy
TAHBSO	total abdominal hysterectomy with bilateral salpingo-oophorectomy
TRAM flap	transverse rectus abdominis myocutaneous flap
VAIN	vaginal intraepithelial neoplasia

Exercise 16.6: MATCH THE FEMALE REPRODUCTIVE ORGAN WITH ITS DESCRIPTION

Column A	Answer
1. labia	I
2. fallopian tube	H
3. hymen	F
4. fundus	G
5. myometrium	D
6. fornix	J
7. prepuce	B
8. fimbriae	A
9. cervix	C
10. Bartholin's glands	E

Exercise 16.7: APPLYING MEDICAL TERMINOLOGY

1. b
2. d
3. a
4. b
5. d

6. c
7. a
8. b
9. d
10. b

Exercise 16.8: PRONUNCIATION AND COMPREHENSION

No answer provided – self-directed study.

Exercise 16.9: CROSSWORD PUZZLE

ACROSS
   1. hysteroscopy
   4. uterine prolapse
   7. colposcopy
   8. hysterectomy
   9. endometriosis
  10. premenstrual syndrome

DOWN
   2. ovarian cyst
   3. fibrocystic disease
   5. aspiration
   6. culdocentesis

Exercise 16.10: ANAGRAMS

   1. mena(r)che
   2. la(b)ia
   3. (o)vary
   4. cervic(i)tis

   5. ovulat(i)on
   6. (f)imbriae
   7. (d)yspareunia
   FIBROID

Exercise 16.11: DISCHARGE SUMMARY ANALYSIS

   1. BSO = bilateral salpingo-oophorectomy; HVS = high vaginal swab; MSU = mid-stream urine; TAH = total abdominal hysterectomy; TCC = transitional cell carcinoma
   2. Mrs Preston has a history of breast cancer in both breasts. The type of cancer she had was oestrogen-receptor positive. This means that the growth of the tumours was stimulated by oestrogen. Oestrogen is released by the ovaries. Therefore, surgically removing the ovaries will lead to a decrease in oestrogen production and may prevent her hormone-positive breast tumours from recurring.
   3. A comorbidity is any disease, disorder or injury that exists in conjunction with another. Comorbid conditions can stand on their own as specific diseases. Their presence will often increase the severity of a patient's overall condition, resulting in a requirement for a greater level of care.
      Endometriosis is a condition where endometrial tissue is found outside the uterus in locations such as the ovaries, fallopian tubes, supporting ligaments, intestine, umbilicus and even in the chest cavity. It is caused when portions of menstrual endometrium pass backwards through the lumen of the fallopian tube into the peritoneal cavity during the menstrual cycle.
      It is important to treat endometriosis to ease the symptoms so the condition does not worsen or interfere with daily life. If endometriosis is not treated it can lead to severe pain, infertility, formation of scar tissue and adhesions. Therefore, treatment will be given to relieve pain, slow the growth of endometriosis, improve the chances of fertility and prevent the disease from recurring.
   4. The medical term for a fibroid is a leiomyoma.
      Many women experience no symptoms at all. However, the likelihood of symptoms increases with age. The most common symptoms include abnormal bleeding such as menorrhagia and metrorrhagia; pelvic pain associated with dysmenorrhoea; dyspareunia; compression of adjacent structures resulting in abdominal distension, frequent urination, constipation and bloating; reproductive dysfunction such as infertility, recurrent miscarriages and premature labour.
      Her medical record states that Mrs Preston experienced menorrhagia and dyspareunia. Menorrhagia is prolonged and/or profuse menstrual bleeding and dyspareunia is painful intercourse.

CHAPTER 17: OBSTETRICS AND NEONATOLOGY

Exercise 17.1: LABEL THE DIAGRAM

1. placenta
2. chorionic villi
3. chorion
4. yolk sac
5. umbilical cord
6. embryo
7. amniotic fluid
8. amnion

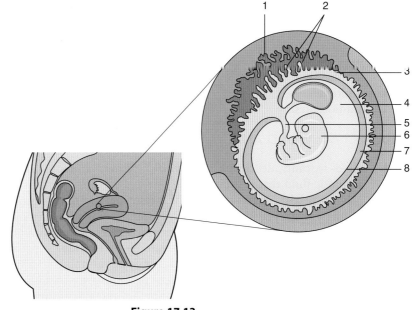

Figure 17.13
The uterus of a pregnant woman

Exercise 17.2: MATCH WORD ELEMENTS AND MEANINGS

Column A	Answer
1. omphal/o	F
2. galact/o	N
3. embry/o	J
4. macro-	M
5. cephal/o	B
6. paed/o	R
7. amni/o	P
8. primi-	O
9. epis/o	L
10. -cyesis	D
11. mening/o	C
12. -icterus	S
13. -rrhexis	T
14. nat/i	A
15. neo-	Q
16. ante-	G
17. terat/o	H
18. -schisis	E
19. fet/o	I
20. part/o	K

Exercise 17.3: VOCABULARY BUILDING

1. nulligravida
2. galactopoiesis
3. antenatal, prenatal, antepartum
4. postpartum, postnatal
5. primiparous
6. pseudocyesis
7. oxytocia
8. omphalitis
9. multipara
10. amniocentesis
11. placenta abruption, abruptio placentae
12. ectopic pregnancy
13. persistent occipitoposterior presentation
14. jaundice
15. spina bifida
16. placenta praevia
17. erythroblastosis fetalis
18. hydrocephalus
19. pyloric stenosis
20. Down syndrome

Exercise 17.4: WORD ANALYSIS AND MEANING

1. oligo- = scanty, deficiency, few; hydr/o = water; -amnios = amnion, amniotic fluid; meaning = amniotic fluid that is scanty
2. pelv/i = pelvis; -metry = process of measuring; meaning = process of measuring the pelvis
3. primi- = first; -gravida = pregnancy; meaning = first pregnancy
4. macro- = large; som/o = body; -ia = process, condition; meaning = condition of large body
5. neo- = new; nat/o = birth; -al = pertaining to; meaning = pertaining to new birth
6. hyper- = above, excessive; -emesis = vomiting; meaning = vomiting (that is) excessive
7. micro- = small; cephal/o = head; -ic = pertaining to; meaning = pertaining to small head
8. perine/o = perineum; -rrhaphy = suture; meaning = suture of perineum
9. chori/o = chorion; amni/o = amnion, amniotic fluid; -itis = inflammation; meaning = inflammation of chorion and amnion
10. gastr/o = stomach; -schisis = split; meaning = split stomach

Exercise 17.5: EXPAND THE ABBREVIATIONS

Abbreviation	Is this obstetric or neonatal?	Expanded abbreviation
APH	O	antepartum haemorrhage
BF	O or N	breastfeeding
DIC	O	disseminated intravascular coagulation
EDC/EDD	O	estimated date of confinement/delivery
HIE	N	hypoxic ischaemic encephalopathy
IUD	O or N	intrauterine death
IOL	O	induction of labour
LGA	N	large for gestational age
NND	N	neonatal death
OT	O	occipitotransverse
PIH	O	pregnancy-induced hypertension
POC	O	products of conception
SGA	N	small for gestational age
SIDS	N	sudden infant death syndrome
TOP	O	termination of pregnancy

Exercise 17.6: CORRECT THE SPELLING AND IDENTIFY THE INCORRECT TERMS

1. cephallic = cephalic; LSSCS = LSCS; fetel = fetal; labur = labour
2. endotracheel intubetion = endotracheal intubation; Intinsive = Intensive
3. wieght = weight; kilograms = grams; 34.4 m = 34.4 cm
4. weened = weaned; ventilater = ventilator; extubayte = extubate
5. spontanous = spontaneous; labuor = labour; gesstation = gestation; ceesarean = caesarean; cesarean = caesarean; feetal = fetal
6. hialine = hyaline; gesstational = gestational; shignon = chignon
7. meetabolic = metabolic; respratory acidiosis = respiratory acidosis
8. caesaren = caesarean; disloccation = dislocation; breach = breech
9. vaccum = vacuum; laybor = labour; post-partuum hemorhage = post-partum haemorrhage; anestetic = anaesthetic
10. labor = labour; artifccial = artificial; syntoccinon = syntocinon; pre-eclampsea = pre-eclampsia; gestaytion = gestation

Exercise 17.7: PRONUNCIATION AND COMPREHENSION

No answer provided – self-directed study.

Exercise 17.8: CROSSWORD PUZZLE

ACROSS

3. Down syndrome
7. placenta abruptio
8. pre-eclampsia
9. episiotomy
10. APGAR score
11. fetalis

DOWN

1. respiratory distress syndrome
2. hyperemesis gravidarum
4. erythroblastosis
5. neuraxial block
6. jaundice

Exercise 17.9: DISCHARGE SUMMARY ANALYSIS

1. PIH = pregnancy-induced hypertension; LSCS = lower segment caesarean section; ARM = artificial rupture of membranes; IV = intravenous; LMO = local medical officer; SCN = special care nursery
2. Pregnancy-induced hypertension (PIH) is a dangerous complication of pregnancy characterised by high blood pressure, oedema due to fluid retention and protein in the urine. It is also called pre-eclampsia. Symptoms include headaches, blurred vision, fatigue, nausea/vomiting, oliguria, photophobia, pain in the RUQ of the abdomen and shortness of breath.
   PIH can cause severe problems for both mother and baby. In the mother, PIH can result in placental abruption, seizures, temporary kidney failure, liver problems and blood clotting problems. In the baby, PIH can prevent the placenta from getting enough blood, resulting in lowered levels of oxygen and nutrition. This can result in low birth weight and a premature birth.
3. Labour is induced if there is more risk in allowing the pregnancy to continue than there is in earlier delivery. At 34 weeks' gestation, Chloe's labour was artificially started due to her PIH. She had a combined induction. Initially Chloe had an ARM performed. This is done by passing a small hook through the cervix. This hook then makes a hole in the membranes, 'breaking the waters'. Simply performing an ARM can be enough to stimulate labour for some women. However, sometimes Syntocinon will be used for induction (or augmentation) of labour. This is given by an IV infusion. Syntocinon is similar to oxytocin, a chemical produced in normal labour that stimulates uterine contractions.
4. An elective caesarean section is usually planned (usually during the antenatal period) and performed prior to labour commencing. An emergency caesarean section is performed as a result of a complication that arises during labour.
5. The babies were born 6 weeks premature and were low and very low birth weights. At that gestational age and weights, it is possible they would have had some developmental problems. They would need to remain in the special care nursery until they put on weight and reached appropriate developmental milestones.

CHAPTER 18: MENTAL HEALTH

Exercise 18.1: WORD ELEMENT MEANINGS AND WORD BUILDING

No answer provided for the medical term – refer to your dictionary for the correct spelling.

Combining forms	Meaning
cycl/o	circle, recurring
hallucin/o	hallucinations, to wander in the mind
iatr/o	physician, medicine, treatment
klept/o	steal
morph/o	form, shape
neur/o	nerve
phil/o	attraction to, love
phor/o	carry, bear
pol/o	extreme
psych/o	mind
schiz/o	split
somat/o	body
xen/o	foreign, strange
agora-	marketplace, open space
cata-	down
electro-	electricity, electrical activity
eu-	normal, good
-lalia	disorder of speech
-leptic	type of seizure
-mania	state of mental disorder, frenzy
-philia	attraction for

Exercise 18.2: WORD ANALYSIS AND MEANING

1. klept/o = steal; -mania = state of mental disorder, frenzy; meaning = a state of mental disorder characterised by stealing
2. geront/o = old age, the aged; -phobia = condition of fear; meaning = condition of fear of old age or the aged
3. hypo- = below, under, deficient, less than normal; chondr/o = cartilage; -iac = pertaining to; meaning = pertaining to under cartilage (of the ribs)
4. dys- = bad, painful, difficult; morph/o = form or shape; -phobia = condition of fear; meaning = condition of fear of bad shape
5. schiz/o = split; -phren/o = mind or diaphragm; -ia = condition of; meaning = condition of split mind
6. neur/o = nerve; -osis = abnormal condition; meaning = abnormal condition of nerves
7. dys- = bad, painful, difficult; -thymia = condition of mind, emotion; meaning = condition of difficult emotion
8. copr/o = obscenity; -lalia = condition of speech; meaning = condition of obscene speech
9. narc/o = stupor or sleep; -leptic = a type of seizure; meaning = a type of seizure (resulting in) sleep or stupor
10. trich/ o = hair; till/o = to pluck; -mania = state of mental disorder, frenzy; meaning = state of mental disorder of plucking hair

Exercise 18.3: VOCABULARY BUILDING

1. hallucination
2. psychiatrist
3. bipolar
4. dysphoria
5. nyctophobia
6. pyromania

7. mental
8. agoraphobia
9. apathy
10. hypnosis

Exercise 18.4: MATCH THE ABBREVIATIONS WITH THE EXPANDED FORM

Column A	Answer
1. AD	G
2. OCD	F
3. MDD	J
4. SSRI	A
5. CBT	H
6. MSE	B
7. ETOH	I
8. SAD	C
9. ASD	D
10. MA	E

Exercise 18.5: MATCH THE THERAPY WITH ITS MEANING

Column A	Answer
1. psychoanalysis	E
2. family therapy	F
3. psychotherapy	G
4. group therapy	A
5. hypnosis	B
6. play therapy	D
7. cognitive behaviour therapy	C

Exercise 18.6: PRONUNCIATION AND COMPREHENSION

No answer provided – self-directed study.

Exercise 18.7: CROSSWORD PUZZLE

ACROSS
1. triskaidekaphobia
3. iatrophobia
5. belonephobia
6. sesquipedalophobia
7. brontophobia
9. gamophobia
10. cynophobia

DOWN
2. acrophobia
4. mysophobia
8. androphobia

Exercise 18.8: DISCHARGE SUMMARY ANALYSIS

1. B_{12} = vitamin B_{12}; EEG = electroencephalogram; MSQ = mental state questionnaire; SMA = sequential multiple analysis; TFTs = thyroid function tests
2. Mrs Harris should be taking 150 milligrams at night.
3. Syphilis serology is performed to determine if there is an organic cause for the depression and seizures. In some patients, tertiary syphilis can result in depression or seizures.
4. The Holter EEG is performed to measure her brain activity over a 24-hour period to assist in diagnosis of a cause for the seizures.
5. Atypical absence seizures are characterised by vacant, staring spells. The person suddenly seems to be 'absent'. It involves a brief loss of awareness, which can be accompanied by blinking or mouth twitching. It presents as a distinctive pattern on a Holter EEG.

CHAPTER 19: ONCOLOGY

Exercise 19.1: MATCH WORD ELEMENTS AND MEANINGS

Column A	Answer
1. blast/o	L
2. rhabd/o	O
3. chondr/o	P
4. meta-	N
5. astr/o	R
6. tele-	Q
7. leuc/o	A
8. -plasia	M
9. onc/o	D
10. cauter/o	T
11. scirrh/o	C
12. pleio-	I
13. mut/a	G
14. cry/o	H
15. brachy-	S
16. papill/o	E
17. fibr/o	J
18. -therapy	K
19. gnos/o	B
20. cac/o	F

Exercise 19.2: CIRCLE THE CORRECT SPELLING

prognosis

metastatic

neurofibroma

anaplastic

adenocarcinoma

cachexia

scirrhoid

sarcoma

carcinogenesis

oncologist

Exercise 19.3: WORD ANALYSIS AND MEANING

1. retin/o = retina; blast/o = embryonic or developing cell; -oma = tumour; meaning = tumour in the embryonic cells of the retina
2. chem/o = drug; -therapy = treatment; meaning = treatment with drugs
3. pleo- = more; morph/o = form or shape; -ic = pertaining to; meaning = pertaining to more shape or form
4. dys- = bad, painful, difficult; plas/o − formation; -ia − condition of; meaning = condition of bad formation
5. immun/o = protection; -suppression = to stop; meaning = to stop protection
6. oste/o = bone; chondr/o = cartilage; -oma = tumour; meaning = tumour of the bone and cartilage
7. brachy- = short; -therapy = treatment; meaning = treatment that is short (generally used to refer to treatment where source of radiation is a short distance from the target)
8. neo- = new; -plasm = growth, formation, substance; meaning = growth that is new
9. onc/o = tumour; -genesis = pertaining to, formation or producing; meaning = pertaining to tumour formation
10. myel/o = bone marrow or spinal cord; -oma = tumour; meaning = tumour of bone marrow

Exercise 19.4: EXPAND THE ABBREVIATIONS

Abbreviation	Expanded abbreviation
ABC	advanced breast cancer
ABMT	autologous bone marrow transplant
ALL	acute lymphoblastic leukaemia; acute lymphocytic leukaemia
BM	bone marrow
Bx	biopsy
Ca	cancer, carcinoma
CLL	chronic lymphocytic leukaemia
DCIS	ductal carcinoma in situ
FAP	familial adenomatous polyposis
FOBT	faecal occult blood test
GIST	gastrointestinal stromal tumour
LMP	low malignant potential
NED	no evidence of disease
NK	natural killer (cells)
PET	positron emission tomography
RAD	radiation absorbed dose
SNB	sentinel node biopsy
SPECT	single photon emission computed tomography
TCC	transitional cell carcinoma
TNM	tumour nodes metastases

Exercise 19.5: APPLYING MEDICAL TERMINOLOGY

1. in situ
2. undifferentiated
3. malignant
4. metastasised
5. well differentiated
6. grade
7. benign
8. neoplasm
9. primary
10. stage

Exercise 19.6: PRONUNCIATION AND COMPREHENSION

No answer provided – self-directed study.

Exercise 19.7: CROSSWORD PUZZLE

ACROSS
1. exenteration
5. cryosurgery
7. Gleason system
9. antimicrotubules
10. fractionation

DOWN
2. radiosensitisers
3. electrocauterisation
4. mixed types
6. metastasis
8. mammogram

Exercise 19.8: ANAGRAMS

1. mali(g)nant
2. (b)iopsy
3. ade(n)oma
4. r(e)mission
5. mela(n)oma
6. (i)nvasive
BENIGN

Exercise 19.9: DISCHARGE SUMMARY ANALYSIS

1. Ca = cancer; CMF = cyclophosphamide methotrexate & fluorouracil; FBC = full blood count; IV = intravenous; q.i.d. = four times a day; WCC = white cell count
2. Haemodynamically stable refers to the fact that the patient's circulatory system functions (e.g. heart rate, blood pressure, pulse) remain stable.
3. Bronchial washing is a procedure performed during a bronchoscopy to irrigate the bronchi. The washings are usually sent to the laboratory for pathological examination.
4. A monophonic wheeze has a single pitch and tone heard over a unique area.
5. The morphological type of a tumour indicates the cells from which the tumour originates. A secondary tumour always has the same morphology as the primary tumour from which it has metastasised. For Mrs Green the morphology of the metastatic tumour was an adenocarcinoma, the same morphological type as the colon cancer. The morphology of her breast cancer was infiltrating ductal carcinoma. Therefore the bronchial secondaries must have metastasised from her colon.

CHAPTER 20: INFECTIOUS AND PARASITIC DISEASES

Exercise 20.1: MATCH WORD ELEMENTS AND MEANINGS

Column A	Answer
1. bacill/o	G
2. -cide	L
3. bi/o	A
4. cocc/o	H
5. crypt/o	N
6. fung/i	O or Q
7. helminth/o	M
8. myc/o	Q or O
9. path/o	P
10. protozo/o	S
11. septic/o	T or B
12. staphyl/o	R
13. strept/o	K
14. tox/o	C
15. vir/o	E
16. -sepsis	B or T
17. -itis	D
18. -form	I
19. anti-	J
20. retro-	F

Exercise 20.2: WORD ELEMENTS AND WORD BUILDING

No answer provided – self-directed study.

Exercise 20.3: BUILDING MEDICAL TERMS

1. rhinitis
2. otitis
3. gastritis
4. hepatitis
5. glossitis
6. dermatitis
7. arthritis
8. gingivitis
9. cholecystitis
10. cystitis
11. vaginitis
12. balinitis

13. colitis
14. appendicitis
15. stomatitis
16. thyroiditis
17. oesophagitis
18. pericarditis
19. bronchitis
20. encephalitis

Exercise 20.4: EXPAND THE ABBREVIATIONS

Abbreviation	Expanded abbreviation
ADT	adult diphtheria tetanus (vaccine)
AIDS	acquired immunodeficiency syndrome
BSE	bovine spongiform encephalopathy
CJD	Creutzfeld-Jakob disease
CMV	cytomegalovirus
C & S	culture and sensitivity
CSF	cerebrospinal fluid
DTP	diphtheria tetanus pertussis (vaccine)
EBV	Epstein-Barr virus
EIA	enzyme immunoassay
ELISA	enzyme-linked immunosorbent assay
HBV	hepatitis B virus
HiB	*Haemophilus influenzae* type b
HIV	human immunodeficiency virus
HPV	human papillomavirus
HSV	herpes simplex virus
IgA	immunoglobulin A
LP	lumbar puncture
MMR	measles mumps rubella (vaccine)
MRSA	methicillin (or multiple) resistant *Staphylococcus aureus*
PCP	*Pneumocystis* pneumonia
STI/STD	sexually transmitted infection/sexually transmitted disease
TB	tuberculosis

Exercise 20.5: VOCABULARY BUILDING

1. bacteriologist
2. septicaemia
3. bactericidal
4. bacteriuria
5. viraemia
6. mycosis
7. microbiology
8. rhinovirus
9. parasitology
10. fungicide

Exercise 20.6: PRONUNCIATION AND COMPREHENSION

No answer provided – self-directed study.

Exercise 20.7: CROSSWORD PUZZLE

ACROSS
3. Hendra virus
4. endoparasite
5. pathogen
7. rubella
9. Ross River fever
10. immunisation

DOWN
1. meningococcal disease
2. aseptic
6. rotavirus
8. helminth

Exercise 20.8: DISCHARGE SUMMARY ANALYSIS

1. BIBA = brought in by ambulance; ICC = intercostal catheter; WBC = white blood cells; ARF = acute renal failure; Ca = cancer; Dx = diagnosis

2. Sepsis is a bacterial infection of the blood, also known as septicaemia, bacteraemia or blood poisoning. It is a serious, life-threatening infection that can worsen rapidly. It is usually caused by infection with *Escherichia coli* (*E. coli*), *Pneumococcus*, *Klebsiella*, *Pseudomonas*, *Staphylococcus* or *Streptococcus*. The bacteria enter the bloodstream as a result of a previous infection, burn, infected wound or other break in the skin. Symptoms include spiking fevers, chills, tachypnoea and tachycardia. The patient can deteriorate rapidly, with shock, hypothermia, hypotension, oliguria and delirium. Septicaemia is a medical emergency requiring urgent hospital treatment such as intravenous antibiotics, oxygen and fluids to maintain the blood pressure.

3. Metastatic breast cancer in the lungs means that Ms Jackson has had a primary cancer in her breast. That cancer has then spread (metastasised) to her lungs, where it is considered a secondary tumour.

4. The symptoms of a pneumothorax or collapsed lung include sharp, stabbing chest pain that worsens on breathing or with deep inspiration; pain that often radiates to the shoulder and/or back; and a dry, hacking cough due to irritation of the diaphragm. If it is a tension pneumothorax, there will be signs of cardiovascular collapse such as dilated veins in the neck, cyanosis, rapid pulse and hypotension. Cardiovascular shock will likely occur.

5. An ICC (intercostal catheter) is a flexible plastic tube that is inserted through the side of the chest into the pleural space. It is used to remove air (pneumothorax) or fluid (pleural effusion, haemothorax), or pus (empyema) from the intrathoracic space.

CHAPTER 21: RADIOLOGY AND NUCLEAR MEDICINE

Exercise 21.1: MATCH WORD ELEMENTS AND MEANINGS

Column A	Answer
1. anter/o	H
2. brachy-	L
3. cine-	P or V
4. cinemat/o	V or P
5. dist/o	B
6. echo-	R
7. fluor/o	U
8. -gram	K
9. -graph	Q
10. -graphy	A
11. iso-	W
12. -ist	X
13. later/o	C
14. -lucent	T
15. medi/o	D
16. -opaque	F
17. proxim/o	I
18. radi/o	Y
19. roentgen/o	J
20. scint/i	G
21. son/o	E
22. therapeut/o	O
23. therm/o	Z

Column A	Answer
24. tom/o	M
25. top/o	S
26. ultra-	N

Exercise 21.2: CIRCLE THE CORRECT SPELLING

venogram
radiolucent
urography
radionuclide
radiopharmaceutical

thallium
brachytherapy
teletherapy
nuclear
scintigraphy

Exercise 21.3: IDENTIFY THE COMBINING FORMS AND MEANING OF MEDICAL TERMS

Medical term	Combining form	Meaning of medical term
cineradiography	radi/o	process of recording a moving x-ray
mammogram	mamm/o	record of the breast
angiography	angi/o	process of recording blood vessels
ultrasonography	son/o	process of recording beyond, excess sound
cardiotocography	cardi/o, toc/o	process of recording heart in childbirth
radiopharmaceutical	radi/o, pharmaceutic/o	pertaining to an x-ray drug
fluoroscope	fluor/o	instrument to view fluorescent or luminous
tomogram	tom/o	record of slices, sections
echocardiogram	cardi/o	record of the reflected sounds of the heart
isothermic	therm/o	pertaining to equal heat

Exercise 21.4: EXPAND THE ABBREVIATIONS

Abbreviation	Expanded abbreviation
AP	anteroposterior
Ba	barium
BE	barium enema
BMD scan	bone mineral density scan
CT	computed tomography
CTCA	computed tomography coronary angiography
CTG	cardiotocography
CXR	chest x-ray
DEXA	dual energy x-ray absorptiometry
DSA	digital subtraction angiography
DXT	deep x-ray therapy
IVP	intravenous pyelogram
MIBI scan	sestamibi scan
MRI	magnetic resonance imaging
MUGA	multiple gated acquisition scan
PET scan	positron emission tomography scan
SPECT	single photon emission computed tomography
SRS	stereotactic radiosurgery
U/S	ultrasound
XR	x-ray

Exercise 21.5: MATCH THE PROCEDURE WITH ITS MEANING

Column A	Answer
1. brachytherapy	G
2. radioimmunotherapy	J
3. thallium scan	K
4. MUGA scan	H
5. cholangiography	B
6. cholecystography	I
7. barium enema	C
8. MRI	L
9. dual energy x-ray absorptiometry	E
10. ultrasound	F
11. echocardiography	A
12. roentgenogram	D

Exercise 21.6: VOCABULARY BUILDING

1. radiopharmaceuticals
2. radioisotopes
3. uptake
4. computed tomography
5. nuclear medicine
6. myocardial perfusion scan
7. radioactive iodine ^{131}I therapy
8. radiotherapy
9. radiology
10. tagging

Exercise 21.7: PRONUNCIATION AND COMPREHENSION

No answer provided – self-directed study.

Exercise 21.8: CROSSWORD PUZZLE

ACROSS

2. thallium
8. radiographer
9. roentgen
10. MRI

DOWN

1. fluoroscope
3. uptake
4. ultrasound imaging
5. radiolucent
6. SPECT
7. gamma rays

Exercise 21.9: DISCHARGE LETTER ANALYSIS

1. This means he was injected with 27.4 mCi (mCi is a millicurie (1/1000 of a curie), which is a unit of radioactivity) of technetium 99 m methylene diphosphonate, which is a radioactive isotope used in nuclear medicine that medical equipment can detect in the human body. It is used to detect bone metastases.
2. Bone scintigraphy, also called a bone scan, is a diagnostic nuclear medicine test in which radioisotopes are injected into the body. The emitted radiation is captured by a gamma camera (also called a scintillation counter) to create two-dimensional images called scintigrams. It is performed to locate abnormalities in bone such as cancers that have metastasised.
3. The scan was performed to assess disease in Mr Dunstan's bones. It takes time for the radiopharmaceutical to be absorbed into the bones in amounts that the gamma camera can detect, hence the 3-hour time delay.
4. SPECT stands for single-photon emission computed tomography. It is a 3D tomographic technique that uses gamma camera data from many projections that can be reconstructed in different planes. The camera builds a computer-enhanced image from the radiation source. Metabolic and physiological

functions of organs such as the brain, heart, liver, spleen and bones are commonly studied using SPECT. It is very similar to conventional nuclear medicine planar imaging using a gamma camera. However, it is able to provide true 3D information.

5. There had been an increase in metastatic disease in Mr Dunstan's bones. The doctors wanted to identify exactly how much disease was present. A SPECT is a very specific procedure that can identify very small lesions in bone – more so than other nuclear medicine techniques.

CHAPTER 22: PHARMACOLOGY

Exercise 22.1: WORD ELEMENT MEANINGS AND WORD BUILDING

No answer provided for the medical term – refer to your dictionary for the correct spelling.

Word element	Meaning
aer/o	air, gas
aesthes/o	feeling, sensation
algesi/o	pain
ana-	up, towards, apart
anti-	against
bacteri/o	bacteria
-cide	killing, agent for killing
contra-	against
cutane/o	skin
emet/o	vomiting
hypn/o	sleep
lingu/o	tongue
-lytic	drug that breaks down
narc/o	stupor
-phylaxis	protection
thec/o	sheath
top/o	place, location
ven/o	vein

Exercise 22.2: IDENTIFY THE COMBINING FORMS AND MEANING OF MEDICAL TERMS

Medical term	Combining form	Meaning of medical term
pharmacologist	pharmac/o, log/o	one who specialises in the study of drugs
toxicology	toxic/o	the study of poisons
antipruritic	prurit/o	pertaining to against itching (refers to a drug)
chemotherapy	chem/o	treatment by drug
bronchospasm	bronch/o	involuntary contraction of bronchial tube
antihistamine	hist/o	nitrogen compound against tissue
iatrogenic	iatr/o	pertaining to formation, producing treatment
mycotoxic	myc/o, tox/o	pertaining to toxic mould and fungus
antipyretic	pyret/o	pertaining to against fever (refers to a drug)
intradermal	derm/o	pertaining to into the skin

Exercise 22.3: MATCH THE ROUTE OF ADMINISTRATION WITH THE DEFINITION

Column A	Answer
1. topical	L
2. transdermal	E
3. otic	H
4. ophthalmic	K
5. enteral	A
6. intra-articular	M
7. subcutaneous	I
8. intramuscular	F
9. intrathecal	D
10. intravenous	C
11. oral	I
12. sublingual	G
13. intraperitoneal	B

Exercise 22.4: MATCH THE DRUG ACTION WITH THE DRUG TYPE

Column A	Answer
1. drug that relieves pain	I
2. drug that induces a loss of feeling or sensation	L
3. drug that relieves mood disorders	E
4. drug that blocks the effect of an allergic reaction	N
5. drug that induces sleep	K
6. drug that opens up the airways	C
7. drug that lowers blood pressure	D
8. drug that increases urine output	M
9. drug that lowers blood cholesterol	O
10. drug that reduces glucose levels	G
11. drug that stops vomiting	A
12. drug that stops blood from clotting	F
13. drug that prevents seizures	H
14. drug that reduces anxiety levels	B
15. drug that treats bacterial infections	J

Exercise 22.5: EXPAND THE ABBREVIATIONS

Abbreviation	Expanded abbreviation
PCA	patient-controlled analgesia
p.c.	after meals
g	gram(s)
b.i.d.	twice a day
q.n.	every evening
NBM	nil by mouth
gtt	drops
MIMS	Monthly Index of Medical Specialties
p.r.n.	as occasion requires, as needed

Abbreviation	Expanded abbreviation
q.4 h.	every four hours
q.6 h.	every six hours
q.d.	every day
q.i.d.	four times a day
stat.	immediately
tab.	tablet
t.i.d.	three times a day
Rx	symbol for prescription or treatment
q.a.m.	every morning, every day before noon
mcg	microgram
IM	intramuscular

Exercise 22.6: APPLYING MEDICAL TERMINOLOGY

1. adverse reaction
2. allergic reaction
3. anaphylaxis
4. idiosyncratic response
5. placebo
6. toxicity
7. side effects
8. dose–response relationship
9. metabolism
10. dependence

Exercise 22.7: BUILDING MEDICAL TERMS

1. pharmacist
2. pharmacotherapy
3. pharmacokinetics
4. pharmacodynamics
5. pharmacy

Exercise 22.8: PRONUNCIATION AND COMPREHENSION

No answer provided – self-directed study.

Exercise 22.9: CROSSWORD PUZZLE

ACROSS
3. dose
4. MIMS
6. contraindication
8. pharmacy
9. subcutaneous

DOWN
1. antipruritic
2. contraceptive
5. pharmacologist
7. intravenous
8. prophylaxis

Exercise 22.10: INTERPRET THE PRESCRIPTION

Drug and dosage instructions	Translated dosage instructions
Zovirax 400 mg t.d.s.	1 400 mg tablet three times a day
Aropax 20 mg q.a.m.	1 20 mg tablet every morning
Warfarin 5 mg noct.	1 5 mg tablet at night
Tagamet 400 mg b.d.	1 400 mg tablet twice a day
Temazapam 10 mg q.h.s.	1 10 mg tablet every night at bed time
Efudix cream 5% 20 g q.d.	apply cream (5% strength, 20 g tube) every day
Ventolin 100 mcg 1–2 inhalations q.i.d.	inhaler or puffer – 1–2 inhalations 4 times a day
Pethidine hydrochloride IMI 50 mg q.d.s.	50 mg intramuscular injection 4 times a day
Flagyl 400 mg b.d. a.c.	1 400 mg tablet twice a day before meals
Ibuprofen 200 mg p.r.n. up to 6 tabs. q.d.	200 mg tablets as required up to a maximum of 6 per day

Picture credits

Chapter 3

Figure 3.3: Based on Salvo SG. *Massage Therapy: Principles and Practice*, Figure 11.18. Saunders, 2007.

Figure 3.6: *Mosby's Dictionary of Medicine, Nursing & Health Professions*, 9th edn, Figure A-5. Mosby, 2014.

Chapter 4

Figures 4.1, 4.6, 4.10a&b: Harris P, Nagy S, Vardaxis N (eds). *Mosby's Dictionary of Medicine, Nursing & Health Professions*, 3rd ANZ edition, p. A-2. Sydney: Mosby, 2014.

Figure 4.2: Thibodeau GA, Patton KT. *Anatomy & Physiology*, 7th edn. St Louis: Mosby, 2010.

Figure 4.3: Griffith HW. *Instructions for Patients*, 5th edn, p. 592. Philadelphia: WB Saunders, 1994.

Figure 4.4: Hansen J, Netter F, & Machado C: *Netter's clinical anatomy*, 4th edn. Figure 1.9 Philadelphia: Elsevier, 2019.

Figure 4.5: Based on LaFleur Brooks M. *Exploring Medical Language*, 6th edn. Mosby, 2005.

Figure 4.7: Thibodeau GA, Patton KT. *Anatomy & Physiology*, 5th edn. St Louis: Mosby, 2003.

Figure 4.8: Leonard PC. *Building a Medical Vocabulary*, 6th edn, Figure 14.17. Philadelphia: WB Saunders, 2005.

Figure 4.9: Stuart Orkin S, Fisher D, Look AT et al. *Oncology of Infancy and Childhood*, Figure 22.8. St Louis: Saunders, 2009.

Chapter 5

Figures 5.1, 5.14: Adkinson NF, Busse WW, Bochner BS et al. *Middleton's Allergy: Principles and Practice*, 7th edn. Mosby, 2008.

Figure 5.2: Leonard PC: *Building a Medical Vocabulary*, 7th edn. Philadelphia: WB Saunders, 2009.

Figure 5.3: Talley NJ, O'Connor S. *Clinical Examination: A Systematic Guide to Physical Diagnosis*, 6th edn, Figure 15.4. Sydney: Churchill Livingstone, 2009. Adapted from Schwartz M. *Textbook of Physical Diagnosis*, 4th edn. Philadelphia: Saunders, 2002.

Figure 5.4: Black J, Hawks J. *Medical-Surgical Nursing: Clinical Management for Positive Outcomes*, 8th edn. Philadelphia: Saunders, 2009.

Figure 5.5: Habif TP. *Clinical Dermatology*, 5th edn, Figure 9.4. Mosby, 2009.

Figure 5.6: Gawkrodger D. *Dermatology: An Illustrated Colour Text*, 4th edn, Figure 7.15. Mosby, 2008.

Figures 5.7, 5.8: Illustrations, Harris P, Nagy S, Vardaxis N (eds). *Mosby's Dictionary of Medicine, Nursing & Health Professions*, 3rd ANZ edition, p. 262. Sydney: Mosby, 2014; photos, Burn Injury Network, NSW Agency for Clinical Innovation.

Figure 5.9: Stevens A, Lowe JS, Ian Scott I. *Core Pathology*, 3rd edn, Figure 23.2. Mosby, 2009.

Figure 5.10: Schwarzenberger K, Werchniak AE, Ko C. *General Dermatology*, Figure 12.1. Saunders, 2009.

Figure 5.11: Callen JP et al: *Color atlas of dermatology*, 2nd edn, Figure 2.59. Philadelphia: WB Saunders, 2000.

Figure 5.12: Marks J, Miller J. *Lookingbill and Marks Principles of Dermatology*, 4th edn, Figure 6.10. Edinburgh: Saunders, 2006.

Figure 5.13: McCance KL, Huether SE: *Pathophysiology: the biologic basis for disease in adults and children*, 4th edn. St Louis:Mosby, 2002.

Chapter 6

Figures 6.1, 6.7: Based on Hutton A. *Medical Terminology for Healthcare: a self teaching package*, 3rd edn, Figure 26. Churchill Livingstone, 2002.

Figure 6.3: Australian Red Cross Lifeblood: *About blood types* 2018 Accessed at https://www.donateblood.com.au/learn/about-blood

Figure 6.6: Perry AG, Potter PA. *Fundamentals of Nursing*, 6th edn. Steps 24 & 29. Mosby, 2005.

Chapter 7

Figures 7.1, 7.2, 7.5: Harris P, Nagy S, Vardaxis N (eds). *Mosby's Dictionary of Medicine, Nursing & Health Professions*, 3rd ANZ edition, p. A-21. Sydney: Mosby, 2014.

Figure 7.3: Applegate E. *The Anatomy and Physiology Learning System*, 4th edn. Saunders, 2011.

Figure 7.4: Cronewett J, W Johnston W. *Rutherford's Vascular Surgery*, 7th edn, Figure 65.4. Saunders, 2010.

Chapter 8

Figure 8.3: Hochberg M, Silman A, Smolen J et al. *Rheumatology*, 4th edn, Figure 180.3. Edinburgh: Mosby, 2008.

Figure 8.4: Zimmermann MB, Jooste PL, Pandav CS. Iodine-deficiency disorders, *Lancet* 372:1251–1262, 2008.

Figure 8.5: Lemmi FO, Lemmi CAE. *Physical Assessment Findings* CD-ROM. Philadelphia: Saunders, 2007.

Figure 8.6: Kanski J. *Clinical Diagnosis in Ophthalmology*, Figure 1.19. Edinburgh: Mosby, 2006.

Figure 8.7: Zitelli BJ, Davis HW. *Atlas of Pediatric Physical Diagnosis*, 3rd edn, Figure 9.23a&c. Gower, 1997.

Chapter 9

Figures 9.1, 9.5, 9.12: © Alila/Fotolia.com.

Figures 9.2, 9.3: Harris P, Nagy S, Vardaxis N (eds). *Mosby's Dictionary of Medicine, Nursing & Health Professions*, 3rd ANZ edition, p. A-13. Sydney: Mosby, 2014.

Figure 9.6: Shiland BJ. *Mastering Healthcare Terminology*, 2nd edn, Figure 10.15a (illustration). Mosby, 2006. Damjanov I, Linder J. *Pathology: A Color Atlas*, St Louis: Mosby, 2000 (photograph).

Figure 9.8: Golman MP, Guex JJ, Weiss RA: *Sclerotherapy: Treatment of Varicose and Telangiectatic Leg Veins*, 5th edn, Figure 9.36. Saunders, 2011.

Figure 9.10: Sellke F, del Nido PD, Swanson S. *Sabiston and Spencer's Surgery of the Chest*, 8th edn, Figure 74.9. Saunders, 2009.

Figure 9.11: A, LaFleur Brooks M. *Exploring Medical Language*, 6th edn, Figure 10.16. Mosby, 2005; B, Ballinger PW, Frank ED. *Merrill's Atlas of Radiographic Positions and Radiologic Procedures*, 10th edn. St Louis: Mosby, 2003.

Chapter 10

Figures 10.1, 10.2, 10.11: Harris P, Nagy S, Vardaxis N (eds). *Mosby's Dictionary of Medicine, Nursing & Health Professions*, 3rd ANZ edition, p. A29 (top figure, bottom figure). Sydney: Mosby, 2014.

Figure 10.3: Thibodeau GA, Patton KT: *Anatomy & Physiology*, 6th edn, Figure 24.33c. St. Louis: Mosby, 2007.

Figure 10.4: Kumar V, Abbas AK, Fausto N. *Robbins and Cotran Pathologic Basis of Disease*, 7th edn. Mosby, 2005.

Figure 10.5: Adam A, Dixon AK, Grainger RG et al. *Grainger & Allison's Diagnostic Radiology*, 5th edn, Figure 15.8. Churchill Livingstone, 2007.

Figure 10.7: Elkin MK, Perry AG, Potter PA. *Nursing Interventions and Clinical Skills*, 4th edn, Figure 14.3. Mosby, 2007.

Figure 10.8: Shiland BJ. *Mastering Healthcare Terminology*, 2nd edn, Figure 11.18. Mosby, 2006.

Figure 10.9: Blamb/Shutterstock.

Figure 10.10: Amy Walters/Fotolia.com.

Chapter 11

Figures 11.1, 11.2, 11.14a&b: Harris P, Nagy S, Vardaxis N (eds). *Mosby's Dictionary of Medicine, Nursing & Health Professions*, 3rd ANZ edition, p. A-33. Sydney: Mosby, 2014.

Figure 11.4: Patton KT, Thibodeau GA. *Anatomy & Physiology*, 7th edn. Figure 25.35. St Louis: Mosby, 2010.

Figure 11.6: Sudhakaran N, & Ade-Ajayi N: Appendicitis in children, *Surgery* 28(1): 16–21, 2010.

Figure 11.7: Kumar V, Abbas AK, Fausto N et al. *Robbins and Cotran Pathologic Basis of Disease*, 8th edn, Figure 18.52. Saunders, 2009.

Figure 11.8: Goldman L, Schafer AI. *Goldman-Cecil Medicine*, 24th edn, Figure 156.1. Saunders, 2011.

Figure 11.9: A, Waugh A, Grant A. *Ross and Wilson Anatomy and Physiology in Health and Illness*, 11th edn, Figure 12.50. Edinburgh: Churchill Livingstone, 2010; B: Sleisenger and Fordtran 2016.

Figure 11.10: Leonard PC. *Building a Medical Vocabulary*, 6th edn, Figure 6.12. Philadelphia: WB Saunders, 2005.

Figure 11.11: Lau WY, Lai ECH, Lau SHY: Laparoscopic Cholecystectomy for Acute Cholecystitis, in *Video Atlas of Advanced Minimally Invasive Surgery*, edited by Frantzides CT. & Carlson MA., Figure 16.10 Philadelphia: Elsevier/Saunders 2013 Pages 139-146.

Figure 11.12: Copyright 1991, Mayo Clinic, Rochester, Minn.

Figure 11.13: Ballinger PW, Frank ED. *Merrill's Atlas of Radiographic Positions and Radiologic Procedures*, 10th edn, exercise G(2). St Louis: Mosby, 2003.

Chapter 12

Figure 12.2: Thibodeau GA, Patton KT. *Anatomy and Physiology*, 5th edn. St Louis: Mosby, 2003.

Figures 12.3, 12.11: Drake R, Vogl AW, Mitchell A. *Gray's Anatomy for Students*, 2nd edn, Figure 8.30a. Churchill Livingstone, 2009.

Figure 12.4: Nicol J, Walker S (eds). *The Language of Medicine*, ANZ edition, Saunders, 2007.

Figures 12.5, 12.10: Monahan FD, Sands JK, Neighbors M et al. *Phipps' Medical-Surgical Nursing: Health and Illness Perspectives*, 8th edn. Mosby 2007.

Figure 12.6: Hall JE. *Guyton and Hall Textbook of Medical Physiology*, 12th edn, Figure 45.1. Saunders, 2010. Redrawn from Guyton AC: *Basic Neuroscience: Anatomy and Physiology*. Philadelphia: WB Saunders, 1987.

Figure 12.7: Black JM, Hawks JH, Keene A. *Medical-Surgical Nursing: Clinical Management for Positive Outcomes*, 7th edn. Philadelphia: WB Saunders, 2005.

Figure 12.8: A, Shiland BJ. *Mastering Healthcare Terminology*, 2nd edn, Figure 12.17. Mosby, 2006; B: Sattenberg RJ, Meckler J, Saver JL, Gobin YP, Liebeskind DS: Cerebral Angiography, in *Stroke: Pathophysiology, Diagnosis, and Management*, 6th edn edited by Grotta J, Albers G, Broderick J, Kasner S, Lo E, Sacco R, Wong L Figure 49.1 Philadelphia: Elsevier 2016 Pages 790-805.

Figure 12.9: Engelborghs, S., Niemantsverdriet, E., Struyfs, H., Blennow, K., Brouns, R., Comabella, M., … Khalil, M: Consensus guidelines for lumbar puncture in patients with neurological diseases. *Alzheimer's & Dementia: Diagnosis, Assessment & Disease Monitoring*, Figure 3.3.1 8(1): 111–126 2017.

Chapter 13

Figures 13.1, 13.6, 13.10, 13.11: Harris P, Nagy S, Vardaxis N (eds). *Mosby's Dictionary of Medicine, Nursing & Health Professions*, 3rd ANZ edition, p. A-44 (top figure). Sydney: Mosby, 2014.

Figure 13.2: Drake R, Vogl AW, Mitchell AWM. *Gray's Anatomy for Students*, 2nd edn, Figure 8.278. Churchill Livingstone, 2009.

Figure 13.7: Thibodeau GA, Patton KT. *Anatomy & Physiology*, 7th edn, Figure 15.31, p. 509. St Louis: Mosby, 2010.

Figure 13.8: Baker et al: Cochlear Implant *Medical Assistant: Integumentary, Sensory Systems, Patient Care and Communication* 2017 Zenith: Elsevier.

Figure 13.9: Malavazzi G and Gomes R: Visco-fracture technique for soft lens cataract removal, *Journal of cataract and refractive surgery* Figure13.9 37(1): 11–2 2010.

Chapter 14

Figures 14.1, 14.2, 14.3, 14.10, 14.11: Harris P, Nagy S, Vardaxis N (eds). *Mosby's Dictionary of Medicine, Nursing & Health Professions*, 3rd ANZ edition, p. A-40 (top figure), p. A-41 (top figure). Sydney: Mosby, 2014.

Figure 14.4: Nicol J, Walker S (eds). *The Language of Medicine*, ANZ edition. Saunders, 2007.

Figure 14.5: Salvo SG. *Mosby's Pathology for Massage Therapists*, 2nd edn, Figure 12.11. St Louis: Mosby, 2009.

Figure 14.6: Young A, Proctor D. *Kinn's The Medical Assistant: An Applied Learning Approach*, 10th edn, Figure 39.3. St Louis: Saunders, 2007.

Figure 14.8: Goldman L, Schafer AI. *Goldman-Cecil Medicine*, 24th edn, Figure 133.1. Saunders, 2011.

Figure 14.9: Marx J, Hockberger R, Walls R: *Rosen's Emergency Medicine: Concepts and Clinical Practice*, 7th edn, Figure 44.12. Philadelphia: Mosby, 2009.

Chapter 15

Figures 15.1, 15.5a&b: Harris P, Nagy S, Vardaxis N (eds). *Mosby's Dictionary of Medicine, Nursing & Health Professions*, 3rd ANZ edition, p. A-38. Sydney: Mosby, 2014.

Figure 15.2: Barthold JS, Hagerty JA. Etiology, diagnosis, and management of the undescended testis, in: *Campbell-Walsh Urology*. 12th edn, edited by Wein AJ, Kavoussi LR, Partin AW, Peters CA, Figure 148-12 Philadelphia, PA: Elsevier 2016.

Figure 15.4: Bonewit-West K. *Clinical Procedures for Medical Assistants*, 7th edn, Figure 11.13. Saunders, 2008.

Chapter 16

Figure 16.1: Lowdermilk D, Perry S. *Maternity Nursing*, 7th edn, Figure 4.7. Mosby, 2006.

Figures 16.2, 16.3, 16.8: Harris P, Nagy S, Vardaxis N (eds). *Mosby's Dictionary of Medicine, Nursing & Health Professions*, 3rd ANZ edition, p. A-36, p. A-37 (top right diagram). Sydney: Mosby, 2014.

Figure 16.4: Wong FWS and Lee ETC: Florid cystic endosalpingiosis presenting as an ovarian cyst in a postmenopausal woman *Gynecology and Minimally Invasive Therapy* Figure 1 (4):170–172, 2015.

Figure 16.6: Pfenninger J, Fowler GC. *Pfenninger and Fowler's Procedures for Primary Care*, 3rd edn, Figure 152.2. Saunders, 2010.

Figure 16.7: Ignatavicius D, Workman ML. *Medical-Surgical Nursing: Critical Thinking for Collaborative Care*, Single Volume, 5th edn, Figure 78.6. St Louis: Saunders, 2006.

Chapter 17

Figures 17.1, 17.13: Based on LaFleur Brooks M. *Exploring Medical Language*, 6th edn. Mosby, 2005.

Figure 17.2: Based on Stoy W, Platt T, Lejeune D. *Mosby's EMT-Basic Textbook*, 2nd edn, Figure 25.2. St Louis, Mosby, 2007.

Figure 17.3: Keith L. Moore KL, Persaud TVN. *The Developing Human: Clinically Oriented Embryology*, 8th edn, Figure 7.11a-h. Saunders, 2008.

Figure 17.4: Slone McKinney E, Ashwill J, Smith Murray S et al. *Maternal-Child Nursing*, Figure 17.9. Saunders, 2000.

Figure 17.6: Moore KL, Persaud TVN, Kohei Shiota K. *Color Atlas of Clinical Embryology*, 2nd edn, Figure 9.11a (Courtesy Dr. A. E. Chudley, Department of Pediatrics and Child Health, University of Manitoba, Children's Hospital). WB Saunders, 2000.

Figure 17.7: Carlson B. *Human Embryology and Developmental Biology*, 3rd edn, Figure 11.38. (Courtesy of M. Barr). Mosby, 2004.

Figure 17.9: Thompson DNP: Spinal dysraphic anomalies; classification, presentation and management *Paediatrics and Child Health* Figure 2 24(10):431–438 2014.

Figure 17.11: Lowdermilk DL, Perry SE, Bobak IM. *Maternity and Women's Health Care*, 8th edn. St Louis: Mosby, 2004.

Figure 17.12: Greer IA, Cameron IT, Kitchener HC et al. *Mosby's Color Atlas and Text of Obstetrics and Gynecology*, Figure 8.34. London: Mosby, 2001.

Chapter 19

Figure 19.5: Frank ED, Long BW, Smith BJ. *Merrill's Atlas of Radiographic Positioning & Procedures*, Volume 2, Figure 23.16b. Mosby, 2007.

Figure 19.6: Courtesy of Peter Farkas, Royal Darwin Hospital.

Chapter 20

Figure 20.1: Zitelli BJ, Davis HW. *Atlas of Pediatric Physical Diagnosis*, 5th edn, Figure 12.1c. Mosby, 2007.

Figure 20.2: Callen JP. *Color Atlas of Dermatology*, 2nd edn, Figure 5.43. Philadelphia: WB Saunders, 2000.

Chapter 21

Figure 21.1: Ballinger PW, Frank ED. *Merrill's Atlas of Radiographic Positions and Radiologic Procedures*, 10th edn. St Louis: Mosby, 2003; LaFleur Brooks M. *Exploring Medical Language*, 6th edn, Table 5.1. Mosby, 2005.

Figure 21.2: A, © Millanovic/Photos.com; (B) Caldemeyer KS, Buckwalter KA. *Journal of the American Academy of Dermatology*. The basic principles of computed tomography and magnetic resonance imaging, Figure 1. Elsevier, November 1999; C(a), Nolte J. *The Human Brain: An Introduction to its Functional Anatomy*, 6th edn, Figure 6.16. Philadelphia: Mosby, 2008. (Courtesy Dr Raymond F. Carmody, University of Arizona College of Medicine); C(b), Mettler F. *Essentials of Radiology*, 2nd edn, Figure 3.22. Philadelphia: Saunders, 2004; C(c), Copyright 2012 Needell M.D. — Custom Medical Stock Photo, All Rights Reserved; C(d), Herring W. *Learning Radiology: Recognizing the Basics*, 2nd edn, Figure 11.15. Philadelphia: Saunders, 2011.

Figure 21.3: Ballinger PW, Frank ED. *Merrill's Atlas of Radiographic Positions and Radiologic Procedures*, 10th edn. St Louis: Mosby, 2003; Hoath SB and Mauro T: Fetal Skin Development in: *Neonatal and Infant Dermatology* 3rd edn. edited by Eichenfield LF, Frieden IJ, Zaenglein A, Mathes E, Figure 1.10 Philadelphia, PA: Elsevier 2015 Pages 1–13.

Figure 21.4: Driscoll CLW MD and Lane JI MD: Advances in Skull Base Imaging, *The Otolaryngologic Clinics of North America*, Figure 8 40(3): 439–454 2007; LaFleur Brooks M. *Exploring Medical Language*, 6th edn, Table 5.1. Mosby, 2005.

Figure 21.5: Ballinger PW, Frank ED. *Merrill's Atlas of Radiographic Positions and Radiologic Procedures*, 10th edn. St Louis: Mosby, 2003; Waldman SD MD, JD and Campbell RSD FRCR: Nuclear Medicine and Positron Emission Tomography, in: *Imaging of Pain*, Figure 4.5 Philadelphia: Elsevier 2011 Pages 11-13.

Chapter 22

Figure 22.1: Sorrentino SA. *Mosby's Textbook for Nursing Assistants*, 7th edn, Figure 24.10. Mosby, 2008.

Figure 22.2: Bonewit-West K. *Clinical Procedures for Medical Assistants*, 7th edn, Figure 11.13. Saunders, 2008.

Index

Page numbers followed by 'f' indicate figures, 't' indicate tables.

A

abdominal hysterectomy, 390
ABCDE, 83t
abdominal ultrasonography, 244t, 259t
abdominopelvic regions and quadrants, 34–37, 36f
abnormal fetal presentation, 403t, 410t
ABO blood group system, 114–116, 115t, 116f
abortion, 403t, 410t, 415t
absorptiometry, 497t
absorption, 244t, 246, 520
acetylcholine, 282
acne, 82t, 87t
acoustic neuroma, 312t, 316t
acquired immune deficiency syndrome (AIDS), 137t, 141t
acquired immunity, 137t, 139–140
acromegaly, 156t, 161f, 161t
acupoints, 534t
acupuncture, 534t
acute bacterial parotitis, 250t
acute bronchitis, 220t
acute cholecystitis, 253t
acute coronary syndrome, 189t
acute kidney disease (AKD), 340t
acute otitis media (AOM), 313t, 314f
adaptive immunity. see acquired immunity
Addison's disease, 156t, 168t
adenoids, 137t, 139
adenomatous goitre, 156t, 163t
adhesiolysis, 244t, 259t
adipose tissue, 84
adrenal cortex, 159, 160t
adrenal glands, 157f, 159, 168, 333t
adrenaline, 158–159, 160t
adrenal medulla, 159, 160t
adrenal virilism, 156t, 168t
adrenocorticotrophic hormone (ACTH), 156t, 158
adverse effect or reaction, 516t
advocacy, 538t
affect, 433t
agglutination, 111t, 115
agranulocytes, 113
alanine aminotransferase (ALT), 263t
albumin, 111t
alcoholic cirrhosis, 254f
alimentary canal, 244t
alimentary system, 242
alkaline phosphatase (ALP), 263t
alkylating agent, 454t, 466t
allergic reaction, 516t
allergic rhinitis, 215t, 219t
allergy, 137t, 141t
allogenic transfusion, 121t
allograft, 97t
alveoli, 215t, 217, 218f, 219
Alzheimer's disease (dementia), 19t, 275t, 282t

American Society of Anesthesiologists (ASA), 522
amine, 156t, 157–158
amnesia, 433t
amniocentesis, 403t, 416f, 416t
amputation, 67t
amygdala, 275t
anaemia, 111t, 117f, 117t
anaesthesia, 522
anaesthetics, 521t
anal fissure, 244t, 258t
analgesics, 521t
anaphylactic reaction (anaphylaxis), 516t
anaphylactic shock, 141t
anaphylaxis, 137t, 141t, 516t
anaplastic, 454t
anatomical position, 34, 35f
aneurysm, 183t, 193t
angina pectoris, 183t, 189t, 190f
angiography, 183t, 197t
angioplasty, 4
anorchism, 360t, 363t
anorexia nervosa, 431t, 440t
antagonism, 516t
anterior chamber, 305, 316t
anterior lobe, of pituitary gland, 160t
anti-alcoholic drugs, 442t
anti-anxiety and anti-panic agent, 431t, 442t
antibiotics and antivirals, 521t
antibody, 111t
anticoagulants, 521t
anticonvulsants, 521t
antidepressant, 431t, 442t, 521t
antidiuretic hormone (ADH), 156t, 158
A antigens, 114
antigen, 111t, 141t
antiglobulin test (Coombs' test), 121t
antihistamines, 521t
antimetabolite, 454t, 466t
antimicrotubules, 454t, 466t
antinuclear antibody test, 67t
antipsychotic (neuroleptic), 431t, 442t
antisocial personality disorder, 440
antiviral drug, 521t
anus, 244t, 248, 258–259
anxiety disorders, 437
aorta, 183t, 186
apathy, 433t
APGAR score, 403t, 416t
apheresis, 121t
aplastic anaemia, 117t
apocrine glands, 82t
aponeurosis, 62t
apoptosis, 454t, 456
appendicitis, 244t, 252t, 253f
appendicular skeleton, 50f–51f, 52, 52t
appendix, 244t, 252–253, 253f
arachnoid membrane (arachnoid mater), 275t, 278

aromatherapy, 534t
arrector pili muscles, 85
arteries, 183t, 186, 187f
    pulmonary, 183t, 186
    systemic, 183t, 186
arteriole, 183t, 186
arteriosclerosis, 183t, 193t
arthritis, 57t, 59t
arthrocentesis, 67t
arthrography, 67t
arthroplasty, 67t
arthroscopy, 67f, 67t
articulation, 57t
artificial insemination (AI), 403t, 417t
ASA Physical Status Classification, 522
asbestosis, 223t
aspartate aminotransferase (AST), 263t
aspermatism, 363t
aspermatogenesis, 360t, 363t
aspermia, 360t, 363t
aspiration, 380t, 388t
assisted reproductive technology/ treatment (ART), 416t
asthma, 215t, 219t, 220f
astigmatism, 306t, 316t
atherosclerosis, 183t, 194t, 195f
athlete's foot, 88t
atonic bladder, 333t, 340t
atria, 185
atrioventricular valve, 183t, 186
attention-deficit hyperactivity disorder, 431t, 434t
audiometry, 316t
auditory meatus, 316t
auditory tube, 316t
augmentation of labour, 403t, 417t
auscultation, 215t, 226t
Australian Department of Health, 518
Australian Health Practitioner Regulation Agency (AHPRA), 534
Australian indigenous medicines, 533
Australian Register of Therapeutic Goods (ARTG), 519, 533
Australian Regulatory Guidelines for Complementary Medicines (ARGCM), 533
autism spectrum disorder, 431t, 434t
autograft, 97t
autoimmune disease, 137t, 141t
autonomic nervous system (ANS), 275t, 281
avulsion, 53t
axial skeleton, 50f–51f, 52, 52t
axon, 275t
Ayurvedic medicine, 533–534, 534t
azoospermia, 360t, 363t

B

B antigens, 114
bacteria, 477t, 478
bacterial analysis, 96t

bacterial infections, 480
bacterial prostatitis, 360t, 363t
balanitis, 360t, 364t
ball and socket joint, 57t
bariatric therapies, 259t
Barmah Forest virus, 484t
Barrett's oesophagus, 244t, 250t
Bartholin's glands, 20t
basal cell carcinoma, 82t, 94t
basophil, 111t, 113
B-cell lymphoma, 143t
B-cells, 137t, 139–140
bed wetting, 341
belching, 250t
benign, 454t, 456t
benign prostatic hypertrophy (BPH),
    360t, 364t
benign tumours, 456, 456t
bias, 538t
bicuspid valve, 186
bile, 244t
bilevel positive airway pressure
    (BiPAP), 230t
biliopancreatic diversion, 260t
bilirubin, 111t, 347t
bilirubin tests, 263t
bioavailability, 516t
biochemistry, 116t
bioequivalence, 516t
bipolar disorder, 431t, 436t
birth weight, 409
bladder, 336
    disorders of, 340–341
bladder calculus, 340t
bladder cancer, 333t, 340t
blastocyst, 405–406
bleeding time, 121t
blinding, 538t
blindness, 306t, 317t
blood
    clotting disorders, 120
    components of, 112
    composition of, 112
    dyscrasias, 117–119
    flow of, 186
    functions of, 112
    leucocytes, 111t, 113–114
    sample analysis, 116
    smear, 113f
    tests, 116t, 121t, 244t, 261t
    transfusion, 115–116, 121t
    types or groups, 114–116, 115t,
        116f
blood-borne diseases, 479
blood cells, 112–115. see also specific
    blood cells
blood poisoning, 485t
blood pressure, 183t, 186
blood urea nitrogen (BUN), 333t, 342t
blood vessels. See also specific blood
    vessels
    pathological conditions of, 193–197
body cavities, 34, 36f
body mass index (BMI), 538t
body systems, 34
bolus, 244t

bone density test, 67t
bone marrow, 111t, 137t
    harvest, 122f
    red, 112
    transplant, 121t, 122f, 464t
    yellow, 112
bone marrow biopsy, 121t, 454t, 462t
bones, 48–56
    abbreviations, 52
    of body, 50f–51f
    combining forms, 48–49
    fractures, 53–54, 53t–54t, 55f
    functions and structure, 52–53, 53f
    new word elements, 48–49
    pathology and diseases, 53–56
    suffixes, 49
    vocabulary, 52
bone scan, 68f, 68t
borderline personality disorder, 441t
bowel cancer, 256t
brachytherapy, 454t, 464t, 465f, 497t,
    505t
bradycardia, 186
brain, 278–279
brainstem, 275t, 279
brain tumours, 285t
brand name, 518
Brand Substitution Policy, 518
breasts, 383, 385f
bronchioles, 215t
bronchiolitis, 403t, 411t
bronchitis, 3, 215t, 220t
bronchogenic carcinoma, 223t
bronchoscopy, 215t, 226f, 226t, 477t,
    486t
bronchus (bronchi), 215t, 219
buckle, 53t
bulbourethral gland, 360t, 363
bulimia nervosa, 431t, 440t
bulk billing, 538t
bulla, 85t
bunion, 57t, 60t
burden of disease, 538t
Burkitt's lymphoma, 19t
burn, 82t, 89t, 90f
    epidermal, 90f
burping, 250t
bursitis, 57t, 60t

C

caecum, 244t
caesarean section, 403t, 418f, 418t
calcitonin, 159
calculi, 333t, 340t
calculus, 333t
cancellous bone, 52t, 53
cancer, 456–462. see also specific types
    in Australia and New Zealand,
        461–462
    causes of, 458, 459f
    grading and staging systems,
        460–461
    tests and procedures, 462–466
    types of, 458–460
    vaccine, 467t
capillary, 183t, 189

capsule endoscopy, 244t, 260t
carbon dioxide, 215t, 217
carbuncle, 87t
carcinogenesis, 454t, 458
carcinoma, 454t, 459t
    basal cell, 82t, 94t
    of breast, 380t, 386t
    of cervix, 380t, 387t
    gastric, 244t, 250t
    of ovary, 380t, 387t
    squamous cell, 83t
cardiac cycle, 183t, 186
cardiac magnetic resonance imaging
    (MRI), 183t, 197t
cardiac muscle, 62t, 65
cardiac nuclear medicine, 505t
cardiac tamponade, 183t, 190t
cardiomyopathy, 183t, 190t
cardiopulmonary bypass, 183t, 198t
cardiovascular drugs, 521t
cardiovascular system, 181
    abbreviations, 184–185
    combining forms, 181–182
    functions and structure, 185–189
    new word elements, 181–182
    pathology and diseases, 189–197
    prefixes, 182
    suffixes, 182
    tests and procedures, 197–201
    vocabulary, 183
cardioversion, 183t, 198t
carpal tunnel syndrome, 275t, 285t
cartilage, 34, 57t
cartilaginous joints, 57, 57t
case control study, 538t
cataract, 307f, 307t, 317t, 319f
catatonic schizophrenia, 436
catecholamines, 156t, 159
cauterisation, 380t, 388t
CD4 T-lymphocytes, 141t
cell body, 275t
cell differentiation, 454t
cell membranes, 32
cells, 32–33, 33f
cellular respiration, 217
cellulitis, 82t, 87f, 87t
central nervous system (CNS), 275t,
    278
    protection for, 278
cephalopelvic disproportion, 419t
cerebellum, 275t, 279
cerebral angiography, 275t, 288f, 288t
cerebral concussion, 275t, 285t
cerebral contusion, 275t, 286t
cerebral palsy, 275t, 283t
cerebral tumour, 275t, 285t
cerebrospinal fluid, 275t, 278
cerebrospinal fluid analysis, 275t, 289t
cerebrovascular accident (CVA), 275t,
    287f, 287t
cerebrum, 275t, 278
cerumen, 314f
cervical screening test, 388t
cervical spine, 37t
chemical digestion, 244t, 246
chemical name, 518

chemotherapy, 465–466, 516t
chest x-ray, 215t, 227t, 477t, 483f, 486t
chickenpox, 483f, 483t
Chinese traditional medicine, 534, 534t
chiropractic, 535t
cholangiography, 244t, 260t
cholecystectomy, 244t, 260t
cholecystitis, 244t, 253t
cholelithiasis, 244t, 253f, 253t
cholesteatoma, 312t, 317t
chorionic villus sampling (CVS), 404t, 418t
choroid, 306, 317t
chromosomes, 33
chronic airways limitation (CAL), 220t
chronic bronchitis, 220t
chronic cholecystitis, 253t
chronic kidney disease (CKD), 338t
chronic obstructive airways disease (COAD), 220t
chronic obstructive lung disease (COLD), 220t
chronic obstructive pulmonary disease (COPD), 215t, 220t
chronic parotitis, 250t
chyme, 244t
cicatrix, 85t
ciliary body, 306, 317t
cineradiography, 497t, 499
circulatory system, 181, 185
circumcision, 360t, 367t
cirrhosis, 244t, 254f, 254t
climate change, 538t
clinical depression, 436t
clinical trial, 538t
clinical trial (research) coordinator, 539t
closed fracture, 53t
clotting, 114, 114f
clotting disorders, 120
cluster, 539t
coagulation, 111t
coagulation (clotting) time, 122t
coccygeal spine, 37t
cochlea, 317t
cochlear implant, 317t–318t, 318f
coeliac disease, 244t, 255t
cognitive behaviour therapy (CBT), 431t, 441t
cohort, 539t
cold chain, 516t
colic, 404t, 411t
collagen, 52t, 83t
collapsed lung, 224t
colon, 244t, 248
colon cancer, staging of, 461f
colonic polyp, 244t, 255t
colonoscopy, 262f
    fibreoptic, 455t, 462t
colorectal cancer, 244t, 256t
colostomy, 261t
colour, 347t
colposcopy, 380t, 388t
combining form, 4, 6–7

combining vowel, 4
comminuted fracture, 54t
compact bone, 52t
complementary medicines, 533–534
complementary therapies, 534
complete fracture, 54t
compliance, 517t
complicated fracture, 54t
compound fracture, 54t
compression, 54t
compulsion, 433t
computed tomography (CT), 68t, 137t, 143t, 244t, 275t, 289t, 333t, 343t, 497t, 499, 499f–500f
    scan of abdomen, 261t
    scan of chest, 215t, 227t
    single photon emission, 497t, 504t
concha, 312, 317t
condyloid joint, 57t
cone biopsy, 389t
cones (photoreceptors), 306
confounding variable, 539t
congenital hypothyroidism, 156t, 164t
congestive cardiac failure, 183t, 191t
conisation, 380t, 389t
conjunctiva, 304, 317t
connective tissue, 33–34
continuous negative pressure ventilation (CNPV), 230t
contagious, 476
continuous positive airway pressure (CPAP), 215t, 230f, 230t
continuous ventilatory support (CVS), 229t
contraindication, 517t
contrast media, 497t
control group, 539t
controlled mechanical ventilation, 230t
corium, 84
cornea, 304–305, 317t
coronal suture, 57t
coronary angiography, 183t, 198t
coronary artery bypass graft (CABG), 183t, 198f, 198t
coronary artery disease (CAD), 183t, 191t
coronary catheterisation, 183t, 198t
coryza, 215t
counsellor, 433t
Cowper's gland, 20t, 363
C-reactive protein, 68t
creatinine clearance test, 333t, 343t
Creutzfeldt-Jakob disease (CJD), 19t
Crohn's disease, 19t, 244t, 256t
crossover study, 539t
cross-sectional study, 539t
cryosurgery, 95t, 380t, 389t, 464t
cryptorchidism, 360t, 364f, 364t
cryptorchism, 364t
CT scan. see computed tomography
culdocentesis, 380t, 389t
curettage, 95t. see also dilation (dilatation) and curettage (D&C)
Cushing's syndrome, 19t, 156t, 168f, 168t
cystic fibrosis (CF), 215t, 221f, 221t
cystitis, 333t, 341t

cystocele, 333t, 341t, 380t, 387t
cystogram, 346f
cystoscopy, 333t, 343f, 343t
cysts, 85t
    ovarian, 380t, 385t, 386f
    pilonidal, 83t, 88t
cutaneous mycoses, 478
cytogenetics, 116t
cytoplasm, 33
cytotoxic antibiotics, 455t, 466t

D

database, 539t
deafness, 313t, 317t
Declaration of Alma-Ata, 539t
Declaration of Helsinki, 539t
deep dermal full-thickness burn, 90f
deep vein, 183t, 186–189
defecation, 244t, 248
defence mechanism, 433t
defibrillation, 200t
degenerative and motor disorders, 282–283
delirium, 431t, 434t
delivery, 407–408, 408f
    forceps, 418t, 419f
    presentation for, 408–409, 408f
delusion, 433t
dementia, 431t, 435t
demographic data, 539t
dendrite, 275t, 281
dengue fever, 477t, 484t
dengue haemorrhagic fever, 484t
dense connective tissue, 34
dental caries, 244t, 249t
deoxygenation, 183t
dependence, 435t, 517t
depersonalisation disorder, 439
depot medroxyprogesterone acetate (DPMA) injection, 380t, 389
depressive disorder, 431t, 436t
dermabrasion, 96t
dermatitis, 83t, 92f, 92t
dermis, 83t, 84
determinants of health, 539t
diabetes insipidus, 156t, 163t
diabetes mellitus, 156t, 167t
Diagnostic and Statistical Manual of Mental Disorders
    5th edition (DSM-V), 433, 433t
diagnostic radiology, 496
dialysis, 333t, 343t
diaphragm, 215t
diarrhoea, 244t, 256t
diastole, 183t, 186
dietary iodine, 159
differentiation, 111t
digestion, 244t, 246
    functions and structure, 246–249
digestive system, 242
    abbreviations, 245
    combining forms, 242–243
    new word elements, 242–244
    organs of, 247f
    pathology and diseases, 249–259
    prefixes, 243

suffixes, 244
vocabulary, 244–245
digital rectal examination (DRE), 360t, 367f, 367t
digital subtraction angiography (DSA), 183t, 198t, 199f
dilation (dilatation) and curettage (D&C), 380t, 390t
diphtheria, 482t, 487t
directional terms, 37–38
disability adjusted life years (DALYs), 539t
dislocation, 57t, 60t
disorders of nerves, 285
disorganised schizophrenia, 436
dissociation, 433t
dissociative amnesia, 439
dissociative disorder, 431t, 439t
dissociative fugue, 439
dissociative identity disorder (DID), 439
distant metastasis, 461
distribution, 520
diverticular disease, 244t, 256t, 257f
diverticulitis, 256t
diverticulosis, 256t, 257f
diverticulum, 244t, 256t
dopamine, 282
Doppler ultrasound, 183t, 199t, 275t, 289t
dose, 517t
dose-response relationship, 521
double-blind trial, 538t
Down syndrome, 20t, 404t, 412t
drug classes, 521–522
drug naming, 518
drugs, 514
    administration of, 519
    anti-alcoholic, 442t
    cardiovascular, 521t
    endocrine, 521t
    gastrointestinal, 522t
    regulation and registration, 518–519
    respiratory, 522t
    terminology of action, 520–521
dual energy x-ray absorptiometry (DEXA), 499
ductus (vas) deferens, 360t, 363
duodenal ulcer, 244t, 251t
duodenostomy, 261t
duodenum, 244t
dura mater, 275t, 278
dwarfism, 156t, 162t

E

ear, 311–312, 311f
ear thermometry, 317t–318t
earwax, 314f
eating disorders, 440
ecchymoses, 120t
eccrine glands, 83t
echocardiography, 183t, 199t
ecology, 539t
ectopic pregnancy, 404t, 410t
eczema, 83t, 93t
effect size, 539t

efficacy, 517t
ejaculatory duct, 360t, 363
elastin, 83t
electrocardiogram, 5
electrocardiograph (ECG), 183t, 199t
electrocauterisation, 464t
electroconvulsive therapy (ECT), 431t, 443t
electrodessication, 95t
electroencephalography, 275t, 289t
electromyography (EMG), 68t
electron beams, 465t
electrophoresis, 111t
electrophysiological study, 183t, 199t
eligibility, 539t
elimination, 244t, 246
ELISA test, 137t, 143t, 477t, 486t
embryo, 406
embryo transfer to uterus, 404t, 416t
emphysema, 215t, 222t
en bloc resection, 464t
encephalitis, 275t, 284t
endemic, 539t
endemic goitre, 156t, 164t
endocarditis, 183t, 191t
endocardium, 185
endocrine, 156t, 157
endocrine drugs, 521t
endocrine glands, 157f, 158, 160t–161t
endocrine system, 154
    abbreviations, 156–157
    combining forms, 154–155
    functions and structure, 157–160
    glands, 157, 157f
    new word elements, 154–155
    pathology and diseases, 161–168
    prefixes, 155
    suffixes, 155
    tests and procedures, 169
    vocabulary, 156
endometriosis, 380t, 387t
endorphins, 282
endoplasmic reticulum, 33
endoscopy, 244t
endotracheal intubation, 215t, 227t
end-stage kidney disease, 340t
enteral, 519t
enteric, 519t
enterostomy, 244t, 261t
entropion repair, 317t–318t
enucleation, 317t–318t
enuresis, 341
environmental determinants of health, 539t
environmental health, 540t
eosinophil, 111t, 113
epicardium, 185
epidemic, 540t
epidemiology, 540t
epidermal burn, 90f
epidermis, 83–84, 83t
epididymis, 360t, 363, 364t
epididymitis, 360t
epidural injection, 419t
epiglottis, 215t, 217
epilepsy, 275t, 284t

epinephrine, 159
episiotomy, 404t, 418t
episodic neurological disorders, 284
epispadias, 360t, 364t
epithelial autograft, 97f
epithelial tissue, 33
epithelium
    olfactory, 317t
    squamous, 83t
eponyms, 19–20
    body structures, 20
    diseases and syndromes, 19–20
    instruments, 20
    procedures or tests, 20
erectile dysfunction, 360t, 365t
eructation, 244t, 250t
erythema, 87t
erythroblastosis fetalis, 404t, 412t
erythrocyte, 111t, 112–113, 217
    in anaemic conditions, 117f
erythrocyte sedimentation rate (ESR), 69t, 122t, 477t, 486t
erythropoietin, 111t
esotropia, 309t
estimated glomerular filtration rate (eGFR), 344t
ethics, 540t
evaluation, 540t
evidence based medicine (EBM), 540t
evidence based practice (EBP), 540t
excisional biopsy, 96t, 464t
excisional debridement, 96t
excision of skin lesions, 96t
exclusion criteria, 540t
excretion, 520
exenteration, 380t, 390f, 390t, 464t
exfoliative cytology, 455t, 462t
exhalation, 215t
exocrine, 156t
exocrine function, 159
exocrine gland, 158
exophthalmia, 164t
exophthalmometry, 169t
exotropia, 309t
experimental study, 540t
expiration, 213
external auditory meatus, 312
external beam radiation (teletherapy), 465t
external beam radiation therapy, 505
external beam radiotherapy, 505t
external beam therapy, 497t
external reproductive structures, 361–363, 362f
external respiration, 217
extracorporeal shock wave lithotripsy (ESWL), 333t, 344t
extranodal lymphomas, 143t
extremely low birth weight, 409
eye, 304f–305f
    functions and structure of, 303–306
eyelashes, 304
eyelids, 304

F

fabricated or induced illness by carers (FIIC), 438t

factitious disorders, 438
faecal immunochemical test (FIT), 261*t*
faecal occult blood test, 261*t*
faeces culture, 244*t*, 261*t*
falciparum malaria, 484*t*
fallopian tubes, 20*t*, 381, 383
family therapy, 431*t*, 442*t*
farsightedness, 308*t*
fascia, 62*t*
fasting blood sugar, 169*t*
Feldenkrais method, 535*t*
female reproductive system, 379
   abbreviations, 381
   benign conditions, 385*t*–386*t*
   combining forms, 379
   fibrocystic disease, 380*t*
   functions and structure, 381–383
   gynaecological disorders, 387–388
   new word elements, 379–380
   organs of, 383, 384*f*
   pathology and diseases, 385–386
   prefixes, 380
   suffixes, 380
   tests and procedures, 388–392
   vocabulary for, 380–381
fertilised ovum, 405
fetal death (deadborn fetus), 409
fetal monitoring, 404*t*, 418*t*
fetus, 406
fetus, in final trimester, 501*f*
fibreoptic colonoscopy, 455*t*, 462*t*
fibrin, 111*t*
fibrinogen, 111*t*
fibrocystic disease, 385*t*
fibroid, 386*t*
fibroma, 386*t*
fibromyalgia, 62*t*, 65*t*
fibromyoma, 386*t*
fibrous joints, 57, 57*t*
field, 465*t*
filtration, 333*t*, 334–336
fissure, 85*t*
flaccid paralysis, 286*t*
flap, 83*t*, 96*t*
flat bones, 52
flatulence, 244*t*, 257*t*
floating kidney, 339*t*
flu, 222*t*
fluorescein angiography, 317*t*–318*t*
fluoroscopy, 497*t*, 499
follicles, 84–85
follicle stimulating hormone (FSH), 156*t*, 158, 361, 382
follicular phase, 382
forceps delivery, 418*t*, 419*f*
forebrain, 275*t*
formed elements, 111*t*
4D scans, 501*f*
fractionation, 465*t*
fractures, 52*t*–54*t*, 53–54
   types of, 55*f*
frontal lobe, 275*t*
fugue, 433*t*
fulguration, 464*t*
full blood count (FBC), 122*t*

full thickness burn, 89*t*
fundoplication, 244*t*, 261*t*
fungal test, 96*t*
furuncle, 83*t*, 87*t*

G

gallbladder, 244*t*, 249, 253
gallstones, 253*t*
gamete intrafallopian transfer (GIFT), 404*t*, 417*t*
gamma camera, 497*t*
gastric banding, 244*t*, 259*t*
gastric bypass surgery (Roux-en-Y gastric bypass), 260*t*
gastric carcinoma, 244*t*, 250*t*
gastric plication, 259*t*
gastric ulcer, 244*t*, 251*f*, 251*t*
gastritis, 244*t*, 251*t*
gastroenteritis, 244*t*, 251*t*
gastrointestinal diseases, 479
gastrointestinal drugs, 522*t*
gastrointestinal endoscopy, 244*t*, 261*t*, 262*f*
gastrointestinal system, 242
gastrointestinal tract, 247*f*–248*f*
gastro-oesophageal reflux disease (GORD), 244*t*, 252*f*, 252*t*
gastro-oesophageal sphincter, 244*t*
gastroschisis, 404*t*, 412*f*, 412*t*
gender dysphoria, 439*t*
gender identity disorder, 431*t*
generalised anxiety disorder (GAD), 431*t*, 437*t*
generic name, 518
genes, 33
genetic modification, 540*t*
genetics, 540*t*
genome, 540*t*
German measles, 482*t*
gestational age, 409
gestational diabetes mellitus, 167*t*
gigantism, 156*t*, 162*t*
glaucoma, 307*f*, 307*t*, 317*t*
Gleason system, 455*t*, 460
globin, 111*t*
globulin, 111*t*
glomerular filtration rate (GFR), 344*t*
glomerulonephritis, 333*t*, 338*t*
glucagon, 156*t*, 159
glucose test, 169*t*, 347*t*
glue ear, 313*t*
goitre, 156*t*, 163*f*, 163*t*
gonadotrophin-releasing hormone (GnRH), 382
gonads, 156*t*, 157–160
gouty arthritis (gout), 57*t*, 60*t*
grading, 455*t*, 460–461
graft, 83*t*, 97*f*, 97*t*
granulocyte, 111*t*, 113
Graves' disease, 156*t*, 164*f*, 164*t*
greenstick fracture, 54*t*
group therapy, 431*t*, 442*t*
growth hormone (GH), 156*t*, 158
fugue, 433*t*
guaiac faecal occult blood test (or haemoccult test), 244*t*

gustation, 315, 317*t*
gynaecomastia, 360*t*, 365*t*

H

habitual aborter, 410*t*
haematocrit, 122*t*
haematology, 109
   abbreviations, 111–112
   blood cells, 112–115
   blood test, 116*t*
   combining forms, 109–110
   functions and composition of blood, 112–116
   new word elements, 109–110
   pathology and diseases, 116–120
   prefixes, 110
   suffixes, 110
   tests and procedures, 121–124
   vocabulary, 111
haematopoiesis, 112
haeme, 111*t*
haemodialysis, 343*t*, 344*f*
haemoglobin, 111*t*
haemoglobin test, 123*t*
haemolytic anaemia, 118*t*
haemolytic disease of the newborn, 412*t*
haemophilia, 120*t*
haemorrhagic disease of newborn, 404*t*, 412*t*
haemorrhagic stroke, 287
haemorrhoidectomy, 244*t*, 262*t*
haemorrhoids, 196*t*, 244*t*, 259*t*
haemothorax, 224*t*, 225*f*
hair, 84–85
hair follicle, 83*t*
half life, 497*t*, 503*t*
hallucination, 433*t*
hard bony tissue, 52
Hashimoto's thyroiditis, 156*t*, 165*t*
Health Act 1956, 481
health care claim, 540*t*
health education, 540*t*
health promotion, 540*t*
hearing
   abbreviations, 310–311
   combining forms, 309–310
   functions and structure, 311–312
   new word elements, 309–310
   pathology and diseases, 312–314
   prefixes, 310
   suffixes, 310
heart, 183*t*, 185–186, 185*f*
   pathological conditions of, 189*t*–193*t*
heart attack, 192*t*
hemicolectomy, 3–4
hemiplegia, 286*t*
heparin, 111*t*
heparinisation, 123*t*
hepatitis, 245*t*, 255*t*
hepatitis A, 255*t*
hepatitis A & B vaccination, 487*t*
hepatitis B, 255*t*
hepatitis C, 255*t*
hepatitis D, 255*t*
hepatitis E, 255*t*

herbal medicine, 535*t*
hereditary spherocytosis, 117*f*
hernia, 245*t*, 257*f*, 257*t*
herniated intervertebral disc, 52*t*, 55*t*
herniorrhaphy, 245*t*, 262*t*
herpes zoster, 483*t*
heterograft, 97*t*
hindbrain, 275*t*
hinge joint, 57*t*
hippocampus, 275*t*
histrionic personality disorder, 441*t*
Hodgkin Lymphoma, 20*t*, 137*t*, 143*t*
holter monitoring, 183*t*, 199*t*
homeopathy, 535*t*
homeostasis, 217
homograft, 97*t*
hormonal agent, 455*t*, 466*t*
hormones, 154, 156*t*, 157–158. *See
    also specific hormones*
    and functions, 160*t*–161*t*
    of pituitary gland, 158, 158*f*
    types of, 157–158
human body, 29
    abbreviations, 32
    abdominopelvic regions and
        quadrants, 34–37, 36*f*
    anatomical position, 34, 35*f*
    bones of, 50*f*–51*f*
    cavities, 34, 36*f*
    combining forms, 29–30
    muscles of, 63*f*–64*f*
    new word elements, 29–31
    planes of, 38, 39*f*
    positional and directional terms,
        37–38
    prefixes, 30–31
    spinal column divisions, 37, 37*f*
    structural organisation, 32–34
    suffixes, 31
    vocabulary, 31–32
human chorionic gonadotrophin
    (hCG) test, 169*t*, 383, 406
human immunodeficiency virus (HIV),
    141*t*
human papilloma virus (HPV) vaccine,
    390*t*, 487*t*
human wellbeing, 540*t*
hyaline membrane disease, 414*t*
hydrocephalus, 275*t*, 288*t*, 404*t*, 412*t*,
    413*f*
hydrocoele, 360*t*, 365*f*, 365*t*
hydroureter, 333*t*, 342*f*, 342*t*
hypercalcaemia, 156*t*
hyperemesis gravidarum, 404*t*, 410*t*
hyperinsulinism, 156*t*, 166*t*
hyperopia, 308*t*, 317*t*
hyperparathyroidism, 166*t*
hypertension, 183*t*, 195*t*
hypertensive heart disease, 183*t*, 191*t*
hypertensive kidney disease, 333*t*, 338*t*
hypertropia, 309*t*
hypnosis, 431*t*, 443*t*
hypnotherapy, 535*t*
hypnotics, 431*t*, 442*t*
hypocalcaemia, 156*t*
hypoglycaemics, 522*t*

hypoparathyroidism, 166*t*
hypophysis, 158
hypospadias, 360*t*, 365*t*
hypothalamus, 156*t*, 158, 275*t*
hypothesis, 540*t*
hypotropia, 309*t*
hysterectomy, 380*t*, 390*t*
hysterosalpingography, 380*t*, 391*t*
hysteroscopy, 380*t*, 391*t*

I

ideation, 433*t*
idiosyncratic response, 517*t*
ileostomy, 261*f*, 261*t*
ileum, 245*t*, 247
immune reaction, 111*t*
immune system, 136
    abbreviations, 137–138
    combining forms, 136
    functions and structure of, 138–140
    new word elements, 136–137
    pathology and diseases, 140–143
    prefixes, 136
    suffixes, 137
    tests and procedures, 143
    vocabulary, 137
immune thrombocytopenic purpura
    (ITP), 120*t*
immunisation, 477*t*, 486*t*
immunochemical faecal occult blood
    test (iFOBT), 261*t*
immunoelectrophoresis, 137*t*, 143*t*
immunoglobulin, 111*t*
immunotherapy, 137*t*, 143*t*, 455*t*,
    466–467
impacted fracture, 54*t*
impetigo, 83*t*, 88*f*, 88*t*
implanon, 380*t*, 389
implantable cardioverter defibrillator
    (ICD) insertion, 200*t*
impotence, 365*t*
incidence, 540*t*
incisional biopsy, 464*t*
incision and drainage (I&D), 97*t*
incomplete fracture, 54*t*
incus, 317*t*
induction of labour, 404*t*, 419*t*
infectious and parasitic diseases, 476
    abbreviations, 477
    combining forms, 476
    modes of transmission, 478–479
    new word elements, 476–477
    notifiable, 481
    outbreaks, control and monitoring,
        479–481
    pathological descriptions, 481–485
    prefixes, 476
    sexually transmissible, 480
    suffixes, 476–477
    tests and procedures, 485–487
    types of infections, 478–481
    vocabulary for, 477
inflammatory and infectious disease, of
    nervous system, 284
influenza, 215*t*, 222*t*
influenza vaccination, 487*t*

informed consent, 540*t*
ingestion, 245*t*, 246
inhalation, 213, 215*t*
injection, angles of insertion, 520*f*
innate immunity, 137*t*, 139–140
inner ear, 312
insight-oriented psychotherapy, 431*t*
in situ, 455*t*
inspiration, 213
insulin, 156*t*, 159
integumentary system, 81
    abbreviations, 83
    combining forms, 81–82
    functions and structure, 83–85
    new word elements, 81–82
    pathology and diseases, 85–95
    prefixes, 82
    suffixes, 82
    tests and procedures, 95–97
    vocabulary, 82–83
intercellular fluid, 138
intermittent mandatory ventilation
    (IMV), 230*t*
intermittent positive pressure breathing
    (IPB), 230*t*
intermittent positive pressure
    ventilation (IPPV), 230*t*
internal radiation therapy, 505*t*
internal reproductive structures, 363
internal respiration, 217
International Non-proprietary Name
    (INN), 518
international normalised ratio, 123*t*
interneuron, 275*t*, 282
interpersonal psychotherapy, 442*t*
intersectoral partnering, 541*t*
interstitial fluid, 137*t*, 138
intracranial haemorrhage, 275*t*, 288*t*
intracytoplasmic sperm injection
    (ICSI), 404*t*, 417*t*
intragastric balloon insertion, 259*t*
intrauterine device (IUD), 380*t*, 389
intrauterine growth retardation
    (IUGR), 404*t*, 413*t*
intrauterine insemination (IUI), 404*t*,
    417*t*
intravenous infusion, 520*f*
intravenous pyelogram, 333*t*, 344*t*
in vitro, 497*t*, 504*t*
in vitro fertilisation (IVF), 404*t*, 417*t*
in vivo, 497*t*, 504*t*
involuntary muscle, 62*t*
iodine, 159
ionising radiation, 497*t*
iridology, 535*t*
iris, 303–306, 317*t*
iron deficiency anaemia, 118*t*
irregular bones, 52
irritable bowel syndrome, 245*t*, 258*t*
ischaemia, 191*t*
ischaemic stroke, 287
islets of Langerhans, 156*t*, 159

J

jaundice, 404*t*, 413*t*
jejunum, 245*t*

jock itch, 88t
joint injection, 69t
joints, 56–61
  abbreviations, 57
  combining forms, 56
  functions and structure, 57
  new word elements, 56
  pathology and diseases, 57–61
  suffixes, 56
  vocabulary, 57
Joliot-Curie, Fréderick, 502
Joliot-Curie, Irène, 502

K

keloid, 85t
keratinocytes, 83
keratoplasty, 317t, 319t
keratosis, 83t, 93t
ketone bodies, 347t
ketone test, 169t, 347t
kidney agenesis, 333t, 338t
kidney disease
  chronic, 338t
  hypertensive, 333t, 338t
  polycystic, 333t, 339f, 339t
kidneys, 333t, 334–336, 336f
  disorders of, 338–340
kidneys, ureters and bladder (KUB),
  333t, 344t
kinesiology, 535t
knee, osteoarthritis of, 59f
kyphosis, 52t–53t

L

labour, 407–408, 408f
labyrinth, 317t
labyrinthitis, 313t, 317t
lambdoid suture, 57t
laminectomy, 69t
Landsteiner, Karl, 115
Langerhans cells, 83–84
laparoscopic cholecystectomy, 260f
laparoscopic vaginal hysterectomy, 390
laparoscopy, 245t, 262t, 380t, 391t,
  455t, 462t
large intestine, 245t, 248, 249f,
  255–258
large loop excision of transformation
  zone (LLETZ), 380t, 391t
laryngitis, 215t, 222t
laryngopharynx, 217
laryngoscopy, 215t, 227t
larynx, 215t, 219
laser photocoagulation, 317t, 319t
LASIK (laser-assisted in situ
  keratomileusis), 317t, 319t
left atria, 185
left atrioventricular valve, 186
left atrium, 183t, 186
left lower quadrant (LLQ), 34
left upper quadrant (LUQ), 34
left ventricle, 183t, 185–186
lens, 306, 317t
leucocyte, 111t, 113–114
leukaemia, 459t
liberation, 520

ligation and stripping, 183t, 200t
limbic system, 275t, 278–279
linear accelerator, 465t
lipid tests, 183t, 200t
listed human diseases, 480
live birth, 409
liver, 245t, 249, 254–255, 254f
liver biopsy, 245t, 262t
liver function tests (LFTs), 245t, 263t
liver scan, 245t, 263t
lobectomy, 215t, 227t, 228f
local hospital networks (LHNs), 541t
long bones, 52
longitudinal study, 541t
lordosis, 52t–53t
low birth weight, 409
lower gastrointestinal series, 245t, 263t
lower respiratory tract, 215t
lumbar (spinal) puncture, 275t, 289f,
  289t, 477t, 486t
lumbar spine, 37t
lung, 215t, 219
lung biopsy, 215t, 227t
lung cancer, 215t, 223t
lung transplant, 215t, 227t
luteal phase, 383
luteinising hormone (LH), 156t, 158,
  361, 382
lymph, 137t
  fluid, 138
lymphadenectomy, 137t, 143t
lymphatic drainage, 139f
lymphatic drainage therapy, 535t
lymphatic system, 136
  abbreviations, 137–138
  combining forms, 136
  functions and structure of, 138–140
  new word elements, 136–137
  pathology and diseases, 140–143
  prefixes, 136
  suffixes, 137
  tests and procedures, 143
  vessels and structures, 138f
  vocabulary, 137
lymph node, 137t, 139, 140f
lymphocyte, 111t, 114, 136, 137t,
  139–140
lymphoedema, 137t, 142f, 142t
lymphoma, 137t, 143t, 459t
lymph vessel, 137t, 139

M

macrocytic anaemia, 118t
macrophage, 111t, 137t
macula, 306, 317t
macular degeneration, 308f, 308t, 317t
macule, 85t
magnetic resonance imaging (MRI),
  69t, 215t, 227t, 245t, 263t, 275t,
  290t, 333t, 344t, 497t, 501, 502f
major depression, 436t
major depressive illness, 436t
malaria, 477t, 484t
male reproductive system, 359
  abbreviations, 361
  combining forms, 359

external structures, 361–363, 362f
functions and structure, 361–363,
  362f
internal structures, 363
new word elements, 359–360
pathology and diseases, 363–366
prefixes, 360
suffixes, 360
tests and procedures, 367
vocabulary for, 360–361
malignant, 455t
malignant hypertension, 195t
malignant tumours, 456
  female reproductive system, 386–387
malleus, 317t
mammary glands, 158
mammography, 380t, 391t, 455t, 462t,
  463f
manic depression, 436t
Mantoux test, 486t
massage, 535t
mastectomy, 380t, 391t
matrix, 85
measles, 482t, 483f, 487t
mechanoreceptors, 316
mechanical digestion, 245t, 246
meconium aspiration syndrome, 404t,
  413t
mediastinoscopy, 215t, 227t
Medicare, 541t
Medicare Benefits Schedule (MBS),
  541t
medication regulation and registration,
  518–519
meditation, 535t
Medsafe, 518
medulla oblongata, 275t, 279
megakaryocyte, 111t
melanin, 83t
melanocyte, 83–84, 83t
melanocyte-stimulating hormone
  (MSH), 158
melanoma, 83t, 95f, 95t
melatonin, 156t, 160
menarche, 381
Ménière's disease, 313t, 317t
meninges, 275t, 279f
meningitis, 275t, 284t
meningococcal disease, 477t, 485t
meningococcal vaccination, 487t
meniscectomy, 69t
meniscus tear, 57t, 60t
menstrual cycle, 381–382, 382f
menstrual phase, 383
mental health, 430
  abbreviations, 432
  combining forms, 430
  disorders, 432–441
  new word elements, 430–431
  prefixes, 431
  suffixes, 431
  therapeutic interventions, 441–443
  vocabulary for, 431–432
Merkel cells, 83–84
meta-analysis, 541t
metabolism, 520

metadata, 541*t*
metastasis (metastases), 455*t*, 457*f*
    common sites for, 458
    distant, 461
metastasise, 455*t*
metastatic, 455*t*, 457*f*
metastatic tumours, 458
microalbumin test, 347*t*
microbiology, 116*t*
microcytic anaemia, 118*t*
microscopy of urine, 347*t*
midbrain, 275*t*, 279
mid-dermal burn, 90*f*
middle ear, 312
migraine, 275*t*, 287*t*
Millennium Development Goals
    (MDGs), 544*t*
MIMS New Zealand, 519
mini-stroke, 287
miscarriage, 410*t*
missed abortion, 410*t*
mitochondria, 33
mitral valve, 186
mitral valve prolapse, 183*t*, 192*t*
mixed type cancers, 459*t*
mnemonics, 21
modified radical mastectomy, 391
Moh's surgery, 96*t*
monoclonal antibodies, 467*t*
monocyte, 111*t*, 114
monoplegia, 286*t*
Monthly Index of Medical Specialties
    (MIMS), 519
mood disorders, 436–437
mood stabilisers, 431*t*, 442*t*
morbidity, 541*t*
morphology, 455*t*, 458
mortality, 541*t*
motor neuron disease, 275*t*
motor neurons, 282
mouth, 245*t*, 246
mucosal, 519*t*
multiple gated acquisition scan
    (MUGA scan), 497*t*, 505*t*
multiple personality disorder, 439*t*
multiple sclerosis, 275*t*, 283*t*
mumps, 487*t*
Munchausen's syndrome, 431*t*, 438*t*
Munchausen's syndrome by proxy,
    432*t*, 438*t*
muscle biopsy, 69*t*
muscles, 61–66, 63*f*–64*f*
    abbreviations, 62
    combining forms, 61
    functions and structure, 62–65
    new word elements, 61
    pathology and diseases, 65–66
    prefixes, 61
    suffixes, 61
    vocabulary, 62
muscle tissue, 33
    types of, 65*f*
muscular dystrophy, 62*t*, 66*t*
musculoskeletal system, 48
    bones, 48–56
    tests and procedures, 67–69

music therapy, 535*t*
mutation, 33
myasthenia gravis, 62*t*, 66*t*
mycoses, 477*t*, 478
myelography, 275*t*, 290*t*
myeloid, 5, 111*t*
    tissue, 112
myeloma, 455*t*, 460*t*
myocardial infarction, 183*t*, 192*t*, 193*f*
myocardial perfusion scan, 497*t*, 505*t*
myocardium, 185
myoma, 386*t*
myopia, 308*t*, 317*t*
myringitis, 313*t*
myringotomy, 317*t*, 319*t*
myxoedema, 156*t*, 165*f*, 165*t*

N

naevus, 85*t*
nails, 85, 85*f*
narcissistic personality disorder, 441*t*
nasendoscopy, 317*t*, 319*t*
nasogastric intubation, 245*t*, 263*t*
National Health Practitioner boards,
    534
National Registration and Accreditation
    Scheme, 534
natural immunity. *see* innate immunity
natural killer (NK) cells, 139–140
naturopathy, 535*t*
necrotising enterocolitis, 404*t*, 413*t*
needle biopsy, 455*t*, 463*t*
neonatal period, 409
neonatology, 402
    abbreviations, 404–405
    combining forms, 402
    definitions related to, 409
    functions and structure, 405–409
    new word elements, 402–403
    pathology and diseases, 409–415
    prefixes, 403
    suffixes, 403
    tests and procedures, 415–419
    vocabulary for, 403–404
neoplasms, 453, 455*t*, 456. *see also*
    tumours
    of nervous system, 285
nephrolithiasis, 333*t*, 338*t*
nephroptosis, 333*t*, 339*t*
nephrotic syndrome, 333*t*, 339*t*
nerve disorders, 285
nervous system, 273, 277*f*
    abbreviations, 276
    central, 278
    combining forms, 273–274
    functions and structure, 276–282,
        276*f*
    neoplasms, 285
    new word elements, 273–275
    pathology and diseases, 282–288
    peripheral, 280–281
    prefixes, 274
    suffixes, 274–275
    tests and procedures, 288–290
    vocabulary, 275–276
nervous tissue, 33

Neuraxial block, 404*t*, 419*t*
neurogenic bladder, 333*t*, 341*t*
neuron, 275*t*, 281–282, 281*f*
neurosis, 434*t*
neurotransmitter, 275*t*
neutrophil, 111*t*, 113
new word elements, 6–8
Nissen fundoplication, 20*t*
nodule, 85*t*
non-alcoholic steatohepatitis (NASH),
    245*t*, 255*t*
non-Hodgkin Lymphoma (NHL),
    137*t*, 143*t*
noninvasive mask ventilation (NIMV),
    230*t*
noninvasive pressure ventilation
    (NIPV), 230*t*
non-receptor mechanisms, 520–521
nonspecific immunotherapies, 467*t*
non-ST-segment elevation myocardial
    infarction (NSTEMI), 192*t*
noradrenaline, 159
norepinephrine, 159
nose, 215*t*, 217, 315
notifiable infectious diseases, 481
nuclear medicine, 496, 497*t*, 502–505,
    503*f*
    abbreviations, 497–498
    cardiac, 505*t*
    combining forms, 496
    new word elements, 496–497
    prefixes, 496
    suffixes, 497
    techniques, 504–505
    vocabulary for, 497
nuclear medicine physicians, 496
nucleus, 33
Nuremberg code, 541*t*
nutritional medicine, 536*t*
nystagmus, 308*t*, 317*t*

O

objective vertigo, 314*t*
oblique fracture, 54*t*
obsession, 434*t*
obsessive compulsive disorder (OCD),
    432*t*, 437*t*
obstetrics, 402
    abbreviations, 404–405
    combining forms, 402
    definitions related to, 409
    functions and structure, 405–409
    new word elements, 402–403
    pathology and diseases, 409–415
    prefixes, 403
    suffixes, 403
    tests and procedures, 415–419
    vocabulary for, 403–404
occipital lobe, 275*t*
oesophageal varices, 245*t*, 250*t*
oesophagus, 217, 246, 250
oestrogen, 156*t*, 159–160
olfactory bulb, 317*t*
olfactory epithelium, 317*t*
olfactory nerve, 317*t*
olfactory system, 315

oncogene, 455*t*
oncology, 453
   abbreviations, 455–456
   combining forms, 453–454
   new word elements, 453–454
   prefixes, 454
   suffixes, 454
   tests and procedures, 462–466
   vocabulary for, 454–455
onychomycosis, 88*t*
oocytes, 381
oophorectomy, 380*t*
open angle glaucoma, 307*f*
open fracture, 53*t*
ophthalmoscopy, 317*t*, 319*t*
opportunistic infection, 478
optic nerve, 306, 317*t*
oral, 519*t*
oral cavity, diseases of, 249–250
oral clefts, 404*t*, 413*t*, 414*f*
oral contraceptive, 380*t*, 389
orbit, 304
orchitis, 360*t*, 365*t*
Organisation for Economic
   Cooperation and Development
   (OECD), 541*t*
organs, 34
osseous tissue, 52, 52*t*
ossification, 52*t*
osteoarthritis (OA), 59*t*
   of knee, 57*t*, 59*f*
osteomalacia, 52*t*, 56*t*
osteopathy, 536*t*
osteoporosis, 52*t*, 56*t*
otitis media, 313*t*, 317*t*
otitis media with effusion (OME), 313*t*
otosclerosis, 314*t*, 317*t*
otoscopy, 317*t*, 319*t*
Ottawa Charter, 541*t*
outbreak, 541*t*
outcome, 542*t*
outer ear, 312
ova, 381, 405
ovarian cyst, 380*t*, 385*t*, 386*f*
ovarian cystectomy, 380*t*, 391*t*
ovarian hyperstimulation, 404*t*, 417*t*
Ovary (ovaries), 156*t*, 157–160, 161*t*,
   381, 383
ovulation, 382–383
ovulation induction, 404*t*, 417*t*
oxygen, 183*t*, 215*t*, 217
oxygenation, 183*t*
oxytocins, 156*t*, 158

P
pacemaker insertion, 183*t*, 200*t*
pain receptors, 316
pancreas, 156*t*, 158–159, 161*t*,
   166–167, 245*t*, 249
pancytopenia, 111*t*
pandemic, 542*t*
panhypopituitarism, 156*t*, 162*t*
panic attack, 437*t*
panic disorder, 432*t*, 437*t*
Papanicolaou (Pap) smear, 20*t*, 380*t*,
   391*t*

papule, 85*t*
paracentesis (abdominocentesis), 245*t*,
   263*t*
parallel study design, 542*t*
paralysis, 286
paranoid personality disorder, 441*t*
paranoid schizophrenia, 436
paraphilia, 432*t*, 439*t*
paraphimosis, 360*t*, 365*t*
paraplegia, 286*t*
parasites, 477*t*, 478
parasympathetic nervous system,
   280–281
parathyroidectomy, 169*t*
parathyroid gland, 156*t*, 159, 160*t*,
   166
parathyroid hormone, 156*t*, 159
parathyroid hormone test, 169*t*
parenteral, 5, 519*t*
parietal lobe, 275*t*
parietal pleura, 215*t*
Parkinson's disease, 20*t*, 275*t*, 283*t*
parotitis, 245*t*, 250*t*
partial thickness burn, 89*t*
partial thromboplastin time (PTT),
   123*t*
participant (subject), 542*t*
pathological fracture, 54*t*
pelvic inflammatory disease, 380*t*, 387*t*
pelvic ultrasonography, 380*t*, 392*t*
pelvimetry, 404*t*, 419*t*
penile cancer, 360*t*, 366*t*
penis, 360*t*, 361–363
Penrose drain, 20*t*
peptic ulcers, 251*t*
peptide, 156*t*, 157–158
percussion, 215*t*, 227*t*
percutaneous, 519*t*
percutaneous endoscopic gastrostomy
   (PEG) tube, 245*t*, 263*t*
percutaneous endoscopic jejunostomy
   (PEJ) tube, 245*t*, 263*t*
percutaneous transluminal coronary
   angioplasty (PTCA), 183*t*, 200*f*,
   200*t*
pericardial cavity, 185
pericardial fluid, 185
pericardial sac, 185
pericardium, 185
perinatal period, 409
peripheral nervous system (PNS), 33,
   275*t*, 280–281
peripheral vascular disease, 183*t*, 195*t*
peristalsis, 245*t*
peritoneal dialysis, 343*t*
pernicious anaemia, 117*f*, 118*t*
persistent occipitoposterior presentation
   (POP), 408
personality disorder, 440*t*–441*t*
pertussis, 477*t*, 482*t*
pertussis vaccinatiom, 487*t*
pervasive developmental disorder, 434*t*
PET, 504*t*
PET/CT, 504*t*
petechiae, 120*t*
PET/MRI, 504*t*

phacoemulsification, 317*t*, 319*f*, 319*t*
phaeochromocytoma, 156*t*, 168*t*
phagocytes, 139–140
Pharmaceutical Benefits Scheme (PBS),
   542*t*
pharmacist, 517*t*
pharmacodynamics, 517*t*
pharmacokinetics, 517*t*
pharmacology, 514, 517*t*. *see also* drugs
   abbreviations, 515–516
   combining forms, 514
   drug administration, 519
   drug classes, 521–522
   drug naming, 518
   glossary, 516–517
   new word elements, 514–515
   prefixes, 515
   registration, 518–519
   suffixes, 515
   terminology of drug action,
   520–521
pharmacotherapy, 517*t*
pharmacy, 517*t*
pharynx, 215*t*, 217, 245*t*, 246
phenylketonuria (PKU), 347*t*, 404*t*
phenylketonuria (PKU) test, 419*t*
phimosis, 360*t*, 366*t*
phlebotomy, 111*t*
phobia, 432*t*, 437*t*, 438
photon, 497*t*
pH test, 347*t*
pia mater, 275*t*, 278
pilates, 536*t*
pilonidal cyst, 83*t*, 88*t*
pilot study, 542*t*
pineal gland, 156*t*, 160, 161*t*
pinna, 312, 317*t*
pituitary gland, 156*t*, 158, 158*f*,
   161–163
   anterior lobe of, 160*t*
   hormones of, 158*f*
   posterior lobe of, 160*t*–161*t*
pivot joint, 57*t*
placebo, 517*t*
placenta abruptio, 404*t*, 410*t*, 411*f*
placenta praevia, 404*t*, 410*t*, 411*f*
plan, 542*t*
planes, of body, 38, 39*f*
plaque, 86*t*, 249*t*
plasma, 111*t*, 112, 114
plasmapheresis, 111*t*
platelet, 111*t*
platelet count, 123*t*
platinum analogue, 455*t*, 466*t*
play therapy, 432*t*, 442*t*
pleura, 215*t*
pleural cavity, 215*t*, 219
pleural effusion, 215*t*, 223*t*
plurals, forming, 18–19
pneumococcal vaccination, 477*t*, 487*t*
pneumoconiosis, 215*t*, 223*t*
pneumonectomy, 215*t*, 228*f*, 228*t*
pneumonia, 215*t*, 224*f*, 224*t*
pneumothorax, 215*t*, 224*t*, 225*f*
policy, 542*t*
poliomyelitis, 275*t*, 284*t*

pollo vaccination, 487*t*
polycystic kidney disease, 333*t*, 339*f*, 339*t*
polymerase chain reaction (PCR), 486*t*
polymyositis, 62*t*, 66*t*
polyp, 85*t*
pons, 275*t*, 279
population health, 542*t*
portal veins, 186–189
positional terms, 37–38
positron emission tomography (PET), 183*t*, 201*t*, 215*t*, 228*t*, 275*t*, 290*t*, 497*t*, 502–505, 504*t*
posterior chamber, 306
posterior lobe of the pituitary gland, 160*t*
post haemorrhagic anaemia, 119*t*
post-herpetic neuralgia, 483*t*
post-term, 409
post-traumatic stress disorder (PTSD), 432*t*, 437*t*
pre-eclampsia, 404*t*, 411*t*
prefix, 4, 7–8
pregnancy, 405, 407*f*
    ectopic, 404*t*, 410*t*
    first trimester, 405–406
    labour and delivery, 407–408, 408*f*
    presentation for delivery, 408–409, 408*f*
    second trimester, 406–407, 407*f*
    third trimester, 407
pregnancy-induced hypertension, 411*t*
premenstrual syndrome, 380*t*, 387*t*
presbyopia, 308*t*, 317*t*
pre-term, 409
prevalence, 542*t*
priapism, 360*t*, 366*t*
primary (1°) health care, 542*t*
Primary Health Networks (PHNs), 542*t*
primary tumours, 458, 460
principal investigator, 542*t*
probability, 542*t*
procidentia, 381*t*, 388*t*
progesterone, 156*t*, 159–160
program, 542*t*
projection radiography, 497*t*
prolactin, 156*t*, 158
prolactin test, 169*t*
pronunciation, 17
proportionate dwarfism, 162*t*
proprioceptors, 316
propulsion, 245*t*, 246
prospective study, 542*t*
prostate, 363
prostate biopsy, 360*t*, 367*t*
prostate cancer, 360*t*, 366*t*
prostate gland, 360*t*
protein marker test, 455*t*, 463*t*
protein test, 347*t*
prothrombin, 111*t*
Prothrombin time test, 123*t*
protocol, 542*t*
proton therapy, 465*t*
pruritus, 87*t*
PSA test, 360*t*, 367*t*

psoriasis, 83*t*, 93*f*, 93*t*
psychiatrist, 434*t*
psychiatry, 430, 434*t*
psychoanalysis, 432*t*, 442*t*
psychological and psychosocial therapies, 441–442
psychologist, 434*t*
psychology, 434*t*
psychopharmacology, 442
psychosis, 432*t*, 434*t*–435*t*
psychotherapy, 442*t*
psychotic disorder, 436*t*
public health, 538, 543*t*
pulmonary angiography, 215*t*, 228*t*
pulmonary artery, 183*t*, 186
pulmonary function tests, 215*t*, 228*t*
pulmonary oedema, 215*t*, 225*t*
pulmonary vein, 183*t*, 186–189
pulse, 183*t*, 186
pupil, 305–306, 317*t*
purpura, 120*t*
pustule, 86*t*
pyelonephritis, 333*t*, 339*t*
pyloric stenosis, 404*t*, 414*t*

Q

quadriplegia, 286*t*
quality adjusted life years (QALYs), 543*t*
quarantinable diseases, 480

R

radiation oncologists, 496
radioactive, 504*t*
radioactive iodine ^{131}I therapy, 497*t*, 502, 505*t*
radioactive iodine uptake test (RAIU), 169*t*
radioactive isotopes, 502
radioactivity, 497*t*
radioisotopes, 503*t*
radioisotope scan, 333*t*, 344*t*
radiologists, 496
radiology, 496, 498–501
    abbreviations, 497–498
    combining forms, 496
    diagnostic, 496
    new word elements, 496–497
    prefixes, 496
    suffixes, 497
    therapeutic, 496
    vocabulary for, 497
radionuclide, 497*t*, 502, 504*t*
radionuclide scan, 455*t*, 463*t*
radio-opaque, 497*t*, 504*t*
radiopharmaceutical, 497*t*, 504*t*
radiosensitisers, 465*t*
radiosurgery, 290*t*
radiotherapists, 496
radiotherapy, 464–465, 505
    techniques, 505
radiotracer, 497*t*, 504*t*
randomisation, 543*t*
randomised controlled trial, 543*t*
random sample, 543*t*
rapid strep test, 477*t*, 486*t*

rate, 543*t*
reabsorption, 333*t*
reading and interpreting terms, 5
receptor, 275*t*
receptor interaction, 520–521
rectal, 519*t*
rectocele, 381*t*, 387*t*
rectum, 245*t*, 258–259
red blood cell count, 123*t*
red blood cell morphology, 123*t*
red bone marrow, 112
reduction and fixation, 69*t*
Reed-Stemberg cells, 143*t*
reflexes, 281
reflexology, 536*t*
refraction, 303, 317*t*
regional lymph nodes, 461
registry, 543*t*
reiki, 536*t*
renal angiography, 333*t*, 345*t*
renal angioplasty, 333*t*, 345*t*
renal biopsy, 333*t*, 345*t*
renal failure, 333*t*, 340*t*
renal ptosis, 339*t*
renal transplantation, 333*t*, 345*t*
renin, 333*t*
reproductive system. *see* female reproductive system; male reproductive system
research, 543*t*
residual schizophrenia, 436
respiration, 215*t*, 217
respiratory distress syndrome (RDS), 404*t*, 414*t*
respiratory drugs, 522*t*
respiratory system, 213
    abbreviations, 216–217
    combining forms, 213–214
    functions and structure, 217–219, 218*f*
    new word elements, 213–215
    pathology and diseases, 219–226
    prefixes, 214
    suffixes, 214–215
    tests and procedures, 226–230
    upper, 218*f*
    vocabulary, 215–216
reticulocyte, 111*t*
retina, 306, 317*t*
retinal detachment, 309*t*, 317*t*
retinoblastoma, 309*t*, 317*t*
retrograde pyelogram (RP), 333*t*, 345*t*
retrospective study, 543*t*
Rhesus (Rh) blood type system, 114–115
rheumatoid arthritis, 57*t*, 59*t*
rheumatoid factor test (RF), 69*t*
Rh factor, 111*t*, 114–115
right atria, 185
right atrium, 183*t*, 186
right lower quadrant (RLQ), 34
right upper quadrant (RUQ), 34
right ventricle, 183*t*, 185–186
ringworm, 88*t*
risk benefit ratio, 543*t*
risk factor, 543*t*

risk management, 543*t*
rods (photoreceptors), 306
Roentgen, Wilhelm Conrad, 498
rosacea, 83*t*, 94*t*
Ross River fever, 477*t*, 484*t*
rotator cuff syndrome, 57*t*, 60*t*
rotavirus, 477*t*, 482*t*
rubella (German measles), 482*t*, 487*t*
rubeola, 482*t*
rule of nines, 91*f*, 91*t*

S

sacral spine, 37*t*
saddle joint, 57*t*
sagittal suture, 57*t*
saliva, 245*t*
salivary gland, 245*t*, 250
salpingo-oophorectomy, 381*t*
sample size, 543*t*
sarcoma, 455*t*, 460*t*
schizoid personality disorder, 441*t*
schizophrenia, 432*t*, 436*t*
school sores, 88*t*
sciatica, 275*t*, 285*t*
scintigraphy, 497*t*, 504*t*
sclera, 304, 317*t*
scleral buckle, 317*t*, 319*t*
scoliosis, 52*t*–53*t*
scrotum, 159–160, 361*t*, 363
seasonal affective disorder (SAD), 432*t*,
    437*t*
sebaceous gland, 83*t*, 158
seborrhoeic keratoses, 93*t*
sebum, 83*t*
secondary (2°) health care, 543*t*
secretion, 245*t*, 246
sedative-hypnotics, 442*t*, 522*t*
sedatives, 442*t*
sediment test, 347*t*
segmental fracture, 54*t*
semen analysis, 361*t*, 367*t*
semicircular canal, 317*t*
seminal vesicle, 361*t*, 363
senses, 301. *see also specific senses*
    tests and procedures, 317–320
    vocabulary for, 316–317
sensory neuron, 275*t*, 282
sepsis, 485*t*
septicaemia, 477*t*, 485*t*
septoplasty, 317*t*, 320*t*
septum, 185
serology, 116*t*
serous otitis media, 313*t*
serum, 111*t*
serum calcium, 69*t*
serum calcium test, 169*t*
serum cortisol test, 169*t*
serum creatine kinase (CK), 69*t*
sesamoid bones, 52
sex therapy, 432*t*
sexual and gender identity disorders,
    439–440
sexual disorder, 432*t*, 440*t*
sexually transmissible infections, 480
shiatsu, 536*t*
shingles, 483*t*

shingles vaccination, 487*t*
Shirodkar suture, 20*t*
short bones, 52
shortsightedness, 308*t*
sickle cell anaemia, 117*f*, 119*t*
side effect, 517*t*
sight
    abbreviations, 303
    combining forms, 301–302
    functions and structure, 303–306
    new word elements, 301–303
    pathology and diseases, 306–309
    prefixes, 302
    suffixes, 303
sigmoidoscopy, 262*f*
silicosis, 223*t*
simple fracture, 54*t*
simple/total mastectomy, 391
single-blind trial, 538*t*
single photon emission computed
    tomography (SPECT), 497*t*,
    502–503, 503*f*, 504*t*
sinoatrial node, 183*t*, 186
sinusoscopy, 317*t*, 320*t*
sinus rhythm, 183*t*, 186
skeletal muscles, 62, 62*t*
skin, 83
    structure of, 84*f*
    symptomatic conditions, 87
skin biopsy, 97*t*
skin cancers, 94–95
skin disorders, 89–94
skin infections, 87–89
skin lesions, 85–86, 86*f*
    excision of, 96*t*
    removal, 95–96
skin test, 97*t*
sleep apnoea, 275*t*, 284*t*
sleeve gastrectomy, 260*t*
slit lamp microscopy, 317*t*, 320*t*
small intestine, 245*t*, 247, 255
smell
    combining forms, 315
    functions and structure, 315
    new word elements, 314–315
    prefixes, 315
smooth muscles, 62, 62*t*
social capital, 543*t*
social cohesion, 543*t*
solar keratoses, 93*t*
somatic nervous system, 275*t*, 280
somatomedin C test, 169*t*
somatosensory system, 316
spastic paralysis, 286*t*
specific gravity test, 347*t*
SPECT/CT, 504*t*
spelling conventions, 17–18
spermatocele, 361*t*, 366*t*
spermatogenesis, 361*t*
spermatozoa, 361, 361*t*
spherocytosis, 117*f*
spina bifida, 404*t*, 414*t*, 415*f*
spinal column, divisions of, 37, 37*f*
spinal cord, 275*t*, 279–280
spine curvature, 53
spiral fracture, 54*t*

spiritual healing, 536*t*
spleen, 111*t*, 137*t*, 139
splenectomy, 123*t*
sponsor, 544*t*
spontaneous abortion, 410*t*
sprain, 57*t*, 61*t*
squamous cell carcinoma (SCC), 83*t*,
    95*t*
squamous epithelium, 83*t*
staging, 455*t*, 460–461, 461*f*
stapes, 317*t*
ST elevation myocardial infarction
    (STEMI), 192*t*
stem cell, 111*t*
    transplant, 464*t*
stent insertion (stenting), 201*t*
stereotactic radiosurgery, 276*t*, 290*t*
steroid, 156*t*, 157–158
stimulant, 432*t*, 442*t*, 522*t*
stomach, 245*t*, 246–247, 250–252
stomach cancer, 250*t*
stomatitis, 245*t*, 250*t*
stool culture, 261*t*
strabismus, 309*t*, 317*t*
strain, 62*t*, 66*t*
strategies, 544*t*
stress echocardiogram, 183*t*, 201*t*
stress exercise test, 183*t*, 201*t*
stress fracture, 54*t*
stress incontinence, 341
striated, 62*t*
stroke, 287
subarachnoid space, 278
subcutaneous mastectomy, 391
subcutaneous mycoses, 478
subcutaneous tissue, 83*t*, 84
subdermis, 83*t*, 84
subdural space, 278
subjective vertigo, 314*t*
substance induced disorders, 435*t*
substance related disorders, 432*t*, 435,
    435*t*
substance use disorder (SUD), 435*t*
suffix, 4, 8
superficial dermal burn, 90*f*
superficial mycoses, 478
superficial vein, 183*t*, 186–189
supportive psychotherapy, 432*t*
suppurative otitis media, 313*t*
surveillance, 544*t*
sustainable development, 544*t*
Sustainable Development Goals
    (SDGs), 544*t*
sweat gland, 83*t*, 158
sympathetic nervous system, 281
symptomatic skin conditions, 87
synapse, 276*t*
synchronised intermittent mandatory
    ventilation (SIMV), 230*t*
syndrome of inappropriate antidiuretic
    hormone (SIADH), 156*t*, 162*t*
synergy, 517*t*
synovial fluid, 57*t*
synovial joints, 57, 57*t*
    types of, 58*f*
synovial membrane, 57*t*

systemic artery, 183*t*, 186
systemic mycoses, 478
systemic radioisotope therapy, 497*t*, 505*t*
systemic vein, 183*t*, 186–189
systole, 183*t*, 186

T
tachycardia, 186
tagging, 497*t*, 504*t*
target group, 544*t*
taste
    combining forms, 315
    functions and structure, 315–316
    new word elements, 315
taste bud, 317*t*
T-cell lymphoma, 143*t*
T-cells, 139–140
technetium (tc)⁻⁹⁹ᵐ sestambi scan, 183*t*, 201*t*
tectum, 276*t*
teeth, 245*t*
tegmentum, 276*t*
telangiectasia, 86*t*
temporal lobe, 276*t*
tendon, 62*t*
term, 409
tertiary (3°) care, 544*t*
testicular cancer, 361*t*, 366*t*
testicular torsion, 366*t*
testis (testes), 156*t*, 158–160, 161*t*, 361–363, 361*t*
testosterone, 156*t*, 159–160, 361, 361*t*
tetanus, 487*t*
tetraplegia, 286*t*
thalamus, 276*t*
thalassaemia, 117*f*, 119*t*
thallium scan, 497*t*, 505*t*
Therapeutic Goods Act 1989, 518, 533
Therapeutic Goods Administration (TGA), 518, 533
Therapeutic Goods Regulations 1990, 533
therapeutic methods, 443
therapeutic radiology, 496
thermoreceptors, 316
thoracic spine, 37*t*
thoracocentesis, 215*t*, 228*t*
thoracoscopy, 215*t*, 228*t*
thoracotomy, 215*t*, 228*t*
threatened abortion, 410*t*
3D scans, 501*f*
thrombin, 111*t*
thrombocyte, 111*t*, 114
thrombolytic therapy, 183*t*, 201*t*
thromboplastin, 111*t*
thymus gland, 137*t*, 139, 160, 161*t*
thyroid function test, 169*t*
thyroid gland, 156*t*, 158–159, 160*t*, 163–165
thyroid-stimulating hormone (TSH), 156*t*, 158–159
thyroxine (T₄), 156*t*, 159
tinea, 83*t*, 88*t*, 89*f*
tinnitus, 314*t*, 317*t*
tissues, 33–34
T-lymphocytes, 160

tolerance, 517*t*
tongue, 245*t*, 315–316
tonsillectomy, 137*t*
tonsillitis, 137*t*
tonsils, 137*t*, 139, 216*t*, 217
topical, 519*t*
topoisomerase inhibitors, 455*t*, 466*t*
total thyroidectomy, 169*t*
touch
    combining forms, 316
    functions and structure, 316
    new word elements, 316
toxicity, 517*t*
toxicology, 517*t*
toxic shock syndrome (TSS), 381*t*, 387*t*
tracer study, 497*t*, 504*t*
trachea, 216*t*, 219
tracheostomy, 216*t*, 229*f*, 229*t*
trachoma, 309*t*, 317*t*
trade name, 518
traditional medicine, 533
tranquillisers, 522*t*
transducer probe, 497*t*
transfusion, 111*t*, 115–116, 121*t*
transient ischaemic attack, 276*t*, 287*t*
transient tachypnoea of newborn (TTN), 404*t*, 415*t*
transplant
    bone marrow, 121*t*, 122*f*, 464*t*
    lung, 215*t*, 227*t*
    renal, 333*t*, 345*t*
    stem cell, 464*t*
Trans-Tasman Mutual Recognition Arrangement June 1997, 519
transurethral resection of prostate (TURP), 361*t*, 367*t*
transvaginal oocyte retrieval, 404*t*, 417*t*
transverse fracture, 54*t*
traumatic disorders, of nervous system, 285–286
tricuspid valve, 186
triiodothyronine (T₃), 156*t*, 159
trisomy, 21, 412*t*
tubal ligation, 381*t*, 389, 389*f*
tuberculin test, 216*t*, 229*t*, 477*t*, 486*t*
tuberculosis (TB), 216*t*, 225*t*
tube thoracostomy, 216*t*, 229*t*
tubular necrosis, 333*t*, 340*t*
tumours, 455*t*, 456–462, 457*f*
tuning fork test, 317*t*, 320*t*
turbinectomy, 317*t*, 320*t*
tympanic membrane, 317*t*
Tympanotomy tube, 314*f*

U
ulcer, 86*t*
    duodenal, 244*t*, 251*t*
    gastric, 244*t*, 251*f*, 251*t*
ulcerative colitis, 245*t*, 258*t*
ultrasonography, 333*t*, 345*t*, 497*t*, 499–501, 501*f*
    abdominal, 244*t*, 259*t*
    Doppler, 183*t*, 199*t*, 275*t*, 289*t*
    pelvic, 380*t*, 392*t*
undifferentiated, 455*t*
universal donor, 115

Universal Health Coverage, 545*t*
upper gastrointestinal series, 245*t*, 263*t*
upper respiratory system, 218*f*
upper respiratory tract, 216*t*, 217
upper respiratory tract infection (URTI), 216*t*–217*t*, 226*t*
uptake, 497*t*, 504*t*
urea, 334*t*
urea breath test, 477*t*, 486*t*
ureter, 334*t*, 336, 342
ureteric colic, 334*t*, 342*t*
ureteric stent, 334*t*, 345*t*
urethra, 336, 342, 361*t*, 363
urethritis, 334*t*, 342*t*
urge incontinence, 341
uric acid, 334*t*
urinalysis, 334*t*, 347
urinary bladder, 334*t*
urinary catheterisation, 334*t*, 345*t*
urinary incontinence, 334*t*, 341*t*
urinary sphincters, 336
urinary system
    abbreviations, 334
    combining forms, 332
    female, 337*f*
    functions and structure, 334–336, 335*f*–336*f*
    male, 337*f*
    new word elements, 332–333
    pathology and diseases, 336–342
    prefixes, 332
    suffixes, 333
    tests and procedures, 342–347
    vocabulary for, 333–334
urine albumin/creatine ratio (UACR), 345*t*
urolithiasis, 338*t*
urticaria, 87*t*
uterine leiomyoma, 381*t*, 386*t*
uterine prolapse, 381*t*, 388*f*, 388*t*
uterus, 383, 406*f*

V
vaccination, 477*t*, 486*t*, 522*t*
vaccine preventable diseases, 480, 482–483
vacuum extraction, 404*t*, 419*t*
vagal blocking therapy, 259*t*
vagina, 383
vaginal hysterectomy, 390
variable, 545*t*
varicella vaccination, 487*t*
varicella zoster (chickenpox), 483*f*, 483*t*
varicocele, 361*t*, 366*t*
varicose veins, 195*t*, 196*f*–197*f*
vascular disorders, of nervous system, 287
vasectomy, 361*t*, 367*t*
vector-borne diseases, 480, 484
veins, 183*t*, 186, 188*f*, 189
    deep, 183*t*
    portal, 186, 189
    pulmonary, 183*t*, 186, 189
    superficial, 183*t*
    systemic, 183*t*, 186, 189
    varicose, 195*t*, 196*f*–197*f*

venae cavae, 189
venepuncture, 123*t*, 124*f*
ventilation perfusion scan (V/Q scan), 216*t*–217*t*, 229*t*
ventilation process, 213
ventilatory support (mechanical ventilation), 229*t*
ventricles, 185–186
ventriculography, 183*t*, 201*t*
venule, 183*t*
verruca, 83*t*, 89*t*
vertebra, 37
vertigo, 314*t*, 317*t*
very low birth weight, 409
vesical calculus, 340*t*
vesical fistula, 334*t*, 341*t*
vesicle, 86*t*
vesicoureteral reflux, 334*t*, 342*t*
vestibular Schwannoma, 312*t*
vestibular system, 312
vestibule, 317*t*
viral parotitis, 250*t*

viruses, 477*t*, 478
visceral pleura, 216*t*, 219
visual acuity test, 317*t*, 320*t*
visual field test, 317*t*, 320*t*
vitamin K deficiency syndrome, 412*t*
vitamins, 522*t*
vitiligo, 83*t*, 94*f*, 94*t*
vitrectomy, 317*t*, 320*t*
vitreous cavity, 306, 317*t*
vitreous humour, 306, 317*t*
voiding cystogram, 346*f*
voiding cystourethrogram (VCUG), 334*t*, 345*t*
voluntary muscle, 62*t*
vulva, 383

W

wart, 89*t*
well differentiated, 455*t*
wheal, 86*t*
white blood cell count, 124*t*
white blood cell differential, 124*t*

word elements, 5–6
word root, 3–4
word structure, 3–5, 5–6
Wrigley's forceps, 20*t*

X

x-rays, 498*f*
    characteristics of, 498
    diagnostic techniques, 499–501
    positioning, 501

Y

YAG laser capsulotomy, 320*t*
years of potential life lost (YPLL), 545*t*
yellow bone marrow, 112
yoga, 536*t*

Z

zoonoses, 480
zygote, 405